Reviews for *Radiology Business Practice: How to Succeed* •••

Radiology Business Practice: How to Succeed is a most thoughtful approach to the business of radiology. Broad in scope, it provides the reader with significant insights into pertinent topics, enabling readers by providing a firm understanding of the strategic elements requisite for success in a competitive environment. The authors have a pragmatic style and a wealth of experience, all of which are easily conveyed in this book. It is a fun read, with key elements that are extremely valuable for those engaged in the practice of radiology.

ROBERT GROSSMAN, CHAIRMAN
DEPARTMENT OF RADIOLOGY, NEW YORK UNIVERSITY

***

Dr. Yousem, of course as everyone knows, has an MBA and his fellows have traditionally been very lucky to learn not only neuroradiology but also the business of radiology. Now he tells us that all of us will have the opportunity to learn the latter subject from him! What a treat.

CHETAN NAYAK

***

I enjoyed reading *Radiology Business Practice: How to Succeed*. It is full of business pearls. I wish I had read it before taking my current job! It is both practical and humerous—like *The World Is Flat* meets *Neuroradiology: The Requisites*.

WILLIAM G. BRADLEY, JR, MD, PHD, FACR
PROFESSOR AND CHAIRMAN, DEPARTMENT OF RADIOLOGY, UCSD MEDICAL CENTER

***

This book is long overdue and without doubt of special interest in today's rapidly changing environment.

MICHAEL YUZ
VALLEY OPEN MRI & DIAGNOSTIC CENTER

***

This well-written book contains an amazing amount of information that should be valuable to all radiology practices, from those in small community hospitals to large academic departments. The level of detail is just right—enough specifics to be useful, but not so much detail as to be overwhelming. The authors write from experience in the specialty and demystify the sometimes murky world of business.

DOUGLAS E. HOUGH, PHD
CHAIR, THE BUSINESS OF HEALTH, CAREY BUSINESS SCHOOL, JOHNS HOPKINS UNIVERSITY

***

Yousem and Beauchamp have compiled a wealth of insights and pearls for the management and leadership of the practice of radiology, and have created a text that not only is enjoyable but also will be an invaluable companion to current and future leaders in the field.

JONATHAN S. LEWIN, MD
MARTIN W. DONNER PROFESSOR AND CHAIRMAN,
THE RUSSELL H. MORGAN DEPARTMENT OF RADIOLOGY
AND RADIOLOGICAL SCIENCE, JOHNS HOPKINS SCHOOL OF MEDICINE

***

A book like this in radiology is long overdue, especially for residents and fellows who need this information before we get out in the real world.

AMISH DAVE, MD
CHIEF, RESIDENT, UNIVERSITY OF TEXAS MEDICAL BRANCH, GALVESTON, TEXAS

RADIOLOGY BUSINESS PRACTICE

How to Succeed

DAVID M. YOUSEM, MD, MBA
Director of Neuroradiology
Vice Chairman of Program Development
Russell H. Morgan Department of Radiology and Radiological Sciences
The Johns Hopkins Medical Institution
Baltimore, Maryland

NORMAN J. BEAUCHAMP, Jr., MD, MHS
Professor and Chair
Department of Radiology
Professor of Neurological Surgery and
Industrial Engineering
President, University of Washington Physicians
University of Washington
Seattle, Washington

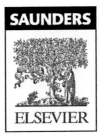

SAUNDERS

ELSEVIER

SAUNDERS
ELSEVIER

1600 John F. Kennedy Blvd.
Ste 1800
Philadelphia, PA 19103–2899

RADIOLOGY BUSINESS PRACTICE: HOW TO SUCCEED   ISBN: 978-0-323-04452-3

Notice

Neither the Publisher nor the Editors assume any responsibility for any loss or injury and/or damage to persons or property arising out of or related to any use of the material contained in this book. It is the responsibility of the treating practitioner, relying on independent expertise and knowledge of the patient, to determine the best treatment and method of application for the patient.

The Publisher

Library of Congress Cataloging-in-Publication Data

Yousem, David M.
   Radiology business practice : how to succeed / David M. Yousem, Norman J. Beauchamp Jr. – 1st ed.
      p. ; cm.
   Includes bibliographical references and index.
   ISBN 978-0-323-04452-3
   1. Radiology, Medical–Practice.   I. Beauchamp, Norman J.   II. Title.
   [DNLM: 1. Radiology–organization & administration.   2. Practice Management,
   Medical–organization & administration. WN 21 Y82r 2008]
   R895.Y68 2008
   616.07′57068–dc22

                                                                2007015848

Acquisitions Editor: Rebecca Gaertner
Editorial Assistant: Elizabeth Hart
Project Manager: Bryan Hayward
Design Direction: Karen O'Keefe-Owens

Printed in the United States of America.
Transfered to Digital Printing, 2011

Working together to grow
libraries in developing countries

www.elsevier.com | www.bookaid.org | www.sabre.org

ELSEVIER   BOOK AID
             International   Sabre Foundation

Editors

David M. Yousem, MD, MBA
Director of Neuroradiology
Vice Chairman of Program Development
Russell H. Morgan Department of Radiology
  and Radiological Science
The Johns Hopkins Medical Institution
Baltimore, Maryland

Norman J. Beauchamp, Jr., MD, MHS
Professor and Chair
Department of Radiology
Professor of Neurological Surgery and
  Industrial Engineering
President, University of Washington Physicians
University of Washington
Seattle, Washington

Contributors

Gautam Agrawal, MD
Cofounder, Vision Radiology
Clinical Instructor, Russell H. Morgan
Department of Radiology and Radiological
  Science
Johns Hopkins Hospital
San Francisco, California

Michelle Bittle, MD
Body Imaging Fellowship Director
Department of Radiology
Harborview Medical Center
University of Washington School of Medicine
Seattle, Washington

C. Craig Blackmore, MD
Professor of Radiology and Adjunct Professor
  of Health Services

Department of Radiology
University of Washington
Seattle, Washington

Martin Bledsoe, MSPH
Administrator
The Russell H. Morgan Department of
  Radiology and Radiological Science
The Johns Hopkins Medical Institution
Baltimore, Maryland

John A. Bonavita, MD
Assistant Professor of Radiology
Department of Radiology
New York University Medical Center
New York, New York

Robert F. Carfagno, MBA, CPA
President and CEO
American Radiology Services, Inc.
Baltimore, Maryland

Felix S. Chew, MD
Department of Radiology
University of Washington Medical Center
Seattle, Washington

Dennis Condon, MSHA, MBA
Director of Operations
Advanced Radiology Consultants
Trumbull, Connecticut

Audrey Drossner, CPA
Partner
SC&H Financial Advisors, Inc.
Sparks, Maryland

James B. Gantenberg, FACHE
Executive Director/CEO
American Society of Neuroradiology
Oak Brook, Illinois

Bob Gayler, MD
Associate Professor, Department of Radiology
The Johns Hopkins Medical Institution
Baltimore, Maryland

Peter Ghavami, MSc
Director of Informatics
HMC Patient Care Services
Harborview Medical Center
University of Washington School of Medicine
Seattle, Washington

Joel A. Gross, MD
Emergency Radiology Fellowship Director
Department of Radiology
Harborview Medical Center
University of Washington School of Medicine
Seattle, Washington

Robin A. J. Hunt
Administrative Fellow
Mayo Clinic
Rochester, Minnesota

Christopher J. Hurt, MD
Department of Radiology
University of Washington
Seattle, Washington

Peter A. Janick, MD, PhD
Lansing Radiology Associates
Okemos, Michigan

Gregory L. Katzman, MD, MBA
John Sealy Distinguished Chair of Radiology
Professor and Chairman
Department of Radiology
University of Texas Medical Branch
Galveston, Texas

Jeffrey C. Langdon, MHA
Administrative Fellow
Duke University Hospital
Durham, North Carolina

Christopher Laubenthal, MBA
University of Washington
Seattle, Washington

Frank James Lexa, MD, MBA
Professor and Country Manager
The Global Consulting Practicum
Adjunct Professor of Marketing
Wharton School, Graduate Division

Clinical Associate Professor of Radiology
School of Medicine
University of Pennsylvania
Philadelphia, Pennsylvania

Andrew W. Litt, MD, FACR
Executive Vice President
Vice Dean and Chief of Staff
New York University Medical Center
New York, New York

F. A. Mann, MD
Harborview Medical Center
University of Washington School of Medicine
Seattle, Washington

Joseph Marotta, MPA, FACHE
Technical Director
Department of Radiology
Harborview Medical Center
University of Washington School of Medicine
Seattle, Washington

Satoshi Minoshima, MD, PhD
Professor of Radiology and Bioengineering
Vice Chair for Research
Department of Radiology
Head, Primate PET Imaging Suite
WaNPRC, University of Washington School
   of Medicine
Seattle, Washington

Julie A. Muroff, JD
Senior Attorney, Office of the General Counsel
U.S. Department of Health and Human Services
Public Health Division, NIH Branch
Bethesda, Maryland

Annemarie Relyea-Chew, JD, MS
Department of Radiology
University of Washington Medical Center
Seattle, Washington

Joseph Robinson
Senior Vice President, Sales and Marketing
Philips Imaging Systems, North America
Bothell, Washington

William P. Shuman, MD, FACR
Professor and Vice Chairman
Department of Radiology
University of Washington School of Medicine
Seattle, Washington

Radiology has grown from an ancillary service often tucked away in the bowels of its host institution into one of the most important medical specialties guiding the progress of patients along the critical pathways that shape their diagnoses and treatments. The quality and efficiency of care delivered in hospitals and in outpatient settings hinge in large measure directly on how well the associated departments of radiology or imaging centers function.

As a consequence of the growth in demand for imaging services, departments of radiology that consisted of dozens of people and had modest budgets 20 and 30 years ago now have hundreds of people and are measured financially in the millions or even tens of millions of dollars. Informal and intuitive management is no longer realistic or competitive. Undocumented models of governance put everyone at undue risk and are no longer acceptable. Third-party payers have upped the ante for meeting the bar for payment, and sophistication and diligence in equal measure to these managed care organizations are required in order for radiology practices to receive what is rightfully theirs. Technology has evolved from the episodic arrival of new marvels to a maelstrom—indeed a blizzard—of innovation that must be evaluated, parsed into priorities, and acquired ... or not. Information systems abound and must be integrated into the larger health care enterprise. Compliance and legal issues face us at every turn.

So the question is, have radiologists and their administrative partners gained management expertise in equal or greater measure to the breadth and scale of the management challenges facing contemporary radiology practices? The answer is almost certainly not, based on the current pathways to leadership and the limited resources available for learning about the specific issues involved in the business of radiology. These limitations extend from the relative dearth of robust formal educational programs for professional and lay managers devoted to the business of radiology to the lack of a suitable contemporary text that tackles the major issues facing managers and leaders of radiology business operations.

Thus it is with enormous pleasure that I help introduce this remarkable book, *Radiology Business Practice: How to Succeed*, edited by two of the outstanding thinkers and leaders in the field, Drs. David Yousem, MD, MBA, of the Johns Hopkins Medical Institution, and Norman J. Beauchamp, Jr., MD, MHS, of the University of Washington. They have teamed up to design, write, and edit a truly remarkable book. *Radiology Business Practice: How to Succeed* is far-encompassing in its material, offers attention to practical detail and theory alike, and mobilizes the substantial experience base of its authors for the benefit of the reader.

Drs. Yousem and Beauchamp have divided their book logically into four parts dealing with leadership and governance, accounting and financial principles, practice management, and legal and legislative concerns. The impressive range of topics covered in each part bespeaks the educational challenges facing new and incumbent managers and leaders.

The editors have invited an outstanding group of contributors to join them in their endeavor. The experience of these contributors can best be described as authoritative. Based on their collective wisdom, *Radiology Business Practice: How to Succeed* promises to fill an important gap in the resources available to all of us who seek to learn more about how to lead and manage in the business aspects of radiology. It can serve equally as text and reference and is likely to find a role as both. It should frequently find its way into the hands of anyone practicing radiology in the academic or private sector, let alone those who have the temerity to tackle management issues in radiology. I also believe this book would be an ideal graduation gift—a guide to success—to all residents and fellows starting out on their new career.

The importance of this valuable new book derives in part from the way people ascend to positions of leadership in the medical world, including radiology. With the exception of a few visionaries who obtain a business degree along the way, most leaders in both private practice and academia rise to their positions by being good at something entirely different—clinical practice and research—and not because they were trained for leadership and management. The same has been true for administrative managers who until recently were typically selected from the ranks of clinically experienced technologists—again, people with positive track records of performance but not necessarily trained to be managers of the business aspects

of radiology. Now anyone with an interest in leadership, management, or a successful radiology practice will have an authoritative and definitive text to which they can turn for guidance.

Going forward, it is likely that leaders and managers will be expected to have more formal training. Larger institutions will see the benefits of this, and radiology groups will be better served with better preparation of their leaders. Hospitals are organizing leadership seminars for mid-career staff, and a number of medical schools have introduced combined programs for training in medicine and business administration. *Radiology Business Practice: How to Succeed* will be an important resource for these new programs.

Drs. Yousem and Beauchamp and their colleagues are to be congratulated for the outstanding new resource they have created for all of us in radiology to use. Anyone whose responsibilities intersect the leadership and management aspects of radiology will be well served to read and reference *Radiology Business Practice: How to Succeed*.

James H. Thrall, MD
Radiologist-in-Chief
Massachusetts General Hospital
Juan M. Taveras Professor of Radiology
Harvard Medical School

One of the great disservices that we exact upon our trainees is sending them out into the "real world" without the skills to understand the business of radiology. The first few years of academic or private practice are a blur of reports no one understands and on-the-job training that influences one's financial situation for years to come. Who teaches young radiologists about employment contracts? Who explains to them the importance of accurate ICD and CPT coding? How can they help in the purchasing of new equipment? Can they influence the profitability of the group they join without an understanding of asset/expense management? Equally unfortunate is the circumstance of finding oneself in a leadership position without the experience or know-how to ensure the success of those who are counting on you. Who insures that individuals new to leadership roles have the skills and traits needed to be effective? It is well demonstrated that the accomplishments that enable one to be selected as the boss are not necessarily the ones needed to stay in the position.

When we started out in our radiology faculty positions, we scarcely knew what an RVU was, having been sheltered from the business side of radiology and consumed with being the best clinical radiologists we could be as well as developing our teaching and research credentials. Relatively early in both of our careers, we came to see that understanding the business of radiology, and contributing to its success, was as important to the mission of impacting the lives of our patients and trainees as being facile with differential diagnoses. This became clear in large part based on our observing the manner in which our Chairman at the Johns Hopkins Medical Institution, Elias Zerhouni, reknown for his business acumen (in addition to a wealth of clinical knowledge and research experience), created an environment for success in all aspects of our mission. Inspired, one of us went on for an MBA while the other got an MHS degree so that we could better understand the health care environment and the ramifications on the business side of the department. We were both fortunate to have our interest, motivation, and fledgling expertise rewarded with leadership opportunities: as Vice Chairman (NJB) and as Neuroradiology Division Chief. In order to ensure our success, Elias enrolled us in the Leadership Development Program of the Medical School.

Importantly, whereas Dr. Zerhouni acknowledged the value of formal training in business, he also felt it was of far greater importance to have mentored on-the-job training. As such, he encouraged us to manage our portions of the departmental expenses and revenue stream as well as to pursue every opportunity to improve efficiency and effectiveness. He accepted early on that we would get as much wrong as we got right but embraced the notion that mistakes provide some of the most teachable moments, even in business.

There were too many teachable moments to count in the first months. Through this period we learned how to "talk the talk," and we learned what questions to ask. We learned to embrace feedback, positive and negative, toward the goal of becoming more effective in our roles. And although it took one of us five years to get the hang of it (DMY) and the other just 18 months (NJB) when he was thrust into the Interim Chairman role, we became comfortable with the business of radiology. It was also during this time that we decided to train together for the Baltimore Marathon. It was during long hours of road work that we reflected on the path to leadership and reached a conclusion better summarized by Nietzsche:

When one has finished building one's house, one suddenly realizes that in the process one has learned something that one really needed to know in the worst way—before one began.

FRIEDRICH NIETZSCHE

Specifically, we came to the mutual conclusion that someone should publish a radiology business book that demystified this aspect of our profession. A book that would shorten the learning curve for those who followed us.

When we mentioned our idea about this book to residents and fellows and colleagues, they would get wide-eyed and enthusiastic: "That's exactly what we need—a practical guide to the business of radiology!" We took the RSNA chairman-to-be courses and the RSNA business courses, became members of the board of radiologist private practice groups, and brainstormed on how to pull off this book. We recognized early on that the combined expertise of two academicians, even with extra three-letter degrees after our MDs, was simply not enough. We decided to edit the book and to recruit experts in academic life and private practice to contribute ... and not just MDs but MBAs and JDs and PhDs. We also decided that this book should be applicable to all health care administrators who deal with or within the practice of radiology.

We were fortunate to assemble a masterful group of contributors. As the chapters rolled in, we were amazed at how adept the authors were in their fields and how lucky we were to have selected the best and the brightest. With each chapter, we grew more and more excited about this book. The tone throughout is familiar, with lots of tables, lists, illustrations, and key "Dos and Don'ts." The final result is a very easy-to-read, definitive guide to the business of radiology.

This book breaks new ground as the first business book in the field of radiology. We believe it will be a valuable tool for those in the specialty who want to succeed. We hope that our lofty aspirations for this contribution are well-founded and that it helps you, the reader, to succeed ... or at least to get up and running that much quicker.

Well it's time for you to dive into the book and unlock the secrets to the radiology business world out there. We hope you enjoy the reading as much as we enjoyed the writing and the editing.

Your hosts,
Norm Beauchamp
Dave Yousem

EDITORS' ACKNOWLEDGMENTS •••

It takes a village, that is for sure! The people to whom I owe a huge debt of gratitude are manifold. Certainly, Norm Beauchamp, my friend and collaborator, was an inspiration and encouraged me to pursue this project. His insights and suggestions elevated the book's quality and helped me with my chapters immensely.

All of the authors were so forthcoming. They met their deadlines, often with days to spare, and created an exceptional product. I express my appreciation to them, and I am sure they will receive individual praise for their valuable insights.

Doug Hough, Chairman of the Hopkins Business of Medicine program, read each chapter and provided an academic businessman's perspective. The medicolegal chapter required the approval of the man who is the expert in our field, Lenny Berlin. Laurie Amell, a lawyer friend, also gave that chapter the thumbs up. We sought the good counsel of friends who live and breathe by the numbers, Chairmen Bill Bradley, Bob Grossman, Jon Lewin, and Jim Thrall. Thanks to all of you.

At Hopkins, I was supported by my Chairman, Jon Lewin, and business administrator extraordinaire, Marty Bledsoe. The brain trust of Bob Gayler, Stan Siegelman, and Bruce Berlanstein gave me encouragement. Within my division, I had the assistance of Drs. Nafi Aygun, Izlem Izbudak, Mike Kraut, Doris Lin, Jay Pillai, Marty Pomper, Dan Sasson, Bruce Wasserman, and Jim Zinreich. My professional standing would not be what it is without my most critical friend, colleague, and research coordinator, Rena Geckle. "She made me!"

I also had support in the office from Elnor Brown, Sue Hayes, Amanda Barnes, Zena Godfrey, and Priscilla Matthews.

At Elsevier, we were privileged to have Meghan McAteer provide the initial go-ahead. She handed us off to the capable team of Rebecca Gaertner and Elizabeth Hart. Liz did the hard work of assembling the chapters, doing a professional edit, inserting some style and grace, and making sure production ran smoothly. I am grateful to Meghan, Rebecca, and Liz for a standout performance.

Finally, four people lived through my incessant carping and chattering about the book's genesis and progression. My children, Ilyssa and Mitch, knew the ins and outs of my dealings with the various authors and tried to take my mind off of it by responding with heavy adolescent issues. Thanks kids. My Mom was always there on the phone, egging me on and telling me she couldn't wait until this book was published. Thanks, Mom. Through the home stretch I met the love of my life, Kelly Beary, who has inspired me beyond the here and now. ILY forever. Thanks for cheering me on and completing me.

DAVE YOUSEM

I hope you find this book helpful in positioning you to have a greater impact in radiology. We are in a field that is transforming the practice of medicine, and it is our responsibility to be as informed as possible to help optimize this contribution. I would like to dedicate this effort to my wife, Kristina, without whom I could not realize my dream of having an impact in medicine. She is an inspiration, a role model, and a partner in the truest sense of the word. I dedicate this to my two sons, Jake and Luke, who brighten my every day with their unlimited potential, insights, kindness, energy, and wonderful races to greet me when I return home every evening. Lastly, I dedicate this to my father and mother, Norm Sr. and Anne Beauchamp, who sacrificed for the benefit of their children and instilled a belief that it was both a possibility and a responsibility to help others.

I acknowledge the great energy and partnership of Dave Yousem. He has been among my very closest friends for over a decade, and we would not have completed this on time without his relentless energy. He has a unique ability to maintain his focus during even the most challenging times. As Dave mentioned, we are both extremely grateful for the team at Elsevier; thanks Meghan, Rebecca, and Liz. Thanks also to Peggy Gordon for producing the book. I would also like to thank my extraordinary leadership team at the University of Washington. During the writing of this book, it has become particularly clear to me how important it is to be surrounded by such outstanding individuals.

NORM BEAUCHAMP

AUTHORS' ACKNOWLEDGMENTS •••

Practice management invariably leads to numbers, bottom lines, and profit margins. At the end, it must come back to the patient. No matter what "performance standards" and goals we try to strive for, at the end there is only the patient's health and well-being. Our patients are mothers, sisters, children, or other loved ones. In all of our decision making, we must place their interests and well-being first. Our performance and goals can be distilled to a single concept: provide the highest quality patient care.

GAUTAM AGRAWAL

I thank my wife for her limitless support for all of my endeavors.

CRAIG BLACKMORE

To the scientists who have developed and continue to enhance our technology. "The greatest mystery is not that we have been flung at random between the profusion of matter and of the stars, but that within this prison we can draw from ourselves images powerful enough to deny our nothingness." Andre Malraux (1901–1976)

MARTY BLEDSOE

Special thanks for help, friendship, and inspiration to Harold Goldman, Robert Grossman, and Howard Pollack.

JOHN BONAVITA

I was pleased when invited to participate in this book. It has been a difficult pleasure over the past 15 years to work in the imaging industry, which is dedicated to improved quality of life as well as saving lives through early detection. Managing change is as good as it gets, but nothing is better than using education and experience to build a healthcare business by creating a culture that focuses on people, including patients, their physicians, and support staff and our own caregivers and support staff. Thanks to all those who have made this their life's work and to my family for their support and encouragement.

BOB CARFAGNO

In memory of William Volk Relyea, MD, 1923–2006.
Thanks,
FELIX CHEW

To my four children, Laura, Jennifer, Emily, and Jacob, who constantly challenge, inspire, and motivate me to go the extra mile.

AUDREY DROSSNER

This working contribution has been refreshing and educational for me. I gave a little, but received a lot. All my professional life has been in academic medical centers, large associations and societies, in both not-for-profit and corporate settings. These hierarchical type institutions create views that are well structured, different from the open, adaptive approach used in small, medium, and large private practices. Those people in these environments have expanded my vision and opened my eyes. Doug Yock, David Seidenwurm, Sal DeSena, and Dave Yousem have expansive, broad views of the newer way to accomplish the important mission of healthcare services in this evolving and rapidly changing world. To them I am indebted, thankful, and now better educated.

JAMES GANTENBERG

Appreciation is expressed to Michael Harris, BSEE, Director of Physics and Engineering, The Russell H. Morgan Department of Radiology and Radiological Science, The Johns Hopkins Medical Institution, for more than 20 years of collegial due diligence in the capital acquisition process.

BOB GAYLER

To Dave and Norm for their patient guidance. To Norm especially for his charismatic stimulation to progress in the game and for his inspirational vision of the big picture. Professionally and personally he will always remain a beacon. To N.H. and S.H. for limitless support. To M.S., T.N., and Y.O. for expanding my horizons. To K.K. for a most generous friendship and societal study. And to S. for the continuing creation of those countless precious memories that I shall cherish for a lifetime and will be the last that dance before my eyes at the end of life's great journey.

CHRIS HURT

Dedicated to Nathan, Aaron, and Beth for their constant support and patience during the many days spent writing this chapter!

PETER A. JANICK

I am tremendously grateful to many who have significantly affected my life. Professionally, I extend immense gratitude to Ben Kuzma, Nick Patronas, Nick Bryan, Eric Russell, Hervey Segall, and Steve Stevens. Academically, MBA team "P2" (Linda Blonsley, Frank Dolce, Peter Foehl, Michele Hilton, Matt Huish, Robert Merrills, Scott Morrill, Ryan Spencer, and Eric Straddeck) compassionately helped me revitalize self-confidence. Personally, my wife Sandra has provided me with life's eloquence. These folks are my greatness.

GREG KATZMAN

Dedicated to all those who have chosen a profession in medicine, teaching, and new discovery. My thanks to you all.

CHRIS LAUBENTHAL

To Frank and Betsy for your encouragement, help, and love from the beginning and to the entire extended Lexa clan for all your support.

To all of the attendings, fellows, residents, staff, and students along the way: I hope that we can preserve and protect our profession so that the next generation will be able to enjoy radiology as much as we have.

To my friends at the Wharton School—I am privileged both to be an alumnus and now to serve with the greatest faculty anywhere.

To Chief, a world class mentor, superb venture capitalist, and a real entrepreneur.

To Alek and Matthew—my special guys—and all my nieces and nephews. You kids are the future and you are my inspiration for building a better world.

To Tanya, my one and only lady love: Thanks for sharing the adventure—I cherish every day.

FRANK LEXA

Thanks to my wife, Sara, and my two children, David and Rebecca, for always supporting me and making my life meaningful. Thanks to William Gold, PhD, for teaching me so much about managed care negotiations.

ANDY LITT

To thank our readers and colleagues, all of whom serve to lead and motivate, perhaps I might borrow from Shakespeare's *Richard II*:
"The purest treasure mortal times afford
Is spotless reputation: That away,
Men are but gilded loam or painted clay."

FRED MANN

I would like to thank Norman Beauchamp for inspiration, David Yousem for insightfulness, Donna Cross for challenges, and my family—Yoshimi Anzai and Erika—for supporting my working style.

SATOSHI MINOSHIMA

I acknowledge my appreciation for the opportunity to work with the radiology community. In particular, I am indebted to my father and mentor, Lawrence R. Muroff, MD, FACR, who has devoted his career to promoting the practice, business, and scholarship of radiology. His insight and support have been invaluable not only to me but also to countless others who have been inspired by his leadership.

JULIE MUROFF

We would like to thank all of the people who were responsible for researching, writing, editing, and correcting this book, especially our wives, Trish Robinson and Veronica Condon. This book is dedicated to those individuals who sincerely want to improve upon the quality of healthcare in the United States and to pursue outstanding radiologic care for all. Those individuals who are reading this for other purposes, please do not read beyond this page. If the constant pursuit of excellence and or a passion for continual education is not burning within you by the end of this book, then we will have failed. There is no passion in mediocrity, and hopefully you will all be able to write new chapters based on your own facilities' success after reading this book.

JOE ROBINSON AND DENNIS CONDON

Thanks to my cat, Indy, for periodically walking on the keyboard of my computer and thus improving the quality of my text and the profundity of my thinking.

I want to thank my boss, one of the editors of this book (N.J.B.), for his continual coaching about how to make the business of academic radiology stronger and for supporting the view that this business strength is our most viable path to a sustainable future. And I want to thank my father, who transmitted to me his interest in the business of medicine.

WILLIAM P. SHUMAN

CONTENTS •••

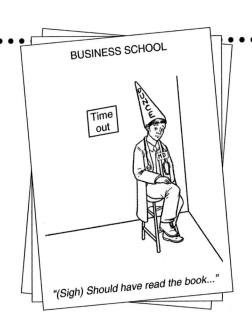

CHAPTER 1

BUSINESS SCHOOL

Time out

"(Sigh) Should have read the book..."

Introduction

David M. Yousem

As the health care environment grows more labyrinthine, there is greater opportunity for effective leaders to establish a marked competitive advantage.

The complexity of health care demands that physician and nonphysician leaders develop an understanding of the business of medicine. This is particularly so in radiology. In the not-too-distant past, it was true that the excess cash flows associated with imaging and image-guided procedures provided a buffer to protect the management neophyte. However, managed care, double-digit imaging growth, increasing competition, multiple points of service, rising capital costs, and ever-increasing operational complexity mandate a depth of understanding that is not routinely acquired during medical school or during the standard educational path taken by nonphysician leaders.

Unfortunately, the only means for learning the business side of the practice of medicine in radiology has been via (1) word of mouth from mentors in the training programs or (2) the "college of hard knocks," as one makes error after error in one's career. There are also the Harvard/Wharton business school offerings which are either too expensive (at $15,000) or too generic (tailored to all medical specialties) to be an "economical" use of one's time as a practicing radiologist or radiology administrator.

Put in a positive frame, one is reminded of Albert Einstein's quote that "in the middle of adversity lies opportunity." We are not referring here to the economic opportunity for us to provide the source code to this understanding in fewer than 300 reasonably priced pages, but rather to the observation we have made that understanding the business of medicine in today's complex environment provides a tremendous competitive advantage. For physicians to truly take control of their practice or their departments, they should understand fundamental business concepts. For business administrators in the health care market there must be specialty- specific knowledge as well.

The truth is that Radiology is Big Business. In most academic hospitals the departments of radiology, pathology, and surgery are the main revenue generators for the institution. Of these, the department of radiology is also one of the greatest consumers of the capital and operating budgets of the institution. Mismanagement of a department that is purchasing $10 million of equipment each year has far-reaching implications. Over 50% of the capital equipment budgets of hospitals often is dedicated to imaging units (although some may be outside the bailiwick of radiology, such as cardiac catheter/electrophysiology labs). The expectation is that these units will then generate revenue, which pays back the investment (usually measured in "years to payback"—see Chapter 11, "Purchasing Capital Equipment") or has a healthy ROI. (In this book ROI means "return on investment," not "region of interest," as in other radiology texts.) Done correctly, imaging can be transformational to patient outcomes and instrumental in securing the needed resources to accomplish institutional goals; when executed poorly, the likelihood of significant economic losses and diminution in quality of care increases.

The danger in not learning business principles in a private practice setting is equally important. Although one may not have hospital administrators, deans, and CEOs scrutinizing the management of resources, the practice partners and each radiologist's livelihood may ride on the quality of financial decisions made. Opening an outpatient imaging center with a CT scanner and MR scanner and a plain film unit involves millions in cash or borrowed capital. With adequate attention to technology and capital planning, business planning and finance, growth promotion, and operational efficiency, the risks can be minimized and the return optimized. Hence the need for a book that can help the physician and nonphysician manager understand the ramifications of these business decisions.

There are also examples, too numerous to count, of physicians entering group practices not understanding the contractual constraints of their first jobs and feeling locked into practices that may be abusive, unyielding, or financially untenable. The rate at which radiologists enter and leave new jobs is quite striking and part of this, no doubt, is due to their inability to adequately assess the quality of the group practice, the contract offered, and the potential for practice growth. These issues are addressed in Chapter 17, "Assessing Growth Opportunities for Your Imaging Practice," and Chapter 23, "Employment Contracts."

APPLICATION OF THIS BOOK TO ACADEMIC VERSUS PRIVATE PRACTICE

The issues that drive an academic practice and those that drive a private practice share some commonalities and some differences.[1,2] However, the designation of an academic university practice as a nonprofit entity should not deceive the reader. Clearly, one of the main goals of not-for-profit and for-profit practices is to make maximum revenue from their existing resources to address their respective missions. There is a tendency to include a greater proportion of non-revenue yet socially necessary services in not-for-profit centers, but as state and federal funding levels decrease, it has become necessary for the not-for-profit centers to pursue an increasing number of net positive clinical ventures.

The distributions of those profits are dramatically different between the two entities. Not-for-profit entities usually plot to achieve a zero balance at the end of the year and will spend the money improving infrastructure, or, in many cases, supporting research or teaching missions or providing annual bonuses to its faculty. To reiterate, the goal of the nonprofit institutions is to maximize profit for the work they are doing to pay for (1) more research opportunities, (2) more resident/fellow positions, (3) more equipment, (4) more seed grants, and (5) more health care to the uninsured or needy, and so on, even though the bottom-line profit at the end of the cycle may register as zero. For-profit entities also distribute income when they achieve a profit, but they may carry over revenue from one year to the next as part of their balance sheet in retained earnings. They may be a publicly held company and need to demonstrate profit for declaration of dividends or to grow the value of the shared equity (i.e., stockholders' value). Again, the goal of the for-profit entity may be to maximize salaries in some cases and in others, particularly when publicly traded, to raise the value of the company stock. So whichever environment you are in, it makes sense to understand the mechanics of how to run a good radiology practice and maximize the revenue obtained from the work you do.

The purpose of this book is not to make capitalists out of radiologists in practice; however, the old joke that the greatest risk to anesthesiologists is that they will get run over in the parking lot by the radiologists already in their cars racing for the golf course could not be further from reality. It is our, admittedly biased, view that radiologists are among the hardest working practitioners in medicine. Our aspiration is that after devouring this book, you should be able to put into action steps that will reduce the money that you leave on the table, improve the fair reimbursement for the hard work that you do, and minimize the needless expenses that chip away at the profit margin.

There is no reason why physicians should not expect to be paid appropriately and maximally for their daily work. Unfortunately, the third-party payers have a business stratagem as well. Their goals are to try to do whatever they can, within guidelines and legal means, to pay the least amount of money per study and to pay only if the studies performed are billed and coded appropriately. After all, they are also in the business of maximizing their bottom line for their shareholders or owners and distributing their own dividend. If they can justify not reimbursing one in every 50 studies that previously they were paying for, for whatever reason, they are already generating a 2% improvement in expense management (see Chapter 10, "Managing Expenses"). The delays that payers create in subjecting physicians to repeated submissions of their bills, that is, the initial denials for various antiquated reasons, create money through the concept of accounts-payable-delaying strategies. You should be able to use them too or to block them from happening to you.

Entrepreneurship in medicine need not be solely the realm of the practice administrators and the venture capitalists (Chapter 20, "Medical Entrepreneurship in Diagnostic Imaging"). The advent of the filmless environment (Chapter 13, "Information Technology Systems"), coupled with the pervasiveness of the Internet and of voice recognition dictation (Chapter 14, "Voice Recognition Dictation"), has spawned the cottage industry of teleradiology (Chapter 19, "Teleradiology in Practice"). In the 21st century you need not be in the same city, state, time zone, country, continent, or hemisphere to be reading the local imaging studies. Thus, to grow the business, you must think in four dimensions. But teleradiology is not the only potential for radiology's growth.

New techniques are being developed every few years. Who would have thought that radiologists would noninvasively be interrogating the coronary arteries at this time (coronary CTA)? Who would have thought that we would be on the brink of visualizing gene expression, protein production, or myoinositol levels with our current molecular imaging and magnetic resonance (MR) spectroscopic techniques? Arteriolar imaging is now possible with 7 tesla MR microscopy. White matter tracts from the cortex to the basal ganglia can be parsed from MR data with relative ease today. We approach psychiatric disease with functional imaging and determine whether there are abnormal connections or activations in patients with schizophrenia. And now we even have a unique nuclear medicine agent, which can detect and quantify beta-amyloid deposition in the brain. We can even predict who will respond to radiation/chemotherapy regimens for head and neck cancer through early evaluation with CT-PET (computed tomography/positron emission tomography) imaging. Through the development of such novel techniques and having a "research mission" in practice (Chapter 5, "Research Mission"), we in radiology have the opportunity to grow or create new businesses if we're smart, and if we have the core knowledge on how to use our prowess. We need to learn.

ORGANIZATION OF THIS BOOK

The book you are reading is divided into four parts: Leadership; Accounting and Finance; Building, Managing, and Growing a Practice; Practice Management; and Legal and Legislative Issues.

Part 1, "Leadership in a Radiology Practice," espouses many principles of effective management of radiology practices from an interpersonal approach. The best leaders adopt a mission and a vision that can be grasped and embraced by all members of the organization, direct a strategic plan that is designed to accomplish that mission, and manage the conflicts and obstacles that may challenge the successful obtainment of the organization's goals. They recognize that leadership skills and traits are essential for success. It is imperative to be able to manage self as well as others. Contributors to the "Leadership" section of the book include chairpersons of academic radiology departments, a CEO of a private practice group, and the executive director of one of the country's largest subspecialty radiology societies. Their perspectives on effective leadership are varied yet applicable to many different settings in your professional and personal life.

To understand business you must understand the vocabulary of finance and accounting. Part 2, "Accounting Basics and Financial Principles," provides the essentials required to be able to decipher the important entries of balance sheets, income statements, and cash flow analyses. Becoming familiar with the terminology used in the business world and being able to understand the concepts involved is the first step to maintaining control of your practice. In some cases you may be able to manage your own professional finances as you manage your personal finances, but when the stakes are as high as they can get in radiology practices, you may opt to hire practice managers for your group. Hiring a practice manager does not have to mean ceding control of your financial future to this person or their team. In fact, it is dangerous if that occurs especially if goals are not aligned properly between team members. This section of the book will allow the physician participant to play an informed active role in practice decisions and allow wise judgments in determining the direction the practice will grow. Accounting basics will be taught by MBA graduates in private practice; however, practice management strategies will be drawn from both the academic and private practice arena from physician leaders.

In Part 3, "Building and Managing a Practice," the infrastructure required for a successful radiology department is explored in the "Nuts and Bolts" section. The second section, "Growing the Practice," includes chapters on how to assess the potential market, advertise, find niches, and reap the benefits from these analyses. Once again these chapters combine theory and practice and will be useful in any practice setting.

Part 4, "Legal and Legislative Concerns," covers the arena of legal and regulatory issues, tying in well with some aspects of practice management, which deal with growth strategies. Most readers will be interested in the primary issues of contractual agreements when starting a new job, risk management, and malpractice issues. In a nutshell, this section will help the reader avoid getting trapped in an unfair contract and, hopefully, also avoid medical litigation for perceived or alleged deviations from the standard of care.

Finally, in the last chapters the authors will draw upon their vast experience of 40 years of swings and misses in the hope of helping all of you avoid some of our growing pains. Although we agree with Benjamin Disraeli's aphorism that all our successes are built upon our failures, there is no reason why your successes cannot build from *our* failings. This is a more personal exploration of potential pitfalls, which can occur as you try to build a thriving practice with enlightened, happy employees and a robust bottom line. Unfortunately, to get to that point, you often have to navigate through shark-infested waters. The oral tradition of passing down horror stories will be carried out in the final chapter, "Learning from Others' Mistakes," which supplies an abundance of admonitions to the unblemished.

We expect that every graduating resident and fellow, every new radiology administrator, every departmental/group practice employee, and every new entrant or partner into a radiology team will read this book and find parts of it fascinating and applicable to their own experience in the world of radiology practice. There will be sections for everyone and, for some, every section will be beneficial. In each chapter we conclude with the top 5 to 10 dos or don'ts as a practical summary of the chapter and guide to practice. This book will unlock the secrets of success in the business of radiology.

REFERENCES

1. Potter SJ: Longitudinal analysis of the distinction between for-profit and not-for-profit hospitals in America. J Health Soc Behav 42(1):17–44, 2001.
2. Sloan FA, Vraciu RA: Investor-owned and not-for-profit hospitals: Addressing some issues. Health Aff (Millwood) 2(1):25–37, 1983.

PART 1

LEADERSHIP IN A RADIOLOGY PRACTICE

Organizational Structure and Governance: Academic, Solo, and Group Practice

James B. Gantenberg and David M. Yousem

THEORY OF GOVERNANCE IN ACADEMIC PRACTICE

Over the past 200 years Americans have seen the health care business grow into a vast industrial complex, with medicine evolving into one of the most powerful professions. The origin, history, and evolution of American medicine greatly impacts today's academic medical center, whose organizational structure has become so complex that it often defies logic.

The health care delivery system was tracked in the 1982 landmark work by Paul Starr, in the Pulitzer Prize–winning book *The Social Transformation of American Medicine*.[1] Starr details the struggles in the complex world of academic medical centers (AMCs), where medical specialties face the onslaught of change as organizations attempt to deal with higher costs, different payment schema, and financial challenges. The administration of the AMC must deal with, at a departmental level, issues regarding equipment costs (capital budget requests), governmental and insurance company oversight (JCAHO, HCFA, and MCO carve-outs), and continued friction between the needs of individual departments within the AMC. Radiology services face these changes more than other specialties of medicine because of their continuous technological advances, the high cost of providing service, and their large revenue stream (second only to pathology departments in most institutions). In addition, although radiology fought well in the turbulent 80s for larger levels of reimbursement dollars for its high-tech studies, it must continue to face these same issues today as new examinations and techniques (i.e., MR spectroscopy, functional MRI, coronary CT angiography, image-guided cryoablation of tumors) are brought to the clinical realm.[2]

ORGANIZATIONAL COMPLEXITY

A traditional managerial policy and organizational chart for a university medical school is shown in Box 2-1.[3] This is the "big picture," with the department of radiology usually a major cog in the wheel. Most chairs of radiology sit prominently on executive and clinical practice committees of AMCs and their professional business representatives also serve prominently on institutional committees. For the purposes of this chapter, however, we will not dissect the AMC but will examine the governance at a departmental level.

At the academic radiology department level, the confluence of teaching, research, and clinical missions creates a new level of (1) "opportunity" (the euphemism for challenge or complexity),

(2) confusion, and (3) the need for coordination of resources. The tripartite teaching, research, and education functions of the AMC radiology department are often subsumed by vice chairpersons appointed by the departmental chairperson. (For the remainder of this chapter, we will refer to male and female chairpersons as "chairs" alone). There may be a vice chair of research, a vice chair of education, and a vice chair of clinical operations. Because all chairs are aware of the adage "no margin, no mission," as well as the admonition that "the one aspect of the job that can most easily get you fired is forgetting about patient care," the chair inevitably must keep a close eye on the clinical operations in the department. Even if that aspect of the job is delegated to another, the chair of radiology must be able to answer to the other clinical chairs regarding issues of patient care, patient safety, and quality assurance. The vice chairs have direct access to the chair and usually have standing meetings with him or her on a weekly basis.

Invariably, an executive committee (EXCOM) plays a large role in the academic medical center. Usually the committee comprises the various division directors of the department, representing either organ systems or modalities, depending on how the department is structured. In most academic settings today, the departments are organized around organ systems, although the divisions of nuclear medicine, interventional radiology, pediatrics, and even ultrasound may cross organ systems. Depending on the size of the department and the need for leadership positions, the department may be divided into both "divisions" (e.g., abdominal imaging) as well as "sections" (e.g., gastrointestinal and genitourinary). At some institutions there is the adage that "if you can't give them more money, give them a title." This leads to numerous capos in the "Radiology Familia." Thus, representation from leadership at a divisional or a section level may be included at the EXCOM. This goes against the business school maxim that a committee greater than 8 to 10 in number will often be ineffectual. However, the strong sense of "buy-in" achieved by participation on the EXCOM outweighs the lack of nimbleness the large committee engenders.

The EXCOM may be a rubber-stamping device used by some autocratic department heads, but, in most cases, it functions as the main decision-making body of the academic radiology department. In the academic arena, the egos usually are such that it would take a supremely confident department chair to hand down dictates to the EXCOM members. It is unlikely that full professors will "go down without a fight" on most decisions. They didn't arrive at their highly regarded status by being passive, and so, while the chair and his or her professional business manager may set the agenda and make recommendations to the EXCOM, most decisions are arrived at by consensus or majority in the committee.

The role of the professional business team in the AMC should be highlighted. Academic medical centers will have business administrators at nearly every level of management in the departments. Because the radiology department is so critical to the success of the AMC from a financial standpoint, there is likely a great deal of collaboration at the billing and collections level between the department and the center as a whole. At Johns Hopkins, because the department feels that collections are better accomplished by professionals who specialize just in radiology current procedural terminology (CPT) and International Classification of Diseases, 9th revision (ICD-9) coding, the members of the business team of nonphysicians number in the dozens and the team is audited but not governed by the institutional financial professionals. Thus, a dichotomy is established.

The other major dichotomy that occurs throughout the AMC in general is the separation of functions into hospital and university divisions. Typically, the AMC has technologists, nurses, front desk personnel, film librarians, escorts, and so forth, all of whom are hospital employees of the department. The faculty, the human resources staff, the administrative support employees, and the research operations office personnel answer to the university side of the chair's office. For example, patient care payments come into the hospital; grants come into the university. In most cases, since the hospitals *own* the equipment, they get paid the technical fees, even for studies funded by grants coming into the university (the professional component, which is retained by the university side, pays for the faculty). Two organizational charts presented by Johns Hopkins illustrate the separation of functions between hospital and university divisions (see Figs. 2-1 and 2-2).[4]

Two lead business administrators are often in an AMC department—one for the hospital and one for the university. This does not mean that AMC departments focus on the university side of the practice and leave the day-to-day running of the hospitals to the Masters of Health Administration (MHAs) and Masters of Public Health (MPHs). Nor do they ignore the greater institutional needs.

Various other committees within an academic department help build consensus around decision making; these committees may be led by the vice chairs. Typical committees in academic settings include some that are unique to that milieu, including the research, promotions, and education committees. Finance, compliance, practice management, and information technology committees may be found in both the academic settings and the nonacademic hospital environment (see below).

Depending on the chair's proclivity for micromanagement, there may be more or less autonomy in the direction of the department's divisions and sections. The day-to-day management of operations may be addressed at this level without the chair's input, but hiring and firing decisions, purchases, and safety issues are usually cleared through the chair. Often the chair establishes guidelines for the various decisions that are made in strategic planning sessions with division heads. The guidelines are as follows:

1. Provide data for decision making by chair
2. Advise and make recommendations for decision making by chair
3. Discuss problem with chair to arrive at joint decision to be executed by division director
4. Advise chair before decision making by division director
5. Inform chair after decision by division director
6. Division director need not inform chair of the decision

Obviously, the greater the confidence the chair has in her or his direct reports, the more likely further decisions will be made autonomously by the chair's delegates.

One of the most important issues from the radiologist's perspective is clarification of roles and responsibility for research, collections, human resources, expenses, budgeting, CPT reimbursement, accounting, credentialing, teaching mission, and marketing. These are defined in AMCs and delegated to business professionals more readily than in freestanding group practices because of the overhead expense they entail. In either setting questions abound. Who will do which tasks? What roles

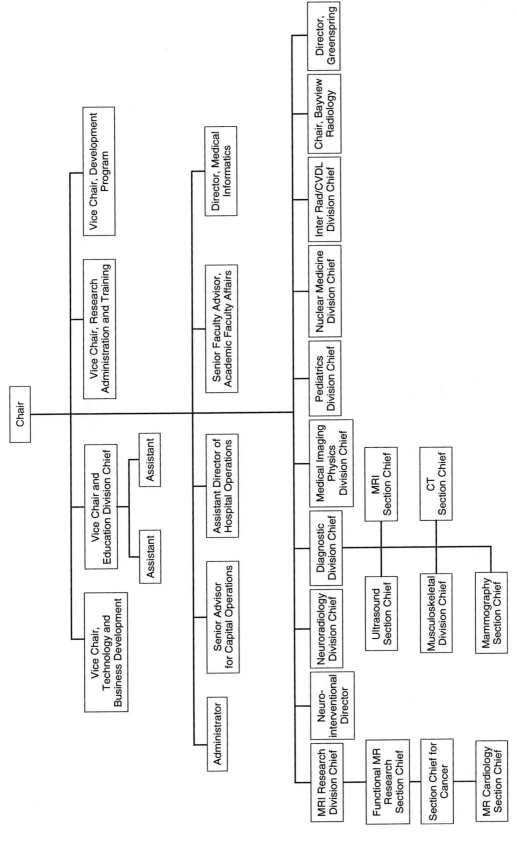

Figure 2-1 Johns Hopkins University and Hospital Department of Radiology. (Courtesy of David M. Yousem, MD.)

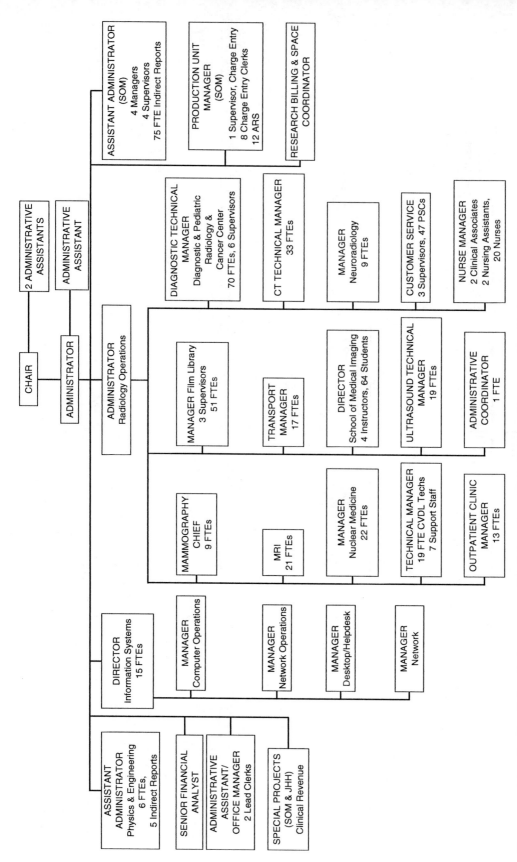

Figure 2-2 Johns Hopkins University Department of Radiology Organizational Chart. (Courtesy of David M. Yousem, MD.)

will the business managers, physicians, administrators, technicians, and staff leaders play? A healthy respect between the physician and business leadership will lead to a successful organization (see Boxes 2-2, 2-3, and 2-4). Thousands of consultants sell management services to AMCs and private practices, often to the tune of $200 million each year, to foster these relationships. The modern business and academic worlds are merging but still have a long way to go. The aim of this book is to help bring about a happy marriage of the two.

BOX 2-2

Radiology Business Manager

JOB TITLE: Radiology Business Manager

DEPARTMENT: Diagnostic Radiology

JOB SUMMARY: At the direction of the Administrative Director, or designee, work collaboratively with the Chairman, Director, and Radiology Section Chiefs as a member of the management team to facilitate the integration, management, and data needs for Radiology, including the outreach programs and research. Manage the departmental budgetary, charge master, billing, reimbursement, coding, compliance, and accounting programs for the Hospital, Clinic, and Radiology research at Dartmouth Medical School and Radiology outreach programs including the Dartmouth Hitchcock Alliance. Conduct programmatic cost analysis for all existing and new programs in the department. Develop and monitor departmental budgets, charge masters, billing and preparation of variance reports, providing recommendations to maintain budget compliance. Manage the reception, financial secretaries, transcriptions, coding specialists, and DWS fiscal personnel.

JOB RESPONSIBILITIES: Manage the departmental fiscal operations, billing systems, coding regulations, financial reporting, insurance and registration process, and research budgets. Maintain a thorough knowledge and command of these areas and integrate that knowledge appropriately into daily operations. Lead the preparation, monitoring, and reporting of operational, revenue, personnel, and capital budgets of the Hospital, Clinic, Dartmouth Medical School, and outreach program for Radiology. Maintain accurate records as they pertain to budgets, billing, and other fiscal programs within the department. Maintain an ongoing evaluation of the Hospital and Clinic Price File (CPT). Recommend new and revised CPT code and Clinic fees to the Department Chairman, Department Director, and Clinic Manager of Codes and Fees. Assist in pricing development for new Radiology procedures with accurate ICD-9 and CPT and revenue codes for Part A and B billing. Monitor expenditures pertaining to purchases, services, and maintenance contracts, and provide feedback and recommendations to the managers concerning budget compliance. Process purchase requisitions and monitor receipt of purchase orders for the department. Prepare graphs, financial feasibility reports, and statistical analyses in any area of departmental programs as directed for the Hospital, Clinic, and Dartmouth Medical School. Provide support, knowledge, and resources to the department Chairman, Director, Section Chiefs, managers, radiologist researchers, and other support staff members in the preparation of documents, reports, statistics, graphs, and surveys for external and internal constituents. Manage Radiology's reception, transcription, billing, and the financial component of the DMS radiology research. Select, direct, monitor, and coach staff members in the areas to work in as a team to create a productive, positive atmosphere for patients and staff. Collaborate with Clinic and Hospital administrative and secretarial staff to assure smooth, productive interactions between these groups and Radiology.

Lead Radiology's Compliance Program as the Compliance Officer to assure the department is in compliance with all federal and state compliance regulations, including: maintaining a departmental compliance program; ensuring staff members understand and abide by ethical standards; ensuring all billing is handled and documented appropriately; fostering open communications in which staff can voice their concerns and/or report noncompliance without fear of retribution. Assume responsibility for the development of ongoing education relating to compliance and ethical standards.

Working with institutional, state, and national resources, take a leadership role to assure pending system changes or that regulatory initiatives are reviewed, challenged, necessary, and, where appropriate, integrated into institutional and departmental operations. Participate with the management team in the development of

Continued

BOX 2-2

Radiology Business Manager—cont'd

departmental goals and process improvement programs that implement these goals and programs into the daily operation of the department. Monitor radiology research and grants and contracts expenditures in conjunction with the principal investigator. Report financial status of grants on a regular basis to the Department Chairman, Department Director, and principal investigator. Collaborate with Dartmouth Medical School and Radiology research administrative staff. Act as departmental liaison with the Hospital, Clinic, and Dartmouth Medical School Business Offices pertaining to areas of responsibility. Maintain membership in related professional organizations, keeping abreast of innovations and changes in the health care environment.

MINIMUM EDUCATION AND EXPERIENCE: Bachelor's degree in accounting or business administration, with 5 years of health care business and/or financial experience, or the equivalent in education and/or experience required. Radiology business management, CPT, and ICD-9 coding and reimbursement experience preferred. Previous experience working with personal computers desired.

© *University of Medicine and Dentistry of New Jersey—website, amended March 30, 2005.*

BOX 2-3

Administrative Director

JOB TITLE: Administrative Director, Diagnostic Radiology

JOB SUMMARY: At the direction of the Chair of the Department of Diagnostic Radiology and in coordination with the administrative direction of the Vice President for Medical Services, be responsible for the management of the department, including (but not limited to) planning, quality assurance, personnel management, and support of academic programs and coordinating Radiology's services within the Hospital, Clinic, and Dartmouth Medical School.

JOB RESPONSIBILITIES: In conjunction with the Chair, Vice President, and appropriate staff input, set goals and objectives for the department and delineate strategies for implementing and achieving goals. Develop and monitor annual and long-range department budgets (Hospital, Clinic, Medical School). Delineate and develop new programs that support department goals and objectives.

In conjunction with the Chairman, be responsible for the quality of all patient care and support activities of the department. Hire, monitor, and evaluate all technical and support personnel with input from appropriate division physician directors. Manage the quality assurance and support activities of the Diagnostic Physicist. Responsible for structuring professional and technical fees and for coding and auditing within third-party payer guidelines. Ensure appropriate and timely quality assurance (QA) activities and documentation, coordinating with the QA Director. Delegate as appropriate. Develop and maintain programs to ensure accreditation, licensure, and a high level of safety in accordance with good practice and state and federal guidelines. Monitor department performance with particular attention to customer satisfaction, market share, and fiscal parameters. Attend Department Director's and other necessary meetings in center institutions and coordinate resources with other departments to achieve department and institution goals. Direct the procurement of supplies and equipment. Evaluate the need for new or modified supplies and equipment to update or accommodate new and existing procedures. Oversee maintenance schedules on equipment and ensure that Radiology's equipment is safe for patients and personnel. Responsible for the cleanliness, sterility, and operation of all equipment, traffic control, and infection control necessary to establish a proper environmental standard for the department. Direct personnel in compliance with safety methods, including disaster and emergency procedures. Work collaboratively with the Chairman/Medical Director, and with Hospital Administration, Finance, and Purchasing in the prospective assessment of technology for the department. Develop a long-range equipment replacement plan which links to the Hospital's strategic plan and presents a basis for becoming a high-quality, low-cost provider of diagnostic imaging services. Participate in state, regional, and national Radiology Administrators organizations. Develop support for ongoing and new interdepartmental education programs, including (but not limited to)

Continued

in-service education and technologist clinical affiliations and department-sponsored regional conference. Perform additional duties and responsibilities as deemed appropriate by the Chair and Vice President.

MINIMUM EDUCATION AND EXPERIENCE: MBA with 5 years of experience in departmental management or the equivalent in education and experience required. Experience in a tertiary care academic Radiology department preferred. Educational and work experience that enables the individual to develop budgets and manage department finances. Familiarity with contemporary computer and radiology management information systems. Certified Radiology Administrator (CRA) preferred.

© *University of Medicine and Dentistry of New Jersey—website, amended March 30, 2005.*

BOX 2-4

Radiology Clinical Operations Manager

JOB TITLE: Radiology Clinical Operations Manager

DEPARTMENT: Diagnostic Radiology

JOB SUMMARY: At the direction of the Administrative Director, Chair, and Clinical Section Chiefs, manage the administrative, informational, quality assurance, regulatory compliance, clinical performance compliance, and operational functions of all patient care sections of the department. Serve as a leader and role model for Radiology employees within the organization and outside the organization. This person shall manage staffing concerns, collaborating on resource utilization, resolving performance management issues, as well as managing clinical activities. It is essential that this individual exhibit leadership behaviors consistent with the DHMC and Radiology mission by collaborating with the Administrative Director, Section Chiefs, institution practice managers/nursing directors, Radiology management team, Radiology nurses and technologists, and Radiology support personnel.

JOB RESPONSIBILITIES: Manage the administrative, informational, quality assurance, regulatory compliance, clinical performance compliance, and operational functions of all patient care sections of the department. Serve as a role model both within and outside the organization by exhibiting leadership behaviors, such as encouraging and involving others, delegating authority, facilitating decision making and building consensus between and within divisions and colleagues. Collaborating with the Radiology management team, and Section Chiefs, manage the clinical Team Leaders and professional staff to ensure compliance with regulatory standards while providing a safe, efficient, and effective Radiology imaging service. Manage imaging equipment assessment needs, acquisition, use, and delivery of service. Apply these responsibilities to clinical and informational components, including all decentralized areas and service. Act in conjunction with appropriate ancillary and nursing departments and hospital committees to collaboratively ensure compliance with standards of care in conjunction with a safe, efficient, and effective radiology imaging service.

Act as a resource and facilitator regarding compliance with both DHMC and radiology-specific policies and procedures. Oversee the evaluation of products, supplies, space, and capital imaging equipment. Make recommendations for change or modification when appropriate. Manage and oversee Radiology's compliance and final documentation of the JCAHO and other mandated clinical certifying agencies (NRC, MQSA) standards. Coordinate the hiring and performance management of professional staff to include technologists, nursing, and support staff. Develop staff scheduling programs to maximize staff and imaging equipment utilization and to minimize overtime.

Work with the Administrative Director, Business Manager, and Asset Manager in developing, implementing, and monitoring the Radiology budget. Exhibit a leadership role in planning, organizing, and developing the department's capital budget specific to each section's needs. Participate in planning, data collection, and the preparation of reports as appropriate. Represent the Radiology department at assigned meetings, and other internal and external activities. Exhibit leadership behaviors and assume a liaison role with other departments to ensure ongoing lines of communication and quality improvement activities. Keep abreast of new developments in Radiology. Champion the continuing education programs of the

Continued

Radiology Clinical Operations Manager—cont'd

department with a focus toward developing and maintaining technologists' and nurses' competencies as identified by the JCAHO, American Registry of Radiologic Technologists, American Radiology Nurses Association, and other continuing education monitoring organizations. Collaborate with the Radiation Safety Officer to ensure compliance with the Department's Radiation Safety Program. Review film badge dosimetry reports, patient-related incident reports, and take appropriate action to assure a safe environment for patients and staff. Mentor supervisory staff and other subordinates in enhancing their management and leadership skills. Perform the duties of the Administrative Director in his/her absence. Serve as a resource to the other departmental managers as appropriate.

MINIMUM EDUCATION AND EXPERIENCE: Radiologic Technologist registered with the American Registry of Radiologic Technologists with a minimum of 5 years' leadership and management experience. Bachelor's degree in Radiology or Business Administration, or equivalent experience required. Excellent communication and interpersonal skills required.

© *University of Medicine and Dentistry of New Jersey—website, amended March 30, 2005.*

PRIVATE PRACTICE GROUP MANAGEMENT

Private group practice has its own challenges. Working in those practices where physicians must double as radiology film readers and practice managers can create friction but can also make the rewards that much greater. Note the functional job descriptions for the academic setting in Boxes 2-2, 2-3, and 2-4 for business managers, clinical administrators, and so forth. These descriptions also apply to group practice, but in the latter one person may do several jobs, with physician and nonphysician personnel sharing responsibilities.[6]

In the 1980s two thirds of U.S. physicians were in solo practice. Less than 40% of physicians now practice alone. Since 1985 more physicians joined group practices than are accounted for by the number graduating from medical schools. Established "solo" physicians are now joining those in small groups, or, more likely, being acquired by large group practices. The scene in radiology mirrors these trends: because start-up expenses are so high it is hard for solo practitioners to go it alone.[5]

From the business side, a solo practitioner today who can handle his or her own finances and contract negotiations is an anachronism. The fragmentation and specialization of services complicating the business of medicine is the driving force toward group consolidation. The insurance industry contributes to the need for large negotiating groups because of its intricate contracts, credentialing requirements, and capitation. The complexity of the medical practice, with OSHA guidelines, practice standards, and human resource specifications, creates more confusion and responsibility at all levels in centers and practice. Throw in managed care contracts, ubiquitous lawyers, debt, and financial uncertainty, and it is not surprising that physicians seek refuge in either academic centers or large group practices. Each offers different advantages and disadvantages, yet both offer above all a form of security. Hence the demise of the Mom and Pop imaging center.

THE GOVERNANCE OF GROUP PRACTICE

The initial formation of group practice, although different from setting to setting and state to state, has some commonalities. Muroff[5] has outlined some sound principles of organization and governance for radiology practices. The first is the development of a viable mission and vision statement, and a business plan. The mission/vision statement clearly defines in simple terms what the group stands for and plans to accomplish. The business plan extends the mission and includes the necessary steps to accomplish goals over a given time frame. The business plan, often formulated by the corporate nonphysician manager, details dates, resources, personnel, and procedures to accomplish the tasks defined by the mission/vision statement.

The next major step is defining the leadership and governance processes. In other words, who will do what. Who are the accountable authorities for the professional, medical side versus the business side of the operation? Sometimes, in small practices, the same person fills both roles. As the group grows, however, special skills are required or cultivated and leaders become more ascendant. The business and the professional sides of the group create the milieu in which strong service goals coincide with strong business principles. Negotiations, collections/billing, and marketing can peacefully coexist with patient, institution, and community relations. The usual leader at this juncture is a physician CEO, not a non-MD administrator business executive.

The development of the group practice is really a lesson in organizational and/or any business ventures. In all medical organizations and practices, success is based on the ability to set vision and solid decision making through a mission statement and a comprehensive business plan. Most groups begin with autocratic governance, which evolves slowly into more democratic structures based on the number of partners, the leadership acumen of the physicians and the actions of the board, and the cooperation of the administrative staff. Power is usually consolidated at the top based on the size of the practice. Shareholders in some group practices with a board of directors may vie for control and ultimate power. Some physicians respond well to the tasks of administration and management, whereas others clearly do not have that expertise. Radiology practice leaders have recognized that one way to obtain buy-in from all parties to achieve a common goal is through empowerment. This strategy is usually actuated through the use of committees such as finance, operations, new business development, and marketing, all of which are clearly critical to the success of the group practice. Moreover, it provides an opportunity to foster leadership talents and interests among the physician and professional corps, as well as a respectful relationship between the physician and executive/administrative leaders.

The structure and composition of practice management committees may vary according to the size of the practice, but the overall intent of the committees is clearly based on the name and the principal responsibilities and activities.

Operations committees deal with personnel, scheduling, HIPPAA regulations, reimbursement, CPS, and other regulatory bodies at local, state, and federal levels. Finance committees deal with compensation, benefits, insurance, business practices for records, coding, and billing. Marketing committees target practice development, advertising, and community awareness. These basic functions are required for every practice, large or small. These principles of effective organization and governance for radiology practice stress competition based on the ability to assess situations rapidly, make solid decisions together, and develop proactive policies, which are adopted by the practice members, the management, shareholders, and owners. Committees work if all members are able to identify with the missions and goals of the group. The hard part is to tailor the committee's function to the desired outcomes and to the problem-solving skills of the individual members. There are no hard and fast rules. Group practice can move more quickly with flexible committee structure, while bigger groups and AMCs often get bogged down, a sure sign of dysfunctional committees. Also, a general understanding of how organizations work enables success. Too many radiologists eschew active involvement in practice governance. They remember their residency years and recall with some pain the cumbersome nature of the bureaucracy at academic hospitals.

With an introduction to the governance principles of nonacademic group practices described above, one can see that there are a number of variables that determine how sophisticated and complex a group's organizational scheme may be. Put simply, a group of radiologists will organize their team based on a number of factors, as listed in Table 2-1.

We recently conducted a survey in which we sought to understand the norms for practice governance addressing some of the factors listed in Table 2-1. The size of the group and, in a related fashion, the ownership, played a major role in how the practice was led. When there were two or fewer members of a practice, the owner(s) ruled without committee structures autocratically with outside or inside nonphysician business administrators who were not involved in strategic planning. If a practice grew, but remained owned by fewer than three individuals, decisions were

Table 2-1 Determinants of Radiology Group Practice Governance Structure

Factor	Impact
Size	Larger number requires greater organization
Hospitals	Often means appointments made as "chairpersons" of the hospital
Partnership/ownership	Owners tend to be autocratic
Business acumen	Comfort with business may mean less professional executives
Buyouts	Venture capitalist management often means nonphysician governance
Desire for C corporation status	Requires more designated officers

From Johns Hopkins University and Hospital Department of Radiology. Courtesy of David M. Yousem, MD.

still often made in an autocratic fashion no matter the number of the hired employee physicians.

Practices with more than two but fewer than 15 radiologists often elected a "president" of the physician group, but they also appointed medical directors or chairpersons for the hospitals they served. Rarely, other "officers" were elected by the group. The president often was not the chairperson/medical director. These practices almost always employed a full-time business manager, more for billing and collections than for leadership functions. Standing committees were unusual (an executive committee was the most common one established) with ad hoc committees appointed as needed for specific projects. Strategic planning was led by the president with input from an executive committee or all members of the physician group. Business administrators' and managers' input to major changes was invited but the physician leadership held the power. Decisions were made by consensus for the most part. If consensus could not be achieved, the majority vote ruled. Minor day-to-day financial decisions were made by the business manager.

Once a group gets to the 15- to 25-member range, there are usually multiple elected officers as well as designated chairpersons/directors at the hospitals. The directors at the hospitals often make decisions by themselves if a small fraction of the group works at that hospital. Executive, finance, marketing, quality assurance, and contracting committees are usually established. Most groups will have full-time business

manager(s) who usually do not play the lead role in strategic planning and business decisions by the group. Often outside consultants are required in addition to the employed business manager for specific tasks/projects. Strategic planning is performed by an assigned committee often at the direction of the president. Consensus is harder to obtain so majority votes are usually required or the elected officers and executive committees bring most decisions to the group for rubber stamp ratification.

The middle- to large-sized groups that have 26 to 50 members often will be organized based on whether physicians are in partnership tracks or not. In these groups a board of directors may be elected in addition to a full complement of officers including president, vice president, treasurer, and secretary. Hospital directors and outpatient center directors may be assigned. Business managers and/or bookkeepers and accountants also are employed.

They usually run the business office autonomously for collections and billings with only reporting authority to the board or executive committee. In addition to the committees mentioned in the 15- to 25-member range, there may be personnel committees to deal with manpower needs or for items such as pension plans/benefits, information technology, and business development. Some groups have committees based on modalities (CT, MR, ultrasound, PET, mammography) led by modality directors and including nonphysician employees. Strategic planning is led by the board (which has elected physician members and possibly nonphysician employees) but occasionally a formal CEO will direct the process with decision making by the physicians. Rarely there are strategic planning retreats (3- to 5-year intervals). Decisions are made by majority rule with the president, the executive committee, or the board having authority to make most decisions that do not personally affect the group members or their wallets (i.e., salary decisions). For hiring/firing or bylaws changes, supermajorities are preferred. Groups these sizes are less likely to hire consultants except for large strategic planning retreats.

The governance for groups of more than 51 physicians may sometimes split into a business management group and a physician group, depending on the ownership of the equipment and the hospital/office-based mix. The less input from hospitals on the group practice the better—it is more likely that the business aspects will be organized by the management employees of the group. The officers, board members, and executive committee members are elected for specific terms and these are coveted positions. It is standard for a CEO to "run his shop" of business-oriented employees, that is, those who help in the billing and collections area. The same board and committee structure is present as with those in the medium-sized group but marketing, finance, and operations and benefits committees are dominated by business professionals with the physicians having majority input in technology, quality assurance, and modality committees. Strategic planning and practice decisions are largely delegated to the EXCOM or board and the rank and file are often the "recipients" of decisions made at these forums. Perceived consensus within the board or EXCOM drives the decision making, similar to a small group. Rarely are votes required because of consensus building in the committee. Consultants are frequently employed for strategic planning at retreats.

It goes without saying that the officers and board members of radiology groups should be democratically elected to their posts and that there should be representation in the committee structures for all types of physicians (partners and nonpartners), business leaders (MBAs and MHAs), support personnel (technologists, front desk workers, site mangers, marketers), and, in some cases, patient representatives. In the words of Richard Gunderman, "If radiology's organizations are to react with sufficient speed, vigor, and acumen to meet . . . challenges, they must ensure that the selection of leaders remains a fully democratic and participatory process. Leadership must never be regarded as a right of passage. . . ."[8]

CONCLUSIONS

Strong leadership within a radiology practice, no matter the size, the setting, or the group's stated mission, is critical to the success of the team. The first step is to determine the goals of the group and the niche that the practice will fill. Create commitment to the mission. Participation in decision making by physicians and nonphysician business leaders must be encouraged as the size of the practice grows for it to flourish. Physicians are not likely to accept a passive role in the determination of their future so the creation of a functional committee structure can serve to empower the members of the group as well as to improve communication between the constituents. Breeding strong leaders in such an environment provides the ability for creating a group's collective historical memory, which enhances good judgments in decision making and prevents repetition of prior mistakes.

Dos and Don'ts of Organizational Structure and Governance	
Dos	**Don'ts**
1. Stress the mission.	1. Rely too much on consultants.
2. Have a well-developed business plan.	2. Rely too much on lawyers.
3. Cultivate leadership throughout the organization.	3. Schedule too many nonconstructive meetings and committees.

Continued

Dos	Don'ts
4. Emphasize short, intermediate, and long-range goals.	4. Proclaim too many top-down decrees.
5. Be inclusive.	5. Forget people skills.
6. Empower the group members.	6. Fear making decisions.
7. Build rapport between professional business staff and physicians.	7. Make decisions in isolation—leaders must also be workers to cultivate empathy.
8. Maintain open and constant communication.	8. Cultivate an "us versus them" mentality.
9. Revisit the mission and vision during strategic planning.	9. Be inert.
10. Remember, democracy rules.	10. Think that profit rules—service does.

REFERENCES

1. Starr P: The Social Transformation of American Medicine. Boston: Basic Books (1982).
2. Fox PD, Wasserman J: Academic medical centers and managed care: Uneasy partners. Health Aff (Millwood) 12:85–93, 1993.
3. Office of the President, University Medical and Dental School, State of NJ website. Amended March 30, 2005.
4. Johns Hopkins University and Hospital Department of Radiology. Courtesy of David M. Yousem, MD.
5. Muroff LR: Implementing an effective organization and governance structure for a radiology practice. J Am Coll Radiol 1:26–32, 2004.
6. Moses H, 3rd, Thier SO, Matheson DH: Why have academic medical centers survived? JAMA 293:1495–1500, 2005.
7. Grigsby RK, Hefner DS, Souba WW, Kirch DG: The future-oriented department chair. Acad Med 79:571–577, 2004.
8. Gunderman RB: Genius of democracy: Implications for the governance of professional organizations. Acad Radiol 9:1119–1121, 2002.

Leadership

Norman J. Beauchamp, Jr.

Leaders take people where they want to go. A great leader takes people where they don't necessarily want to go, but ought to be.

ROSALYN CARTER

ARE GREAT LEADERS BORN OR CREATED?

At a time when so many people are unable to obtain adequate health care, there is a tremendous need for great leaders in medicine. As health care is becoming ever more complex, there is a clear opportunity for leaders to generate a substantial impact. Radiology leadership is particularly challenging because radiology is one of the most rapidly advancing and centrally important specialties (OK, self-aggrandizement is allowed sometimes!). Growth within and interest from outside of radiology in performing diagnostic imaging has fostered a highly competitive environment. Strong leadership is also a necessary competitive advantage for maintaining profitability, as well as recruiting and retaining the best faculty. And how do we define "great" in this context? A "great" leader would be an "effective" one; a leader who can put theory into practice.

Are great leaders born or created? They are born. Therefore, all those without this genetic predisposition should proceed to the next chapter. You know who you are ... turn to page 34. Actually, that was a test to weed out those leadership hopefuls who lacked the fortitude necessary for success (for leaders, perseverance is critical). So, for those of you who remain ... Of course great leaders can be created. Individuals possess differing aptitudes and some will come to the leadership development table with more building blocks than others, but there is irrefutable evidence that leaders can be created. It is the objective of this chapter to help you understand the opportunities and requirements for effective leadership.

WHAT IS A LEADER?

If your actions (or words) inspire others to dream more, learn more, do more and become more, you are a leader.

JOHN QUINCY ADAMS

There are many definitions and descriptions of what a leader is and does. Fundamentally, successful leaders get people to work together toward common goals and help them take part in accomplishing something that they could not do alone. For this reason, stress must be placed on establishing a unifying mission and vision for a radiology department. Leaders help people believe in themselves and in others. They identify talents and establish an environment where those talents and the goals of both the individual and the group can be nurtured. They foster cooperation among individuals, groups, and organizations. They develop the potential of an organization by forming new collaborations and building new synergies.

Being a leader means being a role model and setting an example. A leader is both a teacher and a counselor. An effective leader takes pride in the accomplishments of others and in seeing his or her people receive the credit that is due them and opportunities for growth. A leader is a steward of hope in the face of adversity. A leader takes responsibility for his or her actions with an understanding that those actions affect others.

Being a leader means stepping in when others are unwilling to do so to ensure that a worthy organization is sustained. A leader is bothered by a process that could be done better, and is uncomfortable until that process is optimized, even if it is not "your responsibility." A leader stands up for what is important. Leaders make sure that virtuous goals are always emphasized.

Leadership is overcoming fears. Leadership is occasionally lonely. Leadership is forgiveness of self and of those who are working under you when an expected outcome falls short. Leadership means knowing how to deliver difficult messages to people you care about for the betterment of the organization. Leadership is being able to "transition" (a euphemism for moving someone along, which is itself a euphemism for replacing that person) other leaders when their goals or actions are not aligned with the success of other individuals or of the organization as a whole.

To do something together, we've got to keep our eyes on something bigger than us.

CORNEL WEST

Leadership is clearly many things. Most of all, it is a chance to use your talent and energy to create a scalable impact on the lives of patients, employees, colleagues, and family.

LEADERSHIP DEVELOPMENT

Leadership development begins with distinguishing leadership skills from leadership traits. Leadership *skills* are essentially techniques or practices that leaders apply in advancing a group toward common goals. Examples of leadership skills include being able to generate and communicate a vision, converting that vision to tactics and initiatives, and identifying and delegating tasks to talented individuals who can assist in reaching this vision. Leadership skills are readily taught, both inside and out of the classroom. That this can be learned behavior is fortunate, because developing leaders seldom *show up* with these skills already highly developed.

Leadership *traits* are different. They are essentially behaviors or characteristics that an individual inherently possesses. Leadership traits can be well developed in individuals at a surprisingly early age. These traits include motivation, energy, perseverance, intelligence, self-confidence, fairness, ability to trust others, integrity, and forgiveness. Paramount to all of these traits is the ability to communicate well. While some may consider good communication a skill rather than a trait, it is critically important to be able to consolidate one's ideas and formulate a vision of how to express those ideas to others. Clarity of focus is the trait from which this ability emanates. Although all of these traits can also be formally taught, they often manifest independently of any formal or informal leadership training. Trait-laden individuals are often those identified to pursue leadership opportunities early in their careers. Persons characterized as "born leaders" tend to be those that "present" with advanced leadership traits.

These differences can be illuminated in an historical reflection. Temuchin was an Asian warrior leader who lived about 800 years ago. Many would identify him as a born leader based on the breadth of his leadership traits. These traits were the underpinning of his success. For example, despite significant initial battlefield failings, he persevered. He acknowledged his mistakes and learned from them. He was quick to credit others and he was accepting of contrary beliefs and opinions. He selected leaders based on their honesty and he chose a successor that he felt was most principled.

Despite such traits, he also recognized the need to develop his own leadership skills, such as battlefield tactics and how to implement a merit-based reward system. He actively pursued "formal" military training from a mentor early on. This mentor was one of the strongest Mongolian chiefs at the time. Temuchin treated his mentor with respect, paying close attention to him to gain skills and enhance his traits. Thus, he combined leadership traits with the acquisition of leadership skills.

Today, we know Temuchin by the name Ghengis Kahn.[1] He established the largest contiguous empire in history. Although not necessarily appreciated by his adversaries, he was most certainly effective as a leader. If traits and skills are good enough to enable control of the Mongol horde, clearly a focus on skills and traits is a worthy use of time for an aspiring leader in radiology.

LEADERSHIP TRAITS

One does not have to go back 800 years to determine the impact of leadership traits. McClelland et al studied leaders in 30 organizations. They characterized the traits that differentiated the excellent leaders from the average ones and found those traits to include self-confidence, adaptability, achievement drive, and interest in developing others.[2]

Nothing splendid has ever been achieved except by those who believed that something inside of them was superior to circumstance.

Bruce Barton

Elaborating on this, during my three-year tenure as vice chairman and interim chairman at Johns Hopkins, and my subsequent four years as chairman at the University of Washington, belief in self (self-confidence) is critical. Leadership brings daily challenges. Initially, many of these challenges are new and raw to the neophyte leader. You must have confidence that you are the right person for the position. If you don't believe in yourself, neither will those who work with you.

In addition, fear of failure is a primary driver of stress. While it is true that some level of stress is a normal adaptive reaction to a threat and is an evolutionary mechanism to help us avoid harm, fear of failure in decision making typically leads to maladaptive stress. Such stress leads to aggression and reluctance to cooperate or engage. Stress also impedes your ability to be an effective decision maker and limits adaptability. Make decisions; stand by them when they are good ones, and learn from them when they are poorly conceived or executed.

Put more simply, excessive fear of failure will only lead to more failure. As a leader, you are required to make good decisions every day. Processing of key factors, metrics, key constituent inputs, and prior experiences is essential. Leadership is all about continual learning and responding to change. According to Ed Hallowell, a specialist in learning disabilities, "[t]he most dangerous impediment to learning is fear. Fear shifts us into survival mode and prevents fluid learning and nuanced understanding."[3] Stress prevents the creative thinking and good judgment a leader requires.

Of course, it is easy to "say" be confident and avoid stress. Some guidance may be helpful. When confronting a challenging issue, construct a plan. Once the plan is constructed, compartmentalize it in your mind. In other words, do not carry the problem along with you to your next meeting or any situation in which your complete attention is needed. Do not take the problem home. It can encroach on family life and can keep you from getting the rest you need to approach another new day and new challenges. Once a plan is formulated, stop worrying. Worrying will not help. It will not reduce stress; however, having a well-thought-out plan in place with broad input will. Review is not needed until you have proof that the plan will not work, based on the results of actual implementation. Otherwise, you will find yourself unable to focus on more than a few issues at a time, and your capacity as a leader will be tremendously limited.

Seek input. It is appropriate to seek input in formulating a plan. You should not be ashamed to admit that there are others who are more skilled at dealing with certain issues than yourself. Yes, there are people more knowledgeable than you, the leader, and their advice may be critical to arriving at the best solution. Consult widely with those whose skill sets are positioned to address the challenge. This is a demonstration of capable leadership, not an indication of inability or ineffectiveness. In my leadership efforts, I have constructed an executive committee comprised of the most capable individuals committed to the success of the whole.

Similarly, do not be hypersensitive to input. Being able to receive positive and negative input will ensure that you make the best decision. Trust people. Without trust, you will not attain the synergy needed to achieve real success. There will be times when you will be disappointed. But those will be far less than the times you will be delighted by the efforts people make toward attaining a common goal. You must absolutely trust the people that work for you. I have seen many a talented individual not realize their potential because they saw contradicting opinions as a threat or a criticism or a lack of appreciation.

Do not overreact. Rooke and Torbert emphasize this leadership trait of managing self: "Most developmental psychologists agree that what differentiates leaders is not so much their philosophy of leadership. Rather, it's their internal action logic—how they interpret their surroundings and how they react when their power, their safety is challenged."[4]

Don't take yourself too seriously. As you ascend into higher levels of leadership, recognize that success is not only due to your personal intelligence or uniquely strong work ethic; luck also plays a role. Be cautious about creating an inflated sense of self based on that success—your self-concept will be at risk when you fail, and you may be too slow in giving others credit when successes *do* happen.

Never let your ego get so close to your position that when your position goes, your ego goes with it.

COLIN POWELL

Even when incorporating these approaches for dealing with the challenges of leadership, there will be times in your leadership position when things seem insurmountable. I have found it necessary to remind myself to not put my self-concept on the line based on the results of every action. I cannot stress enough how important this is because many overachievers (if you have an MD, this means you) base their self-concept on the last great thing they accomplished or the most recent feedback, positive or negative, that they received. More simply put, do not hinge your self-concept on a single "grade" from the next "report card." This will limit your ability to truly take risks, because you will be so concerned about failing. Think of yourself as a whole: your entire body of work lies not just in employment, but also at home, and in the community.

In addition, sometimes you will have to do "B" work: knowing when to accept a "B" or a "C" and when to strive for an "A" is one key to being able to sustain multiple tasks in a leadership position. Remember that high-priority, high-impact projects must get your "A" effort and achievement. Reserve "B"s and "C"s for low-level missions. Keeping this in mind will enable you to have the confidence to confront areas of even the greatest difficulty and to remain invigorated in the process.

You will have both successes and failures. Recognize that the next great opportunity is soon to follow and that today's failure will help you realize tomorrow's opportunity. Take stock of progress. Sometimes we look at the number of steps that are ahead of us on the journey and forget to take account of how far we've come. For myself, every day begins with taking stock of how far I have come as well as how far I have yet to go.

A pessimist sees the difficulty in every opportunity; an optimist sees the opportunity in every difficulty.

WINSTON CHURCHILL

Lastly, optimism is also an essential trait in minimizing stress. Challenges should be seen as an opportunity. If you do not believe, then those that are following you will not believe. It does not mean that you hide the challenges from those that you lead; on the contrary, confronting challenges head on can inspire the team to pull together. However, it is your responsibility to generate the optimism necessary to ensure that the team is confident they can succeed in the effort.

Fairness is an important trait. This trait in a leader fosters trust and is a strong predictor of high employee performance. Brockner demonstrated that when there is commitment and communication regarding fairness in policies and procedures, organizations responded with higher performance. In demonstrating fairness one exemplifies integrity. Coworkers will follow a leader with integrity. Process fairness was also shown to foster a culture of innovation.[5]

In 1998, Daniel Goleman published a landmark paper in the Harvard Business Review entitled "What Makes a Leader." He stressed the concept of "emotional intelligence" (EI) as a differentiator of effective leadership. Essentially, EI is the ability to understand one's strengths and limitations and to understand the circumstances that lead to strong emotional reactions in one's self and others. This can be categorized as Self-Awareness, Self-Management, Social Awareness, and Social Skills. This capability enables one to manage self and others more effectively.[6]

Leadership traits and emotional intelligence can be thought of as essentially the same (see Table 3-1): they constitute who you are.

Because of this, advancing your skills in this domain can be particularly challenging because doing so requires you to "modify who you are." The basis for these abilities is formed very early in life and is continually reinforced throughout childhood and early adulthood. Thus, as opposed to learning technical skills, the acquisition of new social and self-management abilities requires a prolonged period of focused attention.

Lastly, it is important to emphasize that individuals without these traits may still garner and succeed in leadership opportunities. They may simply need to have these abilities awakened and then encouraged within themselves. The process is one of evaluation, education, practice, feedback, and redeployment. It is an essential part of any leadership development agenda.

LEADERSHIP SKILLS

Much of this textbook is dedicated to skills that a leader, particularly a business leader in radiology, must possess. These include the use of metrics, practice growth strategies, negotiation techniques, creation of an environment of fairness, and incentives that align with goals, quality improvement initiatives, and use of evidence to

Table 3-1	Leadership Traits		
Self-Awareness	**Self-Management**	**Social Awareness**	**Social Skills**
Emotional self-awareness	Adaptability	Empathy	Building bonds
Self-assessment	Achievement orientation	Organization awareness	Change catalyst
Self-confidence	Conscientiousness		Communication
	Initiative		Conflict management
	Self-control		Developing others
	Trustworthiness		Influence
			Service orientation
			Teamwork

From Goleman D: What makes a leader? Harvard Business Review (November–December 1998).

make medical decisions. However, some additional areas of emphasis should be reviewed.

Any discussion of leadership skills must begin with a reference to Stephen R. Covey's book, *Seven Habits of Highly Effective People.*[7] He presents seven essential behaviors/skills that enable true effectiveness. Summarized in the following list and largely self-explanatory, the book itself explains how to transition desired behaviors into habits (i.e., acquired patterns of behavior) that become nearly involuntary. Admittedly, many of the points are intuitive, but I revisit this book every year and recommend the same for aspiring leaders. Summarized below are the seven habits from Covey's book:

1. Be Proactive—Take personal responsibility for what occurs in life.
2. Begin with the End in Mind—Have a personal mission statement.
3. Put First Things First—Prioritize efforts based not on what is easiest but on what is most consistent with your mission.
4. Think Win/Win—Always seek solutions where both parties can claim success.
5. Seek First to Understand, Then to Be Understood—Take the time to understand the other person's perspective before trying to advance your own.
6. Synergize—Success is best obtained by combining the strengths and abilities of many.
7. Sharpen the Saw—Take time out to educate and rejuvenate.

The concepts integrate well with other behaviors and techniques I have relied upon and have seen commonly employed by highly effective leaders. I discuss these in more detail below.

MISSION, VISION, GOALS, AND TACTICS

Be Proactive; Begin with the End in Mind

An important requirement as a leader is to define the mission and vision of your organization and use this to establish your goals and tactics. This forces and enables you to set priorities and make the critical and tough choices. This formulation requires input from across

the organization and the focused effort of the leadership team.

Let us provide a brief review of mission, vision, values, and tactics. A useful definition of mission is that it is the fundamental reason for being; it is a statement of identity; it stands up over time regardless of changes in industry, technology, and the economy; and it describes the end result. An example of a mission statement is ours at the University of Washington: "To meet the clinical needs of the hospitals we serve, to train the practitioners and the leaders of tomorrow, and to advance the manner in which imaging and imaging sciences improve the human condition."

A vision statement is a compelling picture of future achievements—it is what we are trying to make happen together, what we will be proud to achieve—a stretch. It can change over time (e.g., 5 to 10 years). Here is an example of a vision statement; it is the one for our department: "The UW Department of Radiology is the premier academic radiology program in the nation. Our practice is at the highest levels of measurable success fiscally, clinically, academically, and in our chosen areas of research. Through our involvement at the University of Washington and in WWAMI, we contribute to innovations in clinical practice throughout the region. A key element in our success is the creation and maintenance of a workplace environment that is stimulating, challenging, collegial, and enjoyable for all our physicians and departmental staff."

The core values should be identified for the organization. As demonstrated in Figures 3-1 and 3-2, these values, in the context of the mission and vision, lead to tactics. It is these tactics that will proactively guide the efforts across the organization with incorporated tools to manage change toward the desired end.

TIME MANAGEMENT

Put First Things First

As a leader, it is crucial to manage time effectively. Do not allow a "crisis mentality" to occur. The expedient availability of e-mail has created a situation in which "crises" may be

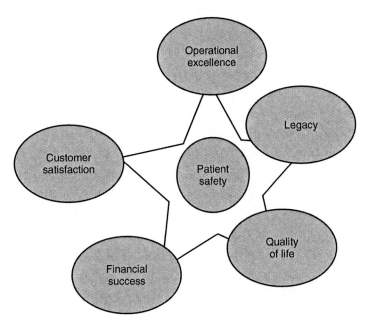

Figure 3-1 Core values.

presented all day long. This results in a reprior-itization of your efforts based on someone else's perception of priorities. As Dr. Covey would instruct us, we must focus on the important, not the urgent and unimportant. He constructs a 2-by-2 box with urgent and nonurgent on the Y axis and important and unimportant on the X axis (Table 3-2).

One should try to avoid and "just say no" to matters in Zone 4, which are unimportant and not urgent. They should not occupy your weekly schedule. Matters in Zone 1 are your crises and they must be dealt with immediately. Issues in Zone 3, which are not urgent but which are important, constitute all of your long-term strategic plans. Covey says that leaders should be spending over 50% of their time in Zone 3 dealing with mission/vision, self-improvement, mentorship/guidance work, and planning for the future. To do so, he recommends that you schedule such thought-provoking reflection into your weekly calendar *first*, to make sure it gets high priority. Otherwise, you will get lost in the minutiae and mundane activities that occupy Zone 2, those things that are urgent but unimportant to long-term success and effectiveness. So first fill your calendar with Zone 3 appointments to ensure you "put first things [the most important ones]

first." "Things which matter most should not be at the mercy of things which matter least." Manage your time for projects you hope to accomplish not on a daily basis but on a week-long or month-long basis, so you don't get bogged down in the unimportant-but-urgent sphere. Sometimes Zone 1 items encroach on the other zones, but these are critical actions that must be taken as well.

THE ROLE OF COMMUNICATION

Think Win/Win

Always seek solutions where both parties can claim success; seek first to understand, then to be understood.

Communicating clearly is the most important charge of a leader. The leader must inspire every individual to take responsibility for creating a better future by effectively communicating and reinforcing that message to all the members of the organization. Thus, success requires both effective communication with small groups or individuals, and across the organization.

In communicating with individuals or small groups, try foremost to be in the moment.

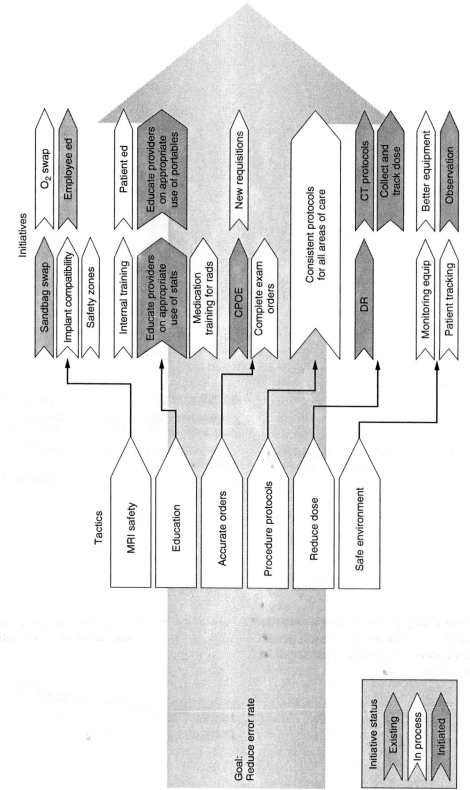

Figure 3-2 Tactical plan: Value patient safety.

Table 3-2 Time Management: Put First Things First

	Important	Not Important
Urgent	Zone 1	Zone 2
Not urgent	Zone 3	Zone 4

From Covey SR: Seven Habits of Highly Effective People. New York: Simon & Schuster, 1989.

Don't be thinking about your last meeting or your next presentation. Listen more than you speak. Time pressures one to cut to the chase. Getting to the wrong place quickly is not expedient. The conversation should be focused on the information that is needed. Open-ended questions can be used to further expand the discussion with closed questions to prompt for discussion. Reflect on what you are hearing. At the end of the discussion, ask the individual to whom you are speaking to summarize key points. Close the meeting delineating required follow-up actions for each member of the conversation.

Clarity in communication is facilitated by a meeting agenda. Request that the individuals meeting with you provide a proposed agenda. This will help them structure their ideas and enable you to review materials that will ensure you are adequately prepared for the meeting. Some advocate an agenda that includes time allotted for each item. As long as you don't become a slave to the timed agenda and cut off discussion prematurely, this is a good idea, particularly if the track record suggests some long-winded discussants. Given a time clock, they may narrow their focus and be succinct. Being punctual and ending the meeting on schedule is an important sign of respect for the people you are meeting with and about to meet with.

A few words of caution regarding verbal and written communication are necessary. If the communication is a positive one, any method will do—write it, say it, sign it—whatever. If it is potentially contentious, the initial communication should be verbal and in person. It will enable you to address any insecurities or concerns that are brought up, as well as to make certain that the intent of the message is clear. More hours are spent unraveling written messages taken out of context, written in anger, or delivered without the benefit of nonverbal cues that can ease the tension of a difficult conversation. A follow-up written summary can then follow as needed.

Never respond in anger to a written communication. E-mail is the worst for this. Remember the 24-hour rule, which is to wait a day before responding to something that really irritates you. Ultimately, use interpersonal communication to build relationships, not destroy them. Gossip should be left to the tabloids. Maintain a forgiving view of others and encourage colleagues to do the same ... always.

Effective communication across the organization is also imperative. This is done both through the selection of an excellent leadership team, as well as personally conveying with clarity the mission, vision, values, and tactics for the organization. The former should receive the highest priority in that a poor leadership team will make the latter irrelevant. The leadership team creates and reinforces the culture of commitment, participation, and pursuit of excellence. It has been said that culture trumps vision every day of the week.

This concept is well supported in the acclaimed book about leadership, *Good to Great*. The author, Jim Collins, reviewed 1,435 companies, looking for those that demonstrated sustained significant improvement over time. It was his observation that real success was dependent on the leadership team, which was shown to be more essential than the strength of the corporate vision, the change management strategies, or the CEOs themselves.[8] Leading companies identified focused, motivated individuals who acted in a disciplined manner.

It is vital that the team consist of individuals with diverse skills that complement the skills of the leader. It bears emphasis that the leader should seek the most highly talented individuals available. A true sign of mediocrity is when leaders surround themselves with "less talented individuals" to make themselves look better by comparison. I have seen this happen all too often among misguided leaders who are ultimately unsuccessful. The individuals selected for the team must be comfortable sharing their opinions and capable of having those difficult conversations with the boss, thereby ensuring that the best decisions are reached.

Identifying such individuals requires careful review. In their classic textbook, Laurence Peter and Raymond Hull introduced the concept of the "Peter Principle."[9] The oft-quoted phrase is that "employees tend to rise to their level of incompetence." The book describes the upward, downward, and lateral movement of individuals in an organization. Peter and Hull share a story regarding an individual who reached a level of incompetence—a line worker who excelled but when promoted to management ceased to perform at a high level. It was not that the job was any more difficult. Rather, the task was simply different and not well suited to the individual's abilities.

The skills that lead one to be successful in a preleadership career do not always translate to becoming an effective leader. Many an accomplished, intelligent individual has finally honed skills to establish high personal productivity but cannot lead a team. I can easily recall two or three highly talented and successful individuals who were unable to shift their focus to that of team builder. They were passed over for less-accomplished individuals who better characterized the abilities needed to attain synergy. To avoid placing individuals on your leadership team who are bound to fail, make sure that they have demonstrated the traits and skills necessary to succeed in a leadership role. Seek objective measures and the opinion of those inside and outside of the department.

Collins does not dismiss the significance of mission, vision, and tactics. He stresses that narrowly focused objectives are essential. In this regard, a leadership team that embraces the vision of the chair or CEO and can convey it to the organization is critical. The leader must communicate this mission precisely to each member of the leadership team and be certain that they are communicating it to their faculty. This is the only way to confirm that the group energy is well understood and focused. Misalignment can be an extraordinary distraction.

MANAGING CHANGE

Synergize

Knowing when and how to manage change is an essential responsibility of a leader. Changes should be made in a coordinated fashion. Change may be internally driven as a result of recognizing that systems are operating at less than their potential. Change may also be mandated as a result of external factors such as reimbursement, new competition, or emerging opportunities. In both circumstances, the response should be anticipatory rather than reactive.

"Change management" (that is, advancing the organization from where it is today to where leadership desires it to be) is best driven by those most familiar with the organization and its goals. Although there are a myriad of organizations that are willing to come and advise your company on how best to proceed, developing internal expertise is crucial.

Give a man a fish and you feed him for a day. Teach a man to fish and you feed him for a lifetime.

AUTHOR UNKNOWN

Tools to assist in change management include Six Sigma[10] and LEAN[11]. In our department, we have formed a collaboration with Industrial Engineering. This brings us content expertise but also helps us continually advance our internal expertise. Moreover, it ensures that changes that are made are consistent with our departmental culture, mission, and vision.

The types of changes that need be managed will be of great diversity in their nature. For example, generating enthusiasm for a collaborative model for image interpretation with physicians in nuclear medicine and body imaging, or transitioning a group from a research to a research *and* a clinical customer focus, will involve different participants, cultures, and jargon. However, the process of change management is essentially the same.

An appealing characterization for change management is maintaining a continual state of issue identification and systems optimization. This allows one to focus on reaping "opportunity," not simply just "responding" to a problem. Thus, rather than doing the latter—with its inherent connotation that someone is underperforming, or doing something wrong—one garners in every circumstance the former, or an "opportunity" for improvement. In this scenario, change is simply moving from current state to improved state. A consistent approach should be used for identifying opportunities, including seeking the input of key customers and constituents with an exchange of ideas. This will facilitate obtaining buy-in, support, and commitment. Transitional steps should be transparent and clearly defined.

Prioritization of what should be changed and on what timeline is an essential management decision. This should be guided by the organization mission, vision, and values, and also take into account required resources and predicted return.

A decision supported by appropriate metrics, as opposed to gestalt, is also key. For example, at my prior institution it was a widely held opinion that physicians directly supervising studies during MRI fostered greater throughput. In fact, this belief was quite rigorously maintained. Modification of this perspective was only possible when a process map, variability measures, and modeling demonstrated that the introduced variability in the process made protocol-driven imaging the only acceptable method. Without a focus on data-driven decision-making, the debate never reached a conclusion.

A similar effect occurred when colleagues in orthopedic surgery were convinced that their challenges in work flow were related to a lack of available X-ray rooms. Using a standard process map, it was clearly demonstrated that the process failing was due to the manner in which new versus returning patients were scheduled within the orthopedics clinic. An additional imaging room would have only brought more expense and continued frustration.

Change is best managed in an environment of perceived fairness. As stated above, process fairness improves performance and fosters innovation. It is not good advice to try to please everyone. It is appropriate, however, to create a process that has the characteristics of fairness and consistency.

E-mail is perhaps the world's best way to procrastinate. Consider delegating e-mail powers to an assistant. She or he can then screen e-mails to determine which ones are high priority. It isn't necessary to fly to every e-mail right away. Allot two times a day to check e-mail and resist the temptation to check back outside of those times.

Leaders also need to know when their dream is detrimental to the success of their organization. In Arthur Miller's play *Death of a Salesman*, Willy Loman illustrates the challenge of living a life full of dreams separated from reality. Good dreams have deep roots in everyday life.[12]

Hope is not a business strategy.

BARRY S. STERNLICHT

If you make decisions based on what you wish is true, you will make some very bad choices. As such, present information to your boss that separates fact from opinion, knowing that opinion is sometimes used to make excuses for underperformance or missing an opportunity.

In closing, a few words about working hard are needed. As the boss, you must work at least as hard as the members of your team. As a team member, you must avoid the tendency to convey to one's boss how "hard you're working." This is a reasonably effective way to prevent one's boss from adding tasks that may benefit your organization and your career advancement.

ACQUIRING LEADERSHIP TRAITS AND SKILLS

Sharpen the Saw

Leadership traits and skills are clearly very important. This has not been lost on business schools and managerial theorists. The approach used by Ghengis Khan is identical to what is emphasized in MBA programs, business journals, and ... outstanding first-edition business of radiology books (shameless self-promotion ... not a leadership trait).

The human capacity to learn and modify behavior is what has made the species flourish. Unfortunately, we also suffer from being somewhat relenting in the pursuit of optimization of self. In seeking to become a highly effective leader, you must focus these innate abilities of learning toward the volitional exercise of seeking to become more effective.

Thus, one essential concept in leadership development is to always be learning. Crucial tools for learning are listening and observation. Learn everywhere and from everyone. Seek leadership lessons in everyday interactions, seeing what works and what doesn't. Observe who does things right, who does things wrong, and how they do them. Learn what is effective and what is not. Study approaches to team building, sharing credit, pursuing goals, and obtaining resources. Evaluate techniques for time management, and managing up and down. (As the terms imply, managing up is how you work with those you report to and managing down is how you work with those who report to you.)

Learn from leaders and nonleaders. In a series of interviews of successful leaders, some of the best guidance came from people often outside the work environment.

Real happiness, he said, comes from striving to do something that isn't easy and succeeding in doing it.
ADVICE TO HENRY M. PAULSON, JR., CHAIRMAN AND CEO OF GOLDMAN SACHS, FROM HIS FATHER

Valuable resources include individuals you barely know, or even family members.[3] For example, I learned a great deal before I left the protections of rural St. Johns, Michigan, by observing the compassion my mother (a mental health therapist) showed in dealing with her patients regardless of their abilities or limitations. The value of being goal oriented was imbued upon me by my father in his work as an electrical engineer.

Also, take advantage of the written experiences and observations of others. The lives of some truly effective leaders are well documented. Learn from spiritual leaders such as Buddha, Ghandi, the Dalai Lama, and Jesus; from political leaders such as Abe Lincoln, Winston Churchill, and Ben Franklin; from business leaders such as Jack Welch and Bill Gates; and from philosophers such as Viktor Frankl. The Art of War by Sun Tzu is a classic that is read by nearly every MBA graduate and should be on the leader's shelf. (Early in my career I was told that one should invest at least 25% of one's reading in nonmedical literature.)

Mentorship is imperative for acquiring leadership skills and traits. One cannot stress enough the need to *seek* strong mentorship. The characteristics of a good mentor are a track record of enabling others, success in obtaining the support of peers and the resources needed to succeed, and, ultimately, demonstrating enjoyment of the process of mentoring.

The best mentors need to be recruited. They seldom come knocking at your door. A successful methodology for the pursuit of mentors is to seek out those to whom you can bring projects of value. An approach that has worked for me is to determine which efforts a potential mentor is most enthusiastic about or is in need of assistance with. Prior to meeting with a potential mentor, undertake preparatory work to become familiar with the topics and issues. Offer to contribute to the project with a request for guidance as needed. Work hard, under promise, and overdeliver. Assuming you did your background work assessing that the individual has a track record of effective mentorship, reciprocity often quickly follows, with the mentee's goals and needs becoming the focus of the relationship.

Note that mentor/mentee relationships do not need to last a lifetime. During my early career, I sought four different primary mentors over eight years. Each was recruited with a goal of working with an individual that possessed the skills I was most in need of developing at that time. It is expected that at some point, the mentee will find it necessary to seek new mentorship to build a growing skill set. A good mentor will not be offended but rather will be enthusiastic about the growth of a student moving on. I have maintained strong friendships with all of my former mentors.

Self-examination is also a very valuable tool for advancing your skills and traits. I have taken to viewing my life as a continual gap analysis, whereby I compare my actual results with my expected results. One should always perform a continual determination of what factors result in outcomes that fall short of expectation.

You should also invite other individuals whose opinions you respect to participate in this gap analysis; that is, seek feedback from others. The business leadership guru Peter F. Drucker stated that although most people feel they know their strengths, they are usually incorrect.

The process of seeking feedback is best done in a formal manner. There is literature on targeting the educational process using a baseline assessment. For example, Robbins et al. introduced a tool that does a baseline assessment of core competencies for leaders, which has been shown to be subsequently effective in targeting skills development. These competencies were categorized into four domains: (1) technical skills (operations, finance, information resources, human resources, and strategic planning/external affairs); (2) industry knowledge (clinical process and health care institutions); (3) analytic and conceptual reasoning; and (4) interpersonal and emotional intelligence.[13]

The only way to discover your strengths and weaknesses is through feedback. Once you know what your strengths are, concentrate on them and put yourself in situations where your strengths can produce results. Then work on improving your strengths. Next, discover what your weaknesses are and work to overcome them. Address your bad habits. It is often the things we *do* or *do not do* that inhibit our effectiveness and performance.

Make time for learning during your day. Going from interaction to interaction without time to reflect assures a blunted path of development. Leadership insights also come from taking time at the end of the day to reflect on conversations you've had, how you've reacted to them, and what was effective and what was not.

Previously, the detriment of stress in terms of learning was presented. Exercise is a good reliever of stress. Good evidence shows that sitting at a desk for several hours decreases mental acuity not only because of reduced blood flow to the brain, but for biochemical reasons as well. Physical exercise also produces an array of chemicals that the brain loves, including endorphins, serotonin, dopamine, epinephrine, and norepinephrine, as well as two recently discovered compounds, brain-derived neurotropic factor and nerve growth factor. You do not have to join a gym to gain the benefit of these compounds—good ol' managing by walking around suffices. If you can find a way to walk up or down a flight of stairs, all the better.

Despite the benefits, there's a tendency to neglect exercise. It is notable that there's a willingness to take medications or to alter diet in the pursuit of good health, but not to exercise. A friend of mine that is an internal medicine physician has taken to prescribing exercise as a requirement of good health. He feels that this assignment is perhaps most relevant to people that are confronted with high-stress, high-pressure leadership roles.

Lastly, remember that what is effective in one environment may not be in another. For example, I received two calls from the vice dean's office during my first month as chair at the University of Washington expressing a concern that I was too confrontational. I had imported a perhaps more East Coast, congruous style of exuberant expression of differences of opinion. I was fortunate to get feedback that my approach would have caused my input to not be as welcomed. I still express my differences of opinion but frame my input in a way that is more consistent with techniques I observed in the effective leaders in my new environment.

SUMMARY

In summary, some leaders are born (or at least predisposed to succeed early on) but most are not. Possession of leadership traits and incorporating them into one's leadership style portends success but does not guarantee it. It is in combination with the acquisition of leadership *skills* that one finds *true success*. Have a mission, a vision, and a plan. Ultimately, believe in yourself and keep a sense of humor.

I want it said of me by those who knew me best, that I always plucked a thistle and planted a flower where I thought a flower would grow.

ABRAHAM LINCOLN

The Dos and Don'ts of Great Leaders	
Dos	**Don'ts**
1. Place great importance on defining the mission and vision of the organization.	1. Lose sight of the greater goals of the organization.
2. Develop good communication skills to espouse the ideals, values, mission, and vision.	2. Micromanage—you need to save time for thought requiring long-range planning.
3. Manage time appropriately to schedule leadership (nonurgent) issues.	3. Delegate the critical-to-success issues and processes unless there is someone better than you to do the job.
4. Be confident and definitive.	
5. Defer to others who have more developed skill sets of funds of knowledge on issues.	4. Perseverate after a failure. Evaluate, learn, but move on.
6. Share the credit for successes.	5. Let a personal issue cloud your good judgment.
7. Mentor others and provide them with growth opportunities.	6. Focus on the failures. Take time to recognize the successes. They are usually more plentiful.
8. Be self-aware. Examine your emotional response to trials and tribulations. Then empathize with others.	7. Forget the people. In the end it's all about the patients, the faculty, and the colleagues.
9. Think win-win.	8. Neglect yourself. We all perform better when we are healthy, exercising, growing individually, and enjoying our life.
10. Celebrate success.	9. Hog the spotlight.
	10. Lose hope. Fail to inspire.

REFERENCES

1. Ratchenevsky P: Genghis Khan. Oxford, UK, Blackwell, 1983.
2. McClelland DC: Identifying competencies with behavioral event interviews. Psychological Science 9(5):331–340, 1998.
3. Hallowell EM: Overloaded circuits: Why smart people underperform. Harvard Business Review (January 2005), pp 55–62.
4. Rooke D, Torbert WR: Seven transformations of leadership. Harvard Business Review (April 2005), pp 67–76.
5. Brockner J: Why is it so hard to be fair? Harvard Business Review (March 2006), pp 122–129.
6. Goleman D: What makes a leader? Best of Harvard Business Review (January 2004), pp 1–10.
7. Covey SR: Seven Habits of Highly Effective People, 15th ed. New York, Simon & Schuster, 2004.
8. Collins J: Good to Great. New York, HarperCollins, 2001.
9. Peter LJ, Hull R: The Peter Principle: Why Things Always Go Wrong. New York, William Morrow, 1969.
10. Pande PS, Neuman RP, Cavanagh RR: The Six Sigma Way: How GE, Motorola, and Other Top Companies Are Honing Their Performance. New York, McGraw Hill Professional, 2000.
11. Jones DT, Roos D, Womack JP: The Machine That Changed the World. New York, Simon & Schuster, 2007.
12. Leadership in literature: a conversion with business ethicist Joseph L. Badaracco, Jr. Harvard Business Review (March 2006), pp 47–55.
13. Robbins CJ, Bradley EH, Spicer M: Developing leadership in health care administration: a competency assessment tool. J Health Manage 46(31):188–202, 2001.

SUGGESTED READINGS

Other useful references for leadership traits include:
Cavallo K, Brienza, D: Emotional competence and leadership excellence at Johnson & Johnson: The emotional intelligence and leadership study. Consortium for Research on Emotional Intelligence in Organizations, Rutgers University, New Brunswick, NJ, 2004.
Hendricks G, Ludeman K: The Corporate Mystic: A Guidebook for Visionaries with Their Feet on the Ground. New York, Bantam, 1996.
Phillips, DD: Lincoln on Leadership: Executive Strategies for Tough Times. New York, Warner Books, 1992.

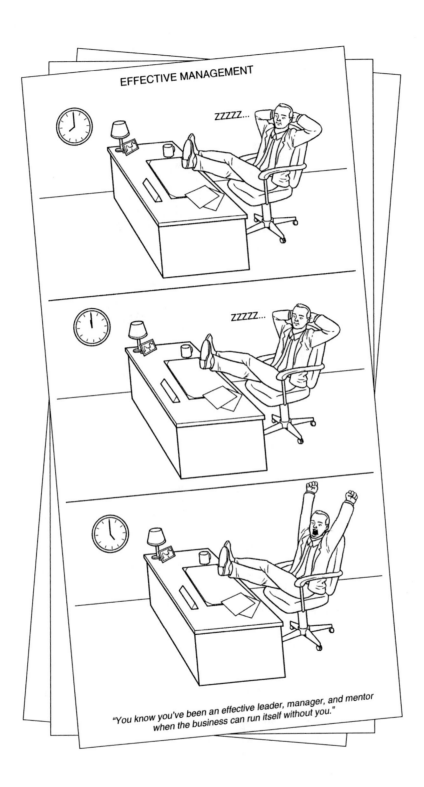

CHAPTER 4

Strategic Planning

Robert F. Carfagno

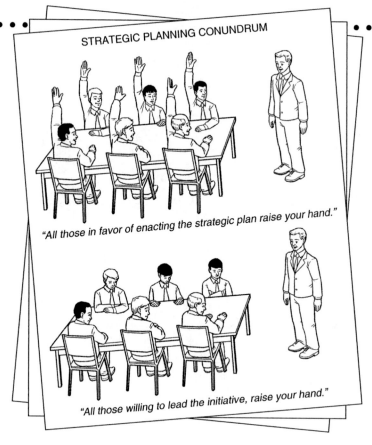

STRATEGIC PLANNING CONUNDRUM

"All those in favor of enacting the strategic plan raise your hand."

"All those willing to lead the initiative, raise your hand."

INTRODUCTION TO STRATEGIC PLANNING IN RADIOLOGY

Radiology has come a long way from the early days when it seemed to thrive in the dark basements of acute care hospitals. It is unclear whether that banishment to the underworld was due to a need to shield X-ray equipment, the need for darkness to develop and read films, or a simple lack of respect for this technology. What is clear now is that imaging technology has undergone dramatic advances over the years and plays an increasingly important role in the early diagnosis of disease and management of patient care. Not only has imaging technology improved as it relates to early and specific identification of abnormalities, but there have also been equally impressive advances in information technology, which have helped speed up the interpretation and transmission of images and reports to referring physicians.

The advent of cross-sectional imaging, interventional radiology, and nuclear medicine have contributed to the fact that in 1995, 34% of radiologic procedures were either relatively new or were in fields that had not previously existed. Computed tomography (CT) and nuclear medicine are major contributors to this advancement.[1]

Although there is every reason to be optimistic about the growth potential of diagnostic imaging services, several factors can have a potential negative impact on a given radiology facility's plan to grow in a profitable fashion. The old days of emerging technologies expanding a retrofit imaging center are gone. The industry is facing increased competition, sharply declining reimbursement rates, increased utilization review and controls from managed health care plans, increased costs, and difficulty in obtaining medical liability insurance, and, as such, requires an entirely new approach to planning and executing successful and profitable imaging center(s). Clearly, this new environment will require today's radiologists to become adept in dealing with change. Despite many years of medical school, residency, and fellowship, one term that does not come immediately to the radiologist's mind is strategic planning.[2]

Quite simply, strategic planning is a tool to aid management in effective decision making. The purpose of strategic planning is to expedite an efficient process of innovation and change within the firm.[3] This becomes increasingly important in a high-growth rapidly changing industry.

Occasionally an idea just seems to take off on its own. Edward de Bono speaks of a young woman's success as a founder of the first marriage bureau in 1939. The idea of bringing two unacquainted people together for marriage was unique and successful despite the lack of a plan on how to achieve it. The venture was successful because its founder had a very good idea and promoted it with energy and a unique style in a field where there was no other competition. The founder also had the good fortune of collaborating with other trustworthy people to help her succeed.

Edward de Bono, who has written extensively on radical approaches to thought—to the way we think—advocates the need for strategic planning. According to him "strategy means putting things in place carefully, and with a great deal of thought. It is the opposite of just waiting for things to happen or taking a flyer."[4]

Extremely successful individuals from Sting (popular musician) to Malcolm Forbes extol the virtues of strategic planning in their biographies. De Bono points out that a strategy is different than a plan. A strategy is not a detailed action list but a broad overview. It provides you with guidelines for making decisions and a long-term view, which encourages risks or even actions that may not make sense in the short term.[5]

March and Simon are responsible for the time-honored text about the theory of formal organizations. The text deals with important issues such as organizational behavior, intra-organizational decisions, conflict in organizations, and performance programs in organizations. The work also dedicates a chapter to planning and innovation in organizations.[6]

According to Alfred D. Chandler, Jr., strategy can be defined as the determination of the basic long-term goals and objectives of an enterprise, and the adoption of courses of action and the allocation of resources necessary for carrying out these goals. Shifting demands, fluctuating economic conditions, changing sources of supply, new developments in technology, and competitors' actions all result in the need for a firm to develop new courses of action to achieve its goals.[7] The importance of strategy cannot be ignored in developing a structure to carry out a plan. Structure can be defined as the design of organization through which the enterprise is administered.

Peters and Waterman, in writing about the keys to successful management, cite seven key criteria for success. One of those is strategy. They also refer to "Leavitt's Diamond" created by Harold Leavitt (Fig. 4-1), which is also a multivariable framework that cites six key variables for success.[8]

Planning is the core capacity developed by firms to adapt to environmental movements. This adaptability is not a purely passive response to external forces, but an active, creative, and most decisive search for conditions that can secure a profitable niche for the firm's business.[9] Strategy, on the other hand, is defined as a coherent set of actions aimed at gaining a sustainable advantage over competition, improving one's position vis-a-vis customers, and allocating resources.[10]

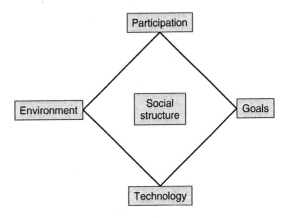

Figure 4-1 Leavitt's diamond multivariable framework for management success. (Modified from Wilson TD: User modelling: A global perspective. Journal of Documentation 2:101, 1999. In Leavitt HG: Applied organizational change in industry: Structural, technological and humanistic approaches, in March, JG [ed]: Handbook of Organizations. Chicago, Rand McNally, 1965.)

WHAT ROLE DOES STRATEGY PLAY IN THE FUTURE OF RADIOLOGY?

There are many advances that have taken place in medicine in the 20th century, but one of the true success stories is diagnostic imaging. Of course, with success comes challenges. Increasing health care costs have caused tightening of health care budgets. Shortages of radiologists and technical staff are exacerbated by the sharp increase in demand. Increases in demand have been fueled by technology advances, patients' increased awareness and demand for the latest technologies, a litigious society in need of tort reform—which has physicians practicing "defensive" medicine—and an aging population (Figs. 4-2 through 4-7 and Tables 4-1 through 4-6).

Much of today's competition in radiology is professional, meaning that sophisticated business people, as well as physicians who previously only referred studies but now own imaging centers, are behind some of the dramatic growth in this field. All of these changing conditions come

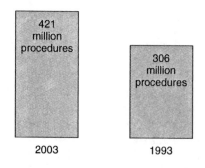

Figure 4-3 Total U.S. medical imaging market.

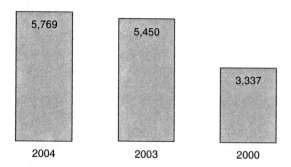

Figure 4-4 Number of centers in United States.

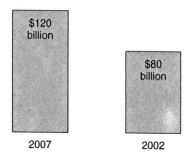

Figure 4-2 U.S. diagnostic imaging, market size.

at a time when technology advances are still occurring at a rapid pace.

This changing market environment highlights the need for radiologists to develop and monitor a strategic plan. While national trends are very important to understand, health care delivery continues to be a local phenomenon so mastering local trends is critical. Clearly, the 21st century will require that the radiologist of the future be not only a skilled "image reader," but also adept in dealing with "managing" in this increasingly complex environment.[11-13]

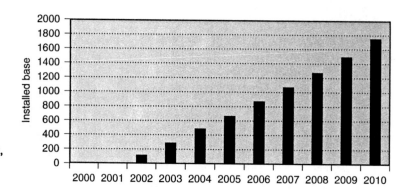

Figure 4-5 PET/CT market, installed base forecasts in United States, 2000–2010.

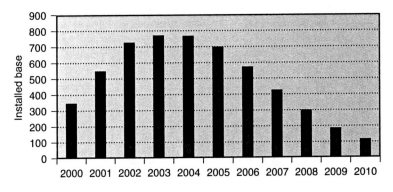

Figure 4-6 PET market, installed base forecasts in United States, 2000–2010. This figure illustrates how PET technology declined with the shift to PET/CT technology. (Data from Frost & Sullivan.)

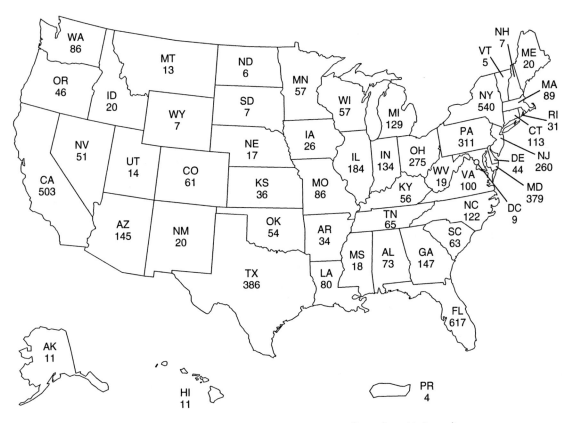

Figure 4-7 National distribution of imaging centers, August 2004. (Data from Verispan.)

BASIC STEPS IN THE CORPORATE STRATEGIC PLANNING PROCESS

Let us review the basic steps in the corporate strategic planning process:

1. Define the vision of the firm.
2. Establish strategic posture and planning guidelines.
3. Develop a mission statement for the business.
4. Formulate business strategy and broad action programs.
5. Formulate functional strategy.
6. Consolidate business and functional strategies.
7. Develop action plans at the business level.
8. Develop action plans at the functional level.

Table 4-1 Total U.S. Medical Imaging Market by Modality (000s)

	2003	1993	% of Growth
X-ray	270,000	231,500	16.6
Nuclear medicine	18,000	7,000	157.1
Ultrasound	60,000	40,000	50.0
MRI	21,000	7,900	165.8
CT	50,579	20,000	152.9
PET	972	—	100.0
Total	420,551	306,400	37.3

Adapted from Frost & Sullivan.

Table 4-4 Center Profile—Equipment

	Full Modality	High-Tech
X-ray/fluoro	3	
X-ray		1
Mammo	3	
Ultrasound	4	
Dexa	1	
Nuc med	1	
PET PET/CT	1	1
CT	1	
MRI	2	1
Total	16	3

Table 4-2 Number of MRI/CT Scanners, 3rd Quarter 2004

	Hospital	Center	Total
CT	5,789	2,730	8,519
MRI	4,816	3,655	8,471
Total			16,990

Adapted from Verispan, IMV Medical Information Division

Table 4-5 PET/CT Market Procedure Volume Analysis in U.S. 2000–2010

Year	Procedure Volumes	Growth Rate (%)
2000	—	—
2001	2,400	—
2002	34,500	1,337.5
2003	105,375	205.4
2004	290,220	175.4
2005	499,440	72.1
2006	857,088	71.6
2007	1,211,539	41.4
2008	1,473,482	21.6
2009	1,714,192	16.3
2010	1,959,879	14.3

CAGR (2003–2010): 51.8%
Adapted from Frost & Sullivan-2003 base year

Table 4-3 Center Profile

	Full Modality	High-Tech
Size	15,000 sq ft	4,000 sq ft
Equipment	16 pieces	3 pieces
Cap ex	$8–10 mil	$4 mil
Volumes	75,000	25,000
Revenues	$11–14 mil	$4–8 mil
Staff FTEs		
Physician	3	1
Tech	20	7
Support	20	4

9. Allocate resources and define performance measurement for management control.
10. Budget at the business level.
11. Budget at the functional level.
12. Consolidate budget and approve strategies and operational funds.

Table 4-6   Trends

Imaging volumes double next 10 years

Regional consolidation of fragmented industry

Shift from hospital to office

Huge growth noninvasive CTA

Collaboration of cardiologists and radiologists

High growth in molecular imaging (physiology vs. anatomy)

Technology and IT solutions
   Dayhawk/nighthawk
   Imaging access
   Filmless environments

THE VISION OF THE FIRM

A firm's vision is typically articulated by its CEO, the purpose of which is to:

1. Communicate the reason that the enterprise exists, including corporate purpose, business scope, and competitive leadership.
2. Set the ground rules for the relationship between the firm and its stakeholders: employees, customers, shareholders, suppliers, and the communities where the firm operates.
3. State broad performance objectives as related to growth and profitability.

The vision should be a unifying theme for all organizational units and serve as a source of inspiration for managing daily activities.

A FIRM'S STRATEGIC POSTURE AND HOW TO GET THERE

A firm's vision is typically updated in five-year intervals. It should be translated into guidelines that enable the development of strategic proposals for the businesses and major functions of the firm. The inputs for this process are the vision of the firm, a diagnosis of the past and future general health of the industrial sectors relevant to the business in which the firm is engaged (environmental scans), and internal scrutiny at the corporate level. This latter input involves a broad evaluation of the human, financial, productive, physical, and technological resources available to the firm: now, in the past, and in the future.

The output from this process is a set of qualitative strategic thrusts and quantitative performance objectives. The strategic thrusts are the primary issues that the firm must address in the next three to five years to establish a healthy competitive position in its key markets. For example, suppose that one critical issue for a radiology firm is a shortage of radiologists. A thrust demanding development of recruitment and retention strategies will create a burst of energy to focus on this issue. The performance objectives are quantitative indicators that relate to the overall financial and nonfinancial goals of the firm.

While there is no universal set of indicators that firms use to express their performance objectives, some beneficial measurements are as follows:

- Growth rate (What is our expectation for increase in procedure volumes?)
- Profit ratios
- Return on revenues
- Return on equity
- Capital investment (% of revenues)
- Debt to equity ratio
- Dividend payout
- Employee retention and satisfaction
- Patient satisfaction

DEVELOP A MISSION STATEMENT FOR THE BUSINESS

The mission of the business is similar to the vision statement at the firm level, and should be expressed in terms of products, market, geographical scope, and competitive uniqueness (Table 4-7).

As an example, multiple business units in a radiology firm would each require separate mission statements as follows:

- Fixed-site imaging locations
- Teleradiology division
- Overnight services
- Daytime services

Table 4-7 Example of Mission Statements for Business Units of a Radiology Firm

Radiology Business Units	Example of a Mission Statement
Fixed-site imaging locations	Alpha Radiology Services is dedicated to providing superior fixed-site diagnostic imaging services to medical practices for the purpose of providing optimal patient care. We place quality and value first in all that we do.

Teleradiology services
   Overnight
   Daytime
	Teleradiology services is a team of dedicated professionals providing superior remote interpretive imaging services to radiology practices and hospitals with which we are affiliated. We successfully serve by placing quality first in all that we do.

Mobile-imaging business	Mobile rad services provides superior mobile magnetic resonance imaging (MRI) services to hospitals with which we are affiliated.
Billing division	Radiology billing management services is dedicated to providing the industry's highest quality billing and collection services to the radiology practice that we serve.

- Mobile-imaging business
- Billing division

The vision and mission are very important to the firm as well as the individual business units. They have to be more than just statements. How do we effectuate them? The culture of a firm should be built around these statements. One way to promote them is to post them all over the office. Discuss them at the beginning or ending of staff meetings. Company stationery, business cards, websites, brochures, flyers, and other collateral might also display them. Repetition is key. If your vision and mission statements revolve around quality, all strategic and tactical activity should reinforce that.

FORMULATE BUSINESS STRATEGY AND BROAD ACTION PROGRAMS

A business strategy is a set of well-coordinated action programs aimed at securing a long-term sustainable advantage. Once again, each business unit must perform a thorough analysis regarding past and future business positions in terms of both the external environment and internal scrutiny, each as previously defined.

FORMULATE FUNCTIONAL STRATEGY

Functional managers in a radiology environment include location office managers, departmental modality managers, call center managers, and various others. In a decentralized firm (meaning that much of the authority and empowerment resides with field staff), functional managers are directly involved in the development of their functional strategies, which unite with the overall vision and mission.

In a business that operates under a centralized management system (i.e., much of the planning, control, and decision making takes place at a corporate level), the functional managers should be involved in review and analysis of business plans that are proposed by the corporate staff.

CONSOLIDATE BUSINESS AND FUNCTIONAL STRATEGIES

This next critical step requires review of all business and functional programs at a corporate level. This process should include all key executives who have responsibility for shaping the strategic direction of the firm. The best venue for this is an offsite location where attention can be totally dedicated to the process (Table 4-8).

Table 4-8 Sample Action Program Format for Radiology Practice

Objective: Radiologist Productivity and Capacity

Initiative: Recruitment

Initiative Champion	Initiative Team	Statement of Objective	End Result Statement	Key Action Items	Responsible Individuals	Interdependencies	Dates	Resource Requirements

The items addressed should include but not be limited to:

1. Resolve conflicts. In a process as complex as this it is not uncommon to have unresolved differences between business and functional managers. This can be an appropriate forum in which to debate and resolve such differences.
2. Balance the business portfolio of the firm. This includes:
   • Consider short-term profitability versus long-term development needs.
   • Evaluate trade-offs for risk and reward.
   • Seek balance in the sources and uses of funds.
3. Define the availability of strategic funds, the debt policy, and maximum sustainable growth. This step is also designed to help determine the amount of funds available to support investment in capital assets, working capital increases, as well as other expenditures on business development.
4. Preliminary review of proposed action plans is essential for resource allocation. All business firms have limits to the resources available to carry out action plans. This is a very organized method to work through this process.
5. Reflect on and review the vision and mission to make sure the priorities set at the local level match the greater purpose of the firm. Never lose sight of why the company exists and what its objectives are. Do the action plans reinforce the vision or are they peripheral to those goals?

DEFINE AND EVALUATE SPECIFIC ACTION PROGRAMS AT THE BUSINESS AND FUNCTIONAL LEVELS

These should be concrete action items that can be monitored in quantitative terms. These are the tactical plans that typically are carried out with measurable impact in 12 to 18 months. The definition of the action programs should include:

• Description of action item
• Stated priority of high, medium, or low. High priority is reserved for those items that are critical to maintain or advance the competitive

position. Medium priority is reserved for those items for which postponement will adversely affect competitive position. Low priority are optional projects, which could enhance competitive position, if funds were available
• Costs and benefits estimates
• Manpower requirements
• Timetables to complete tasks
• Person/people responsible to complete task
• Process to monitor progress and completion

ALLOCATE RESOURCES AND DEFINE PERFORMANCE MEASUREMENTS FOR MANAGEMENT CONTROL

This critical step requires top managers to make a final evaluation of the proposals originated at the business and functional levels. Recognizing once again that all firms have a limited amount of resources (money and people), this balancing and prioritizing is critical to the success of the plan.

The process begins as follows:

• Determine total funds for supporting broad and specific action programs presented.
• Deduct funds required for investment, debt service, other legal commitments, and funds already allocated to previously authorized ongoing projects.

These steps will define the remaining pool available. The remaining funds should be appropriated based on review of the following:

• Analysis of the correlation of requests for funds and strategic direction of the business unit (Does the allocation support the overall mission?)
• Value creation of the proposed programs
• Ability to develop performance measurement programs for the broad and specific action items

STRATEGIC AND OPERATIONAL BUDGETING: THE FINAL CYCLE OF STRATEGIC PLANNING

After the strategic programs have been approved and resources allocated, the commitments should be translated into detailed operating budgets.

These steps require heavy functional management involvement at a local level and approval of final consolidated budgets by top management.

ADVANTAGES OF STRATEGIC PLANNING

Strategic planning is a powerful tool that enhances management's ability to make decisions in a forward-thinking fashion. Several critical reasons to adopt this process include:

1. The planning process will assist in the unification of corporate directions. Recall that the process begins with the firm's vision, works through establishing the mission of each business, acknowledges core functional competencies, and mobilizes managers in the direction of shared objectives.
2. Segmentation of the firm is enhanced. This process plays a vital role in balancing organizational strategy and organizational structure, through alignment of shared concerns and shared resources throughout the firm.
3. The planning process helps a firm become skilled in long-term thinking. Managers often get caught up in routine day-to-day activities. This can result in a total focus on operational issues, without regard to those issues that will likely have an impact over the long term. By having a formal planning process, key managers will be forced to think about and plan around the strategic direction of the business.

The planning process can be educational. A formal strategic planning process can help develop management competency in turning objectives into reality.

PITFALLS OF STRATEGIC PLANNING

As in any organized process, the advantages need to be weighed against the disadvantages. It may be more appropriate in this case to say that there are certain pitfalls that should be guarded against.

1. Avoid a process that becomes too unrealistic. Do not allow planning to become an end in itself. This can be avoided by:
   - Establishing a three- to five-year cycle for a full review of the corporate mission, vision, and overall strategic planning process with minor upgrades to strategies and programs in the interim years.
   - Focusing on the business units each year that require more attention due to significant changes to internal organization or environmental (external) conditions.
   - Selecting a planning theme each year that will require the attention of all key managers. Some examples include teleradiology opportunities, new technology or modalities, value-added services to referring physicians, patients, or insurance payers.
2. Failing to integrate the planning process with other key management systems. As previously mentioned, do not treat planning as an isolated activity conducted by a heavy planning department. The process should engage key managers of the firm and improve the identification and execution of organizational tasks.
3. Use of a calendar-driven process excluding potential for opportunistic or program-period planning. While the time management benefits of a calendar-driven system cannot be denied, the need for planning outside the date-specific approach, triggered by unexpected events or the need for program initiatives to be generated any time during the year, should not be ignored. [14]

One goal of the strategic planning process is to create a long-term sustainable competitive advantage for a firm. According to Michael Porter, there are three generic competitive advantages a firm may gain: cost leadership, product differentiation, or focus. These all speak to a firm's relative position within its industry. A well-positioned firm will likely earn above-average profits thus gaining a sustainable competitive advantage. Gaining a competitive advantage is the heart of any strategy.

In a cost-leadership strategy the firm strives to become the low-cost producer in its industry. Low cost can involve a number of sources, including economies of scale, proprietary technology, or preferential access to raw materials. For the firm to use its cost leadership as a means to yield higher-than-average returns, it must achieve product parity (or close) relative to its competitors. If it does not achieve product parity, the firm will have to sell products or services at a discount, which will erode profits. In radiology, this may mean a large-scale screening coronary CTA center, which is able to charge patients at a minimum, creating a market for a totally out-of-pocket expense business.

A differentiation strategy involves a firm attempting to be unique in its industry. The uniqueness can be along some criteria that are widely valued by buyers. It chooses one or more product attributes that many buyers in an industry perceive as important, and then attempts to meet those needs. If the firm is successful, they will be rewarded with a premium price. The firm will be successful, if the premium price received exceeds the extra costs incurred to be unique. In a radiology practice this might be effectuated as an ultrasound-guided, 3-D model of a 24-week fetus for proud mothers. Another example of a differentiation strategy could be a practice that uses only fellowship-trained, specialty radiologists (musculoskeletal, neuro, and nuclear medicine) to provide superior quality reads to its referring physicians.

The third generic strategy is focus. The firm that chooses this strategy focuses on a segment in the industry and tailors its strategy to servicing that segment to the exclusion of others. By optimizing its strategy for the target segments, the firm (i.e., focuser) seeks to achieve a competitive advantage in its target segment, even though it does not possess a competitive advantage overall. The focus can be on cost leadership or differentiation.

In Baltimore, one entrepreneurial radiologist achieved this by being the outpatient center for dialysis catheter placement and maintenance. All he did every day was provide and maintain access for dialysis shunt catheters. Another example of a differentiation focus strategy in radiology is a firm that provides only unique high-tech services, such as mobile 3.0 tesla MRI and CT-PET to its referring physicians and patient populations.[16]

To form a competitive strategy it is very important to relate a company to its environment. This involves understanding the level of its competition.

The state of competition in an industry depends on five basic competitive forces:

1. Rivalry among existing firms
2. Threat of new entrants
3. Threat of substitute products
4. Bargaining power of suppliers
5. Bargaining power of buyers

Let's look at some examples of these competitive forces at work in the diagnostic imaging industry.

RIVALRY AMONG EXISTING FIRMS

The number of outpatient imaging offices has significantly increased in the past five years. This can be attributed to two main reasons:

1. Hospitals and referring physicians are looking for ways to increase their ancillary cash inflows. They see attractive returns on investment in imaging equipment.
2. Entrepreneurs see an opportunity to make adequate returns on their investment in imaging equipment.

As the number of imaging sites and thus capacity increases, the rivalry among firms has also increased. This condition has given increased leverage to buyers (third-party payers), which will be discussed later.

Rivalry takes many forms, using tactics like price competition, advertising, product line extensions, technical upgrades, and increased customer service. In most industries, competition moves by one firm have a noticeable effect on its competitors and thus may incite retaliation or efforts to counter the move. An example of this occurring in the radiology industry follows:

Firm A updates its fleet of MRI, CT, and PET scanners to the latest technology. This very expensive move is perceived as a threat to Firm B. Worried about loss of referrals to Firm A, Firm B matches this move.

THREAT OF NEW ENTRANTS

New entrants in an industry bring new capacity. This can have a negative impact on price and thus have a reducing effect on profitability. The threat of entry to an industry depends on the barriers to entry that are present. If barriers are high the threat of entry is low.[17]

There are seven major sources of barriers to entry:

1. Economies of scale
2. Product differentiation
3. Capital requirements
4. Switching costs
5. Access to distribution channels
6. Cost disadvantage independent of scale
7. Government policy

Economies of scale deter entry by forcing the entrant to come in at large scale, risking reaction from existing firms, or come in at small scale and accepting a cost disadvantage, neither of which is a desirable option.

Product differentiation means that established firms have brand identification and customer loyalty. This deters entry by forcing entrants to spend heavily to overcome existing customer loyalties.

Heavy capital requirements create a barrier to entry, particularly if the capital is required for risky or unrecoverable up-front advertising or research and development. This is a major barrier unique to imaging centers that focus on MRI, CT, or PET services.

Another barrier to entry is created by the presence of switching costs, that is, one-time costs facing the buyer when switching from one supplier of products to another. If the costs are high then the new entrant must offer a major improvement in cost or performance for the buyer to switch loyalties.

A barrier to entry can be created by the new entrant's need to secure a distribution channel for its product. If logical distribution channels for the product have already been served by an established firm, the entrant may have to offer price breaks and cooperative advertising allowances which will reduce profits.

Established firms may have cost advantages not replicable by potential entrants no matter what their size and attained economies of scale. Some examples are: proprietary product knowledge, favorable access to raw material, or favorable locations.

The last major source of entry barriers is government policy. Government can limit or even foreclose entry into industries with such controls as licensing requirements or environmental controls.

The most significant barriers to entry in radiology in the past have been capital requirements, product differentiation, and government policy. Investment in high-tech imaging equipment costs millions of dollars. This barrier has been partially removed as vendors have offered creative financing that requires less down-payment dollars, financing for fit out, and payment skips in the early months of operations as equipment volumes ramp up. Purchases by physicians who have a built-in stream of referrals have also removed this as a potential barrier. Another barrier in radiology is product differentiation. There are many long-established relationships between referring doctors and radiologists. These referral patterns can be broken with better technology offerings as well as service improvements. Lastly, government licensing issues such as Certificates of Need (CON) can prevent new entrants. Currently, these exist only in a few states.

The bottom line is that the barriers to entry in the diagnostic imaging industry, which were once monumental, have sharply eroded in the past five years and as a result there are many new outpatient centers.

PRESSURE FROM SUBSTITUTE PRODUCTS

This is really not an issue for the overall imaging industry, but it is true that within radiology, multidetector CT angiography has eroded some of the marketing position previously held by MR angiography and duplex sonography. Some serologic tests and genetic assays may ultimately serve as effective screening techniques that heretofore were in the domain of imaging (e.g., prostate-specific antigen screening for prostate cancer or HD gene testing for Huntington's disease).

BARGAINING POWER OF BUYERS

Buyers compete with the industry by forcing down prices, bargaining for higher quality or more services, and playing competitors against each other, all at the expense of industry profitability.

This is occurring extensively in the imaging industry. As the number of providers sharply increases and the number of third-party payers (buyers) decreases, prices (reimbursement rates) have sharply declined. HMO products, such as capitation, promise volume for price concession. These need to be carefully analyzed before any of these deals are accepted. At the same time, radiologists may use this same strategy for getting better pricing for their IT PACS/RIS systems or imaging equipment purchases. Buying in bulk for a large group may also aid in competitiveness.

BARGAINING POWER OF SUPPLIERS

Suppliers can exert bargaining power over industry players by threatening to raise prices or reduce the quality of purchased goods and services.

The more likely recent impact in radiology is rapidly changing technology that is not well communicated in advance to buyers, thus causing premature product obsolescence of equipment that is relatively new. Questions about new products or new planned releases should be extensive. Nonobsolescence packages may be critical to maintaining a technological advantage in the market.

INTRODUCTION TO BUDGETING IN RADIOLOGY

Strategic planning thinking has evolved over several decades and has passed through various stages of development. The five major stages are:

- Budgeting and financial control
- Long-range planning
- Business strategic planning
- Corporate strategic planning
- Strategic management

There is no one right way to plan. A firm will have an appropriate planning system in place when its degree of planning competence matches the degree of complexity of the firm's businesses, as well as its internal culture.

The purpose of this section is not to focus on a detailed review of the differences, merits, and limitations of each of the stages but to recognize the complexity of the topic and gather some insight on one of the earliest and most important stages of strategic planning thinking.

The most basic concept of systems management lies in budgeting and financial control. The concepts emerged many years ago to enable management to monitor the increasing number of activities developed by a firm. It is important that both of these formal procedures make up an integral part of administrative functions used by managers to run a company and that they be closely related to the development of overall strategies in the company.

Let us first define the budgetary process. Budgeting represents projections of revenues and costs typically related to a one-year period. The consolidated budget of a firm consists of all those activities that need to be monitored for healthy development of a firm's business to occur. Financial performance is at the heart of every business enterprise. Profit is not the only objective that a firm might pursue, but if neglected, a lack of profitability will adversely impact all other objectives of a firm.

Managers, especially the CEO, consider profitability to be a central area of concern. Well-designed and implemented budget and financial control systems are helpful for the definition, monitoring, and achievement of profit goals. While the importance of the "annual budget" should be recognized, we must avoid the trap of achieving short-term profits at the risk of failing to develop the business for the long term. It is important that we do not inadvertently weaken our asset base by placing too much emphasis on short-term return on investment (ROI). This can be caused by milking capital assets past their useful lives at a time when one should be making necessary investments to preserve long-term competitive standing. Exercise caution not to mortgage the future for a hefty ROI in the upcoming one-year period.

So, how does one avoid this dilemma? The simple answer is to be certain that ROI should not be a goal unto itself, but rather established as a by-product of strategic direction. Financial performance in the short and long term must be conditioned by strategic commitments.[15] (See also reference 9.)

This is a very real issue in the radiology business. Improved ROI can easily be achieved in the short run by avoiding the expensive replacement of obsolete equipment. This will do wonders for financial performance in the short term as profits continue on a fully depreciated asset base. However, failure to upgrade equipment for technological advances will likely result in lost market share to competitors who have lower ROI in the short term, but better long-term prospects for profitable growth by investing in advancing technology. The key to a successful balance of long- and short-term goals is the development and communication of the business strategy and translation of strategic commitments into meaningful financial indicators.

One means to ensure that the strategic commitments are properly communicated is to adopt a formal strategic planning system. This next section is dedicated to a review of the budget process in a radiology firm. It addresses some of the intricacies of the process as well as issues of format and content.

THE BUDGETING PROCESS

The budgeting process always begins with a look at the recent past. There is no better predictor of future trends than to understand how the key variables, which drive revenues and expenses, have changed in the past. Of course, this is only one component of setting the future to a "quantifiable plan." Other changes in the internal and external environments can have an impact on prior trends.

For example, let's assume growth in net revenues of MRIs has been 12% in each of the past two years, ending 2004 and 2005. This growth has resulted from a 10% growth in market size and a 2% increase in reimbursement rates. Before merely setting the MRI net revenues growth rate at 12% for 2006, you should check on projected market growth trends for MRI volumes as well as projected changes to reimbursement rates. Projected market growth

trends can possibly change from year to year, which can be ascertained via market research publications such as those published by Frost and Sullivan, Booz Allen, and Verispan. Medicare and other third-party payers use published fee schedules to communicate their reimbursement rates. These schedules can be reviewed to help anticipate the impact of rate changes on next year's revenues.

To emphasize the point in this example, both market growth trends and reimbursement rate changes can differ from year to year. Efforts must be made to determine anticipated changes for the upcoming year. Every budget cycle should begin with the "top line" question: What are we budgeting next year for revenues? To understand this we need to analyze two major components: volumes and reimbursement rates.

NET REVENUES

The net revenue section of the budgeted income statement (Table 4-9) should be broken into three line items:

- Fee-for-service net revenues
- Capitated net revenues
- Other net revenues

Volumes typically will drive our expenses but to understand their impact on revenues we have to understand how projected changes in volumes relate to "capitated" versus "fee-for-service" business. Fee-for-service net revenues are the more straightforward category. These are a by-product of modality volumes and reimbursement rates. Each procedure performed is reimbursed at a preestablished rate. Rates will most likely vary depending on the payer. In projecting volumes for fee-for-service business, what are the right questions to ask? The list includes but is not limited to:

- What is the projected market growth for each modality by payer?
- Are there any limitations on our site's ability to handle the projected market growth?
- Are we adding new equipment capacity that might enable us to grow in excess of market growth rates?
- Have we improved infrastructure such as scheduling or registration capability, which

Table 4-9   Consolidated Income Statement

Net Revenues
    Fee for Service
    Capitation
    Other
        Total Net Revenues

Expenses
    Provision for Uncollectible Accounts
    Physician Salaries
    Physician Benefits
    Contract Labor and Professional Radiology
        Total Physician Costs
    Employee Salaries and Benefits
    Office, Computer and Linen Supplies, Forms
    Licenses and Permits, Subscriptions
    Medical Supplies, Film, Contrast
    Rent and Facility Expenses (excluding
      telephone)
    Telephone
    Equipment Rental
    Purchased Services
    Repairs and Maintenance
    Service Contracts
    Allocation of Billing
    Info Services Expenses
    Allocation of Transcription
        Total Operating Expenses

Nonoperating Revenues and Expenses
    Interest Income
    Other Income/(Expense)
        Total Nonoperating Revenues and Expenses

EBITDA (Earnings Before Interest, Taxes,
Depreciation, and Amortization)

Depreciation and Interest
    Amortization
    Depreciation
    Interest
        Total Amortization, Depreciation, and
        Interest
EBT (Earnings Before Taxes)

Income Taxes

Net Income

• Has an existing major referring group or practice left our territory?

Capitated revenues are determined on a completely different basis. An imaging provider is contracted to provide all the imaging needs of a certain number of patient lives as presented by a payer. In exchange for this commitment the provider will receive a fixed payment per patient life per month, regardless of how much care is given. Below is an example of a capitated contract:

Imaging Provider, Improv, owns and operates 20 facilities throughout the state of Maryland. Third-party payer, 3rd Pay, has contracted with Improv to provide imaging services for 50,000 patients on a capitated basis for $10 per member per month (pmpm). Regardless of how many studies Improv performs on these capitated patients, it will receive $500,000 per month (50,000 x $10) or $6 million annually for the provision of these services. This may represent the typical capitated case, but it is also possible to receive a capitated contract that has a "carve-out" for high-tech studies such as MRI or PET studies. By "carve-out" one might mean (in another scenario) that the insurer will not pay for those studies at your facility or it may mean that in addition to the capitated payment there will be an additional fee-for-service for every MRI or PET study performed. Another variation can have payment "corridors," which will retroactively adjust total amounts paid if imaging volumes are below or above certain thresholds.

Once we have completed our analysis of these elements of revenues we should build a model designed to project volumes from the "bottom up" that specifies numbers by modality for each office location. The modality totals will be summarized by the payer and appropriate reimbursement rates will be applied to arrive at net revenues. The "other net revenues" category could include fees derived from billing or management services.

NET REVENUES SUMMARY STATEMENT

The total net revenues include capitated and fee-for-service volumes as well as income derived from other sources, such as billing fees or

correspondingly could increase our ability to grow above market or historical rates?
• Do we have access to a new group of physicians that are going to refer patients to us?

management services. Critical analyses of projected volumes as well as reimbursement rates are necessary to properly estimate future year revenues. Tables 4-10, 4-11, and 4-12 illustrate examples of volume and rate projections.

Step one in the revenue budgeting process is to thoroughly analyze the recent prior year's volume and rate components as they relate to both capitated and fee-for-service contracts.

Table 4-10   Table of Volume Projections for Year 2006, Modality, and Locations

NAME	QTR 1	QTR 2	QTR 3	QTR 4	Total
Business Days	64	64	63	63	254
Diagnostics					
Location 1					
Location 2					
Total diagnostics					
Volume per day					
CT Scans					
Location 1					
Location 2					
Total CT scans					
Volume per day					
Ultrasound					
Location 1					
Location 2					
Total ultrasound					
Volume per day					
Nuclear Medicine					
Location 1					
Location 2					
Total nuclear medicine					
Volume per day					
Mammography					
Location 1					
Location 2					
Total mammography					
Volume per day					
DEXA					
Location 1					
Location 2					
Total DEXA					
Volume per day					

Continued

Table 4-10   Table of Volume Projections for Year 2006, Modality, and Locations (Cont'd)

NAME	QTR 1	QTR 2	QTR 3	QTR 4	Total
MRI					
Location 1					
Location 2					
Total MRI					
Volume per day					
PET Scans					
Location 1					
Location 2					
Total PET scans					
Volume per day					
Total Scans					
Location 1					
Location 2					
Total scans					
Volume per day					

Table 4-11   Table of Volume Projections by Location and Modality

	2004 Actual	2005 Actual	2006 Projected
Location 1			
Diagnostics			
CT scans			
Ultrasound			
Nuclear Medicine			
Mammography			
MRI			
Fluoroscopy			
DEXA			
PET/CT scans			
Total			

Table 4-12   Table of Reimbursement Rate Assumptions by Payer and Modality

	X-ray	CT scans	Ultrasound	Mammo-graphy	MRI	Fluoro-scopy	DEXA	PET/CT scans
	$	$	$	$	$	$	$	$
Charge rate								
Medicare								
Medicaid								
Capitated HMO*								
Blue Shield								
Commercial								
Worker's compensation								
Self-pay								
Average gross reimbursement (before bad debt)								
Average net reimbursement (after bad debt)								

Based on average HMO and capitated rates at the offices.

EXPENSES

In a similar fashion to revenue projections, volumes by modality by office will be the key component in the expense budgeting process. Each modality should represent a department for which detailed line item costs are projected. The key expense items will include salary and benefits for technical, clerical, and other support staff; medical supplies; facility costs including rent, maintenance, etc.; office supplies, telephone, equipment rental, repairs and maintenance, equipment service contracts, billing, information services, transcription, and purchased services (see Table 4-9).

Purchased services include (but are not limited to) items such as: accounting, insurance, advertising, bank fees, business travel, contributions, seminars, employee training and development, legal assistance, and consultants.

One additional major expense to be accounted for is physician costs. This line item will include the cost of physicians' salaries and all benefits paid on their behalf. These benefits will include (but not be limited to) items such as: health care costs, business allowances, retirement plans, and medical liability insurance. The physician costs section should include any physician services purchased on a contractual basis (e.g., nighthawks, moonlighters).

There also needs to be a section in the income statement that accounts for equipment depreciation and interest on the debt used to fund the purchase of equipment. This can be a very significant expense as it costs millions of dollars to equip an imaging facility. We will learn more about that in the subsequent Capital Expenditures Budget section, which discusses the "capital expenditure" cycle as it relates to the budgeting process.

Now that we have identified the various expense categories to be captured in the income statement, let's review how the budgeting process works for the quantification of next year's expenses. We will use projected volumes for the upcoming year to begin the expense cycle (see Table 4-10).

Separate departmental budgets should be prepared for the following modalities: X-ray/fluoroscopy, ultrasound, mammography, DEXA, nuclear medicine, CT, MRI, and PET. Each of these modalities requires separate technologist staffing and has separate requirements for expense line items such as facility space, medical supplies, equipment depreciation, physician support, etc. Once the departmental budgets are complete, they are ready to be consolidated.

There are certain expense items that need to be budgeted for the facility as a whole and then "allocated" to the departments based on criteria such as space utilization or level of activity (volumes are usually the key measurement). Examples of these types of expenses include (but are not limited to) office manager, rent and facility expenses, billing costs, transcription, front desk, and film library costs.

An imaging system that consists of multiple office locations that include a corporate infrastructure will also include costs at a central location for items such as: accounting, human resources, and central operations, which will be budgeted in total and then allocated back to the individual office locations.

EXPENSES SUMMARY STATEMENT

There are several key things to consider when completing the expense portion of the budgeted income statement:

- Begin the process with volumes that have been projected for each modality.
- Identify the proper expense line items to be budgeted in detail for each modality on a departmental basis.
- Determine which line items will be budgeted on a direct departmental basis versus those that will be estimated for the entire facility and allocated back to the departments.

- Identify any support costs that will occur at a corporate level and then be allocated back to individual offices.

CAPITAL EXPENDITURES (CAPEX) BUDGET

The diagnostic imaging business is people and capital intensive. These represent the two largest cash outlays required to support the business. As such, there is a high baseline investment to be made in these two areas and thus very careful planning is required in both areas.

For discussion purposes, let's assume that we are dealing with a full modality imaging center: typically that means X-ray, fluoroscopy, ultrasound, mammography, DEXA, CT, MRI, and PET. If we were building an imaging center from scratch, we would need capital not only for equipment, but also a substantial amount of capital to "fit out" the facility. It could require up to $8 million to equip a full modality imaging center, including fit-out costs of close to $2 million. "Fit–out" is defined as the cost to prepare facility space for operation of an imaging business (e.g., shielding, lead-lining walls, information technology (IT) lines). This type of transaction could be financed in several different ways including operating leases and/or capital lease purchases, either of which can be financed through a bank, leasing company, or the finance arm of a vendor.

Major capital decisions such as these will depend on typical return on investment (ROI) analyses, which include a detailed assessment of how to service the debt as well as what profits are available after servicing that debt. A key assumption includes projections of volumes and revenues that will be produced as well as the operating costs required to achieve the projections. This ROI analysis is a "mini-budget process" for each piece of equipment being purchased. The analysis might also include a decision as to whether to include all or only some modalities. Other factors also influence this decision, such as the need to be a full-service provider for a given third-party payer or geographic population.

Other than building full or partial modality imaging sites de novo, the major part of the

CAPEX cycle is dedicated to a determination of what additional new equipment, replacement equipment, and/or equipment upgrades are needed. It is therefore helpful to summarize proposed equipment purchases into the following categories:

- Replace for quality purposes
- Replace for patient safety reasons (a big JCAHO directive)
- Add for additional capacity
- Add new modality for existing location
- Upgrade to existing equipment
- Add new location
- Required due to regulatory change.

Ultimately, all equipment must pay for itself on a full-cost allocated basis, but sometimes an upgrade or replacement is required strictly for quality purposes where there is no incremental financial return (e.g., upgrade to digital radiography from plain radiography).

BUDGET REVIEW PROCESS

It is always advisable to include field personnel in the budgeting process. Office and modality managers (department and technical) and marketing staff should be the key drivers of volume projections. This enables the firm to consider feedback directly from referring physicians and evaluate capacity for growth.

Once the budget consolidation process is complete for an office, there should be a critical review of the income statement and all key assumptions prior to presentation as part of a final plan.

CAPACITY ANALYSIS

Analysis of capacity should be an integral part of the budget review process. Each modality will have various budgeted slots based on time required to complete a study. Most time slots vary from 10 to 30 minutes, depending on the modality, although multidetector CT scan time slots are quickly approaching this minimum. Hours of operations will then determine how many procedures can be performed in a given workday. It is also necessary to determine if

the office will maintain hours on the weekend. This can usually be profitable for high-tech studies at low break-even volumes but is not sustainable for low-tech studies at low volumes.

Capacity analysis should also include assessment of potential incremental volumes, revenues, and costs that will occur if hours are expanded from existing hours of operation. In a people- and equipment-intensive business with such high fixed costs, utilization of excess capacity represents a big financial opportunity.

CAPACITY ANALYSIS SUMMARY STATEMENT

Capacity analysis for a given office consists of two separate analyses. The following steps need to be performed for each modality:

- Determine maximum number of procedures that can be performed based on time required for each study and the current number of hours of operation (current capacity).
- Determine maximum number of procedures that can be performed based on the most practical hours that we would expect patients to be willing to have these procedures performed (practical capacity).
- Compare current actual volumes to these two benchmarks to quantify excess capacity and provide volume information needed to quantify potential revenue, costs, and profit data.

SHORT-TERM INITIATIVES

Each year's financial plan (operating budget) should be accompanied by a qualitative plan which, if achieved, will result in a high probability that the financial goals will be met. Let's review the key questions that should be addressed, who should address them, and how the plan should be communicated throughout the organization.

In the diagnostic imaging world, which has become swamped with competitors of all types, key drivers of growth for referring physicians and patients revolve around quality and service. The most effective means to translate focus on these issues to a productive plan is to have key staff members meet at an offsite location for several days and put themselves in the mindset of their customers and patients, referring physicians, and third-party payers. This represents a large and diverse set of customers, each with different needs, and as such, should be considered separately.

From the perspective of each of these groups, ask yourself the question "What are the 'best practices' related to each key area of service to these constituents?" The next step is to evaluate how your practice performs relative to these "best practices." Be honest. The purpose of the exercise is constructive not punitive. This is not a vehicle to punish the staff for shortcomings. The purpose is to identify "gaps" and potential for improvements that consequently can have a big impact on pleasing the customers. Happy customers will result in continued growing relationships from a volume standpoint, which is the ultimate goal.

Some key functions in the diagnostic imaging field include (but are not limited to) the following:

- Patient scheduling
- Patient registration
- Study performance
- Image interpretation
- Physician radiologists' report preparation and communication

As they relate to patients and referring physicians, all of the above functions are going to be rated on efficiency and time consumed.

Third-party payers want their patients and providers who use radiology services to be "satisfied at a reasonable cost." An integral part of this evaluation process should be to gather feedback directly from the customers. This is a relationship business and nothing can take the place of "responding" to customers' needs and requests.

If this part of the process is ignored, our customers will exercise one of the many options they have. And that means losing a valuable patient or referring physician and having "bad press" circulate about us in the marketplace.

Let's look at the scheduling function to identify how this process can produce an initiative designed to yield improvements in this area.

The appointment to have a diagnostic imaging procedure performed may be scheduled by the patient or the referring physician. As it relates to this function, they both desire the same thing: ease of scheduling the appointment. To assess how we fare related to this function from a customer perspective, we must have a telephone system that will allow us to measure key metrics such as average speed of answer (ASA), abandoned calls, length of calls, percent of time calls are answered within target time, and number of outliers from some target number (e.g., calls that take longer than 60 seconds to answer).

These are just examples of key metrics but by understanding our customer's expectations, we can measure our performance and set a plan to improve. It is critically important to be very specific in identifying who will do what by when, to achieve set goals.

Another important decision when working on annual "initiatives" involves deciding who will participate in the process. Old-school thinking gives responsibility for this type of activity to the management team. A much better approach is more "participatory" and includes as many frontline field staff as possible. This makes great sense. First of all, they know better than anyone what is occurring and how we can make changes to achieve better results. They will appreciate being asked their opinion, be honest about what changes are realistic, and then make it happen. Don't underestimate how important it is to have field staff included in your brain trust when choosing whom to include in this process.

Let's take a moment to discuss the area of key metrics in reviewing these annual (short-term) initiatives. What are the key drivers of the diagnostic imaging business? To further our discussion, below is a list of key metrics for some of the functions previously listed for a diagnostic imaging business. Before we review the list, let's define what a key metric is. Remember, our goal in setting initiatives is to make sure the desired outcome is measurable.

We previously visited some of the key metrics in the scheduling function: what about patient registration, diagnostic imaging study performance, image interpretation, and report preparation? Patient registration should be measured as the time from when the patient first arrives until they are sent to the imaging technologist to have their study performed. How quickly is the patient greeted upon arrival? Preregistration can also help to make the registration process more efficient, including making certain that the patient is properly prepped and that they bring all necessary prescription and insurance paperwork with them. All of these details will make the process of registration run more smoothly. The goal here is to minimize patient wait time, which is ultimately impacted by how efficiently things go in the back (imaging departments).

The key metrics for the registration function might be:

- What percentage of time does a patient arrive on time, properly prepared, and with all the right paperwork?
- What are the average as well as distribution of wait times for a patient to be received by the imaging department?

Study performance begins with prescribed time slots and a schedule of patients to be scanned throughout the day. Studies like MRI, mammography, ultrasound, and PET will usually be performed based on a schedule, but it is not uncommon for a high number of patients to walk in for plain X-rays and even some of the higher-tech modalities. Staying on a schedule can be very difficult in an office handling up to 300 patients a day, but it is important for patient satisfaction. Measuring performance in this area will be key to long-term success. Key metrics include receiving a patient efficiently and completing the patient's imaging procedure on time.

The end product of an imaging study is the physician's report. Report turnaround (RTA) is measured from the time a study begins until the time the report is sent to or received by the patient's referring physician. This function encompasses five critical steps:

- Physician reads the images once study is complete
- Physician dictates reports as to findings and impression
- Report is transcribed
- Report is verified and signed by physician
- Report is delivered to referring physician

Technology has played a huge role in expediting this part of the process. Major efficiency gains have occurred in the past five years to streamline the activity around these steps. Physicians no longer have to read films; they are able to interpret digital images on high-quality monitors. Rather than moving doctors around, teleradiology enables movement of images at high speeds, to enable remote reading of specialty studies. Voice recognition software can significantly reduce the time and cost of report transcription. The technology also exists to send reports and images electronically to referring physicians. However, despite the advances in technology, it is still key to measure all of the steps in the report generation cycle.

Three other important points to consider are: (1) how to manage the process of establishing initiatives, (2) assigning leadership and a team to each initiative, and (3) making sure that the organization has adequate resources to complete the tasks.

Since the process will involve a cross-section of staff from diverse functions in the organization, there will be an opportunity for competing forces to become parochial in identifying and prioritizing gaps and resource use. Using an outside facilitator with experience in this type of process is highly recommended. This also provides an independent resource in ascertaining that the final list of initiatives is achievable. Initiative overload is a surefire formula for disaster. Lack of execution and achievement creates a very discouraging environment for a group that is focused on performance and ensures that the financial goals, which are driven by the qualitative plan, will be missed.

Finally, every initiative needs to have a committee of people to help accomplish the goal. Once again, a blend of functions as well as staff at the mid-management and the field level make up the ideal team to ensure execution. The deeper into the organization we go in developing and executing these initiatives, the more likely it is that we will succeed.

In conclusion, radiology has become a very complex business. The increased competition, declining reimbursement, and increased complexity in obtaining appropriate payment for service rendered require a true focus on where your business is going and how it will get there. Strategic planning is the tool to enable efficient and effective decision making, innovation, and sustainability.

Dos and Don'ts of Strategic Planning

Dos	Don'ts
1. Use an outside facilitator to conduct the process and be sure that action plans are accompanied with timelines and responsible parties.	1. Limit the process to managers only.
2. Involve staff across all functions and levels of the business (executive, field level, and management).	2. Allow egos or personal agendas to drive the process.
3. Support vision and mission statements with proper planning and action items.	3. Emphasize short-term gains over necessary investments, which will drive sustainable competitive advantage.
4. Obtain a clear understanding of the industry environment—past, present, and future trends.	4. Overextend cash flows.
5. Review anticipated changes in technology carefully before making final CAPEX plans and purchases.	5. Ignore a plan once developed.

REFERENCES

1. Margulis A, Sunshine J: Radiology at the turn of the millennium. Radiology 214:15–23, 2000.
2. Chan S: The importance of strategy for the evolving field of radiology. Radiology 224:639–648, 2002.
3. Lorange P: Corporate Planning: An Executive Viewpoint. 1980, p 1.
4. De Bono E: Tactics: The Art and Science of Success. 1984, p 143.
5. Ibid, pp 141–151.
6. March J, Simon H: Organizations. 1958, pp 172–210.
7. Chandler AD, Jr: Strategy and Structure. 1962, p 16.
8. Peters TJ, Waterman RH, Jr: In Search of Excellence, Lessons from America's Best-Run Companies. Harper & Row, 1982, pp 9–11.
9. Haux AC, Majluf NS: Strategic Management: An Integrative Perspective. 1984, pp 1–9.
10. Ibid, p 94.
11. Hillman B: Medical imaging in the 21st century. Lancet 350:731–733, 1997.
12. Poudevine G: Planning the Radiology Department of the Future. Radiology Manage 2000.
13. Hillman B: The past 25 years in medical imaging research: A memoir. Radiology 214:11–14, 2000.
14. Haux AC, Majluf NS: Strategic Management: An Integrative Perspective. 1984, pp 41–71.
15. Dearden, J: The case against ROI control. Harvard Business Review 49(3):124–135, 1969.
16. Porter M: Competitive Advantage: Creating and Sustaining Superior Performance. 1985, pp 11–16.
17. Porter M: Competitive Strategy: Techniques for Analyzing Industries and Competitions. 1980, pp 3–29.

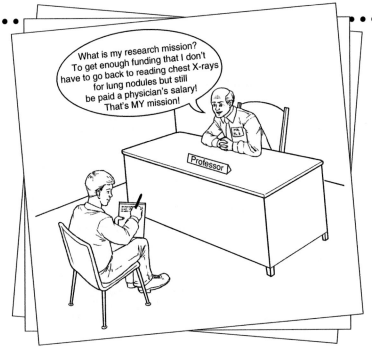

CHAPTER 5

Research Mission

Satoshi Minoshima

INTRODUCTION

Traditional academic missions of medicine are clinical care, research, and education. Through these missions, we attempt to make significant improvements on current and future health care and the well-being of patients. It is not necessarily easy to estimate the contribution of each mission toward our eventual goal. However, a simplistic view of each contribution can be described as follows: one outpatient clinician may be able to see patients through daily clinical work—maybe ten thousand patients through his or her entire career—depending on the volume of the clinic. Working in an academic institution and providing education and teaching to trainees and inside and outside colleagues, one physician may be able to transmit his or her knowledge through the medical care provided by those trainees and colleagues, eventually benefiting a large number of patients. If research produces a significant outcome, such as the critical understanding of the pathophysiology

of a disease, an innovative technology for accurate diagnosis, effective treatment, the most cost-effective use of imaging technology for a large population of patients, and so on, research can potentially change our medical practice. Thus, the contribution of research goes far beyond individual physicians, institutions, and nations. For these reasons, research is a critical mission of our academic radiology practice.

RADIOLOGY RESEARCH

The field of radiology research is diverse. Traditional radiology research has focused on observation and descriptive findings of medical disorders using radiological devices. Another field of radiology research is to establish new imaging technologies for appropriate clinical applications. Such research endeavors have been supported by strong engineering and physics expertise in the field of radiological sciences. It is important to recognize that academic radiology departments typically provide positions not only for MD physicians, but also for a relatively large number of engineers, physicists, and scientists holding PhDs. Collaboration between physicians, physician scientists, engineers, and basic scientists becomes an important element to the success of radiology research.

Due to increasing health care expenditures over the past few decades, approval for new imaging technologies and reimbursement for clinical practice using such technologies comes under careful scrutiny. This actually gives us an opportunity to reexamine not only our clinical practice, but also the research missions. Radiology researchers commonly use radiological techniques to study biology and diseases, investigate imaging methods, and establish more effective diagnostic and interventional techniques, and so on. Their hope is to improve patients' outcomes either by providing more accurate diagnosis for treatment decision making or by providing insights into disease processes or biological mechanisms to help develop better treatment methods. If treatment outcomes guided by research discovery or new imaging practices prove to be better than prior strategies, such new techniques will be submitted for approval by governmental agencies for disseminated use and, thus, facilitate better clinical practice.

This "innovation cycle" of imaging technology and implementation has been summarized in Figure 5-1. It is increasingly clear that to get a new radiological discovery and innovation to be accepted in our medical practice, we have to demonstrate beneficial outcome combined with available treatments. Thus, imaging research and treatment developments are closely related in this cycle. One way to facilitate this link is to study carefully diseases and biology using radiological devices and generate a better understanding of disease processes that in turn lead to improved diagnostic methods and treatment developments. Both observational and mechanistic research approaches to studying "disease" attempt to accomplish this goal in the traditional approach of radiology research (see Fig. 5-1, *solid arrow A*).

Parallel to these approaches, a new way to use radiological devices is to directly facilitate drug and other therapeutic developments (see Fig. 5-1, *dashed arrow B*). This line of investigation often falls into the category of clinical or phase trials. In this research, investigators may not necessarily come up with their own hypotheses or discoveries. Rather, they facilitate developments of new interventions by providing radiological findings as surrogate markers for trials.

Both traditional research and trials are important components of radiological research. If we are successful in supporting effective treatments and therapeutic developments for better

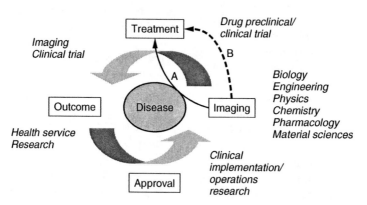

Figure 5-1 Radiology research and innovation cycle of imaging technology and implementation. **A,** Traditional imaging research is to study "disease" using imaging technology, better elucidate pathophysiology, provide more accurate diagnosis, help guide optimal treatment, and evaluate response, all aiming at ultimate improvement in patient outcome. **B,** Additional pathway of imaging research is to help direct therapeutic developments by using imaging technology, such as providing surrogate end points (biomarkers) for clinical trials to facilitate drug development. Diverse fields of radiology research can been seen at different stages of the cycle.

patient outcome, our imaging practice will flourish in the future through approval of new treatments and imaging technology. Individual investigators are typically specialized to each component of the innovation cycle (see Fig. 5-1, e.g., physics, disease-specific research, health service research). However, an understanding of the entire cycle allows investigators to position themselves in the big picture of radiology research and contribute more effectively to the eventual goal of patient care and imaging practice.

HIERARCHY OF CLINICAL RESEARCH AND EVIDENCE

In our era of "evidence-based medicine," approvals for new imaging technology and translation of research outcome to clinical applications are reviewed systematically based on existing evidence in the literature. Clinical implementation of imaging technology and imaging research outcomes requires stringent processes of governmental review and approval (see Fig. 5-1), including that of the Food and Drug Administration (FDA) and Centers for Medicare and Medicaid Services (CMS), both of which reside within the U.S. Department of Health and Human Services (DHHS). As our critical mission of research is to make eventual improvement in patient care an outcome, it is essential for clinical investigators to aim for producing high-quality evidence through imaging investigations.

The hierarchy of clinical research and evidence can be seen in relation to study designs (Fig. 5-2). Those studies that are designed to produce high-quality evidence are typically ranked at a higher hierarchical level and have greater potential to make an impact. Also, this type of research typically requires significant resources, funding, and time commitment. Investigators at the different levels of their academic career engage in clinical research at different levels of the hierarchy. Observational studies such as case reports, case series, and case control studies can be done without specific research funding: well-designed observational studies can potentially produce outcomes comparable to randomized controlled trials.[1]

In contrast, it is difficult to perform large cohort studies, despite their observational nature, or prospective randomized control trials without funding and/or departmental financial or infrastructural support. Investigators typically start from a lower hierarchical level, develop their own research questions, use initial observational data to apply for pilot funding (if available), develop further research questions and data, and then apply for larger funding and engage in prospective experimental studies such as randomized controlled trials. Observational research has been prevalent in radiology research, and transition from unfunded observational research to funded prospective research is admittedly challenging. Eventually, successful career development in research comes down to investigators' passion, energy, and persistence in making this transition. However, appropriate mentorship, initial department support for academic time and

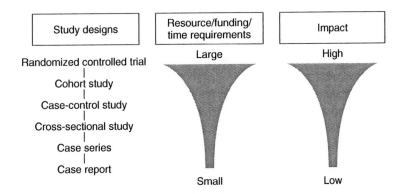

Figure 5-2 Hierarchy of clinical research. The diagram describes different study designs typically employed in radiology research and the impact of outcome relative to the resource and funding requirements.

start-up resources and funds, and departmental research infrastructure can make the transition more feasible for many. The National Institutes of Health (NIH) and other funding agencies are providing more funding opportunities for clinical-trial-type research, along with an emphasis on translational research.

Investigational research is an iteration of hypothesis generation, preliminary investigation, funding, extended investigation, publication, and technology transfer when it is applicable (Fig. 5-3). Hypothesis-driven, mechanistic investigations are the core of the investigator-initiated research in R01, R21, and R03 mechanisms of NIH funding. Basic science research as well as biology and disease-specific research often falls in this category. Due to increasing competition, the average age of a faculty member receiving her or his first R01 grant is over 40 years old. Investigators engaging in this type of research initially start with small-scale research, often in the established group of researchers, with funding from institutional grants, training grants, small pilot grants, or existing research funding in the group. Sufficient demonstration of preliminary results and proof of independent investigation are essential for successful R01 funding. The R21 grant can be used effectively to support the development of initial preliminary data for subsequent R01 funding applications.

Funding is the beginning of research, but not the goal of the research endeavor. Research funding without significant outcome or productivity does not fulfill our research mission. This notion should be kept in mind if faculty incentives are determined in part based on research activities. Some departments provide principal investigators with a percentage of their direct costs as an annual bonus. This may be an incentive for getting more research dollars but not necessarily for manuscript productivity, mentorship, relevant science or faculty development, or leadership. The best bonus plans for researchers reward all the components of a successful research enterprise, not just grant procurement.

RESEARCH FINANCE

The pursuit of organizational missions needs to be supported by sound finance and infrastructure.

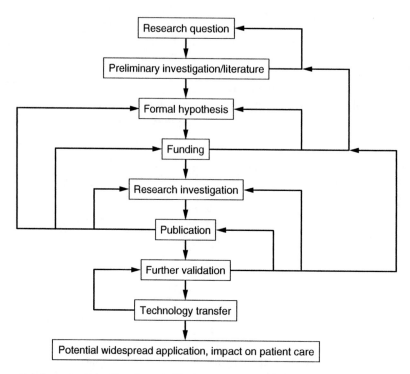

Figure 5-3 Investigative research. The diagram illustrates a typical iteration of research development from the initial research question to widespread application.

Adapted from Gazelle GS, Dunnick NR: Subsidizing radiology research. Acad Radiol 9:195–197, 2002.

BOX 5-1

Source for Research Finance

- Clinical revenue
- Indirect revenue from grant funding
- Corporate partnerships
- Philanthropy (gift, donation)
- Intellectual property (patent, licensing)
- Endowment, tenure line from organization

The research mission of radiology practice cannot be pursued without adequate financial management. Without sustainable financial support, it is difficult to maintain research activity and achieve eventual goals and contributions. Radiology departments have become an enterprise with operational finances in the tens of millions of dollars, where strategic allocation of research finances becomes critical, though not necessarily straightforward.

Several venues of finance can support research activity in radiology departments (Box 5-1). Clinical revenue generated by the radiology department has been a traditional source for research dollars, in particular for research activity that is not funded by grants and resources through a regular grant mechanism.[2] In biomedical industries, the amount of investment in research and development from the company's overall profit is one of the critical benchmarks to gauge their well-being and future growth. For example, the top 10 pharmaceutical companies invested 11% to 18% of their annual income in research and development.[3] The amount of investment in research is a fine balance between clinical and research productivities. If too much of the revenue is spent on research without a clear strategic plan, this will impact departmental finances. Should that revenue be better allocated for faculty salaries and faculty retention in a competitive job market? If you lose personnel, the remaining faculty members have to work harder to keep up the clinical revenue and may lose their academic time or interest. This will further deter academic faculty candidates from being attracted to the program, and the research mission will suffer over the long term from a lack of academically minded members in the department. Similarly, if too much of the revenue is spent to keep the faculty salary level competitive with that of private sectors, faculty members will have to work harder to come up with more clinical revenue and will consequently lose their research time and productivity, and the program again becomes unattractive to academic radiologists. Thus, the research investment needs to be determined upon careful and strategic balance between clinical activity and research productivity along with the organization's mission. One common difficulty is to establish metrics to measure research productivity and to demonstrate its benefits relative to other radiology missions particularly in financial terms.

Research discoveries and innovations often start with careful observation and initial applications without definitive funding. However, translation of these initial observations to widespread acceptance and applications requires financial support to pursue more rigorous investigations. As the mission of research is to contribute eventually to global health care, it is critical to obtain funding to pursue research projects. To support growing biomedical research, the NIH has tripled research funding during the past two decades (Fig. 5-4), although a recent scale back in the last year or two has occurred in the current U.S. administration.[4] At the same time, the number of grant submissions has increased significantly, and the success rate is in decline as a consequence. The traditional funding mechanism for the independent investigator, the R01 grant is still considered to be central, but it is becoming increasingly more difficult for junior investigators to obtain R01s. NIH provides various funding mechanisms for different levels of research and research investigators. However, overall NIH funding for biomedical research also suffers from budgetary cutbacks. In the early 1990s and again in 2005, there were incidences of overall funding decline from NIH, which created chaotic responses from biomedical research communities.

Although the recent decline may be transient, it is highly desirable to diversify the research portfolio to include both federal and nonfederal funding to sustain the research mission in radiology practice. Nonfederal funding sources include research funding from nonprofit organizations, industry funding, professional societies (such as RSNA), and pilot grants from the parent university. Other research funding comes from gifts and donations. Philanthropy is recognized as an important funding source for

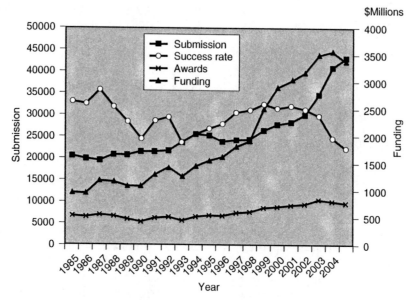

Figure 5-4 Trends in NIH funding and awards. The graph is generated from the data available at http://grants1.nih.gov/grants/award/award.htm.

radiology research.[5] Funding through philanthropy requires great effort in communication, understanding of mutual interests, and a clear demonstration of research excellence. These can be coordinated through the development office of the university or organization, but also often through personal interaction and communication with potential donors. Research leadership can facilitate such communication by screening potential opportunities for investigators.

If successful research programs result in the generation of intellectual properties, patents and licensing can be potential and sustainable sources of research support. Radiological research often involves technical developments (e.g., hardware, software, contrast materials) and innovative applications (application patents). These can be protected by patents and licensed to interested industries. From the viewpoint of the research mission, research innovations will not benefit widespread clinical practices unless these technologies and discoveries are distributed through established channels such as the industrial marketing network. Thus, technology transfer creates a win-win situation for investigators, organizations, and eventually, patient care. To facilitate this process, the technology transfer office becomes a key partner for both the execution of the research mission and the education of faculty members in an academic university setting.

We invite several lecturers from the technology transfer office, specifically for our radiology department, concerning patent/licensing, invention disclosure, application process, policies and guidelines, and opportunities, in addition to their regular lecture series in the university. These lectures facilitate interactions between faculty members and the technology transfer office through individual and group meetings. Our department tripled the number of invention disclosures in two years and became one of the top 10 departments of innovation disclosures in the university. Financial translation of these disclosures is yet to be seen.

OPPORTUNITIES

As described in Figure 5-1, radiology research encompasses multidisciplinary fields of research. The field is expanding with technical developments and new applications. Despite some difficulties in the fulfillment of the research mission in the current radiology environment, imaging research brings continuing excitement and new opportunities to radiology operations.

Synergy across Missions

Synergy between clinical care and research can enhance both research and clinical missions of the academic operations. This synergy can be established at multiple levels. Unique collaborative research programs can contribute to the excellence of patient care, which consequently distinguishes their radiology operations from others. Close collaboration between imaging and clinical (treatment) teams (see Fig. 5-1) not only facilitates the research innovation cycle, but also promotes imaging referrals from clinicians who closely collaborate with imaging physician-scientists. Strong physician-scientists are more attracted to institutions where cutting-edge research can be performed, and a productive research environment can be a great incentive to those faculty members. Funded research projects that use clinical imaging resources can bring not only indirect cost to the department, but also guaranteed collectables to the facility if an appropriate research charge is established. The synergy can even be enhanced by a federal funding opportunity such as a Specialized Program of Research Excellence (SPORE) grant, which promotes translational research involving basic, clinical, and population investigators.

Translational research is bidirectional. Clinical collaborations generate critical research questions for both clinical and basic imaging investigators. At our institution at the University of Washington, several basic science imaging investigators communicate well with clinicians inside and outside the radiology department, develop new collaborative research projects, and obtain successfully external funding. The academic radiology operations can provide various platforms (conference, interdisciplinary lectures, and incentives) to facilitate such communications and interactions.

Molecular Imaging

Owing to significant advancements in molecular medicine and bioengineering techniques during the 1990s, imaging technology is evolving into more disease-specific, biology-specific approaches. Some of this research has been coined as "molecular imaging." Although there is no unified consensus on how to define molecular imaging, the term is most often applied to imaging research that aims to unveil specific biological and pathologic events that stem from genetic, proteomic, metabolic, or cellular processes. Molecular imaging can provide information not only for basic science investigations but also for clinical diagnosis, therapeutic

evaluation, and prognostic evaluation. The foundation of molecular imaging is a strong engineering development such as PET-CT,[6] high-field MRI, optimal imaging, and small animal imaging in conjunction with specific probe developments such as new radiotracers, paramagnetic nanoparticles, and optical tracers.

Since the development of new therapeutic drugs is moving toward molecular and mechanistic designs, imaging specific to such molecules and biological processes is well suited for in vivo evaluation of therapeutic responses. Some molecular imaging technologies, such as PET-CT combined with the commercially available radiotracer [F-18]fluorodeoxyglucose (FDG) have been already incorporated into our clinical practice, which has created great enthusiasm from both radiology practices and industries. These costly examinations are often scrutinized for governmental reimbursement. The approval of such technology is based on improved outcomes and evidence established around the technology. Effective implementation of the new technology in radiology practice can also be a matter of research. This completes the innovation cycle indicated in Figure 5-1. Other new imaging developments, such as new pulse sequences for MRI and new contrast agents for MRI and ultrasound, are sometimes viewed under this umbrella of molecular imaging. These research endeavors involve multidisciplinary groups of researchers and clinicians, which in turn help to generate creative research ideas in a synergistic fashion.[7]

The establishment of new imaging technologies has been a traditional strength of radiology research. Success in the new era of radiology research depends critically on collaboration with expertise centered around imaging technology, biology, and medicine. New imaging technology, such as molecular imaging, provides opportunities for radiology investigators to lead such projects and facilitates a cultural change within the radiology research environment.

Imaging in Basic Sciences

Through the exercise of molecular imaging technology, the recognition of imaging technology in the field of basic sciences has increased significantly. There is an increasing demand for imaging of small animals and large animals, with eventual translation to human subjects.

Animal imaging research, in particular high-resolution cross-sectional imaging, has been facilitated by the initial development of microPET[8] in the mid 1990s. Since then, the development of high-resolution, animal-capable scanners such as MRI, optical imaging, microCT, and animal single-photon emission computed tomography (SPECT) imaging have provided precious opportunities for diverse investigators to use imaging as a tool for their research projects. This enthusiasm has created opportunities for radiology investigators to interact with basic scientists, analogous to clinical radiologists interacting with clinicians in the clinical care setting. Research imaging expertise established in the radiology department not only assists our own research investigators, but also creates research synergy with investigators throughout the medical school and beyond. Strategic development of such basic science imaging expertise in academic radiology is a great opportunity for radiology research. It can position a radiology department as an essential player in biomedical research, which will certainly influence the dean's view of the department as suggested by the 2002 American College of Radiology (ACR) Intersociety Conference.[5] If radiology leadership does not make the most of this opportunity, other enthusiasts will certainly take this lead.

Translational Imaging Research

Radiology imaging is inherently suited to "translational" research. "Bench to bedside" has been a recent roadmap in NIH initiatives. Large center grants have been granted to facilitate translation of basic science discoveries and technologies to clinical applications. As described above, imaging technology can be applied to animals *and* humans, thus enabling translations of basic biological findings and technologies to potential clinical applications on the same platform. The term "translational imaging research" initially appeared in Medline around the late 1990s. Since then, there has been a rapidly increasing number of reviews and commentaries published about this new imaging research emphasis in various fields of medicine.[9-11] Imaging can now elucidate basic biological processes and pathophysiology in animal models as well as in humans, facilitate new diagnostic methods, and help develop more effective treatments

through accurate and specific diagnoses and treatment response evaluation in vivo.

The thrust of imaging research (see Fig. 5-1, *solid arrow A*) has afforded us many possibilities and opportunities to promote translational research. In parallel, there is great enthusiasm to use imaging findings as a "surrogate" end point for clinical trials in pharmaceutical industries, which is being supported by several FDA/NIH "biomarker" initiatives.[12,13] Potentially, in vivo imaging findings can replace clinical end points—which for both time and financial reasons are difficult to obtain—and facilitate therapeutic developments. Major pharmaceutical industries are developing their own imaging research capabilities to facilitate translation of preclinical research to early phase trials, but imaging of clinical patients often relies on radiology practice. To facilitate therapeutic trials (see Fig. 5-1, *dotted arrow B*), research use of a clinical imaging facility can become an opportunity for radiology practice when the balance between clinical care and research activity is met productively.

Investigative Research

In various scientific meetings outside radiological societies, there are many investigators who use imaging as an investigational tool to study biology and diseases. Many scientific and medical societies organize sessions devoted to imaging research, and these outside investigators are often funded by research grants. Although traditional radiology research has many strengths in technological development and clinical applications, hypothesis-driven mechanistic investigations of biology and medical disorders are still open opportunities for both basic and clinical radiology investigators.

Just as surgeons may operate on patients as a part of their clinical work, but may also study target diseases using molecular technology in their laboratory, radiologists can apply imaging technology not only for clinical workup, but also to investigate diseases and biology. Many investigators outside of radiology practice may or may not have sufficient access to high-end imaging instrumentation or imaging expertise to effectively establish experimental protocols and data analysis. Radiology researchers are sitting on a wealth of investigational devices and imaging expertise, and other investigators crave access to these and are successfully receiving the funds to use such tools. Through a paradigm shift and a bit of cultural change, radiology investigators may be able to tap into the wide-open fields of biological and medical investigations using their own radiological devices.

To take a lead in the medical investigation of diseases using imaging devices, collaboration with specialty clinicians becomes essential, because radiologists typically do not directly manage patients. A certain number of radiology investigators can be successful in these types of investigations and may compete for grants outside of radiology-specific funding opportunities.

CHALLENGES AND PERSPECTIVES

When pursuing research missions in radiology practice, we face several challenges ranging from finance to the general culture of radiology practice. There have been numerous discussions around these issues, and solutions are not necessarily straightforward.[14]

Culture in Radiology

Regardless of the nature of radiology research, if academic radiology does not engage in research and development, we will create a vacuum in our future: "Today's research is tomorrow's practice."[5] Due to the diminishing margin of clinical revenue and increasing salary levels, radiologists are expected to work harder, and therefore have limited time for research. Radiology departments are often seen as a "service" department in both the clinical and research arenas. Radiologists may feel comfortable providing a service, but often lack research initiative based on their original ideas and critical thinking. Without these, it is difficult to sustain a viable research program. Technically inclined departments also limit research and funding opportunities. Traditional radiology research frequently employs a descriptive approach, but hypothesis-driven research, which funding agencies typically reward, has been limited in part due to a lack of research, education, and enthusiasm. With limited time and financial support, clinical practice and research engagement tend to create a conflict. Even though members are interested in research, there may not be enough resources or infrastructure to support such enthusiasm. These

issues need to be addressed through multiple venues. Some of them require a cultural change of the current radiology research environment and research education for future generations.

The significant cultural changes can be introduced by the recruitment of new faculty members. Strategically identified candidates can strengthen research programs. Also, the recruitment is an opportunity for the department to acquire additional resources through a school or organization. In the current era of interdisciplinary research, such recruitment can be done as a joint effort by collaborating departments, an effort that also flourishes in a collaborative research environment.

Although cultural change and leadership alone do not solve all the issues we face in radiology research, they can effectively create a positive atmosphere where investigators can exercise their creative thinking and engage in research investigations. Clear indication of our radiology missions by leadership becomes critical when somewhat conflicting practices such as clinical care versus research conduct become an issue at a tactical level.

Mission Statement

The establishment of a research mission statement is a good way to clarify the eventual values and goals of the organization. One example of such a statement is "to improve radiological and medical practice through innovative and collaborative research investigations" and sets the tone for investigational research organizations. Another example, more suited for clinical institutions, might be "to promote state-of-the-art imaging technology for patient care through clinical research and trials." Some institutions may also have an umbrella mission statement defined by a parent organization (such as a university or an institution), or a statement that focuses their mission on a unique patient population or disease prevalence.

The mission statement is typically defined when the organization is first created to meet a particular need. However, the statement needs to be reviewed periodically and revised, if necessary. It needs to be updated and relevant to the organization so that operations can stay on track. (There are many articles available about how to develop missions and mission statements as an organization.)

As evident from the above examples, traditional radiology mission statements (patient care, research, and education) are interrelated. One successful academic institution states, "Our primary mission is to provide high quality compassionate care to patients through the use of medical imaging. We advance the frontiers of medical science by integrating our clinical expertise with research, and we strive to pass on our knowledge through excellence in teaching."[15] This statement clearly indicates synergy across traditional missions as a great strength of the organization. Understanding these interrelated missions at the executive committee level makes radiology operations more robust and sustainable.

Resource Allocation and Investment

Many departments struggle with limited resources, space, and finances to fulfill academic missions of radiology operations. With a clear mandate from the leadership of the organization, resource allocation can be prioritized according to the mission statements created by the organization. Academic radiology departments that are closely tied to a specific field of research (such as a cancer center) may be able to prioritize resources around a unified theme of the research. However, academic institutions typically support diverse research interests among faculty members and divisions, and often department leaders are asked to support different types of research and investigators. Naturally, then, the mission statement of academic institutions is often inclusive and sufficiently broad, not outlining specific research goals that can be used to prioritize operational decisions including resource allocation.

One traditional way to allocate resources for a maximum research outcome is to identify investigators with a track record of grant funding, research publications, and research education (graduate students, residents, fellows) and invest resources to further enhance their research programs. These investigators are proactive enough to seek out multiple external fundings to keep their research activities going and also often use department investments most effectively. Department leaders can encourage junior faculty members to work in their programs so that they can be mentored and supported indirectly through the departmental investments. This is particularly effective when those investigators

are open to internal/external collaborations and research mentorship. Nevertheless, potential problems may include heterogeneous department support, potentially resulting in resentment among faculty members, and difficulty in strategizing departmental research as a whole. As well, the policy may not support small yet unique and critical research or start-up research. Internal competition for research apparently supports the theory of "survival of the fittest," which may work well in a large prestigious organization where highly talented investigators are competing for research productivity. Another common way to identify resources that benefit a large number of investigators and research programs within the department is to invest these resources in the general mission of the organization. The concept is referred to as a "shared resource" investment. Many radiology research projects depend on high-end instruments that are often too costly to be funded by a single investigator or funding source. Shared resource and high-end instrumentation grants from the NIH, the National Center for Research Resources (NCRR), and the National Science Foundation (NSF) can fund a few million-dollar instruments. However, the department and institution can potentially fund more expensive or extensive resources through a collection of multiple funding sources (clinical revenue reserve, corporate partnership, donation) for multiple research projects and investigators. Both operational and financial arrangements should be established around these resources at the departmental and organizational level (e.g., operations committee, cost recharge center). Specific research can then be facilitated by individual funding support and other specific measures, such as research education and mentorship.

Resource allocation for unfunded research, start-up research, or research somewhat peripheral to the overall mission of the organization has to be discussed at the executive research committee level. Resources then need to be allocated based on strategic planning, including how to convert unfunded to funded research, as well as how to allocate pilot funding for start-up projects within the department. Since resources and funding are almost always limited in academic radiology operations, resource allocation without strategic planning can become a conflict at the tactical level. Although so-called "emergent strategic planning" still is a major operational mode for day-to-day operations, a project-by-project discussion of resource and budget allocation often creates more confusion and inconsistency over time. Therefore, strategic planning is necessary to allocate the set of resources and budget for the above types of research based on general missions and goals of the department.

Bottom-up Versus Top-down Approach

Research cannot flourish through a solely top-down approach. Given that research excellence eventually comes down to an investigator's talent, recognition of an individual's strengths in leadership and a bottom-up approach are critical to the successful research establishment. There are many excellent examples in which great research programs were started by individuals who had the talent and energy to pursue their goals. Persistence in pursuit of those goals is probably the most critical factor for the success of a research endeavor ("10% inspiration, 90% perspiration"). Identifying such individuals within an organization and providing appropriate support is the core of the bottom-up approach. Naturally, the recruitment of such individuals at both faculty and training levels is an opportunity for an organization to elevate research activity. Thus, strategic recruitment of faculty members and trainees is desirable, particularly when resources are limited for multiple missions. Leadership also needs to recognize that grant funding is the beginning of research and a tool to conduct research for eventual contribution to science and patient care (see Fig. 5-3).

Under financial stress and limited resources in current radiology practice, obtaining grants becomes the first priority, since it is a metric on which we can easily rely. Often, the mission of research is secondary because research outcome and contribution may not be easily appreciated in quantitative metrics. Many major discoveries in medicine are said to have been accomplished without funding, which will hopefully change in 21st-century medicine. Careful observation is the beginning of research for the greater contribution to science. Since radiologists are traditionally good at observation, leadership within radiology can create a culture in which they can move from observation to investigational operations.

Faculty Engagement

Keeping faculty engaged in research is sometimes challenging. Clinical faculty members are facing increasing demand in clinical care, teaching, and administration. Thus research can become a secondary priority even in academic departments. Research faculty members bring great research expertise to the department; however, they may not be integrated into overall departmental research activity and may become isolated in their own research space. Even though such environments can make individual research faculty members productive in their respective fields of research, there may be even greater opportunities if they work collaboratively with other members in the department or other clinical departments in multidisciplinary research. In a recent survey in our department, "collaboration within the department" was ranked as one of the top three factors for securing grant funding.

In addition to the considerations for faculty research time, research infrastructure, and finance, it is useful to provide opportunities for faculty members to exchange conversations and information and to be updated and involved in research operational decision making and implementation. This falls into a team-building strategy, and there are many discussions around this issue in business management and organization. Leadership skills contribute to successful team building and individual engagements. One way to keep faculty members on board is to have monthly or bimonthly faculty research meetings and provide information pertinent to research operations, including research developments, grant awards, and finance. Our department organizes a monthly faculty research meeting around noon that has been well attended by research faculty members. Clinical faculty members have difficulty attending a research meeting at this time, but depending on the topics and location of the meeting, attendance can be substantial. Researchers are highly critical, analytical, and sophisticated, and, if the right amount of information and direction is provided for discussion, they often come up with effective and unique solutions to the issues. This is a part of the importance of the bottom-up approach in research operations as described previously. Increasing the number of research-related conferences, such as Research Grand Rounds, can be an effective way to facilitate communication among investigators and introduce ongoing research projects to one another. Our researchers are also invited to interview radiology resident candidates and give a lecture on an overall research activity in the department using a set of slides submitted by faculty members. We use department online surveys for research operational improvements and guide strategic planning and tactical translation.

Role Model

The traditional academic role model still plays an essential part in the research establishment. In the bottom-up approach to research operations, researchers often seek advice from successful research investigators and look to model their own research approach after that of established colleagues. If an academic department chair can fulfill this role, it is ideal given that the chair can operate in both mission and strategic frameworks. However, as radiology practices and issues grow within the academic operations, the chair may not be able to be a role model for all academic missions. Delegation of such roles to the vice chair of research or research directors who operate more closely in research practice is an effective way to facilitate the research environment.

Basic Science Faculty in Radiology

Because radiological research often involves expertise in engineering, physics, and basic sciences, radiology departments appoint a relatively large number of PhD faculty members. These researchers are vital to radiology research and provide imaging expertise to other departments that do not have such immediate access. Supporting these members in radiology research practice requires both operational and financial considerations. Despite the research expertise that PhD faculty members bring to the department, collaboration and communication between physician scientists and PhD investigators within the department may be limited. Traditionally, nuclear medicine research is an effective model of collaboration in which physician scientists, imaging physicists, and radiochemists work together for the mutual goals of radiotracer imaging research. PhD investigators specific to radiology section operations, for example, an MRI physicist for neuroradiology or engineers for interventional radiology, facilitate

research programs within respective fields. Since radiology is a clinical department and typically does not have classroom teaching assignments, supporting PhD investigators requires financial considerations. Even though many PhD investigators are often self-funded in radiology, the department needs to provide gap funding, bridge funding, and research resources. Several options for funding of engineers and basic scientists in radiology include joint appointments in basic science or engineering departments, involvement in clinical medical physics operations, research service operations, and industrial collaboration. Some of these options also facilitate better collaboration between PhD investigators and others in radiology practice.

Interrelated Missions of Academic Radiology

The three academic missions in radiology—clinical care, research, and education—interplay operationally and financially. Both clinical and translational research use clinical resources that are often operated under the hospital management. To facilitate research use of clinical resources, both clinical and research productivities have to be maximized for the mission of the program. Leaders who understand both the mission and operations have to take a lead in discussion and negotiation to establish a clinical research environment. One of the challenges is to demonstrate research productivity and contribution to the institution in operational and financial terms.

A strong research institution is attractive to patients. Successful implementation of research outcomes to clinical operations establishes institutional excellence. Competitive, potential clinical faculty members and trainees can be attracted to the program through research and an environment conducive to research. One thing to keep in mind is that a lack of research is one reason academic faculty members may be lost to the private sector.[16]

The value of research education as part of a radiology residency program has been discussed extensively. Research education for trainees exists not only to teach research techniques—such as experimental designs, manuscript writing, and grant writing—but also to establish an academic radiology environment where trainees can exercise the desire to stimulate intellectual thinking with conversations in both clinical and research settings. Interestingly, the size of radiology resident programs and the number of fellows are significantly associated with research productivity.[17] A good understanding of interrelated academic operations is essential for radiology leaders who wish to achieve overall success in the radiology program and its missions.

CONCLUSION

In this chapter, the research mission in radiology practice has been discussed from the viewpoint of opportunities and challenges. Many excellent strategic discussions of radiology research can be found in the references.

Dos and Don'ts in Developing a Research Program	
Dos	**Don'ts**
1. Recognize synergy across radiology academic missions. 2. Capture new research opportunities. 3. Diversify funding sources. 4. Promote cultural change. 5. Balance between bottom-up and top-down approaches.	1. Fail to align with the mission of the institution. 2. Do research in a vacuum with no clinical or multidisciplinary input. 3. Consider grant funding the "end"; rather, think of it as a means to an end. 4. Start up with a lack of support in funds, equipment, resources, time, and mentorship. 5. Create small fiefdoms or silos; instead, focus on collaborative, shared research.

REFERENCES

1. Concato J, Shah N, Horwitz RI: Randomized, controlled trials, observational studies, and the hierarchy of research designs. N Engl J Med 342:1887–1892, 2000.
2. Gazelle GS, Dunnick NR: Subsidizing radiology research. Acad Radiol 9:195–197, 2002.
3. SCRIP Pharmaceutical Company League Tables (2005).
4. Data from National Institutes of Health, Office of Extramural Research, 2006.
5. Dunnick NR: Opinion. Report of the 2002 Intersociety Commission meeting: Radiology 2002—today's research is tomorrow's practice. AJR Am J Roentgenol 180:925–928, 2003.
6. Townsend DW: A combined PET/CT scanner: The choices. J Nucl Med 42:533–534, 2001.
7. Chan S, Gunderman RB: Emerging strategic themes for guiding change in academic radiology departments. Radiology 236:430–440, 2005.
8. Cherry SR, Gambhir SS: Use of positron emission tomography in animal research. ILAR J 42:219–232, 2001.
9. Koo V, Hamilton PW, Williamson K: Non-invasive in vivo imaging in small animal research. Cell Oncol 28:127–139, 2006.
10. Matthews PM, Honey GD, Bullmore ET: Applications of MRI in translational medicine and clinical practice. Nat Rev Neurosci 7:732–744, 2006.
11. El-Deiry WS, Sigman CC, Kelloff GJ: Imaging and oncologic drug development: J Clin Oncol 24:3261–3273, 2006.
12. Frank RA, Galasko D, Hampel H, et al: Biological markers for therapeutic trials in Alzheimer's disease: Proceedings of the biological markers working group; NIA initiative on neuroimaging in Alzheimer's disease. Neurobiol Aging 24:521–536, 2003.
13. Biomarkers and surrogate endpoints.: Preferred definitions and conceptual framework. Biomarkers Definitions Working Group. Clin Pharmacol Ther 69:89–95, 2001.
14. Alderson PO, Bresolin LB, Becker GJ, et al: Enhancing research in academic radiology departments: Recommendations of the 2003 Consensus Conference. Acad Radiol 11:951–956, 2004.
15. Thrall JH: Massachusetts General Hospital, available at http://www.massgeneralimaging.org/.
16. Taljanovic MS, Hunter TB, Krupinski EA, et al: Academic radiology: The reasons to stay or leave. Acad Radiol 10:1461–1468, 2003.
17. Itagaki MW, Pile-Spellman J: Factors associated with academic radiology research productivity. Radiology 237:774–780, 2005.

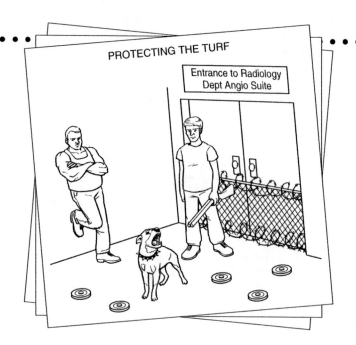

PROTECTING THE TURF

Entrance to Radiology
Dept Angio Suite

Turf Issues in Radiology

Norman J. Beauchamp, Jr.

INTRODUCTION

Declare the past, diagnose the present, foretell the future; practice these acts. As to diseases, make a habit of two things—to help, or at least to do no harm.

GALEN

Imaging has transformed the practice of medicine. A panel of Nobel Prize recipients identified MRI and CT as among the top five most impactful advances of the 20th century. A primary threat to the contribution that imaging can make to the health benefit of society is inappropriate use and substandard practice. Success in addressing either will require the detrimental impact of *turf* issues to be better understood and controlled. It is for this reason that a chapter on *turf* issues is particularly germane to a book on the business of radiology.

A nonmedical use of the word "turf" can be traced back to the 1950s as a "territory claimed by a gang." Turf has come to be used in medical language as an area of practice that is the purview of a specific group.[1] Incursions into another's territory can be driven by financial gain, entitlement, peer pressure such as training standards, or in response to concerns of becoming obsolete. Similarly, these incursions may be in response to unmet clinical need, seeking more comprehensiveness of care or a sincere belief that a better patient outcome will result. There is a tendency to ascribe the former more pejorative motivations when it is one's territory being encroached on and the latter when one is in the group laying claim to a new area of practice. Such is the way of all human conflicts and their justifications.

In my approaching this issue, ascribing ill intent to my fellow physicians by specialty grouping has never been satisfying to me. Among my closest friends are cardiologists and surgeons who show no less commitment to helping those in need than do my colleagues in radiology of whom I am most proud. I have found it to be more effective and appropriate to focus on doing what is best for the patient. As such, targeting the detrimental behaviors, whether ascribable to an individual physician or a group, is the appropriate emphasis. We must keep the patient, not the specialty per se, as our core value with a continual emphasis on optimizing quality and safety and reducing cost. (See Dos and Don'ts section near the end of this chapter.) This approach is the only one that is relevant to payers, legislators, administration, and, what is most important, the patient.

TURF ISSUES AND THE IMPACT ON QUALITY, SAFETY, AND SERVICE

Using this approach, the path forward becomes clearest and the most defensible. Sun Tzu, in the book *The Art of War*, said it best, "You can ensure the safety of your defense if you only hold positions that cannot be attacked." One cannot question a position that is focused on quality, service, access, and cost control. Fortunately, as will be demonstrated, this path is also completely aligned with radiology maintaining a dominant role in diagnostic imaging and imaging-guided intervention. For these reasons, a great deal of this chapter is focused on making the case for the central role of radiology and providing the reader the evidence needed to be effective in presenting this case locally and nationally. The chapter closes with strategies that can supplement the quality, safety, and cost arguments for those unfortunate circumstances where maintaining what is in the best interest of the patient is an inadequate driver of appropriate physician or leadership behavior.

Hippocrates is the icon for the ethical practice of medicine. It is for this reason that graduating physicians take an oath committing to the goals he defined in the 4th century B.C. It is remarkable that this 2400-year-old oath identified the importance of specialization to ensure the best interests of the patient. To quote, "I will not cut for (kidney or bladder) stone, even for patients in whom the disease is manifest; I will leave this operation to be performed by practitioners, specialists in this art." Losing sight of the value of specialization is a true threat to

quality of care and an issue that often gets lost in turf battles.

Radiology brings needed subspecialty focus to imaging and medicine. The deficiencies to quality are particularly manifest in radiology when nonradiologists interpret diagnostic images in the absence of sufficient training. A number of studies of quality comparing radiologists to nonradiologists have been undertaken. Eng and colleagues quantified diagnostic performance of radiologists, radiology residents, emergency department faculty, and emergency department residents.[2] The authors used a measure referred to as the area under the receiver operator curve (ROC). An ROC curve is a plot of sensitivity versus (1-specificity). The area under the curve has been used to assess the diagnostic accuracy of a test.[3] An area of 0.5 is equivalent to a random guess and 1.0 is a perfect diagnostic study. Each group interpreted 120 radiographs, 50% of which contained a clinically important imaging finding. The area under the curve for the radiology attending physicians was 0.15 greater than for emergency department attending physicians; radiology residents scored 0.08 better than emergency department physicians; and the radiology residents outperformed the emergency department residents by 0.13. In a similar study, E. J. Potchen and colleagues used a standardized set of chest radiographs comparing board-certified radiologists, radiology residents, and nonradiologist physicians. The respective areas under the curve were 0.86, 0.75, and 0.66.[4] Once again, radiology attending physicians and radiology residents substantially outperformed nonradiologists.

Reports of diminished accuracy have also been reported outside the radiology literature. Alfaro and colleagues reviewed the concordance of interpretation of CT scans comparing ED physicians and radiologists.[5] The ED physician was discordant to that of the radiologist physician 38.7% of the time. Of the 555 total cases reviewed, 11.4% of the missed interpretations by ED physicians were considered major including 25 new infarcts, 10 mass lesions, 8 cases of cerebral edema, 6 contusions, 4 subarachnoid hemorrhages, 1 epidural and 1 subdural hemorrhage. In a similar study by Walsh-Kelly et al., 14% of Pediatric Emergency Department studies were misinterpreted by the ED personnel.[6]

As demonstrated, there are clear discrepancies in quality of interpretation and these discrepancies are unequivocally linked to training. A radiologist undertakes four years of training in image interpretation with the vast majority of trainees continuing on for an additional year of subspecialty fellowship training. Wechsler et al. demonstrated major and minor discrepancies when comparing the interpretation of residents and fellows to attending radiologists. The magnitude of the discrepancies decreased as training progressed.[7]

Levin and colleagues have also demonstrated that inadequate training results in poor outcomes.[8] They point out that the opportunity for nonradiologists to receive adequate training is truly limited. Specifically, formal training in the United States is all essentially hospital-based. Greater than 90% of plain films, neurologic MR and CT scans, and nonobstetric ultrasound studies in hospitals are performed by radiologists. This affords little opportunity for other specialties to attain the needed training to provide equivalent levels of image interpretation proficiency. In fact, the majority of nonradiologists do not receive training beyond reviewing the imaging studies of the small number of patients being carried on their clinical service. This is considerably different from the rigorous exposure to imaging that radiology residents receive as they undertake increasing responsibility in the daily interpretation of 50 to 100 studies a day. In the apprentice format that is radiology training, every study the trainee reviews is also reviewed by an attending physician with correct interpretations reinforced and incorrect interpretations corrected.

This limitation has also been recognized by nonradiologists. J. M. Porter, a noted vascular surgeon, commented that to be an independent endovascular proceduralist, a radiologist undergoes no fewer than five years of training. He states to expect even the most dexterous vascular surgeon to attain similar skills, including catheter skills, and understanding the safe application of ionizing radiation and contrast media, is simply "nonsense."[9] Similarly, in a 2004 editorial, the editor-in-chief of the *Journal of the American College of Cardiology* opined that "we ought to guard against providing services for which we have little experience. We invite criticism if we undertake to perform procedures

for which we have had little training, scant experience, or very low volumes. We should avoid obtaining equipment for our offices for which there is little demonstrated need or advantage."[10] It is imperative that prior to participation in endovascular therapies an equivalent training program be completed.

The issues regarding quality are further exacerbated by losses in quality of images obtained when not overseen by a radiologist.[11] Radiologists are required to learn imaging physics, radiation, and MRI safety. They must be conversant in imaging quality assurance and quality control processes to receive board certification. For example, in a study of 1,086 radiographs obtained in radiologists' offices versus that of orthopedists, family practitioners, podiatrists, and chiropractors, a blinded review demonstrated that radiology facilities had the lowest percent of technically inadequate films (12%) and that nonradiology facilities had a concerning level of images of inadequate quality ranging from a low of 13% to a high of 82% inadequate. A similar finding was made by Hopper et al. identifying a 28% inadequacy of film quality when obtained by a nonradiologist compared to a 3% inadequacy for radiologists.[12]

These quality measures have been incorporated into pay for performance initiatives with a demonstrated return in terms of quality and cost. Verrilli and colleagues summarized the results of a health plan that performed on-site inspections of imaging facilities to determine whether a facility met standards of care.[13] Of 1,004 imaging sites inspected, 197 (20%) failed to remedy the violation, and 106 (10%) failed with fundamental and serious deficiencies. The failure rate also varied with specialists and was highest for chiropractors and podiatrists. Notable additional findings were that groups refusing voluntary review of their facility had the highest failure rate and that by implementing this quality program, there was a 2% decline in total imaging expenditures. This return was a 10 to 1 return on investment for the health plan, demonstrating that enforcing quality standards is better for the patient and is cost effective.

Moskowitz et al. also evaluated cost and quality and demonstrated that the use of imaging privileges restricting the imaging performed by nonradiologists could lead to substantial improvements in quality and decreases in cost. He demonstrated a decrease in radiation dose and a decrease in cost with a greater than 20% reduction in the number of radiographic examinations. Finally, there were zero deficiencies in the inspection of radiology offices as opposed to significant deficiencies of equipment, equipment maintenance, or documentation of the examinations performed in 78% of nonradiologists' offices.[14]

Lastly, there is a risk in terms of the detrimental impact on resident and fellow training. There are radiology training programs that have diminished exposure to a variety of diagnostic studies and procedures that they will be called on to perform. These include fetal ultrasound, cardiac imaging, musculoskeletal MRI, and neurointerventional and endovascular interventional procedures. A significant lapse in any one area can make a training program less appealing and can negatively impact the ability to recruit and retain the faculty responsible for the education of the trainees. In two surveys published in *JACR*, greater than 50% of program directors and over 90% of the responding residents felt that their training program was adversely affected due to turf issues.[15,16]

In summary, the preceding emphasized the remarkable extent to which turf, self-referral, and lack of subspecialty focus diminish the contribution imaging can make to patient care as a function of inadequate safety and quality. In consideration of the Institute of Medicine's identification of over 100,000 lost lives as a result of medical errors and lack of safe practice, constraining self-referral and inadequate training must be emphasized if we are to bring the value our patients deserve. Of all the "defenses" to prevent turf incursions, this is the one that is unassailable.

TURF ISSUES AS AN UNNECESSARY DRIVER OF COST

If you're not greedy you will go far, you will live in happiness too ... like the oompa ... loompa ... doom-pa-dee-do.
FROM *CHARLIE AND THE CHOCOLATE FACTORY*

Another substantial risk to the ability of imaging to contribute to improvement in patient care is the escalating cost of health care and the substantial efforts to constrain all costs, with a particular emphasis on limiting imaging costs. Imaging is the fastest driver of cost in health care with a growth rate of approximately 2.5 times that of other medical services. CT and MRI exceeded the nonimaging growth rate by greater than 4 times. The annualized growth for PET-CT is estimated to be more than 20% per year for the next five years. It is therefore correct that imaging costs are a focus.

This growth is in the setting of an increasing proportion of the population uninsured or underinsured and of an industry trend to put a greater burden of the cost of health care on the patient. As such there are multiple efforts to constrain its use, particularly in the inpatient setting by hospital leaders, without adequate emphasis on identifying where imaging brings value and where it does not. In considering growth, it is important to segment into appropriate growth and inappropriate growth. To make appropriate decisions regarding cost containment, this delineation is essential.

In regard to desirable growth, there are innumerable instances where imaging is being demonstrated to remove cost from medicine. For example, the early use of diffusion and perfusion MRI in the setting of acute stroke can demonstrate whether or not there are regions of tissue at risk for infarction. When no at-risk tissue is demonstrated, a patient can avoid an obligatory intensive care unit stay for monitoring. The same is true when a patient with acute chest pain can undergo a "triple rule out" CT differentiating between PE, aortic dissection, or myocardial infarction. This can lead to correct triage potentially obviating a critical care stay or to a more expeditious discharge from the ED. Lastly, a PET-CT can ensure that patients are appropriately triaged to surgical and nonsurgical arms of treatment by basing conclusions related to nodal status on infiltration with metabolically active tumor as opposed to nonspecific enlargement.

The aging of the population is an unavoidable driver of imaging use, and is in fact a reflection of effective health care that has led to successful aging. The median age of the population has increased 4% since 1990, and the U.S. population has more than quadrupled in the 20th century. Of the 300 million population,

27 million are older than 65. The common diseases affecting the aging population include stroke, heart attack, and cancer, which have a substantial dependence on imaging for diagnosis and treatment planning. Thus, an aged population is a significant and justifiable driver of cost secondary to required imaging.

The irrational funding mechanism currently in place for health care is also a driver of cost in medicine and imaging in particular. Specifically, from an economics standpoint, outside of medicine, price controls supply and demand. As such, when price trends toward zero, demand will grow unrestrained. Conversely, escalating costs lead to decreasing demand. This is referred to as "price elasticity." However, the presence of third-party payers and governmental funding has created a situation in which medical demand is minimally impacted by cost. Health care is price inelastic. This is exacerbated by patients' expectation that they are entitled to the best that modern medicine can offer and with unlimited access. Increased access has been demonstrated to correlate with increased use.[17] If you build it, they will come.

Patient-driven demand is also a factor in growth. Self-directed medical care greatly expanded during the 1990s with direct-to-patient marketing for such procedures as lung, cardiac, and colon screening studies. To an extent, patients taking greater ownership of their health care decisions is a good thing. Examples include seeking CT colonography and whole body screening.

A much bigger problem is the inappropriate drivers of imaging growth. Self-referral is defined as a physician who refers patients for certain health care services to entities with which the physicians or their immediate family members have a financial relationship. A financial relationship can be either an ownership interest or a compensation arrangement, and can be direct or indirect.

Such practices not only limit or eliminate competitive alternatives in the health care services market, resulting in overuse of health care procedures, but also may increase costs to the health care system, and may adversely affect the quality of health care.[18]

To determine the impact of self-referral on the growth of imaging, Rao and Levin reviewed cardiac nuclear scans between 1998 and 2002. The overall use rate per thousand Medicare beneficiaries went up by 43%. Separating that out, use rates among radiologists went up by 2%, while among cardiologists they rose by 78%. In another evaluation, Levin et al. also reviewed imaging claims based on Medicare Part B claims. Between 2000 and 2003, it was demonstrated that radiologists' imaging increased 14% versus nonradiologists' 42%. In a review of the published literature by Kouri et al.,[19] the relationship between self-referral and use became apparent. Self-referral accounts for 60–90% of nonhospital radiography and sonography. Self-referring nonradiologists are between 1.7 and 7.7 times more likely to order an imaging study as nonself-referring physicians.[20–23]

A more direct examination was performed by Hemenway et al. of 15 physicians running ambulatory centers who were initially salaried employees. Subsequently, a policy was instituted that shifted them to bonus pay in proportion to generated revenues. In response, use of lab services increased 23% and radiology use increased 16%. The total charges per month, adjusted for inflation, grew 20%. This further demonstrates how every organization is structured to get exactly the results it is getting. As such, the wages of the seven physicians who regularly earned the bonus rose 19%.[24] Florida has taken a lead in evaluating the impact of self-referral. In 1992, the state determined that in imaging centers where the physicians had an ownership stake, there were higher rates of use and charges. In addition, the physician-owned facilities were geographically located in higher-income communities. Lastly, it was determined that 48% of the imaging done was by self-referral.

As might be anticipated, our nonradiology colleagues have a different perspective on the value of self-referral. For example, it has been stated that on-site imaging for a multispecialty group provides more expedient care as well as more convenient care. Moreover, the additional costs of lost days of work are minimized with one-stop shopping and should be factored into any economic analysis of cost. (Parenthetically, an analysis of Medicare claims has demonstrated that same-day imaging may occur as infrequently as 3% of the time in the setting of nonradiologist imaging.) Lastly, physicians have to transcend conflicts of interest on a daily basis in all areas of medicine, and this can be as successfully accomplished with imaging.

Unfortunately, the data are too compelling that self-referral is a conflict of interest that is not effectively managed by physicians. The response has been inadequate to control costs and ensure quality. Whenever the "physician heal thyself" mechanism fails, the government feels compelled to lend its hand to it. These government regulations are wonderfully summarized in the chapter by Dr. Katzman (see Chapter 26), but an overview is provided here for completeness.

"Stark" laws are two separate guidelines that are targeted to limit self-referral for Medicare and Medicaid patients. Stark I forbade self-referrals for clinical services under Medicare.[25] Stark II extended the restriction to include additional services such as imaging, applied these restrictions to both Medicaid and Medicare, and also sought to limit some of the exemptions to self-referral allowed in Stark I.[26] A concern regarding the Stark laws is the remaining in-office exemption for ancillary services and prepaid health plans. This enables physicians to be exempt when they provide services subject to the Stark law as part of their office practices. Specifically, a physician practice can own their own CT, MRI, PET, or ultrasound, self-refer their patients, and evaluate the images obtained even if they have no documented training. As such, the current regulations are inadequate to limit a practice that is demonstratively not in the best interest of the patients. More concerning is that maintaining this exemption has been an area of active emphasis of nonradiologists. In June 2004 the AMA House of Delegates passed a resolution brought forward by nine specialty societies. The resolution sought the support of the AMA to oppose any and all federal and state legislative and regulatory efforts to repeal the in-office exception to physician self-referral laws.

Closing the in-office exemption has been a major effort of the American College of Radiology (ACR). Maryland instituted a self-referral law that restricts self-referral to a health care entity in which the practitioner has an equity stake. This specifically delineates CT, MRI, and radiation therapy devices. Although this has been on the books since 1993 with no enforcement, to the state's credit, the Maryland Board of Physicians is revisiting the enforcement

of this policy in response to payer concerns about an orthopedic practice performing their own MRI scans.[27]

The government has also put in place anti-kickback regulations. A kickback is defined as a return of a percentage of a sum of money, typically as a result of pressure, coercion, or a secret agreement. In imaging, an example of a kickback would be receiving payment from an imaging center in return for referring a patient. Whereas a Stark violation will result in fines, a kickback violation can result in fines, exclusion from federally funded care, and prison time. The law has generally been applied to broker-style arrangements, whereby an individual offers remuneration to another individual for the purpose of recommending or referring an individual for the furnishing or arranging for an item or service. In an anti-kickback statute analysis, it is immaterial whether remuneration induces one in a position to refer or recommend. It is sufficient that the remuneration may induce one to refer or recommend. The anti-kickback provisions also provide a "safe harbor" whereby referrals are induced but the anti-kickback law is not broken. It is our responsibility to report such violations.

In a January 2007 report in the Chicago *Tribune*, there was an allegation that 20 Chicago-area radiology centers created incentives for referrals by providing illegal kickbacks to referring doctors. The claim was that the physicians paid the centers a reduced rate but charged the insurance company a higher rate. The referring doctor could allegedly keep the difference. This was said to have been done using a "sham" lease arrangement. Specifically, the referring physician allegedly paid a lease rate of $400 but billed the patient's insurer $1,000 for nothing more than the patient referral. The lawsuit states that the defendants violated the Consumer Fraud and Deceptive Business Practices Act, Illinois' anti-kickback law, and the Insurance Fraud Prevention Act.

Nongovernmental payers are also joining the battle against self-referral. They are doing this through pre-authorization programs requiring that criteria for appropriateness be met. They are requiring ACR certification of the imaging facility, privileging of the providers, quality and service indicators, and demonstration of cost control through appropriate use and quality. The pay-for-performance initiatives that are now upon us will initially reward higher-quality centers with improved reimbursement, but ultimately not meeting these standards will result in diminished reimbursement. They have also introduced some limitations for reimbursement of studies that are self-referred.

Unfortunately, another effort at controlling costs is to limit the financial return for imaging studies without consideration of whether it meets quality standards or is indicated. The rationale behind such an approach is that if the driver of inappropriate use is the potential to earn revenue, the best countermeasure is to decrease the revenue potential. However, this thinking is misguided for a number of obvious patient care reasons that will be summarized.

First, there may be a paradoxical effect that results in lower-quality, higher-quantity imaging. It is likely that well before self-referral is effectively curtailed, entrepreneurial physicians will have long succeeded in maintaining a substantial return. They will seek higher throughput or decreased investment in technology. In addition, straight line cuts are not beneficial in any business. Both the valuable and the not valuable are reduced. Imaging done right is transformational in terms of decreasing morbidity, decreasing length of stay, and expediting appropriate therapy. Arbitrary reduction will not be good for patient care.

Moreover, despite increasing costs of health care, our hospitals remain in peril due to decreasing margins. Imaging, done correctly, generates a margin through increased revenue and decreasing expenses. The expense decrease is secondary to decreased length of stay, lessened morbidity, and more expedient implementation of appropriate therapy. Cuts in reimbursement have been shown to impact quality. Loss of profitability will require at some point decreased investment in infrastructure or operations. Reductions in reimbursement in California resulted in a reduction of services. This reduction was greatest in the service of Medicaid and uninsured patients.[28] Decreases in reimbursement from Medicare also have been shown to increase 30-day mortality of AMI patients.[29] Lindrooth et al. measured changes in nurse staffing at hospitals related to potential declines in reimbursement through the BBA. Hospitals that were most susceptible to the provisions of the BBA experienced a decline in RN staffing ratios at about twice the rate of the hospitals that were least susceptible to the BBA. Increasing nurse workload at a time of increasing complexity is not the direction in which health care should go.[30]

STRATEGIES FOR MINIMIZING THE DETRIMENTAL IMPACT OF TURF WARS

It is clear that we must be more strategic in guiding the response to escalating costs for imaging. There are many ways we can more effectively target cost. As a specialty we must keep the focus where it belongs, on restricting low-quality image acquisition and low-quality image interpretations as well as the *inappropriate* drivers of cost. We must ensure that high-quality standards are maintained for all imaging facilities. For example, the FDA mammography quality standard act mandated it for breast imaging. The ACR provides accreditation criteria and we must be aggressive in seeing to it that all sites of practice, radiologists or nonradiologists, meet these standards. We must also encourage radiologists to embrace maintenance of certification and certificates of subspecialty certification. We must establish credentialing standards for the number of procedures a person needs to perform under supervision before they can be an independent practitioner. We should encourage, not dissuade, the pay-for-performance initiatives that will hold imaging facilities and imagers to an appropriately high standard.

We need to be conversant in the costs of self-referral and the mechanism to limit this. We need to be vocal in our conversations with administration internal and external to our hospitals and be active in conversations with third-party payers. We should participate or contribute funds to the ACR to support lobbying efforts to close the Stark in-office exemption. We must report violations of Stark and anti-kickback laws. In so doing, we will keep the emphasis on quality, safety, and cost and what is ultimately in the best interest of patients.

In considering how to navigate turf issues, one also must consider models for working with nonradiologists. Opportunities for collaboration occur with diagnostic imaging as well as image-guided intervention. The first approach is to "hold the line" and limit all efforts of other departments to participate in the turf of radiology. Success in this approach is best done by being able to document and demonstrate that when it comes to imaging, radiology is the best. Essentially it is living the quality and cost and safety argument. This effort provides great customer service to the patient and the referring physician. It requires excellence in supply management, radiation safety, image interpretation, and getting information where it is needed when it is needed and by whom it is needed. It requires a true understanding of costs and being able to demonstrate the added cost of duplication of resources. (In fact, as will be elaborated, this emphasis is important independent of the model followed.)

In addition, one should be conversant on the detrimental impact that not providing some level of protection for radiology turf can have in terms of the patient care mission for the entire hospital. For example, prior to my arrival my current institution experienced an unwanted integration of nonradiologists into the interventional lab. The IR physicians felt that without control over self-referral their ability to maintain a successful and gratifying practice would not be attainable. The majority of the faculty in IR departed. This devastated the institutional ability to provide care for transplant, trauma, and cancer.

It is my belief and experience that preventing all areas for collaboration is not sustainable. For example, model one is challenged in specific areas where involvement is felt to be essential for the survival of a given specialty. Perceived risk of obsolescence will inspire an unrelenting response from nonradiologists. In neurosurgery and vascular surgery, for example, it is deeply held that endovascular intervention is a key component of their training programs and essential to their future practice. In such circumstances, ensuring a leadership role for radiology is better than imaging and image-guided procedures occurring outside of the control of radiology.

Imaging and image-guided intervention occurring outside of radiology is model two. In model two, other departments pursue their own imaging-related programs, but do not have access to radiology resources. A benefit of this approach is that the radiologist is not reminded as directly on a daily basis that nonradiologists

are actively involved in "radiology turf." Out of sight, out of mind. The radiology department also ensures that the business it oversees is done in a quality-focused cost-effective manner with similarly trained, similarly oriented faculty enabling better standardization, lower cost, and greater throughput. In this model the radiologist must modify his/her practice to ensure an adequate inflow of patients. Radiology must develop strong marketing and reach out directly to primary care physicians and patients.

The disadvantages of this model are numerous. Whereas patients who come to your institution and receive imaging done by radiology are ensured quality care, it is unacceptable not to maintain consistent quality for all individuals needing imaging services at your institution. There is unnecessary duplication leading to loss of needed economies of scale in terms of staffing, supplies, and imaging equipment. There is also a duplication of skills required that shifts the focus of interventionalist away from being a dedicated proceduralist. To maintain the flow of patients, the radiologist must put more energy into establishing and maintaining a clinic in which are evaluated those patients referred for suspected vascular disease who have undergone minimal workup. A number of these patients will not require a diagnostic imaging study nor an interventional procedure. An iteration of the second model is to hire a vascular surgeon or cardiologist to work in your group or department. This model can work very well in terms of not requiring your IR physicians to develop noninterventional clinical skills equivalent to those of a surgeon or cardiologist. If the individual you hire does not maintain ties to his or her specialty department, however, there will still be detrimental duplication of services and poor use of resources.

This takes us to a third model. In this model, nonradiologists become involved in imaging and image-guided intervention but they do this with a great degree of cross-department partnership and radiology oversight. Specifically, a nonradiologist can be jointly hired with funding provided by percent FTE spent in the respective departments. For example, I partially fund a cardiologist to read cardiac nuclear studies and cardiac stress tests. His revenue when he is doing imaging accrues to radiology, and when he is seeing patients in the clinic, accrues to cardiology. We are doing collaborative research and he educates both the cardiology and the radiology trainees. This provides a wonderful level of synergy and the educational outlet that is required for cardiology in terms of training, and, as we develop skilled practitioners, a few will similarly join our practice.

A fourth model is to commit to a true collaboration: radiologists, cardiologists, and vascular surgeons from different departments working together to optimize clinical evaluation, patient access, quality of care, cost effectiveness, and training and research. In this model, it remains important for radiology to oversee the capital acquisition, operation, and maintenance of the interventional suite. We have established an endovascular center that follows this model. The center has a physician leader who is the director of interventional radiology. The group has a leadership team consisting of a designee from IR, vascular surgery, and cardiology. Radiology oversees the training of the vascular surgeons and cardiologists to ensure that appropriate clinical standards are met. The group performs monthly q/a and q/c meetings so that patients get the best in care.

In this model, restrictions must be placed on self-referral. In the initial iteration of our endovascular center, no self-referral was allowed. All cases were referred to a center with distribution of a case to the physician assigned to the angiography lab (see Appendix 6-1). As the collaboration evolved, the model for how we dealt with self-referral was modified. Based on input from the members of the vascular center, it was felt that as long as it could be demonstrated on a monthly basis that each participating department was performing an equivalent number and type of cases, self-referral was not a threat to any of the departments. It simply requires the nonendovascular proceduralists in cardiology and vascular surgery referred to the center. The benefit is that those vascular surgeons and cardiologists who could perform endovascular interventions could also care for their patients from initial interaction to successful treatment.

One challenge to this model is aligning incentives with the desired behavior of referring patients to the center. For example, if the Department of Surgery compensates its faculty based on the surgeon's profit and loss statement, this is a tremendous motivation for self-referral. It is important to be able to demonstrate that participation in the center ultimately improves their productivity. For example, participating in performing endovascular procedures may only be possible if one is a member of the center—no participation, no chance for productivity. We also track referral sources so that our nonradiology colleagues can see that a number of procedures come to the center by way of radiology referrals following MRA or CTA and as a result of our superior marketing efforts. Another response would be to pool funds to better align financial incentives. For example, a "section of endovascular" could pool revenue and expenses from each department's contributing physicians with bonuses distributed equally to all members of the section. Another response is for the participating departments to limit the at-risk component of compensation. In this model, leadership has to ensure that productivity remains high and the group is committed to its overall success.

Of tremendous importance to success in model four is the people and trust. I was fortunate that the division chief of cardiology, the chair of medicine, and the chair of surgery were individuals of integrity who were able to trust that by ceding some control to radiology, they would in the long run gain more than if we all competed. When the model was first introduced, it was very restrictive in that the primary goal was to prevent people from feeling taken advantage of. We needed to reestablish trust, and over time we relaxed some of the restrictions. The result was that we now have a highly collaborative team that has brought together not only the clinical skills but the research and educational talents of three departments. We co-recruit with interdepartment input on candidates. We seek input from all members of the committee. We all work hard to convey that we are a team committed to each other. Ultimately, I believe this to be the best solution in that it maintains the patient as the core value and meets the needs of important constituents. The whole ends up greater than the sum of its parts, as demonstrated in Figure 6-1.

In addition to correctly establishing models for collaboration and focusing on quality, cost, and safety, we must continue to innovate. Radiologists who have been out of training for only a decade are now performing procedures and using diagnostic tools that were barely

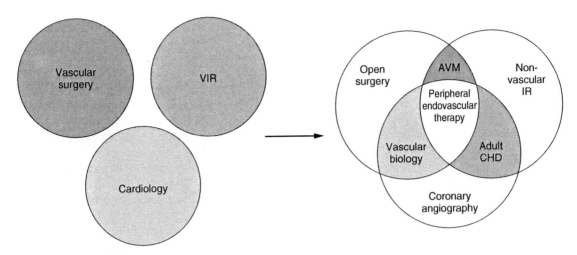

Figure 6-1 A collaborative model for endovascular therapy. (Courtesy RT Andrews, Director of Endovascular Center, University of Washington School of Medicine; Section Chief, Interventional Radiology, Department of Radiology, University of Washington.)

considerations when they were in training. PET-CT, PACS, 3T MRI, Stent grafts, and molecular medicine are examples of but a few of the tools. We can get so caught up in laying claim to the present that we are at great risk if we do not invest in discovering the future. We must do more research to determine where imaging brings value and where it does not. We must ensure that we emphasize outcomes research. We must pursue operations research to optimize the cost effectiveness of what we do. In reviewing the funding both from the NIH and from our radiological societies, we can see that the funding we need to address what is so essential to our future is inadequate. Remember, no mission, no margin. If we do not demonstrate how to get this right we will not have the revenue to fund the very important initiatives in molecular medicine and minimally invasive intervention.

If innovation is important to preservation of the specialty, we need to ensure that it is adequately funded. At present, this is becoming increasingly difficult for the academic departments to continue to subsidize. The past paradigm of shifting revenues from clinical profitability to the research mission is becoming increasingly challenging. Both private practice and academics need to be committed to supporting those individuals dedicated to innovation. This can occur in many ways. For example, many private practice physician leaders contribute to the academic mission by way of educational contributions at society meetings or by contributing clinical or teaching effort to their local radiology training program. Private practice groups contribute to radiology society research funds; funding fellowship programs aligns our efforts with private practitioners. Done correctly, there is both an immediate and a long-term gain. For example, my department has a private practice collaboration where the private group funds a fellow who will have a predisposition to join one of our groups and strengthen ongoing collaborations. We also benefit from a local community that contributes their time to teach our residents; among them are some of our best teachers. Student and volunteer faculty alike are enriched by this exchange and the faculty gains more time for research.

And at last the locusts did descend. They settled on every tree and on every blade of grass; they settled on the roofs and covered the bare ground. Mighty tree branches broke away under them, and the whole country became the brown-earth color of the vast, hungry swarm.

Things Fall Apart, by Chinua Achebe

At this point in the chapter, it has been demonstrated that the optimal is for radiologists to maintain control over imaging and image-guided interventions using a quality, safety, and cost rationalization with development of collaborations based on where it brings value to the patient. I have used this model effectively and so too have many of my fellow department chairs. It is also true that sometimes the facts don't matter—at least to those in a position of decision making. Specifically, despite the demonstrable benefits to the patient and the bottom line, leadership does not support radiology. When this occurs, there are a number of approaches that can be employed.

First, take advantage of opportunities to negotiate for regaining or retaining "turf." An ideal time to accomplish this is when negotiating for the position of department chair or in accepting a hospital contract that may be less appealing to other radiology groups. For example, prior to my arrival at my current institution, the relationship between radiology and surgery was very dysfunctional. It was clear to me that in order to reestablish an effective training program and a clinically capable radiology department, a complete realignment in endovascular procedures would be required. I made it clear that I could not accept the chairmanship without this being addressed. Although it was clear to the dean that there would be some transitional pain involved with this realignment, he also realized that any person capable of leading the department would make a similar request. Taking such a posture in negotiations may mean walking away from a position that might still be very appealing, but if an individual is not willing to step away from personal benefit for the good of the department, then he or she should not be seeking a leadership position in the first place.

I have been fortunate that the chairman of surgery and medicine as well as the division chief of cardiology have stood by the commitments made when I joined the institution. I am also aware that there are others who face greater challenges than I. At my former institution, I accepted the role of interim chair. Within the first weeks of my appointment, I was invited to meet with a chairman from a different department. Although I anticipated being the recipient of insights from a colleague understanding the challenges I would face as an interim chair, I was instead informed that he was prepared to help me transition a major component of noninvasive imaging to his department. I thanked him for his "generosity" but made him aware that I did not share his perspective. In this instance, my response was to emphasize to the dean how inappropriate it would be for another department to take advantage of a position of "weakness" in radiology, that is, a leadership

transition, and conveyed to him that enabling this to proceed would speak poorly for the culture of the institution and would make the recruitment of a future chair challenging. In this instance, I was fortunate that the dean concurred with my sense of fairness and supported not forcing change in a time of transition.

There might be a time when one is no longer effective in helping the hospital CEO or the dean understand the importance of maintaining a strong department of radiology. In this instance, it might be time to step aside as a leader. Clearly, this should not be in the context of providing an ultimatum of "my way or the highway." Effective leaders do not offer to fall on their sword; they try other tactics. However, when one loses the ability to preserve what is clearly in the best interest of the patient and the institution, it is time to allow for an incoming leader to return to the negotiating table.

Once you accept the responsibility of leading the department, make certain you have the resources necessary to hire the best people. This resource commitment could be a block grant from the dean or CEO, or a simple confirmation of substantial reserves or departmental profitability. In academics, "the best" means an individual recognized as the leading innovator or technically most gifted in the field. This person can be an MD or a PhD. In private practice, it is providing areas of subspecialty expertise, particularly in areas where nonradiology specialists, such as neurologists, seek to compete.

In addition to recruiting the best, be the best and demonstrate that you are. Do not find yourself short on staff so that you cannot maintain excellence in access, quality, and cost. Create a staffing grid to project growth, and be proactive in hiring the individuals needed. Establish objective quality and safety measures that demonstrate that you are as good as you say you are. Useful measures can include cost/relative value units (RVUs), fluoroscopy time, room use, case number to qualify for performing a procedure, certificate of added qualifications, ACR, RADPEER, and ACR standards. Maintain excellent quality assurance logs and M&M documentation. Fight on quality, but to do so, you need outstanding data as evidence.

Establish a standard for equivalent responsibilities for all those participating in providing a service. For example, in the case of nonradiologists performing vascular ultrasound during the day, the same group should be required to cover the service 24/7, or at least to participate in the call with radiology. This is simply a matter of professionalism. Those unwilling to follow this model should not be allowed to participate. Garnering support for this position, if a call to professionalism is not successful, might mean charging an added fee to the hospital if the radiology is going to cover nondesirable service hours. Make it clear to the administration that this incremental cost is unnecessary in a model where the burden is shared.

In addition, it should not be possible for nonradiology departments to want to participate in the profitable aspects of a service and to forego the less profitable. For example, practitioners who want to perform Stent grafts must also be available to perform fistula declots. Let administration know that it will not be possible for the department of radiology to provide less profitable services such as mammography and pediatric radiology if the more lucrative aspects of radiology are parceled to other services. Mammography, for example, is a particularly valuable service that is not easily done by others. There are very clear quality standards that are not easily met, the financial return is limited, the legal liability is great, the availability of mammographers is outstripped by demand, and access to breast imaging screening studies is now becoming an accepted pay-for-performance requirement that practice plans will have to meet.

Provide local examples that demonstrate the cost of unnecessary duplication. The costs include maintaining duplicate supplies, technologists, and technical support. This can be identified a priori to dissuade a poor leadership decision or monitored so that actual costs of duplication can be tracked and perhaps lead to the reverse of a poor decision. During my period as interim chair, a proposal was made to establish a completely duplicate leadership structure in catheter lab oversight. We provided a model of the costs. Unfortunately, the leadership made the appeal that complete independence was needed to maintain the morale of the group seeking this level of independence. The predicted result was subsequently realized with loss of money on purchases, service, supplies, techs, administrative costs, and so on. It is likely that the hospital will revisit this now that they are seeing the cost of maintaining "morale."

Provide a comprehensive imaging option to capture the business. For example, being able to perform a triple rule-out with spiral CT enables excluding dissection and PE but also enables participation in coronary vessel narrowing. Nonradiologists would have a difficult time being as comprehensive. This comprehensive assessment provides better throughput. One-stop-shopping efforts can be used to our advantage.

Don't oversell the profit in your business. If the money is the sole motivator, a reality check will deter those financially motivated. For example, the University Health System Consortium has recently reported that succeeding on the professional fees alone is nearly impossible for a department of radiology. The return is on the facility side, which goes to the hospital unless the physicians have an equity stake in the equipment. In most academic practices, there is no or limited access to technical fees. Lastly, given the profits are on the facility side, make it clear that radiologists understand how to optimize the return on investment for capital equipment and that ultimately these hospital profits support the infrastructure of the entire institution.

Partner in win-wins. If you are losing or have lost cardiac scoring, for example, establish the policy of having radiologists review the lungs and mediastinum for the cardiologists. Share the RVUs. But negotiate for your trainees to learn cardiac calcium scoring from the experts, as part of the bargain. Similarly, seek to understand the actual goal of other departments in terms of wanting to participate in imaging services. Although it may all be an issue of revenue, it may also be a need to ensure that their trainees get exposure to imaging and image-guided intervention. This can be done without relinquishing turf.

In most hospital systems, the profitability of the hospital is contingent on highly effective operations in radiology. In assuming my role as department chair, it was my belief that to obtain the very best "turf" protection meant becoming the most profitable department in the institution as soon as possible. Having attained this, I have found the hospital leadership very responsive when I express concerns of risks to this profitability when imaging is not coordinated by radiology. In a time of decreasing margins, protecting margins is a compelling argument.

In conclusion, turf issues that lead to the performance of lower-quality imaging and intervention are to the detriment of the patients whom we have taken an oath to serve. We have summarized the compelling quality, safety, and cost reasons why imaging and image-guided intervention need to be done primarily by radiologists. It is perhaps most healthy to be nonjudgmental, take a leadership role in radiology, and make sure the *patient* remains your core value. Ensure adequacy of training as well as site certification and contribute to advancing. Lastly, in pursuing what is best for our patients, we will find that there are times when strategies *beyond* emphasizing what is best for the patient need to be implemented.

Dos and Don'ts Strategies for Maintaining Turf	
Dos	**Don'ts**
1. Emphasize the quality, safety, revenue, and cost savings arguments in rationalizing the central role of the radiologist in diagnostic imaging and image-guided intervention.	1. Use the entitlement argument for why radiology should oversee imaging services. Nobody cares what you feel you are entitled to, except perhaps your mother.
2. Be facile with the facts that support the quality and safety that radiologists bring to imaging and image-guided intervention.	2. Burn bridges with clinical services. In the end they refer more work to you than just the items that span the common turf.
3. Be aware that the value contributed to patient care through the rigorous training undertaken by radiologists is espoused by those inside and outside of radiology.	3. Underuse the credentialing and certification bureaucracy in creating barriers to entry that are reasonable and that clearly are designed to ensure quality care.
4. Establish strong credentialing policies as a part of your delineation of privileges. Rigorous training requirements are a barrier to entry of those who do not have the patient as their primary focus.	4. Be reluctant to turn in and report people who violate Stark rules or are flagrant self-referrers. In the end, you are improving health care.
5. Be conversant regarding the detrimental impact of turf wars on training of radiologists. Many of the incursions into radiology turf occur in the name of training requirements for nonradiology specialties.	5. Allow certificate-of-need applications to pass without your scrutiny. If the market is saturated, new entrants that will just hurt business should not get free passes.
6. Keep legislators, payers, and administrators aware that radiologists are not the biggest drivers of growth in imaging costs.	6. Get short staffed. Keep staffing levels robust and have succession plans handy so that there are no gaps in service or quality if a radiology key player moves on.
7. Understand Stark and anti-kickback rules. Report violations.	7. Be reluctant to share your concerns with vendors. A short-term increase in sales by targeting nonradiology customers will ultimately foster growth.

APPENDIX 6-1. UW MEDICINE CENTER FOR ENDOVASCULAR THERAPY

Overview

The UW Medicine Center for Endovascular Therapy shall be a multidisciplinary specialty group dedicated to the diagnosis and elective treatment of vascular disease using minimally invasive, percutaneous, image-guided, endovascular techniques. Examples of these techniques include, but are not limited to, catheter-directed angiography, percutaneous transluminal angioplasty, embolization therapy, catheter-directed thrombolytic therapy, and endovascular repair of aneurysmal disease. Recognizing the value of different but overlapping skill sets, the Center shall combine the skills of interventional radiologists, interventional cardiologists, and endovascular-trained vascular surgeons.

Goals

1. To identify patients who would benefit from endovascular interventions and to provide those patients with the highest level of clinical care during such procedures.
2. To train physician providers in the techniques of endovascular interventions.
3. To apply to endovascular interventional therapy the scientific efforts necessary to continually improve and refine its techniques and outcomes.
4. To establish the University of Washington as an international leader in such techniques.

Scope

The Center shall oversee all endovascular interventions undertaken within the UW Medicine system, with the following limited exceptions:

- Interventions within the coronary arteries and those involving the valves and chambers of the heart, which shall be managed by interventional cardiology.
- Intracranial interventions and those within branches of the external carotid artery, which shall be managed by neurointerventional service.
- Prenatal umbilical vein catheterization for transfusion, which shall be managed by the Department of Obstetrics and Gynecology.

Governance

Overall operation of the Center, including clinical care, shall be under the direction of the Director of Endovascular Therapy in partnership with hospital administration. The Director of Interventional Radiology will also serve as the Director of Endovascular Therapy. Departmental stakeholders shall be represented by Associate Directors for Endovascular Therapy for Medicine, Radiology, and Surgery, each of whom shall be appointed by their respective departments. Together with the Director of Endovascular Therapy, this group shall be referred to as the Executive Committee, and shall meet on a monthly basis, chaired by the Director of Endovascular Therapy. The Executive Committee shall advise the Director on matters pertaining to the clinical practice within the Center and work with hospital administration (e.g., the nonphysician Manager of Endovascular Therapy) to oversee Center operations. The Manager of Endovascular Therapy will in turn manage nonphysician employees, coordination of billing, and daily nonclinical operations.

An Oversight Group will be convened which will be chaired by the Vice-Dean for Clinical Affairs. Additional members of the group will include the Chairs of Medicine, Radiology, and Surgery; and the Chief Operating Officers and Medical Directors of UWMC and Harborview Medical Center. *Ex officio* members of the Oversight Committee shall include the Director and Associate Directors of the Center and the administrative manager of the Endovascular Center. This body shall meet on a quarterly basis (or as frequently as appropriate).

Clinical Participation

Participation in endovascular procedures shall be limited to members of the Endovascular Center. Physician participation in the Center for Endovascular Therapy shall be made available as needed to meet the clinical demands of the Center. Participation shall be limited to individuals who

- have a current license to practice medicine in the State of Washington;
- have an appointment in the Department of Medicine, Radiology, or Surgery;
- have undergone formal training in radiation physics, radiation biology, and radiation safety;
- have obtained clinical privileges in the Center for Endovascular Therapy at the University of Washington Medical Center and/or Harborview Medical Center (attached) that bear the signature of the Director of Endovascular Therapy and the Chairman of the Department in which the individual has a primary appointment; and
- meet the ongoing clinical practice requirements discussed below.

Clinical Practice Requirements

All members of the endovascular group shall

- accept into their practice, and provide treatment for, any patient requiring endovascular therapy in accordance with UW Medicine and hospital policies for service and access;
- participate in the identification, evaluation, and longitudinal management of patients undergoing endovascular therapy, including (but not limited to) outreach programs, community lectures, and similar activities, pre-and post-procedure care clinics, and inpatient care;
- be subject to and participate in a uniform program of quality assurance, including pre-, peri-, and post-procedural surveillance. Variables recorded during each endovascular case shall include (but not be limited to) procedural time, fluoroscopic time, patient absorbed dose, contrast type and volume, and equipment used. In addition, any attempted procedure that fails or is converted to an open repair shall be documented. Short- and long-term outcomes for diagnostic and interventional procedures shall also be tracked. All of the data derived from this program shall be reviewed on a regular basis in the context of a combined morbidity and mortality conference. Any physician member of the Center who performs in the lowest quintile for the group in any category during four of the preceding 12 months shall, at the discretion of the Director of Endovascular Therapy, be required to seek

additional training or discontinue his or her participation in the Center; and
- participate in the training of all endovascular fellows, independent of the physician's own departmental appointments.

Operational Considerations

- Each of the three represented departments shall participate fully in the clinical activities of the Center, with each department performing, on average annually, one third of elective endovascular cases. This distribution will allow for similarity in terms of types of cases and RVUs. Departmental distribution of cases shall be reported to the Oversight Committee at least quarterly.
- Scheduled endovascular procedures shall be performed in a dedicated angiographic suite, assigned in blocks of an entire clinical day, rather than by specific case, to one of the three services sharing duty in the Endovascular Center. These daily blocks shall be distributed on a rotating basis. No service shall undertake elective endovascular procedures except on days during which that service is assigned to the endovascular suite, unless specifically approved by the Director of Endovascular Therapy. On its assigned days, each service shall be responsible for all cases undertaken in the endovascular suite, including the smooth and efficient operation thereof. Unanticipated delays in the progress of scheduled endovascular cases shall not routinely result in overtime operation of the room. Thus, should scheduled cases threaten to exceed the allocated time, they shall be rescheduled or redistributed to other procedure rooms and be performed by the interventional radiology service.
- The scheduling of individual physician members' participation in endovascular procedures shall be the responsibility of the associate director of the department assigned to the endovascular suite on a given day. (Note to reviewers: this change is suggested to eschew daily discussion among all associate directors; this is clearly a responsibility, not just an opportunity.)
- No department shall seek "extra days" to accommodate an oversupply of participating members under its jurisdiction or inefficiencies that prevent the group from finishing cases in a timely manner.

- Unscheduled, emergent, and "on call" endovascular cases shall be performed by the interventional radiology service, unless these occur during or as the direct result of a procedure being undertaken by a member of the Center, in which case they may be performed by that person in whatever location is clinically appropriate.
- Scheduling of patients for treatment in the Center (including those undergoing surgical exposure in the operating room for endograft placement) shall be coordinated through a single point of contact in the Center. Non-emergency endovascular cases will be added to the daily schedule in a balanced fashion so that on any given day there will be no more than two additional endovascular cases relative to other days that week. For example, it will not be acceptable to add a second case on a specific day of the week until there are single vascular cases already added to the other days of the week. Exceptions to this can be granted at the discretion of the Director of the Endovascular Center.
- Physicians who participate in the Center may perform endovascular procedures on those patients whom they have personally seen and evaluated in clinic, or for whom they have previously provided care. This mechanism of occasional "self-referral" shall not result in any one department of the Center performing more than one third of all endovascular procedures on a quarterly basis and shall not result in any one participating practitioner referring to specific participating service more than 25% of the cases evaluated by him or her.
- Referral by nonparticipating physicians of patients for treatment shall be accommodated on a first-available basis, without a treating service being specified (i.e., directed referral for treatment shall not be accepted).
- The operation of fixed angiographic equipment used for peripheral endovascular therapy, and the direction of employees operating that equipment, shall be under the jurisdiction of the Department of Radiology.

Financial Considerations

The technical fee for each procedure performed under the jurisdiction of the Center shall accrue to the hospital Radiology Department in the facility in which the procedure is undertaken. Professional salaries for all participants shall be determined by, and shall be paid by, the department in which the operator has his or her primary appointment. All professional fees generated by each participant shall accrue to his or her primary department.

Acknowledgments

Thanks to Bob Bree, Professor of Radiology at the University of Washington and a true scholar in issues related to imaging quality and utilization, who generously shared materials he had gathered regarding these issues. In addition, it is important to recognize Drs. David Levin and Vijay Rao. They have ensured that the radiology community is well informed on the detriments secondary to inappropriate incursion on turf. Their work has been frequently referenced and should be reviewed by those seeking greater insight. Lastly, I would like to acknowledge Bruce Hillman as one of the first radiologists to recognize the magnitude of this topic. His Visiting Professor Lecture at the University of Washington provided a wonderfully comprehensive overview, on which I have relied to ensure completeness in addressing this issue.

REFERENCES

1. http://www.etymonline.com.
2. Eng J, Mysko WK, Weller GE, Renard R, et al: Interpretation of emergency department radiographs: A comparison of emergency medicine physicians with radiologists, residents with faculty, and film with digital display. Am J Roentgenol 175(5):1233–1238, 2000.
3. Hanley JA, McNeil BJ: The meaning and use of the area under the ROC curve. Radiology 143:29–36, 1982.
4. Potchen EJ, Cooper TG, Sierra AE, Aben GR, et al: Measuring performance in chest radiography. Radiology 217(2):456–459, 2000.
5. Alfaro D, Levitt MA, English DK, Williams V, et al: Accuracy of interpretation of cranial computed tomography scans in an emergency medicine residency program. Ann Emerg Med 25(2):169–174, 1995.
6. Walsh-Kelly CM, Melzer-Lange MD, Hennes HM, Lye P, et al: Clinical impact of radiograph misinterpretation in a pediatric ED and the effect of physician training level. Am J Emerg Med 13(3):262–264, 1995.
7. Wechsler RJ, Spettell CM, Kurtz AB, Lev-Toaff AS, et al: Effects of training and experience in interpretation of emergency body CT scans. Radiology 199(3):717–720, 1996.

8. Levin DC, Rao VM: Turf wars in radiology: The quality of interpretations of imaging studies by nonradiologist physicians—a patient safety issue? JACR 1(7):506–509, 2004.

9. Porter JM: Vascular surgery residency training curriculum. J Vasc Surg 12(1):79–83, 1990.

10. DeMaria AN: Self-referral in cardiology. J Am Coll Cardiol 43(8):1500–1501, 2004.

11. Edmiston RB, Levin DC: Film quality assessment varies among specialties. Diagn Imaging 14(7):37–39, 1992.

12. Hopper KD, Rosetti GE, Edmiston RB, et al: Diagnostic radiology peer review: A method inclusive of all interpreters of radiographic examinations regardless of specialty. Radiology 180(2):557–561, 1991.

13. Verrilli DK, Bloch SM, Rousseau J, Crozier ME, et al: Design of a privileging program for diagnostic imaging: Costs and implications for a large insurer in Massachusetts. Radiology 208(2):385–392, 1998.

14. Moskowitz H, Sunshine J, Grossman D, Adams L, et al: The effect of imaging guidelines on the number and quality of outpatient radiographic examinations. Am J Roentgenol 175(1):9–15, 2000.

15. Shortsleeve J, Herring W: The impact of self-referral on radiology residency training programs. JACR 2(5): 415–417, 2005.

16. Venkatesan AM, Shetty SK, Galdino GM, Davila JA, Lawrimore TM: The impact of professional turf bettles on Radiology resident education: perspectives from the radiology class of 2005. JACR 3(7):537–543, 2006.

17. Oguz KK, Yousem DM, Deluca T, Herskovits EH, et al: Effect of emergency department CT on neuroimaging case volume and positive scan rates. Acad Radiol 9(9):1018–1024, 2002.

18. American College of Physicians: Florida. http://www.acponline.org/chapters/fl/ref_law.htm

19. Kouri BE, Parsons RG, Allport HR: Physician self-referral for diagnostic imaging: Review of the empiric literature. Am J Roentgenol 179:843–850, 2002.

20. Hillman BJ, Joseph CA, Mabry MR, et al: Frequency and costs of diagnostic imaging in office practice—a comparison of self-referring and radiologist-referring physicians. N Engl J Med 323(23):1604–1608, 1990.

21. Levin DC, Rao VM: Turf wars in radiology: The overutilization of imaging resulting from self-referral. JACR 1(3):169–172, 2004.

22. Levin DC, Rao VM: Turf wars in radiology: Other causes of overutilization and what can be done about it. JACR 1(5):317–321, 2004.

23. Hillman BJ, Olson GT, Griffith PE, et al: Physicians' utilization and charges for outpatient diagnostic imaging in a Medicare population. JAMA 268(15): 2050–2054, 1992.

24. Hemenway D, Killen A, Cashman SB, Parks CL, et al: Physicians' responses to financial incentives: Evidence from a for-profit ambulatory care center. N Engl J Med 323(12):836–837, 1990.

25. Omnibus Budget Reconciliation Act of 1989 (OBRA, 1989).

26. Omnibus Budget Reconciliation Act of 1993 (OBRA, 1993).

27. Maryland Board of Physicians online: Available at www.mbp.state.md.us/index.html.

28. Dranove D, White WD: Medicaid-dependent hospitals and their patients: How have they fared? Health Serv Res 33:163–185, 1998.

29. Shen Y-C: The effect of financial pressure on the quality of care in hospitals. J Health Econ 833:1–27, 2003.

30. Lindrooth RC, Bazzoli GJ, Needleman J, Hasnain-Wynia R: The effect of changes in hospital reimbursement on nurse staffing decisions at safety net and nonsafety net hospitals. Health Serv Res 41(3): 701–720, 2006.

PART 2

ACCOUNTING BASICS AND FINANCIAL PRINCIPLES

CHAPTER 7

The Vernacular of Accounting

Audrey Drossner

Sales and revenue mean the same thing.

Profits, earnings and income mean the same thing.

Now, revenue and income do not mean the same thing.

Costs are different from expenses.

Expenses are different from expenditures.

Sales are different from orders but are the same as shipments.

Profits are different from cash.

Solvency is different from profitability.[1]

This chapter is intended not to turn you into an accountant but to give you the tools necessary to evaluate opportunities for your radiology practice. It will give you the terminology you need to know the right questions to ask and how to interpret the answers. The idea is not for you to learn to compile the information but instead to have the knowledge needed to interpret the materials, to recognize the important financial statements, and to know the

principles on which the information in the statements was based.

Two major authorities regulate accounting. First, for the financial part, there is the Financial Accounting Standards Board (FASB). Second, for tax accounting, there is the Internal Revenue Service (IRS). Frequently, you will notice that a tax return does not mirror the financial statements because of the separate and independent accounting systems. Adjustments must therefore be made to financial statements to prepare an accurate tax return; these are referred to as book/tax adjustments.

The financial accounting industry operates based on a complex set of rules and opinions that allow for multiple interpretations leading to many different conclusions. Both the Securities and Exchange Commission (SEC) and the American Institute of Certified Public Accountants (AICPA) recognize that FASB has the authority to set the standards. These standards, made up of rules and opinions, are known as the Generally Accepted Accounting Principles

(GAAP) system, containing five separate categories. The top category has the most authority. The higher in the hierarchy, the more weight is given to the rule.

GAAP Hierarchy[2]

A. Statements of Financial Accounting Standards (FASB)
  • FASB Interpretations (FASB)
  • Accounting Principles Board Opinions (APB)
B. Technical Bulletins (FASB)
  • Industry Audit and Accounting Guides (AICPA)
  • Statement of Position (AICPA)
C. Consensus position. Emerging Issues Task Force (FASB)
  • Accounting Standards Executive Committee Practice Bulletins (AICPA)
D. Accounting Interpretations (AICPA)
  • Staff Implementation Guides (FASB)
  • Industry Standards
E. Statements of Financial Accounting Concepts (FASB)
  • Federal Accounting Standards Advisory Board Statements, Interpretations, and Technical Bulletins (BASB)
  • Issue Papers (AICPA)
  • Technical Practice Aids (AICPA)
  • Government Accounting Standards Board Statements (AISB)
  • Pronouncements of other professional associations and regulatory agencies, and accounting textbooks and articles.

It is important to differentiate bookkeeping from accounting. Bookkeeping is the recording of the economic events that took place in a chronological, detailed manner so that the accountant can make sense of the information. This is a painstaking process. The entries made by the bookkeeper are generated from source documents, such as invoices, statements, receipts, checks, and any documentation of a transaction. From these source documents summaries are prepared. Generally there is a cash receipts journal, a cash disbursements journal, and a general ledger where all the entries are posted. The posting of entries to the general ledger is where you hear the terms *debits* and *credits* (debits are on the left and credits are on the right). Accounting, on the other hand, takes the information the bookkeeper has recorded and tries to make financial sense out of it. Accountants prepare multiple financial reports and calculate performance measurements so that other parties can get a clear understanding of what has happened.

The best way to follow this chapter is to do so with a copy of the various statements I will refer to in hand so you can see the components of the financial documents. Copy them now and join me in the next paragraph (Boxes 7-1 and 7-2).

STATEMENT OF FINANCIAL CONDITION: THE BALANCE SHEET

The first financial statement is called the statement of financial condition, more commonly known as the balance sheet. This statement is created at a specific point in time (one specific day) and will tell you where you stand financially as of that date. This date also corresponds with the last day of the period of time covered by the income statement (to be discussed later). The statement of financial condition is also referred to as the balance sheet because it is made up of two columns that balance and equal each other. The left side includes the assets and the right side includes the liabilities and retained earnings. These two sums always equal each other.

$$Assets = Liabilities + Retained\ Earnings$$

Both the assets side and the liability side of the balance sheet are split between current and noncurrent. A current asset or liability is defined as being an asset or liability that can be liquidated or will come due in the next 12 months. If, for example, you have an equipment loan, the debt would be bifurcated between the current amount that is due over the next 12 months and the balance, which would be classified as long-term debt. The importance of segregating the current and long-term assets and liabilities is so that certain ratios can be calculated. These ratios help you value the company from a liquidity standpoint. A ratio is simply an abbreviated expression of numbers. It reduces two large numbers to a more readily comprehensible form. For instance, it is easier to understand

BOX 7-1

Radiologists R We
Consolidated Balance Sheet
12/31/XXXX

December 31, XXXX

ASSETS	Consolidated
Current Assets	
Cash and cash equivalents	$1,500,000
Patient accounts receivable, net	17,900,000
Accounts receivable—other	2,951,000
Prepaid expenses	1,311,000
Total Current Assets	23,662,000
Property and Equipment, net	46,000,000
Goodwill and Intangible Assets, net	21,700,000
Other Assets, net	3,750,000
Total Assets, net	$95,112,000

> Radiology practices are capital intensive.

LIABILITIES AND STOCKHOLDERS' EQUITY	
Current Liabilities	
Current portion of long-term bank debt	$800,000
Current portion of long-term capital leases	5,250,000
Current portion of long-term notes payable	367,000
Accounts payable and accrued expenses	11,500,000
Total Current Liabilities	17,917,000
Long-Term Liabilities	
Deferred compensation	3,500,000
Long-term bank debt, net of current portion	50,450,000
Long-term capital leases, net of current portion	10,200,000
Long-term note payable, net of current portion	367,000
Accrued other, net	1,272,000
Deferred tax liability	9,900,000
Total Long-Term Liabilities	75,689,000
Stockholders' Equity (deficit)	
Common Stock	100
Retained Earnings	1,505,900
Total Stockholders' Equity (deficit)	1,506,000
Total Liabilities and Stockholders' Equity	$95,112,000

> Radiology practices are highly leveraged.

BOX 7-2

Radiologists R We
Consolidated Income Statement
1/1/XXXX–12/31/XXXX

	Total Consolidated	
NET REVENUES		Fees on credit increase accounts receivable on the Balance Sheet.
Fee for Service	$ 91,800,000	
Other	800,000	
Total Net Revenues	92,600,000	
EXPENSES		
Provisions for Uncollectible Accounts	0	
Physician Salaries	17,500,000	
Physician Benefits	5,300,000	
Contract Labor and Professional Radiology	6,400,000	
Total Physician Costs	29,200,000	
Employee Salaries and Benefits	18,500,000	Expenses, when incurred, increase accounts payable on the Balance Sheet.
Office, Linen, and Computer Supplies, Forms	400,000	
Licenses and Permits, Subscriptions	294,000	
Medical Supplies, Film, and Contrast	4,475,000	
Rent and Facility Expenses (Excluding Telephone)	570,000	
Equipment Rental	380,000	
Service Contracts	6,200,000	
Total Operating Expenses	60,019,000	
NONOPERATING REVENUES AND EXPENSES		
Interest Income	15,000	
Total Non-Operating Revenues and Expenses	15,000	
EBITDA	32,596,000	Depreciation expense increases accumulated depreciation, lowering property and equipment net on the Balance Sheet.
AMORTIZATION, DEPRECIATION, AND INTEREST		
Amortization	1,630,000	
Depreciation	9,700,000	
Interest	5,600,000	
Total Amortization, Depreciation, and Interest	16,930,000	
EST	15,666,000	Net income is added to retained earnings on the Balance Sheet.
INCOME TAXES	5,640,000	
NET INCOME	$ 10,026,000	

"3 to 1" than "$416,839.42 to $138,945.33." Below is an example of a current assets (working capital) ratio:

$$\text{Working Capital} = \frac{\text{Current Assets}}{\text{Current Liabilities}}$$

This is an indicator of how liquid the company is. Usually you want to see a 2 to 1 or better ratio. On the "Radiologists R We" balance sheet (see Box 7-1) the ratio is low, 1.32 to 1.

Assets

The assets generally included in the current assets section are cash, accounts receivable (amounts due from patients—see "Accounts Receivable," Chapter 9), and inventory. There is a second ratio called the quick assets ratio (or asset test ratio) that is similar to the current assets (working capital) ratio, with the exception that inventory is excluded from current assets:

$$\text{Quick Assets Ratio} = \frac{\text{Current Assets} - \text{Inventories}}{\text{Current Liabilities}}$$

Inventory is usually the least liquid current asset. In balance sheets in which inventory is significant this ratio is more important to assess.

For a radiology practice, receivables are usually the most significant component of current assets. If the accounts receivable are listed as net receivables (as opposed to "gross receivables"), this implies that there has been an allowance for the bad debts. This is an estimate of the amount that is believed to be uncollectible. For financial statement presentation, an allowance is set up based on an aging schedule or percentage of sales in which, for tax purposes, the direct write-off method is used.

Deferred assets are another current asset that includes payments made in the current year for expenses of the next year (prepaid expenses). The following year the asset is reclassified from the balance sheet (credit) and expensed on the income statement (debit).

Another category on the balance sheet is intangible assets. The most commonly included items for a radiology practice are the value of covenants not to compete and goodwill (these are the values assigned to the practice's reputation upon acquisition). For tax purposes, intangibles created as a part of an acquisition are amortized (written off as an intangible asset investment over the projected life of the asset) over 15 years.

The last category is the company's fixed assets, also known as their property, plant, and equipment. Fixed assets are used to produce income and are not for sale. Fixed assets include buildings, machinery, equipment, and furniture. When fixed assets are shown (net amount), this means the depreciation has already been deducted from the historical cost. All fixed assets, with the exception of land, are depreciated (reduction of the value of an asset as a result of wear and tear, age, or obsolescence) over their useful life. There are several methods for depreciating equipment that are discussed later under Budgets.

It is important to realize that a lot of information is not included on the face of many financial statements but instead is disclosed in the footnotes of financial statements, such as contingent pension liabilities. A thorough examination of the footnotes is therefore required when analyzing the value of a practice. Another drawback of balance sheets is that the assets are recorded at cost, rather than at current market value. As such, balance sheets do not reflect the increase or decrease in value of fixed assets owned by the practice (e.g., appreciation on the office building and land owned by the practice or the decrease in value of older and obsolete office equipment).

Liabilities

On the liability side of the balance sheet, debts are recorded as current or noncurrent liabilities. Debt that is payable within the next 12 months, along with accounts payable and accrued expenses, are all listed as current liabilities. Liabilities include debts and accounts payable, such as amounts owed to suppliers. The largest liabilities for a medical practice are debt for equipment purchases and accounts payable (see "Managing Expenses," Chapter 10). There is also a category for accrued expenses, which are items that have been properly expensed but have not been paid for. Examples are salaries, legal fees, and taxes. As you incur profit, you need to accrue the taxes that will be due on that profit. The final category of liability is the stockholder's equity or shareholder's equity.

INCOME STATEMENT

The income statement summarizes the income and expense items for a period of time, not at a specific date like the balance sheet. The net of the income less the expenses is referred to as the bottom line, or the profit of the entity. Sometimes it is referred to as EBITDA (earnings before interest, taxes, depreciation, and amortization) or EBT (earnings before taxes). These subtotals are shown on the "Radiologists R We" income statement (see Box 7-2). Other terminology used for profits is net earnings or net income. The net income reported on the income statement is added to retained earnings under the stockholder's equity section of the balance sheet's liabilities.

STATEMENT OF CASH FLOWS

The statement of cash flows (or sources and applications statement) summarizes the inflows and outflows during the period specified. It shows which financial transactions created cash and which financial transactions used cash, taking you from the beginning cash balance on the balance sheet to the ending cash balance. Also shown is the conversion of net income from the income statement to the amount of cash flow from operating activities. The statement of cash flows is critical to assessing the immediate needs of the company with respect to liquid assets, needs such as paying salaries or purchasing stock. If there is no money readily available a company cannot survive. If the ups and downs of cash flows are predictable, a strategy of securing short-term loans in certain periods can make sense. Think, if you will, of all of the retail shops that make 40% of their revenue between Thanksgiving and Christmas. They may be flush with cash in November and December but have trouble making payroll during the slow months of April and May. This is a dramatic example of how examining cash flows in a cyclical business can prevent potential disasters.

The three statements—the balance sheet (or statement of financial condition), the income statement, and the statement of cash flows—are the basic statements used to financially evaluate a business.

The financial statements prepared by the accountant usually summarize all the information in totals instead of giving the detailed activities. They are prepared for a specific period based on the needs of the group. Usually, those periods are monthly, quarterly, and annual summaries. A budget is prepared prior to the beginning of the year, and updated throughout the year, so you can gauge how you are doing.

BUDGETS

The budgeting process is very important as it allows you to set goals in financial terms that become the benchmark against which you can compare your actual performance. Budgets help you identify whether any deviations ("variances" is the term often seen on the financial statements) from what was expected were due to revenue or specific expense fluctuations. Any large fluctuations are referred to as "red flags." A budget should be considered a practical action plan, not a straight jacket or "pie in the sky" wish. Budgeting is for internal use only and is used to forecast results against which actual results can be compared. It is a way to formulate your goals as part of a business plan and also provide a yardstick for evaluating performance.

You can prepare annual budgets and long-term budgets. There are multiple ways to create budgets. Models include rolling forecasts, prior year plus a percentage increase, and bottom-up budgets, just to name a few. A good model will let you know what segments of your practice are succeeding and what segments may need to have some process changes.

When creating a budget, many of the components are a function of other components, which allows you to look at "what if" calculations. For example, if you wanted to see what would happen to profit if revenues were 20% higher or 20% lower (a "sensitivity analysis"), you would have your variable costs calculated as a function of revenues. For each additional unit of revenue from reading a film, for example, there would be a corresponding increase in cost for information technology and other direct expenses. Your budget should thus allow you to determine which types of film studies have greater profit margins. Profit margin is the ratio of operating

Table 7-1   Fixed Asset Depreciation Schedule

	Original Purchase Price	Years of Useful Life	Annual Depreciation Charge	Net Book Value Year 1	Net Book Value Year 2
Building	$3,000,000	20	$150,000	$2,850,000	$2,700,000
Land	1,000,000	Unlimited	0	1,000,000	1,000,000
Equipment	350,000	7	50,000	300,000	250,000

income to revenue (sales), and trends in profit margin may be more important than revenue trends. Most budgets only forecast down to the operating income (profit), which is referred to as EBIT (earnings before interest and taxes).

$$\text{Profit Margin} = \frac{\text{Operating Income}}{\text{Revenues}}$$

Revenues in budgeting are a function of volume. For each procedure performed (case read) you multiply by the expected fee. Expenses are slightly more difficult and are usually separated between fixed and variable expenses (also referred to as marginal or incremental costs). Variable expenses are a function of revenues and increase and decrease in proportion to those revenues. Fixed expenses do not vary with revenue volume and are incurred just to keep the practice open. The largest fixed costs in a radiology practice are salaries, benefits, rent, and insurance. By analyzing a practice in this way, you can make decisions about equipment. For example, each practice needs to decide whether to buy, lease, or pay a "per click charge." In the first few years while you are building volume, the per click charge may be the most advantageous. You can run your budget calculating the per click charge under different volume assumptions, or a "quantitative" measurement. If you believe the equipment will shortly become obsolete, this is a "qualitative" reason for paying the per click charge. Both quantitative and qualitative measurements must be weighed in making decisions. You can next calculate the costs of purchasing your own equipment. On the income statement you generally enter a depreciation expense amount equal to dividing the original cost by the useful life, thereby yielding an equal amount of depreciation annually (Table 7-1).

Depreciation is one of the major areas where book reporting (income statement) and tax reporting differ. For tax purposes, depreciation is generally deducted on an accelerated basis. This gives you the tax benefit early and increases cash flow (Table 7-2).

By combining tax depreciation schedules, bonus depreciation and expensing options can rapidly reduce the actual cost of equipment. There is an IRS Section 179 expense allowance of $108,000 for 2006, but this amount is scheduled to be reduced by $25,000 for 2008. Therefore, you always need to be aware of what current tax legislation applies. Another example of legislative changes would be the adjustment for the tax credit for hybrid vehicles. The credit is scheduled to be reduced by 50% from $3,150 to $1,575 when the manufacturer sells 60,000 vehicles. The date of this change is obviously uncertain, therefore you need to annually evaluate which tax laws will benefit you and your practice.

If you have to borrow to finance the acquisition of equipment, you need to expense the interest in preparing your budget and in making

Table 7-2   General Depreciation Systems Schedule

If the Recovery Year Is	5-Year
1	5.00
2	38.00
3	22.80
4	13.68
5	10.94
6	9.58

your comparison. If you pay for the purchase with cash, you need to calculate your opportunity cost (the amount you would have earned on the principal) and subtract this amount when computing your real economic profit.

ACCOUNTING ENTITIES

Financial statements need to be prepared for an accounting entity. One of the first things one needs to choose is the entity type under which one is going to record transactions. Generally speaking, you have three types of entity structures in the private practice arena: (1) a C corporation, (2) a partnership/pass-through entity, and (3) a sole proprietorship. Under the Internal Revenue Code, a regular corporation is called a C corporation. C corporations file annual income tax returns and pay tax on their taxable income. Their stockholders then pay a second tax on any dividend distributions from the C corporation. Therefore, a C corporation is subject to double taxation, first at the corporate level and again at the shareholder level. Many businesses thus choose to organize as a pass-through entity, such as a partnership, S corporation (see the next section), or limited liability company (LLC) to avoid this double taxation. Each of these entities files annual tax returns but they do not pay income taxes. Instead, the return issues what is known as a Form K-1 to each investor reporting their percentage share of each type of income or deduction. The investors in turn report their share of income and deductions on their individual returns. Therefore, the tax is only on the investor level and not the entity level.

S Corporation

For a corporation to qualify as an S corporation, it must elect to be treated as such and must meet certain criteria. For example, an S corporation may only have one class of stock (no common and preferred stock), must be limited to 75 or fewer shareholders, and must obtain unanimous approval from the shareholders for the S corporation election. All shareholders have limited liability under the S corporation structure, meaning only their investment in the corporation is at risk. For example, if the S corporation is successfully

sued, only assets of the corporation are available for collection. The individual shareholders generally cannot be forced to contribute their own assets in satisfaction of the judgment.

Partnership

Partnerships can be structured as general or limited partnerships. They are similar to S corporations in that both types of partnerships must file an annual income tax return. The partnership itself does not pay any income tax liability, however. It issues a Form K-1 to each partner reporting that partner's share of income and deduction items. All members of a general partnership are general partners, while a limited partnership has both limited partners and at least one general partner. Like shareholders in an S corporation, limited partners are liable for debts of the partnership only up to their investment. General partners remain fully liable for all partnership debts and may be forced to contribute additional assets to satisfy any judgments or debts. An advantage of the partnership structure is that it is much more flexible than an S corporation. Any number or type of investors can become partners and the partnership agreement can provide for customized payouts to each individual partner. For example, if one partner is contributing the majority of the working capital, the agreement can provide that this partner will receive a preferred payment until he or she has been fully reimbursed.

LLC

Limited liability companies are a hybrid type of entity that borrow many features from the corporate structure and many from the partnership structure. An LLC with more than one member can elect to be taxed as a C corporation (with double taxation) or as a partnership (taxation only at the investor level). An LLC with only one member can elect to be taxed as a C corporation or as a "disregarded" entity, meaning the sole member reports all items of income and deduction directly on his or her personal return. No separate LLC return with a Form K-1 would be required. Like the S corporation or limited partnership, the LLC members are liable for LLC debts only to the extent of their investment. There is no requirement that a member have general liability for LLC debts—all members should have limited liability. An LLC can have any number or type of investors, and the LLC operating agreement has the flexibility to provide for preferred returns to certain shareholders if needed.

In many states, professional practices are not allowed to organize as regular corporations, partnerships, or LLCs. These states have created separate entities for the organization of a professional practice, known as professional associations (PAs), professional corporations (PCs), or professional limited liability companies (PLLCs). All shareholders or investors must be licensed by the state body governing that particular practice, such as the state medical board. They are taxed just like a regular corporation or pass-through entity and they do provide liability protection for business-related debts and accidents on the premises. They may also protect one shareholder from being personally liable for the malpractice of another. They do not, however, protect a shareholder from his or her own malpractice, thus the separate system from the near total liability protection of a regular corporation, partnership, or LLC is gone.

Now that you have selected an accounting entity, the accountant can report the financials. The next choice to be made when starting to prepare financial statements is whether they will be on the cash or accrual basis. If a business has any type of inventory, there is no choice and the entity must use the accrual basis. Accrual basis accounting does a very good job of accurately matching expenses against revenue. The revenue is recognized when the sale is complete, not necessarily when the cash or the order is received. When the cycle of revenue recognition is complete, the revenue is recorded and is matched with the cost associated with that revenue.

INSURANCE

It is also essential to have your practice adequately insured. Beyond malpractice insurance you should consider an umbrella policy, disability insurance, and key-man life insurance. If you are in a multipartner practice, key-man life insurance can fund any buyouts at death. Many medical practices have a buy/sell agreement in place that is funded with life insurance owned either by the entity or by the other doctors. When a doctor dies, the life insurance is paid to the entity or to the other doctors in the practice. The buy/sell agreement requires the entity or doctors to then purchase the deceased doctor's interest in the practice from his or her estate. Thus, the surviving spouse or other heirs can be compensated for the deceased doctor's contribution to the practice.

Absent a buy/sell agreement, you may still want to protect your surviving spouse or other heirs from the cessation of income produced by your practice. If you are purchasing life insurance on your own for this reason, you should consider establishing an irrevocable life insurance trust (ILIT), preferably to apply for and buy the policy. If you own the policy on your own life, the insurance proceeds will typically pass income tax–free to the beneficiaries. The proceeds will be fully includible in your gross estate, however, and thus subject to estate tax. If the ILIT purchases and owns the policy, the insurance proceeds should not be included in your estate as you would not own the policy. You may also contribute an existing policy to the ILIT, but you must then survive three years to get the exclusion from your estate. There are other considerations, including cash surrender value on premium payments.

Another common "mistake" made in insurance planning is to deduct disability insurance premiums on your income tax return. While this would result in short-term tax savings, it is generally recommended that you do not deduct the premiums for disability insurance. If the premiums are deducted when paid, any proceeds payable as a result of your disability would be taxable as ordinary income. Paying the premiums on an after-tax basis would allow you to take disability payments income tax–free.

RETIREMENT PLANS

You should also consider the tax-deferral benefits of establishing a retirement plan. There are essentially two types of retirement plans available, defined benefit plans and defined contribution plans. The traditional defined benefit plan is generally funded by the entity and pays a certain amount of income for life upon retirement, such as a pension plan. Because of funding requirements and the high cost of maintaining a pension plan, these are not generally used as a medical practice benefit. There are certain defined benefit plans that are practical and advantageous in certain situations, so if you are in a small practice with young administrative staff you should discuss your options with your financial advisor.

Defined contribution plans (401ks, 403bs, and SEPs), on the other hand, are funded by you through salary deferrals (with possible contributions from the entity for matching or profit sharing). You elect that a certain amount of your salary each pay period is to be invested for retirement. In many cases you can deduct the contribution on your income tax return and not pay tax on any of the income or growth until you begin taking distributions. Of course, there is no guarantee that either a defined benefit or defined contribution plan will provide adequate income for retirement. Again, factors including ages of the employees, salary levels, and the number of employees in a practice will impact the choice of a retirement plan. Prepare a census (each employee's age and salary information) and present this to your advisor and he or she should be able to assist you in developing the retirement plan that is best for you.

PRACTICE VALUATION

What is a radiology practice worth? The simple answer is that it is worth what an unrelated buyer is willing to pay. This price is defined as the fair market value. If you are in the process of buying or selling a practice, you should obtain a valuation from an independent third party. Valuations are used to determine the fair market value of a privately held entity when considering a sale, negotiating agreements between partners, or when funding a buy-sell agreement with insurance. There are different levels of valuation reports ranging from a mere calculation of value to an opinion of value. The level of the report required depends on the purpose of the valuation.

There are three basic valuation methodologies that are used in valuing a privately held entity: (1) the *asset* method, (2) the *income* method, and (3) the *market* method (the market method is discussed further under Discounted Future Earnings Value). Each method considers different factors in the calculation of value, and therefore the method or methods ultimately used should be chosen based on the specific circumstances of the entity valued.

The *asset* method involves an analysis of the entity's assets over its liabilities. The fair market value of the entity is based on the difference between the fair market value of the entity's assets and liabilities. This method does not consider the operating earnings of the company and is typically used to value family limited partnerships holding real estate, entities holding significant hard assets, or entities liquidating.

The *income* method relies on the past or future earnings of the entity. The two primary income methods are capitalization of earnings and discounted cash flow (DCF). Under the capitalization of earnings method, the average annual historic earnings of the entity are capitalized using an appropriate capitalization rate to arrive at a value. The capitalization rate is no more than a multiplier used to convert a defined stream of income to a present value. This method is appropriate when the entity has a long track record of consistent performance and is not experiencing a growth trend.

2006	$400,000
2005	350,000
2004	300,000
2003	250,000
2002	200,000
Total (divided by 5)	$1,500,000
Average Earnings (x 10)	$300,000
Capitalized Earnings	$3,000,000

The DCF method bases the value of the company on the present value of its projected future earnings, plus the present value of its terminal value. The projected future earnings and terminal value are discounted using an appropriate discount rate. This method is appropriate when the entity is experiencing tremendous growth and has forecast its income stream into the future. The following example assumes base net earnings of $400,000, a 10% growth rate and a 4% discount rate:

2007	$440,000
2008	484,000
2009	532,400
2010	585,640
2011	644,204
	$2,686,244
Discounted at 4%:	$2,403,960

97

DISCOUNTED FUTURE EARNINGS VALUE

The third basic valuation method used in valuing a privately held entity is the *market* method, which relies on a comparison of what other similar entities have sold for in the past. This method uses recently sold businesses to develop market multiples that are then applied to the subject entity. The multiples can be based on EBITDA, net income, cash flow, or other financial statistics but are typically derived from income. The range runs from lower multiples indicating a high degree of risk to high multiples where there is minimal volatility.

In the purchase or sale of a practice, the appropriate valuation method to be used is always a matter of negotiation. For tax purposes as well, there is no individual method of valuation that is accepted by the IRS. The Treasury Department issued Revenue Ruling 59–60 which enumerates the fundamental factors that must be evaluated when preparing a valuation. These factors include the type of business, economic outlook of the particular industry, book value, earning capacity, and intangibles (including goodwill). To determine a reasonable value for sales or for tax purposes, multiple methods must be considered. The different methods would yield a range of values from which an average value could be calculated.

SUMMARY

Accounting has many terms, financial statements, and ratios. As a doctor, you are not only treating patients, you are an independent business owner on whom your family and employees rely. A good understanding of financial information is therefore essential and will keep you apprised as to your financial stability. This knowledge can also help you identify growth opportunities, such as potential mergers with or acquisitions of other practices. Just like with your investment portfolio, you cannot afford to rely completely on a trusted advisor to interpret the data and make all the crucial financial decisions for you.

Dos and Don'ts of Accounting	
Dos	**Don'ts**
1. Evaluate technology and obsolescence as well as cost in determining whether to buy or lease.	1. Rely solely on historical data.
2. Use multiple methods to value a practice.	2. Focus on the net income.
3. Read all financial statement footnotes.	3. Pass over income tax incentives.
4. Consider relevant ratios.	4. Disregard potential cost savings and economies of scale.
5. Consult financial professionals for assistance.	5. Ignore red flags.

REFERENCES

1. Ittelson TR: Financial Statements—A Step-by-Step Guide to Understanding and Creating Financial Reports. Career Press, 1998.

2. Thomsett MC: Annual Report 101: What the Numbers and the Fine Print Can Reveal about the True Health of a Company. New York, American Management Association, 2007.

The Resource-Based Relative Value Scale

Martin Bledsoe, Robin A. J. Hunt, and
Jeffrey C. Langdon

INTRODUCTION

Since the Medicare bill was signed into law by President Lyndon B. Johnson in 1965, the federal government has undertaken various approaches for reimbursing hospitals and physicians for their provision of care. Implementing a payment mechanism that is both equitable among providers and operated within monetary constraints is not an easy task. As our nation's largest health care payer and provider, Medicare has understood the problems inherent with several of the historical reimbursement methods. In 1992, after several years of study and modifications, the federal government instituted the current reimbursement method—the Resource-Based Relative Value Scale (RBRVS).

This chapter provides an evolutionary overview of the RBRVS, discusses its general workings and relative value unit derivation, presents the dimensions of the RBRVS payment structure, and provides a detailed look at actual payment calculations.

HISTORY OF MEDICAL CARE REIMBURSEMENT IN THE UNITED STATES

Usual, Customary, and Reasonable Charges

Prior to the implementation of the RBRVS, Medicare's reimbursement was based on usual, customary, and reasonable (UCR) charges. The following explains the rationale behind each component of a UCR charge as well as other terms that are important to understanding billing:

Usual (U) Charges: The average charge that the providing physician charges for the service.
Customary (C) Charges: The average amount charged by physicians in the same specialty and locality.
Reasonable (R) Charges: The maximum amount that the insurer is willing to pay for the procedure.

Billed Amount: The amount charged for a service before discounts are applied.

Deductible: The amount of money patients are required to pay each year before insurance companies pay for medical care. It may range in magnitude according to the insurance plan.

Discount: A percentage below the billed amount that the provider agrees not to charge the patient.

Allowed Amount: The amount health plans agree to pay after UCR charges and/or discounts are applied.

Insurance companies determined the amount paid to physicians by collecting data on UCR charges. The payment to the provider was the amount equal to the lowest charge out of the three. Some physicians were given the option to participate in contracts with insurance companies that stated the UCR rate would be considered full payment, thus relieving patients from responsibility for the remaining balance. In cases where the physician did not participate with this sort of an agreement with insurance companies, patients were responsible for any additional costs over the UCR rate given to them by insurance companies.

UCR charges experienced a great deal of criticism. Not only were they considered difficult to administer but they were also inflationary. Because they were linked to historic charges, costs increased with no control methods to enforce containment. In addition, they were biased in favor of specialists and surgeons. Because there was no standardized method to update charges, the rate system became increasingly irrational.

As health care costs continued to rise, it became clear that the UCR charge system was an ineffective mechanism to control health care spending because future charges were heavily dependent upon current charges and the incentive was to constantly increase charges. Therefore, high charges were transferred from year to year.

In addition to the problem of contributing to inflation in health care spending, UCR charges were also unreliable in predicting the amount of reimbursement. In most cases, patients and providers were unaware of the reimbursement amount until it was received.

Furthermore, charges were highly dependent on resource use favoring technical procedures including surgery, laboratory, and radiology services. General services began to suffer from comparatively low reimbursement. As medical costs began to increase with the complexity of procedures, so did the need for a new or improved method of reimbursement.

Evolution of RBRVS

In an effort to develop a new method of reimbursement that was more effective than the current UCR charge methodology, the Health Care Financing Administration (HCFA)—now known as the Centers for Medicaid and Medicare Services (CMS)—initially contacted the American College of Radiology (ACR) to develop an alternative system. Although the ACR submitted a methodology, in the end HCFA supported a system developed by Dr. Hsiao from the Harvard School of Public Health. The system was based on his Resource-Based Relative Value Scale Study. The purpose of the study was to develop a fee structure based on the consumption of resources. By determining the physicians' resource requirements for work, and measuring them in a standardized fashion, the Hsiao study created a reimbursement method that allowed for comparison of costs between physicians, regardless of specialization.

To accurately measure the work entailed in procedures, the Hsiao study focused on three key metrics: (1) physician work, (2) costs associated with maintaining a practice, and (3) opportunity costs. The physician work included any time spent before, during, and after a procedure with intensity of effort taken into consideration. Costs were inclusive of operating and supply costs. Because no consistent method of reporting data existed among specialties, after receiving physician input, Hsiao developed a comparison scale to ensure cross-specialty alignment. This meant that for the first time the work of a radiologist could be compared to that of a surgeon.

In addition to developing new metrics, the Hsiao study also concluded that the UCR charge method did not accurately reflect resource consumption. For example, regardless of the level of provider education or experience, invasive and imaging services were reimbursed a higher rate than patient management and evaluation services. However, the most important result of the Hsiao study was a resource-based relative value scale (RBRVS) that allowed comparison of work and resources for all procedures, regardless of the specialty performing them.[9] Within each specialty, procedures were assigned a numerical value of Relative Value Units (RVUs) to represent the amount of work involved. Further detail regarding the calculation and derivation of RVUs is covered later in this chapter.

RBRVs

On January 1, 1992, CMS introduced the current system, RBRVS, which was a modified version of the proposed system in the Hsiao study. In CMS's system, each procedure or service was classified by a Current Procedural Terminology (CPT) code that was used nationwide and had an assigned number of RVUs, based on physician work, practice expense, and malpractice expense. Because CMS is the largest third-party payer in the U.S., its system served as the precedent in developing policies and procedures. Other nongovernmental third-party payers adopted the same or similar CMS methodology. Private payers often target payments at a defined percentage less than or more than the CMS payment.

The impact of using RVUs to define reimbursement alleviated prior concerns that specialty services received a higher rate of reimbursement than primary care services and established charges according to the required work and resources needed. The result of the new fee schedule was an increase in primary care reimbursement, and a decrease among some specialty service reimbursements. In addition, this system allowed comparison of services between specialties and estimation of reimbursement. Most importantly, it established a single national payment methodology through CPT coding and defined RVUs for procedures and physician encounters.

RVUs not only help to compare procedures or services across disciplines, but they also provide physicians with common productivity metrics. As a result, physicians are able to compare the number of RVUs at work to determine how they spent their time, as well as to assess the complexity of their exams and procedures. Although it is now possible to compare the work of a neuroradiologist to that of an interventional radiologist or pediatrician through RVUs, the education level of the provider is not taken into consideration. When using RVUs to benchmark productivity between physicians, the RVUs are often adjusted to reflect the percentage of time the physician is clinically productive. This can be based on a per-clinic session, or on hours of clinical work. In academic medical centers, adjustments are often made by full-time equivalent (FTE) to account for time spent in research, since individuals funded through grants do not spend the same percentage of effort at clinical work as unfunded physicians. Hence, the RVUs for a person whose salary is 50% funded by the NIH would be expected to be half those of another physician performing the same work on a full-time basis. This physician would be considered to be 50% of an FTE or, as usually stated, 0.5 FTE.

While the RBRVS resulted in more accurate relative reimbursement, there were still concerns regarding the fairness of the system. Debate continued about the equity reimbursement across specialties. Furthermore, some critics noted that RVUs did not always take changes to the health care market or environment into consideration. They also did not effectively allow for differences in case complexity, in circumstances in which physicians performed the same procedures on different patients requiring varying amounts of time due to widely variable clinical presentations. Finally, RBRVS does not provide any measurement of the quality of patient care or patient satisfaction.[7]

The system is sometimes criticized within radiology subspecialties since, as designed, the RVUs are not perfectly "relative." A radiologist reading plain films full time will not generate as many RVUs as a radiologist reading MRIs or CTs full time. Since both contribute equally to the job of doing the radiology group's work, sometimes an adjustment factor is applied when benchmarking productivity. Recently published adjustment factors are 50% for Interventional Radiology, 58% for CT and MRI, and 130% for nuclear medicine. Table 8-1 shows how these adjustments would be made for some commonly used CPT codes. This same group of CPT codes will be used repeatedly as an example throughout

Table 8-1   Adjusted RVUs to Be Used for Workload Benchmarking

	CPT Code	Total Professional	Productivity Adjustment	Adjusted Productivity
Chest PA and lateral	71020	0.30	100%	0.30
Upper GI	74240	0.95	100%	0.95
Barium enema	74270	0.95	100%	0.95
Head CT without	70450	1.17	58%	0.68
Chest CT with contrast	71260	1.70	58%	0.99
Abdominal CT with contrast	74160	1.75	58%	1.02
Pelvic CT with contrast	72193	1.59	58%	0.92
RUQ ultrasound	76705	0.81	100%	0.81
Pelvic ultrasound	76705	0.81	100%	0.81
MRI brain with and without	70553	3.24	58%	1.88
MRI cervical spine without	72141	2.20	58%	1.28
MRI lumbar spine without	72148	2.04	58%	1.18
Nuclear bone scan, whole body	78306	1.19	130%	1.55
PET of whole body with CT#	78816	3.47	N/A	N/A
Abdominal aortogram and run-off	75605	1.58	50%	0.79
Bilateral ECA angiogram	75662	2.31	50%	1.16
KUB	74241	0.95	100%	0.95

Adapted from Lu Ying, Arenson RL: The academic radiologists productivity: An update. Acad Radiol 12:1211–1225, 2005.

this chapter. It is important to remember that these adjustments are useful in comparing the workload between subspecialty radiologists, but the adjusted RVUs are totally unrelated to actual payment mechanism.

RVU DERIVATION

The Importance of CPT Codes

The first step in assigning RVUs to a procedure or service is defining a CPT code. Used nationwide, CPT codes are standardized across disciplines, allowing effective communication between parties. Most procedures or services within every discipline have a unique CPT code.

The system allows submission of a generic code for "radiology procedure not otherwise specified." In this case, a charge is submitted and payers make a judgment about paying the charge on a case-by-case basis. However, for the vast majority of procedures that do have codes, this method eases classification. Nevertheless, CPT coding and determination of RVUs are complex. Within a practice, accurate coding is critical to maximizing the level and timeliness of reimbursement. In many cases, descriptions for procedures are similar, but so specific that the wrong codes are sometimes used when billing for procedures. As a result, each year coding errors result in reimbursements that are either too high or low. Medicare considers it each provider's responsibility to submit CPT codes that most accurately reflect the actual procedure performed. Failure to do so can be considered fraud and can be associated with fines that far exceed the amount of the incorrectly received reimbursement. Not only must the codes be accurate, they must be supported with documentation in the body of the image interpretation. If the CPT code for a two-view chest study is submitted, the report must clearly say that the physician reviewed two views of the chest. Simply reviewing findings without documenting the type of study being reviewed places the radiologist at risk for the practice of accepting payment for CPT codes that could not be supported by documentation, a potentially fraudulent practice.

The first CPT codes were developed by the American Medical Association (AMA), and only contained codes for selected procedures; radiology codes were not included in this original group. Subsequent updates included a transition from four-digit to five-digit codes, and eventually included internal medicine, radiology, and other diagnostic and therapeutic procedures. CPT codes eventually evolved to cover thousands of medical procedures, and are classified into three categories:

1. Category I codes consist of a five-digit number with a specific description of the procedure or service. In general, the procedures and services marked by these codes are consistently performed and are considered to be the most current and widely used. They are tied to the RVUs that define payment.
2. Category II codes comprise performance measurement codes. Data collection and quality-of-care measurements are facilitated through the use of these codes, which are associated with procedure outcomes or compliance. An example of a Category II code is "assessment of tobacco use." Although these codes are useful in evaluation, their use is not mandated.
3. Category III codes differ from those of Categories I and II because they are temporary, do not have RVUs associated with them, and are used for emerging technologies. They may be used as part of the FDA approval process or to substantiate widespread use of a new technology. They are codes that are not yet approved by CMS for

payment. Because there are no RVUs associated with these new codes, payment is at the discretion of nongovernmental carriers. CMS states that "[i]t is not reasonable for private insurers to categorically deny payment for CPT Category III codes since they are effectively more specific, more functional versions of unlisted codes which many payers cover with appropriate documentation." Often, after a year of use, RVUs are assigned to Category III codes, and they then become a new reimbursable Category I code. If they are not adopted after five years, Category III codes are deleted.

Code Requirements

The AMA maintains and approves all codes through the CPT Editorial Panel and CPT Advisory Committee. The CPT Editorial Panel consists of physicians who are nominated by the AMA or third-party payers. The panel's purpose is to maintain the current codes by making any necessary changes. The CPT Advisory Committee comprises physicians associated with AMA House of Delegate societies, which includes the American College of Radiology and cites the following objectives as described by the AMA:

1. Advise the CPT Editorial Panel on correct procedural descriptions for coding.
2. Support services or procedures under consideration for codes to the CPT and Editorial Panel.
3. Suggest CPT revisions.
4. Facilitate education and publication, maintain knowledge of coding concerns.
5. Educate members on the usefulness of CPT codes.

Because Category I, II, and III codes differ as to the type of procedure or service they represent, as well as their intended use, the requirements for each group vary. The AMA sets the following criteria for a Category I code:

- The Food and Drug Administration (FDA) must approve each service's or procedure's use of drugs.
- The service or procedure is used nationwide.
- Clinical efficacy has been proven through peer-reviewed U.S. literature.

- Prior use of the procedure or service has not taken place, and the code is not encompassed in another procedure or service.
- The procedure or service is not an unusual event associated with a current or previous procedure or service.

As mentioned earlier, Category II codes are associated with quality and performance measurement. Therefore, the Performance Measures Advisory Group focuses on the following (as stated by the AMA) when considering a procedure or service for Category II:

- A national organization has developed evidence-based measurements for the procedure or service through health outcomes.
- The measurements consider risk and cost and are commonly used in the health care environment.

Whereas Category I codes have specific requirements, Category III codes are not held under stringent requirements. However, procedures or services must meet the following criteria, as described by the AMA:

- A current protocol must be available.
- Specialties must be in favor of the procedure or service.
- Publications supporting the procedure or service in the form of peer-reviewed U.S. literature must be accessible.
- U.S. clinical trial documentation must be available proving the effectiveness of the service or procedure.

Category III codes are released on January 1 and July 1 of each year, and may be used six months after release.

Evaluation and Management (E&M) Codes

Evaluation and management (E&M) codes were also introduced as a complement to CPT codes. E&M codes are used by most physicians for office visits that include various levels of history and physical examination, as well as developing treatment plans and otherwise making decisions about a patient's care. CMS provides specific guidelines for selecting the various E&M codes. These are most relevant in radiology to the practice by interventional radiologists who see

Table 8-2 Office Visit RVUs		
	New Patients (99201–99205)	**Established Patients (99211–99215)**
Level I	.97	.57
Level II	1.72	1.02
Level III	2.56	1.39
Level IV	3.62	2.18
Level V	4.60	3.17

Adapted from Medicare resource-based relative value scale (RBRVS), January 2006.

patients in clinics or who spend lengthy periods in interviews, examinations, and counseling sessions with patients about their therapeutic options. The RVUs for new patients are established at a rate higher than those for previously seen (established) patients. Some examples with their associated RVUs follow. Level I exams are quick and simple, compared to Level V exams, which include complete histories and physicals, as well as making complex treatment decisions and coordinating care with other providers or agencies. All aspects of the history, physical, treatment decision, and coordination with other providers must be documented to justify the use of the code.

Table 8-2 is accurate for patients seen in a "non-facility" such as a freestanding office visit. It represents all components of the professional fee RVU. The total is less if the visit takes place in a "facility" (e.g., a hospital) but, in that case, the hospital and not the physician could charge the practice expense component of the RVU. There will be a review later in the chapter of the three components of the RVU.

Updating Codes

As medical technology continues to evolve, procedures and services often change as well. While some Category I codes are no longer used and are deleted, many Category III codes advance to Category I as new technologies are adopted. In an effort to maintain effectiveness, codes are continually updated on an annual or biannual basis. In an effort to encourage necessary code changes, the AMA provides code change request forms. Forms require specific information as to why current codes are not sufficient, description of the procedure, work involved, and typical patient, as well as peer-reviewed literature that explains the purpose of the procedure or service as well as its efficacy.

The process of determining a CPT code for a procedure or service is very detailed, and encompasses several activities and sometimes years of work. Once a procedure or service has received an accurate CPT code, RVUs are assigned by the AMA-assigned committee, which, as noted above, is appointed by the ACR.

UNDERSTANDING THE RESOURCE-BASED RELATIVE VALUE SCALE (RBRVS)

Key Abbreviations

- CMS—Centers for Medicare and Medicaid Services
- CPT—Current Procedural Terminology
- HCFA—Health Care Financing Administration
- GPCI—Geographic Practice Cost Indices
- MFS—Medicare Fee Schedule
- NPI—National Provider Identifier
- RBRVS—Resource-Based Relative Value Scale
- RBRVU—Resource-Based Relative Value Unit
- RVU—Relative Value Unit
- UPIN—Unique Physician Identification Number

Overview

We have now established a basic understanding for the rationale behind the Centers for Medicare and Medicaid Services (CMS) (formerly Health Care Financing Administration [HCFA]) and the introduction of the resource-based relative value scale (RBRVS). Before moving on to the remainder of the chapter, which focuses on applications of that scale, we should note that to receive payments from CMS for services, physicians must apply for and receive several unique identifiers. UPIN (Unique Physician Identification Number) and NPI (National Provider Identifier) are examples. Processing the applications can take

several weeks. To allow time for this procedure, physicians should begin the credentialing process with their employer well before they intend to begin generating professional fees.

You should thoroughly comprehend the financial payment mechanisms under which you and your business entity—whether a private group practice or a large academic health care system—will be reimbursed for the provision of services. In the constantly evolving health care environment, you should have a solid grasp of the principles of the RBRVS. Without a working knowledge of the underlying structure behind clinical revenue streams, you will be at a disadvantage when trying to actively manage your service line(s) or business. Difficulties will arise when trying to collaborate with management personnel to increase market share through service expansion, improve profitability to cover operating and capital expenditures, negotiate third-party contracts, or enhance your personal wealth.[4] Many year-end bonuses paid to physicians are weighted based on the resource-based relative value units (RBRVUs) generated during the fiscal year under consideration. Radiologists' productivity is often measured using the clinical RBRVUs generated. The justification for this basis of measurement is that the RBRVS system is a proxy (subject to the limitations previously noted for the difference between modalities) for the amount of effort or resources consumed in providing the specific imaging service. Maybe the most compelling reason for developing a comprehensive understanding of the RBRVS system is that our nation's largest health care payer, the federal Medicare system, uses a Medicare Fee Schedule (MFS) system based on RBRVUs to pay physicians. Since most other large third-party payers typically follow the lead of Medicare, they too are paying health care providers based on varying forms of the RBRVS scale.

RBRVS Structure[2]

Prior to discussing and walking through an actual RBRVU payment calculation, let's first take a look at the structure of the payment system. The structure of the RBRVS payment system breaks down the overall global payment into two distinct components: a technical component and a professional component (Fig. 8-1). Based on a sampling of radiology

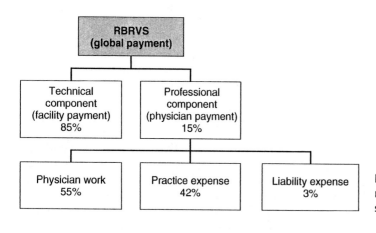

Figure 8-1 Schematic of the resource-based relative value system (RBRVS).

codes using the 2006 MFS within the Los Angeles, California, Medicare locality, the technical payment averages around 85% of the total compensation, while the professional fee makes up the balance, or approximately 15%. In Table 8-3, you will note that the exact mix of professional and technical reimbursement depends on the combination of procedures performed in a practice. A practice with a higher mix of X-ray studies will have a lower technical percentage, while a practice performing predominately cross-sectional studies will have a higher technical percentage. While we have yet to discuss the exact calculations, this table provides an illustration of the global payment breakdown for the Los Angeles sampling. Now you understand why it is so advantageous to *own* the equipment in radiology; although it varies by modality, the vast majority of the global fee is in the technical component. This is evident from and shown in Table 8-4, where the professional component ranges from a low of 11% to a high of 38%.

Technical Component

The technical segment is payment for expenses that are not directly related to the physician's effort. Technical reimbursement is intended to cover costs attributed to the facility where the care is provided, equipment for the imaging study, and technical staff associated with producing the diagnostic and/or therapeutic image. If the physician is providing the service in a hospital or hospital-based facility, the technical payment is received and booked as hospital revenue. The hospital or hospital-based facility finances the building and infrastructure for patient care, purchases the capital equipment for the imaging studies, and employs the technical staff assisting with the procedures. Therefore, they receive the revenue to help cover their expenditures. When the care is provided in a hospital or hospital-based facility, the facility submits a Medicare Part A claim to capture their technical revenue, and the physician submits a Medicare Part B claim for the professional component. This is often a source of confusion to patients who do not understand why they get two bills for every imaging examination: the bill they receive shows the 80% that Medicare paid, and the 20% that the patient will pay (unless the 20% is covered by another insurer). This 80/20 split is reflected on both the bill for the technical fees and the bill for the professional fees, so it is not surprising that many patients are perplexed by their bills. This confusion is mitigated somewhat if the facility is freestanding, because both the technical and professional payments would be made by Medicare Part B under the global payment.

Professional Component

The professional segment is payment directly received by the physician for her or his resource inputs into the health care encounter. The professional payment is divided into three subordinate components: physician work, practice expense, and malpractice insurance (detailed in the following sections). Because the costs of health care continue to escalate, when Congress convenes to pass the annual

Table 8-3 Global Payment Breakdown for Procedure Sampling from Los Angeles, CA, Medicare Locality

Los Angeles, CA GPCIs 2006 Conversion Factor	Work 1.041 $37.8975	PE 1.156		MP 0.954	Professional Component				
	CPT Code	Global Payment	Technical Fee	Work	Practice Expense	Malpractice Expense	Total Professional	Prof/ Global
Chest PA and lateral	71020	$41.02	$28.91	$8.68	$3.07	$0.36	$12.11	30%
Upper GI	74240	105.85	67.47	27.22	10.08	1.08	38.38	36
Barium enema	74270	117.68	79.30	27.22	10.08	1.08	38.38	33
Head CT without	70450	265.42	218.17	33.53	12.27	1.45	47.25	18
Chest CT with contrast	71260	395.51	326.82	48.92	17.96	1.81	68.69	17
Abdominal CT with contrast	74160	386.97	316.30	50.10	18.40	2.17	70.67	18
Pelvic CT with contrast	72193	380.52	316.30	45.76	16.65	1.81	64.22	17
RUQ ultrasound	76705	98.39	65.71	23.28	8.32	1.08	32.68	33
Pelvic ultrasound	76705	98.39	65.71	23.28	8.32	1.08	32.68	33
MRI brain with and without	70553	1,281.33	1,150.44	93.11	34.17	3.62	130.89	10
MRI cervical spine without	72141	606.70	517.83	63.12	23.22	2.53	88.87	15
MRI lumbar spine without	72148	657.17	574.78	58.39	21.47	2.53	82.39	13
Nuclear bone scan, whole body*	78306	245.22	197.14	33.93	12.70	1.45	48.08	20
PET of whole body with CT†	78816	1,390.28	1,250.00	98.63	37.68	3.98	140.28	10
Abdominal aortogram and run-off*	75605	646.02	582.23	44.97	16.65	2.17	63.79	10
Bilateral ECA angiogram*	75662	675.74	582.23	65.49	25.85	2.17	93.51	14
KUB	74241	107.16	68.78	27.22	10.08	1.08	38.38	36
Total		7,499.39	6,408.13				$1,091.26	
	Technical		85%			Profes	15%	

Adapted from http://www.cms.hhs.gov/apps/ama/license.asp?file=/physicianfeesched/downloads/rvu06c.zip.
*Additional codes for injection or surgical procedures will be generated with these.
†Not covered through CPT/RVUs, APC #154 reimbursement set at $1,250 in 2005.

Table 8-4 RVU Components for Selected Commonly Performed Procedures

	CPT Code	Technical Component	Professional Component				
			Work	Practice Expense	Malpractice Expense	Total Professional	Professional Percent of Global
Chest PA and lateral	71020	0.66	0.22	0.07	0.01	0.30	31%
Upper GI	74240	1.54	0.69	0.23	0.03	0.95	38%
Barium enema	74270	1.81	0.69	0.23	0.03	0.95	34%
Head CT without	70450	4.98	0.85	0.28	0.04	1.17	19%
Chest CT with contrast	71260	7.46	1.24	0.41	0.05	1.70	19%
Abdominal CT with contrast	74160	7.22	1.27	0.42	0.06	1.75	20%
Pelvic CT with contrast	72193	7.22	1.16	0.38	0.05	1.59	18%
RUQ ultrasound	76705	1.5	0.59	0.19	0.03	0.81	35%
Pelvic ultrasound	76705	1.5	0.59	0.19	0.03	0.81	35%
MRI brain with and without	70553	26.26	2.36	0.78	0.1	3.24	11%
MRI cervical spine without	72141	11.82	1.6	0.53	0.07	2.20	16%
MRI lumbar spine without	72148	13.12	1.48	0.49	0.07	2.04	13%
Nuclear bone scan, whole body*	78306	4.5	0.86	0.29	0.04	1.19	21%
PET of whole body with CT[†]	78816	?	2.5	0.86	0.11	3.47	
Abdominal aortogram and run-off*	75605	13.29	1.14	0.38	0.06	1.58	11%
Bilateral ECA angiogram*	75662	13.29	1.66	0.59	0.06	2.31	15%
KUB	74241	1.57	0.69	0.23	0.03	0.95	38%

From http://www.cms.hhs.gov
*Additional codes for injection or surgical procedures will be generated with these.
[†]Not covered through CPT/RVUs, APC # 1514 reimbursement set at $1,250 in 2005.
[‡]Note: All RVUs are for 2006. The 2007 deficit reduction act decreased some values.

Medicare budget, they often try to reapportion funds between government programs, thus controlling spending on health care. The same concept applies in the RBRVS payment system. If malpractice costs begin rising as they have in recent years, RVUs for the malpractice insurance component may be increased commensurate to the rising insurance premiums. In an attempt to stay budget neutral, the federal government will often offset the RVU increase in one area with a decrease in another. In this case they may lower the RVU value of the physician work due to the increase in the malpractice insurance RVUs.

Physician Work

As noted in Figure 8-1, physician work constitutes the majority, or approximately 55%, of the total relative value of each professional payment. It represents the physician resource input in providing the service, which averages about 8.25% (55% of 15% = 8.25%) of the overall charge for the study when adding in the technical fee. In broad terms, physician work encompasses professional costs related to the time, training, skill, and intensity or stress of the particular service provision. When considering the time aspect of the physician work, it includes the preservice, intraservice, and postservice efforts. Through this measurement, the setup time, actual patient encounter, and postprocedure activities are all noted. This methodology makes it clear why efficiency is the linchpin under this payment methodology.

No additional payment is received if additional time is taken to set up a procedure room, perform an imaging study, or dictate a case and consult with the patient. One cannot add an E&M code for time in proximity to the performance of a procedure; an exception might be a clinic visit a week in advance of the regularly scheduled visit may be acceptable for use of a separate E&M code.

Practice Expenses

The second largest portion of the professional payment—practice expense—averages around 42% of the 15% charged under the professional component, hence, 6.3% of the global fee. RVUs in this category have been assigned to reflect the practice expenses consumed in providing care. Office supplies, utilities, labor, expenses associated with billing and collections, as well as rent are examples of practice expenses. It may help to think of practice expenses as those that are general operational expenditures required for daily operations.

Malpractice Insurance

The smallest portion of the professional payment, approximately 0.45% of the combined professional and technical RVU, is the malpractice fee. This amounts to 3% of the total professional RVU and is attributed to malpractice insurance. As implied by its name, this payment is made to help offset professional liability expenses. Although malpractice premiums have been skyrocketing over the past decade, the RBRVU system has not been modified to reflect these recent increases in premium expense.

Geographic Practice Cost Indices

After the relative value units have been assigned to each of the components listed above, they are adjusted to account for the variability in the cost of living across the different Medicare localities throughout the United States. This adjustment is called the geographic practice cost index (GPCI). On a national basis, the GPCI will equal 1.0. If the cost of living in a particular region is higher than the national average, then the GPCI for that area will be higher than 1.0. Conversely, geographic regions with costs below the national average will be assigned GPCIs less than 1.0.

As a reference, we've included Table 8-5, which presents GPCIs for 2006 by Medicare carrier and locality. As you might expect, there is significant variation between geographic regions within the United States.

Conversion Factor

The relative value units by themselves do not constitute a payment system. The relative values must be converted into dollars. A conversion factor (CF) is a multiplier that is used to convert the relative values assigned to each procedure code into monetary dollar figures. This national CF is set on an annual basis by Congress when they work on the Medicare

Table 8-5   GPCIs by Medicare Carrier and Locality*,[8]

Carrier	Locality	Locality Name	Work GPCI	PE GPCI	MP GPCI
00510	00	Alabama	1.000	0.846	0.752
00831	01	Alaska	1.017	1.103	1.029
00832	00	Arizona	1.000	0.992	1.069
00520	13	Arkansas	1.000	0.831	0.438
31140	03	Marin/Napa/Solano, CA	1.035	1.340	0.651
31140	05	San Francisco, CA	1.060	1.543	0.651
31140	06	San Mateo, CA	1.073	1.536	0.639
31140	07	Oakland/Berkley, CA	1.054	1.371	0.651
31140	09	Santa Clara, CA	1.083	1.540	0.604
31146	17	Ventura, CA	1.028	1.179	0.744
31146	18	Los Angeles, CA	1.041	1.156	0.954
31146	26	Anaheim/Santa Ana, CA	1.034	1.236	0.954
31140	99	Rest of California[†]	1.007	1.053	0.733
31146	99	Rest of California[†]	1.007	1.053	0.733
00824	01	Colorado	1.000	1.014	0.803
00591	00	Connecticut	1.038	1.170	0.900
00903	01	DC + MD/VA Suburbs	1.048	1.250	0.926
00902	01	Delaware	1.012	1.018	0.892
00590	03	Fort Lauderdale, FL	1.000	0.988	1.703
00590	04	Miami, FL	1.000	1.046	2.269
00590	99	Rest of Florida	1.000	0.934	1.272
00511	01	Atlanta, GA	1.010	1.089	0.966
00511	99	Rest of Georgia	1.000	0.872	0.966
00833	01	Hawaii/Guam	1.005	1.111	0.800
05130	00	Idaho	1.000	0.868	0.459
00952	12	East St. Louis, IL	1.000	0.939	1.750
00952	15	Suburban Chicago, IL	1.018	1.115	1.652
00952	16	Chicago, IL	1.025	1.126	1.867
00952	99	Rest of Illinois	1.000	0.872	1.193
00630	00	Indiana	1.000	0.906	0.436
00826	00	Iowa	1.000	0.868	0.589

Table 8-5   GPCIs by Medicare Carrier and Locality*,[8]—Cont'd

Carrier	Locality	Locality Name	Work GPCI	PE GPCI	MP GPCI
00650	00	Kansas[†]	1.000	0.878	0.721
00660	00	Kentucky	1.000	0.854	0.873
00528	01	New Orleans, LA	1.000	0.946	1.197
00528	99	Rest of Louisiana	1.000	0.847	1.058
31142	03	Southern Maine	1.000	1.013	0.637
31142	99	Rest of Maine	1.000	0.886	0.637
00901	01	Baltimore (Surr. Cnties), MD	1.012	1.078	0.947
00901	99	Rest of Maryland	1.000	0.980	0.760
31143	01	Metropolitan Boston	1.030	1.329	0.823
31143	99	Rest of Massachusetts	1.007	1.103	0.823
00953	01	Detroit, MI	1.037	1.054	2.744
00953	99	Rest of Michigan	1.000	0.921	1.518
00954	00	Minnesota	1.000	1.005	0.410
00512	00	Mississippi	1.000	0.839	0.722
00740	02	Metropolitan Kansas City, MO	1.000	0.975	0.946
00523	01	Metropolitan St. Louis, MO	1.000	0.955	0.941
00523	99	Rest of Missouri[†]	1.000	0.802	0.892
00740	99	Rest of Missouri[†]	1.000	0.802	0.892
00751	01	Montana	1.000	0.844	0.904
00655	00	Nebraska	1.000	0.875	0.454
00834	00	Nevada	1.003	1.043	1.068
31144	40	New Hampshire	1.000	1.027	0.942
00805	01	Northern NJ	1.058	1.220	0.973
00805	99	Rest of New Jersey	1.043	1.119	0.973
00521	05	New Mexico	1.000	0.887	0.895
00803	01	Manhattan, NY	1.065	1.298	1.504
00803	02	NYC Suburbs/Long Island, NY	1.052	1.280	1.785
00803	03	Poughkpsie/N NYC Suburbs, NY	1.014	1.074	1.167
14330	04	Queens, NY	1.032	1.228	1.710
00801	99	Rest of New York	1.000	0.917	0.677
05535	00	North Carolina	1.000	0.920	0.640

Table 8-5 GPCIs by Medicare Carrier and Locality*,8—Cont'd

Carrier	Locality	Locality Name	Work GPCI	PE GPCI	MP GPCI
00820	01	North Dakota	1.000	0.860	0.602
00883	00	Ohio	1.000	0.933	0.976
00522	00	Oklahoma	1.000	0.854	0.382
00835	01	Portland, OR	1.002	1.057	0.441
00835	99	Rest of Oregon	1.000	0.925	0.441
00865	01	Metropolitan Philadelphia, PA	1.016	1.104	1.386
00865	99	Rest of Pennsylvania	1.000	0.902	0.806
00973	20	Puerto Rico	1.000	0.698	0.261
00524	01	Rhode Island	1.045	0.989	0.909
00880	01	South Carolina	1.000	0.893	0.394
00820	02	South Dakota	1.000	0.876	0.365
05440	35	Tennessee	1.000	0.879	0.631
00900	09	Brazoria, TX	1.020	0.961	1.298
00900	11	Dallas, TX	1.009	1.062	1.061
00900	15	Galveston, TX	1.000	0.952	1.298
00900	18	Houston, TX	1.016	1.014	1.297
00900	20	Beaumont, TX	1.000	0.860	1.298
00900	28	Fort Worth, TX	1.000	0.989	1.061
00900	31	Austin, TX	1.000	1.046	0.986
00900	99	Rest of Texas	1.000	0.865	1.138
00823	09	Utah	1.000	0.937	0.662
31145	50	Vermont	1.000	0.968	0.514
00973	50	Virgin Islands	1.000	1.014	1.003
00904	00	Virginia	1.000	0.940	0.579
00836	02	Seattle (King Cnty), WA	1.014	1.131	0.819
00836	99	Rest of Washington	1.000	0.978	0.819
00884	16	West Virginia	1.000	0.819	1.547
00951	00	Wisconsin	1.000	0.918	0.790
00825	21	Wyoming	1.000	0.853	0.935

Adapted from http://www.e-mds.com/support/customer_support/gpci_updates.html.
*For 2005 and 2006 if the work GPCI falls below a 1.0 index, the work GPCI equals 1.0.
†States are served by more than one carrier.

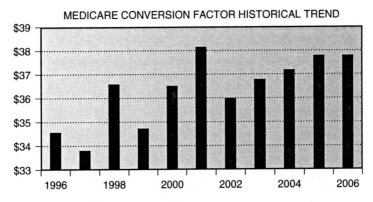

Figure 8-2   Ten-year historical trend of Medicare conversion factors (1996–2006). (American Medical Association, adapted from http://www.ama-assn.org/ama1/pub/upload/mm/ 380/cfhistory.pdf.)

budget. Simplistically, the math looks like this:

Payment = Total GPCI Adjusted RVUs × CF

One RVU does not equal one dollar. One RVU equals the dollar value assigned to the CF for that particular fiscal year. For example, the CF assigned for 2006 is $37.8975. Therefore, one RVU would equal $37.8975 during the 2006 Congressional budget year (Fig. 8-2). The next section reviews exact payment calculations and provides the details behind this example.

RBRVS Payment Calculation

As previously mentioned, the RBRVS is used both by Medicare and many third-party payers. Our case example is based strictly on federal Medicare payments. Complexities can result if third-party payer methodology was used because they typically base their payments on a variation (percentage) of the RBRVS system.

Case Example: Let's operate under the premise that you are an academic radiologist practicing in the state of Wisconsin. Jane Doe is a Medicare-insured, 93-year-old female who has been referred from her community physician for a diagnostic pelvic X-ray examination due to a recent fall. She presents at your hospital-based outpatient facility, the radiological technologist produces and processes the pelvic radiograph, and you subsequently read and dictate the case. Thankfully, no fractures or

artifacts are noted. With the assistance of her daughter and a wheelchair, Jane Doe returns home with mild discomfort and bruising.

Under the RBRVS, how much revenue will be received for Jane Doe's episode of care? How will it be apportioned between you, the academic physician, and the hospital-based outpatient facility in Wisconsin where you are practicing?

Jane Doe's medical record is sent to the hospital billing department where coders document her care and assign it to Current Procedural Terminology (CPT®) code 72190. Using the CPT code book, purchasing reimbursement software, or referring to one of the many free Internet websites, you can determine the number of RVUs assigned to each component (work, practice, malpractice) of CPT code 72190 (Box 8-1).

Physician Medicare Part B Payment Calculation[3,5]:

A. Work RVU × GPCI

B. Practice RVU × GPCI

C. Malpractice RVU × GPCI

Total RVUs (A + B + C)

National Conversion Factor $

Medicare Payment = $(A + B + C)

Applying the general formula to our case example, you can see that the total allowed Medicare professional fee is $10.39, geographically

---

BOX 8-1

CPT 72190 X-ray Exam of Pelvis—Professional Fee (RVU Modified)

Medicare Locality Wisconsin CPT Code 72190 CPT Description X-ray exam of pelvis Conversion $37.8975 Factor	Geographic Practice Cost Indices (GPCI) for Wisconsin		
	Work RVU	Practice RVU	Malpractice RVU
	1.000	0.918	0.790

Step 1: Geographically adjust the Relative Value Unit (RVU) components:

A.	Work RVU 0.21	×	Work GPCI 1.000	= 0.21
B.	Facility PE RVU 0.07	×	Practice GPCI 0.918	= 0.06426
C.	Malpractice RVU 0.01	×	Malpractice GPCI 0.790	= 0.00079

Step 2: Add the adjusted RVU components of Step 1 (A+B+C). Round to fourth decimal:
Total Geographically Adjusted RVU = 0.2743

Step 3: Multiply the Total Geographically Adjusted RVU by the appropriate
Conversion Factor:

National Conversion Factor $37.8975	×	Total Geographically Adjusted RVU 0.2743	Total Professional Medicare Fee Schedule = $10.39

Adapted from Medicare Part B Billing Guide, ingenix,® 2003.

adjusted for Wisconsin in 2006 (see Box 8-1). As a reminder, this amount will be split—80% paid by Medicare and 20% paid by either the patient or another insurer. The detailed formula presented above applies to all Medicare RBRVS payment calculations. As previously demonstrated, the only difference from the above reimbursement and that of other CPT codes is the differing RVUs assigned to each CPT and the GPCI adjustment, based on Medicare locality. The calculation for the technical fee follows and is similar, but the RVUs differ (Box 8-2).

Applying the general formula to our case example, you can see that the total allowed Medicare technical fee is $25.65, geographically adjusted for Wisconsin in 2006. Once again this amount will be split—80% paid by Medicare, 20% paid by either the patient or another insurer. At times, providers refer to the "global payment." This is the combined

fee for the professional and technical components. Medicare Part B providers that are freestanding imaging centers must bill the global fee. In the example above, it would be the combination of the two numbers in the lower right-hand corner of Boxes 8-1 and 8-2; the professional fee of $10.39, plus the technical fee of $25.65, for a global fee of $36.04.

Finally, you should be aware that Medicare claims will not be paid without an ICD-9 (International Classifications of Diseases, 9th revision) code. These codes, which for the most part correspond to diagnoses, must be appropriate for the particular examination performed. A payer usually will not approve payment for a chest study if the diagnosis submitted is ankle trauma. The ICD-9 coding system is not technically a part of RBRVS, but is a very necessary component of billing and collections.

BOX 8–2

CPT 72190 X-Ray Exam of Pelvis—Technical Fee

Medicare Locality	Wisconsin	Geographic Practice Cost Indices (GPCI) for Wisconsin		
		Work RVU	Practice RVU	Malpractice RVU
CPT Code	72190	1.000	0.918	0.790
CPT Description	X-ray exam of pelvis			
Conversion Factor	$37.8975			

Step 1: Geographically adjust the Relative Value Unit (RVU) components:

A.
Work RVU		Work GPCI	= 0.0
0.0	×	1.000	

B.
Facility PE RVU		Practice GPCI	= 0.61506
0.67	×	0.918	

C.
Malpractice RVU		Malpractice GPCI	= 0.0316
0.04	×	0.790	

Step 2: Add the adjusted RVU components of Step 1 (A+B+C). Round to fourth decimal:
Total Geographically Adjusted RVU = 0.6767

Step 3: Multiply the Total Geographically Adjusted RVU by the appropriate Conversion Factor:

National Conversion Factor		Total Geographically Adjusted RVU	Total Professional Medicare Fee Schedule
$37.8975	×	0.6767	= $25.65

SUMMARY

This chapter reviews the basics of physician reimbursement under the federally directed resource-based relative value system. Federal and state governments, third-party payers, and professional societies are in constant search of improving reimbursement methodologies. Alterations in reimbursement structures and systems—to keep pace with increasing health care costs—are a continual process.

Dos and Don'ts of the Resource-Based Relative Value Scale

Dos	Don'ts
1. Be sure your billing is done under the auspices of an imaging billing professional. The RBRVU and ICD-9 coding systems are complex and change annually. Risks of "getting it wrong" are lost collections, on the one hand, and fraudulent (even unintentional) billing, on the other.	1. Assume that because you are being paid, your billing practices are compliant with regulations. When and if incorrect billing practices are discovered, it is not unusual for an audit to review several years' worth of prior claims and assess treble damages.

Dos & Don'ts of the Resource-Based Relative Value Scale	
Dos	**Don'ts**
2. Be sure you spend some of your practice income on educating your billing staff annually. 3. State the views you are reviewing in your report to justify the CPT code that will be submitted. 4. Favor cross-sectional work, to the extent you can control the mix. Cross-sectional work carries more RVUs than plain film work. 5. Use RVUs to evaluate radiologists' productivity within a subspecialty that trends year to year.	2. Presume you don't need a compliance expert to review your documentation and billing practices—you do! 3. Use RBRVUs to compare productivity between imaging subspecialties without adjusting the RVUs. 4. Count on maximizing practice income by avoiding the expense of a professional billing staff, who have some certification of their expertise in radiology billing and coding practices. 5. Assume the RBRVU and CPT guidelines are static. Instead, become involved in professional societies that you consult, and have input into the political decisions that define changes in reimbursement.

REFERENCES

1. Available at http://www.aapmr.org/zdocs/hpl/rbrvs_historical.doc.
2. Grimaldi PL: RBRVS: How the new physician fee schedule will work (resource-based relative value scale payment system). Healthcare Financial Management Magazine 45(9):58–59.
3. Available at http://www.ama-assn.org/ama/pub/category/2292.html. 2007 RBRVS. What is it and how does it affect pediatrics?
4. Freeman LN: Resource-based relative value scale dictates revenue stream: Physician work, practice expense, professional liability insurance play key roles in reimbursements. (Pay close attention.) Ophthalmology Times (December 15, 2003), p 37.
5. Medicare Part B Billing Guide: Rules, values, and edits for the physician office. ingenix® St. Anthony Publishing/Medicode, 2003.
6. Available at http://www.cms.hhs.gov.
7. Moorefield JM, MacEwan DW, Sunshine JH: The radiology relative value scale: Its development and implications. Radiology 187:317–326, 1993.
8. Available at http://www.aap.org/visit/rbrvsbrochure.pdf.
9. Hsiao WC, Dunn DL, Verrilli DK: Assessing the implementation of physician-payment reform. N Engl J Med 328:928–933, 1993.

SUGGESTED READINGS

American College of Emergency Physicians Reimbursement Committee. The Fundamentals of Reimbursement: What Every Graduating Resident Should Know Before Starting Practice. Available at http://www.acep.org/webportal/PracticeResources/issues/reimb/

American Medical Association, http://www.ama-assn.org/.

Becker E, Dunn D, Braun P, Hsiao WC: Refinement and expansion of the Harvard resource-based relative value scale: The second phase. Am J Public Health 80(7): 1990.

Centers for Medicare and Medicaid Services, http://www.cms.hhs.gov/default.asp.

CPT Process—How a Code Becomes a Code. American Medical Association. Available at www.ama-assn.org/ama/pub/category/3882.html.

Federal Register, http://www.gpoaccess.gov/fr/index.html.

Grimaldi PL: Medicare fees for physician services are resource-based. J Health Care Finance 88(17):2002.

Johnson SE, Newton WP: Resource-based relative value units: A primer for academic family physicians. Fam Med 34(3):172–176, 2002.

Kulesher RR:: Medicare—the development of publicly financed health insurance: Medicare's impact on the nation's health care system. Health Care Manager 24(4):320–329, 2005.

Lee PR, Ginsburg PB: Building a consensus for physician payment reform in Medicare. West J Med 149:352–368, 1988.

Lu Y, Arenson RL: The academic radiologists productivity: An update. Acad Radiol 12(9):1211–1225, 2005.

Maxwell S, Zuckerman S, Aliaga P: Effects of the implementation of resource-based practice expense relative value units under the Medicare physician fee schedule, 1998–2002. A study conducted for the Medicare Payment Advisory Commission by The

Urban Institute 2005 pp 1–28. Available at http://www.medpac.gov/publications

Medicare RBRVS 2006: The Physicians Guide (published annually).

Sunshine JH, Burkhardt JH: Radiology groups' workload in relative value units and factors affecting it. Radiology 214:815–822, 2000.

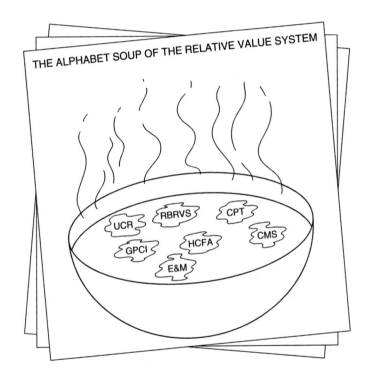

CHAPTER 9

Accounts Receivable

Norman J. Beauchamp, Jr., and Christopher J. Hurt

INTRODUCTION

The concept of accounts receivable (AR) is not novel to modern-day radiology or even health care. Indeed, in early European civilization, sponsors would send goods via ship to far-off lands. While the ships were at sea for a year or more, the goods would be considered AR. When seafarers returned from sea at a future time, with money attained from the delivery of the goods to afar, the account would be settled. What we see is that there has been a transaction. This is the essence of business. Goods, services, and properties are exchanged for goods, services, property, *and* money.

Centuries later, the similarities to the U.S. health care system are striking. Back in the day, the sponsor, who had already released his goods, might receive full payment, no payment, or anything in between. The magnitude of the return was impacted by numerous variables, such as the competence and honesty of the intermediary (the captain), good negotiation skills, supply, and regional policies. Importantly, not getting cash back could well put the ship's sponsor "out of commission." Due to the risk of obtaining a poor return and the need to ensure it was optimized, it behooved the sponsor then, and now, to do everything possible to maximize the return and keep track of the account until payment was obtained.

Understanding and optimizing your accounts receivable management must be among your highest priorities. In this chapter, we will strengthen your understanding of accounts receivable. Topics include the importance of AR to the bottom line, AR measurement and management, AR reduction strategies, bad debt, collection agencies, and AR factoring.

Accounting principles are given a more thorough review in Chapter 7. A succinct review is provided here to facilitate the discussion of accounts receivable. In addition, suggestions for further reading are supplied at the end of the chapter.

DEFINITION AND ACCOUNTING REVIEW

Accounting refers to the process of recording and summarizing business transactions, as well as interpreting their effects on the business. These transactions, and the current financial position of the company, are captured at a point in time on a balance sheet (Box 9-1). The components of the balance sheet are assets (what a business owns), liabilities (what a business owes), and the difference between the two (i.e., the owners' equity, or value of the company).

Goods and services can be purchased using cash or credit. Cash is ideal in that it immediately becomes an asset that can be used to fund operations, provide new capital, and pay dividends. In a business that deals purely in cash at the time of a transaction, there is no need for AR. However, most radiology practices scan patients on an open account basis with the agreement that the patient's insurers, or the patient, will pay for the scans in the future. Accounts receivable is the accounting record that monitors the request and the receipt of payment from a customer for the goods or services provided. It will ultimately be converted into some amount of cash. As such, AR falls into the category of assets, that is, the business owns them and there is clearly a value.

BOX 9-1

Balance Sheet for Jakenluke Imaging as of December 31, 2006

Assets	Liabilities
Current Assets • Cash • Accounts Receivable • Inventory	**Current Liabilities** • Accounts Payable
Noncurrent Assets (Fixed Assets) • Property, Buildings, Imaging Equipment • Less-Accumulated Depreciation	**Fixed Liabilities** • Loans • Issued Debt
	Owner's Equity

LIQUIDITY

Cash truly is best. Ease of conversion into cash is referred to as liquidity. A company with no liquid assets cannot pay its operating expenses or its monthly creditors. A company operating at a loss that has enough cash each month for accounts payable, salaries, and so forth, will survive, through start-up support or periods of capital investment. Lastly, as will be expanded below, even in financially stable times, the more cash is in your hands, the more it can be accruing interest or providing for more opportunities for your organization. Accordingly, the principle of converting revenue, that is, profit, into cash as soon as possible, should be of utmost interest. AR management is truly key to thriving as a successful radiology practice.

Let us take as an example an isolated one-person radiology practice with a throughput of 100 patients per day. AR takes 110 days to collect. Suddenly, throughput shoots to 200 patients per day. Wages for doubling radiology technologist and other support staff coverage must be immediately paid. Supply costs for intravenous access, film, processor chemicals, contrast dye, and so on, must be paid in 30 days. In this scenario with *immediate* accounts *payable*, the practice will be bankrupt before the 110 days it takes to collect the accounts *receivable*.

COST OF ACCOUNTS RECEIVABLE (NONCASH SALES)

In the United States, being overly disparaging about credit would do a disservice to a true driver of economic growth. Credit is important in that for all businesses it increases the buying capacity of customers. For instance, if I buy a computer with a credit card, the computer store can decide if, by extending me credit (which results in a receivable), an economic benefit is attained (i.e., improved sales), leading to improved margins and therefore profit. If I am a shady character, however, with a poor credit history, the computer store may decide, prudently but albeit much to my dismay, to deny me extension of credit, for fear of never getting their money (i.e., lack of economic benefit).

In health care, such a conscious decision to extend or not extend credit is much more limited. We have a moral obligation to care for the uninsured and underinsured. Our ability to control the partnership with third-party payers is limited. The limitations in this regard are such that AR should not be considered a method to enhance profitability.

There is a financial penalty for noncash sales (Box 9-2). Any of you who have lent money to a "pal" realize that being owed money is not equivalent to being paid money. The same is true in health care, whether the debt owed to you is from an individual, a commercial payer, or a government payer. The moment you do not receive full cash payment at the time of delivery of service, you begin to lose money. This loss of money can be categorized as (1) the time value of money, (2) opportunity costs, (3) predictability costs, (4) financing costs, (5) morale costs, and (6) costs due to payment less than the "credited" value charged for the service.

The time value of money essentially means that a dollar in hand today is worth more than a dollar in hand in the future. Imagine your wealthy grandmother said she would give you either $250,000 today or $250,000 in five years. You would obviously pick the former option. By simply investing the money, you could accrue interest and ensure that by year 5, the amount of money available to you would far exceed $250,000. The "excess" is the time value of money. Until that money is in your hands, it is a "non-performing asset." In business with receivables in the

million-dollars-plus range, these numbers become substantial. The following is a demonstration of the calculated return at an interest rate of 5%, compounded annually for five years:

$$\text{Future Value} = \text{Original Amount}$$
$$\times (1 + \text{interest rate per period})^{\#periods}$$
$$= \$250,000 \times (1 + 5\%)^5$$
$$= \$319,070 \ (\text{return} = \$69,070)$$

Unrealized cash locked in AR cannot be used to invest. For instance, there are investments that have a greater return than standard investing vehicles, such as certificates of deposit or stocks. In radiology, an example of this type of investment would be a scanner. This investment would result in obtaining improved production capacity, allowing increased revenue and ultimately translating into profits. This rate of return would exceed what the local bank can do for you. The incrementally greater return is referred to as the opportunity cost.

Predictability cost is the expense resulting from imprecise forecasting of cash receipts. Mistakes here can lead to failure to keep to budget, to meet deadlines, to tend to accounts payable, and so forth. This may require creating new budgets, the process of which engenders administrative costs.

Financing cost refers to costs associated with credit lines or other regular funding used to smooth erratic cash flow associated with collection cycles. Bank credit is often not available to practices, due to perceived health care instabilities, which require more costly financing options.

There is also the harder to characterize but very important subject of morale cost. If AR is not going well, a practice may shift from income-generating projects to tasks designed to minimize losses, leading to further cash shortage. There will be diminished incentive for employees to produce, in that the reward is not as predictable. There will be loss of confidence in leadership. A practice that cannot grow, or even maintain its current status, can lead to staff turnover, work stress, and a gloomy pessimism that stymies the very drive needed to improve financial performance.

BOX 9-2

Financial Penalty for Noncash Transactions

1. The time value of money
2. Opportunity costs
3. Predictability costs
4. Financing costs
5. Morale costs
6. Cost due to payment less than the "credited" value charged for the service

---

Another cost of credit is the cost due to receiving less payment than the "credited" value charged for a service. This occurs for a number of reasons, two of which commonly occur and are easy to quantify: low self-pay collections and denial of payment by insurance companies.

Less easy to track but also costly are loss of submitted charges, underpayment, delayed payment, and the expense of resubmission of bills. It has been estimated that ineffective revenue cycle management leads to losses of 3% to 5%. For a 400-bed hospital, this can be in the range of $10 million. Let's drive this home with a little data. A 2001 survey from the Commercial Collection Agency section of the Commercial Law League of America found that the probability of collecting a delinquent account drops quickly with time: after 90 days a practice has an approximately 73% chance of collecting; by six months, the collection rate drops to 50%.[1]

On the expense side, pursuing payment for AR is associated with substantial administrative costs. These costs include generating billing statements, following bills until paid (or written off), and collection commissions. Even the best-run practice should expect that collection costs run 3 to 4 cents for every dollar collected.

Thus, accounts receivable should be viewed as, at best, a nonperforming asset or worse, a negatively performing asset. It imposes costs on the practice: collection losses, administration costs, morale costs, and payment less than credit. In each circumstance, AR will overstate eventual cash returned. The total amount of accounts receivable at a given time point is a function of the volume of care provided that is not immediately paid for in cash, and the average length of time between sales and collections.[2]

REVENUE CYCLE/AR PROCESS OVERVIEW

The revenue cycle is the process of obtaining cash in exchange for care initially funded with credit. The revenue cycle includes preauthorizations to ensure appropriateness of the test and ability to pay, performing the indicated procedure, and coding that procedure so that an appropriate bill can be generated. An accounts receivable is initiated at the time a bill for services is generated.

Practices usually submit claims within 24 to 72 hours following outpatient encounters, and within 72 hours after inpatient discharge dates. A practice waits for validation of the discharge diagnosis (by medical records), which can delay the claim submission. Waiting for this validation is prudent, as it ensures the most accurate information from the medical records department. Unfortunately, the information needs of the medical records department (i.e., the hospital) and the radiology practice often differ requiring data retrieval, thus furthering delay of claim submission. The period from service rendered to bill submitted is referred to as the "charge lag."

Charges are held in submission until a claim is completed. Cash payments from payers return slowly, on the order of months, dictated most often by payer cash flow agendas, unless contractually arranged. Patients with large balances may arrange special payment plans, resulting in payments spanning many months, which often are not paid in full.

When payment finally arrives, payers normally include a document reflecting contract adjustments or a statement of what the payer is willing to pay. This information is then posted to the AR documentation. Bad debt and charity care is care given by hospitals but not paid for by the patient. Hospitals provide care regardless of an individual's ability to pay. Entries to this documentation that reflect bad-debt write-offs are typically not made until two to three months of seeking payment after the date of service. New charges increase the balance, while cash, contract adjustments, and bad-debt write-offs reduce the balance.

Thus, the fate of an accounts receivable can be put in two groups: (1) exams paid at the fee negotiated by the practice and payer and (2) exams paid at an amount less than expected by the practice, with the balance a potential bad debt or adjustment. The ideal outcome group is the first one, whereby payment is received per the negotiated fee, with the only difference between fee and cash received being the adjustment. No balance remains.

When payment is less than expected, all significant balances should be invoiced to patients. Certain balances may be so small that it is not cost effective to pursue them. Such small accounts should not be sent to collection agencies to pursue the payer. Other accounts are significant and should be sent to collection.

A good deal of the AR in this debit balance group likely will end up being written off. Included will be primary payer balances being pursued from patients, accounts challenged by payers due to lack of precertification or coding problems, and care related to events such as accidents resulting in physical injury, legal claims, or workers compensation, which can take years to resolve.

Lastly, there will be a small group where money is actually owed to the patient. This group is referred to as the credit balance group. The amount of refunds is generally small and may represent oversight. Possible causes include duplicate payments, overcharges, or erroneous data entry of noncash credits.

MEASURING AR

The importance of AR management to the success of your radiology business should be clear. Moreover, you can't manage what you don't measure. Along these lines, the Radiology Business Managers Association (RBMA) sought to establish a standard set of metrics, founded on commonly used performance indicators in U.S. radiology practices. Based on their analysis, they established eight key AR performance indicators for radiology practices in the United States (Box 9-3). These useful measures can be categorized as measures of time to convert billings to cash and the rate of collection relative to charges.

Days in accounts receivable is a measure of time to collection. The indicator is defined as total AR balance divided by average daily

---

BOX 9-3

RBMA Key Factors for Tracking AR

AR days outstanding
AR aging percentage over 120 days
Adjusted collection percentage (ACP)
Total write-offs as a percentage of gross charges
Total write-offs as a percentage of adjusted charges
Bad-debt recovery as a percentage of collection
Agency write-offs
Collection expense percentage
Billing cost per procedure

---

billings. Average daily billings are the average monthly gross charges divided by 30 days:

Total Accounts Receivable Calculation :

Monthly Gross Charges = \$3,000,000

Average Daily Charges = Monthly Gross Charges/30 days
= \$100,000 per day

Total Accounts Receivable = \$6,000,000

Days Accounts Receivable = Total Accounts Receivable /Average Daily Billing:

\$6,000,000/\$100,000/day = 60 days

A lower number typically indicates faster collection of outstanding balances.

Prompt claim filing after accurate patient demographic data collection, with immediate follow-up of claim denial, will ideally keep AR days low. A comparison to a standard benchmark is useful. The RBMA annually surveys radiology practices regarding accounts receivable performance. The acceptable standard is to keep days in AR under 60 (Box 9-4). In a 2003 survey of national radiology practices the mean days in AR were 63.74 days for professional billing and 77.33 days for global billing. These improved to 56.11 and 55.54 days in 2004, respectively. Such improvement is likely due to the increasing vigilance of radiology practices (in terms of AR), as well as more robust AR management systems, which use electronic claim filing and payment posting. The Centers for Medicare and Medicaid Services (CMS) is, in 2007, at the forefront of electronic billing.

There will be variation based on the payer mix of your practice, so benchmarks alone won't suffice. It is important to monitor the changes in the data for your practice. Control charts can be used to monitor variation over time, plotting adjusted collected percentage versus time, with upper and lower control limits statistically calculated. Combined with benchmarking, it will be possible to detect when there is worsened performance. AR days should be monitored for each of your different payer groups, for example, Medicaid, Medicare, Commercial, and Managed Care, as well as the total days in AR for your entire payer mix.

Too many AR days may indicate troubled collections, lax credit policies, conservative collection

---

BOX 9-4

RBMA Accounts Receivable Standards

- <60 gross AR days
- 80% of AR <90 days
- <17% total AR at 91–180 days
- <3% total AR at >180 days
- >95% accurate registration acquisition
- <5% electronic claim edit failure
- Monthly AR collections > 100% of monthly average of prior 2 ~ 3 months of net revenue
- DNFB (discharged but not final billed) <2 gross AR days beyond facility's criteria for bill-hold days
- Facility's bill-hold days <4 days for outpatient and <3 days for inpatient services
- Number of rebilled claims <5% of number of claims filed for the month
- Accounts requiring claim correction should not be on Medicare remote terminal >1 day, unless additional documents or medical records are needed, which should be followed to ensure timeliness
- Bad-debt expense <4% of gross revenue (contingent on self-pay revenue percent)
- Credit balances <1 day of gross revenue and <30 days in age
- Denials <5% of number of claims submitted for a month

Prior to service, preregistered patients' benefits should be verified, authorizations and certifications should be obtained, and patient should be advised of financial obligations. The percentage of over-the-counter payments in relation to the total self-pay revenue for the month should be tracked.

---

practices, or payer withholding of payment. You should determine when poor performance is internal to your organization or related to the performance of the payer; in either case, try to resolve the issue to lower the AR days.

It is worth noting that the payers have no incentive to pay promptly. The principle of the time value of money applies to them as well. The longer the money is in their hands, the better for them. As discussed in Chapter 22 ("Contracting with Managed Care Organizations"), contractual language as well as a commitment to partnership can facilitate fair practices. In addition, 5 CFR Part 1315, published in the Federal Registry, September

29, 1999, and effective October 29, 1999, mandated that departments and agencies need to pay commercial obligations and to pay interest penalties when payments are late. This is referred to as the Prompt Payment Act. The specifics of this Act can be found in the Federal Registry.[3] Suffice it to say, the government is attempting to hold itself accountable and there is recourse.

Time to convert bills into cash can also be measured by aggregating the bills into "duration outstanding" time bins. AR management systems have been developed with excellent segmentation properties. The first step is to break AR down by age. Age categories typically are: 0 to 30 (current), 31 to 60 days overdue, 61 to 90 days overdue, 91 to 120 days overdue, 120 to 180 or more days overdue. Subsequent categorization by account age and individual payer should also be done, as it allows trend identification. Compiling can be done by account size to identify particularly large accounts that deserve more prompt attention to maximize return. An appropriate goal is to have 80% of AR less than 90 days, less than 17% total AR at 91 to 180 days, and less than 3% total AR at more than 180 days.

You must make every effort to optimize this collection percentage. In the past, this could be monitored by looking at collections as a function of gross charges. However, it is now accepted that gross charges well exceed what can be anticipated even with a highly effective AR process. There are a number of expected deductions from gross charges that are unrelated to the effectiveness of billing, making it more appropriate to monitor net collections. Such anticipated deductions from gross charges include contractual agreements and payer allowables.

Let us use a somewhat typical example to provide clarity. You must first correct your charges to what the payer is obliged to pay. This obligation varies by payer and includes negotiated contract adjustments, government fee schedules, and refunded overpayments. For example, if you charge $70 per RVU but Medicare allows only $35, you would have an effective AR process if you recovered $34 (>97%). Thus, AR should be valued at the amount a payer is obliged to pay (net charge), not at the charge (gross) value;

such valuation allows improved comparison of revenue to AR. For this reason, collections are usually calculated at a net collection rate.

The RBMA recommended collection rate metric is the adjusted collected percentage (ACP). ACP is defined as adjusted collections divided by adjusted charges multiplied by 100. Adjusted collections are payments received less refunds and returned checks, while adjusted charges are gross charges less total adjustments. The metric discards monies not expected to be collected. Basically it's money you got versus payment you thought you'd get.

The RBMA survey (2004) provides expected results. These results are separated into ACP for profession billing in a hospital setting versus global billing for an imaging center. Median results were 90.8% for global versus 85.1% for professional billing. Outsourcing billing resulted in slightly better results for both professional and global billing. Specifically, the mean ACP for professional billing in a hospital environment improved collections approximately 2% when outsourced. Outsourcing global billing increased collection percentage over 10%.

A number of other indicators deserve monitoring. Total write-offs as a percentage of gross charges, which can be significantly affected by patient mix, should be monitored. For this indicator, appropriate categorization of adjustments and write-offs is requisite for accuracy. Write-offs expressed as percentage of adjusted gross charges should also be calculated, as this added together with ACP should be 100%.

The next indicator is refunds plus returned checks as a percentage of gross charges. If the patient is prematurely billed before the payer has paid, more refunds will be needed, leading to higher administrative costs. If refunds plus return rates exceed 1%, bills are being submitted prematurely.

Collection expense as a percentage of adjusted collections is a useful measure of productivity. To assess this indicator, consider allocation of collection expenses to include costs of dual-duty employees who work part-time on collection and part-time on other nonrelated tasks.

Billing cost per procedure is another indicator, calculated as collection expense divided by the number of procedures billed for the corresponding period. Similar to collection expense percentage, accurate tracking of collection expense

allocation is essential. Volume and extent of administrative work (e.g., insurance verification, need for seeking authorization, information collection at time of service, etc.) all obviously affect this indicator.

Once the measures are obtained, they need to be compiled in a manner that answers the necessary questions. AR must be able to be compiled by date of service, as well as billing date, which determines how long it has been since a claim was filed and insurance company efficiency. Compiling by payment date gives a date of last account activity, provides input for secondary payer filing, and enables financial class to be changed. Categorizing by account age and individual payer allows for trend identification, as well as collection period reduction. Compiling by account size can also be useful to identify particularly large accounts that deserve more prompt attention to maximize return. Unbilled account analysis is also useful, as it may ascertain why an account has not been billed, typically due to some element of missing information. By identifying trends here, it may be possible to increase efficiency of initial information capture.

By tracking by month of service, you can examine continuity, seeing which payers make up the majority of gross charges. A significant change in gross percentage for a payer may indicate the need for investigation, but such a change can result from change in a particular examination volume. Examining alterations in the group whereby payment is received in full as negotiated may also prove useful. In particular, watch changes in average cash per examination, which, again, may result from examination mix differences, but perusal of such changes may identify other more undesirable trends.

AR SYSTEMS

A hospital-based radiology practice will create 25 to 50 times the number of new patient accounts than the busiest referring physician group. Such volume necessitates automated advanced computer systems. Most systems are constructed such that payment is expected on submission of a claim to a payer. A busy practice may submit claims to over 100 different payers.

A robust AR system brings together all transactions related to AR for a given month. The system should capture and refine information, create patient accounts, file claims, bill self-pay balances, and complete adjudication of accounts in a timing pattern easily defined. That way, you can measure consistency and compare parameters on a monthly basis.

AR OUTSOURCING

No doubt the overriding goal of a radiology practice should be patient care. Nonetheless, the second goal is collecting payment after services have been rendered. No money, no mission. Collection is accomplished with either internal or outsourced billing.

The decision to internally manage or outsource billing is debatable. A centralized billing program has the potential to decrease cost through economies of scale in contracting, HR services, computer interfaces to third-party payers, and a compliance office. At my institution, we are a part of a centralized practice that enables such savings. However, our department has its own internal coders to ensure subspecialty expertise and develop a relationship that fosters an effective interaction with the faculty. If the practice is participating in a centralized practice plan, this is strongly advised.

It has been shown that return is enhanced when billing is outsourced. Before outsourcing, you should understand what goals the practice wants the outsourcing group to accomplish. The contract should detail services to be provided, performance standards, service costs, confidentiality agreements, termination means, and insistence on regulatory adherence.

Determining the right price to pay can be tricky. A vendor should deliver the system at a fixed monthly percentage rate based on receipts, not charges. Avoid any vendor that offers a standard processing rate. A desirable vendor will determine the rate based on the practice's exam volume, estimating the number of new accounts per year, which determines staffing, supply, and system needs. The vendor will then estimate cash value of an average account, based on knowledge of payer reimbursement schedules. The mix of inpatient and outpatient accounts will alter the examination number per account, on average, but a properly designed interface between AR and hospital information systems will likely render this difference in the examination number moot. The vendor will calculate the pay rate per new account to cover direct expenses, as well as, of course, to generate profit.

AUDITING AR SYSTEMS

AR system auditing is performed to check billing efficiency and integrity. Radiology billing has unique factors in that there is no control over ordering exams, no direct access to patients, and dependence on hospitals for clinical/demographic information. Audits can be exceedingly expensive, far greater than any other medical specialty, especially for radiology systems, given the vast number of accounts.

Traditional manual auditing of an AR system would sample about 10% of accounts. By constructing a database with relevant fields, auditing becomes relatively easy. If the database includes payer-specific codes and contracted fees, then payer-specific collection performance can be tracked. A variance report can be produced when payment is less than the negotiated fee.

DECREASING AR

To decrease AR, a systematic approach is desirable, rather than aggressive quick fixes. To achieve such an approach, let's examine factors that impact the return on AR.

When looking at the revenue cycle, it is useful to create a process map from scheduling to the final zero balance, so that trouble spots can be identified. This can also underscore the role of each individual in the revenue cycle. Approach the problem as a "quest" for why AR is delinquent, searching from registration to medical records, billing, collection, and final data processing. By beginning with the billing department, you can see how all other departments interact by way of billing to affect the revenue cycle.

Reports of denied claims, billing productivity, quality insurance, and electronic edit failures are necessary. If the number of denials exceeds established standards, this should prompt review to evaluate the cause. Dispute of arbitrary and capricious denials could recover significant revenue. Billing productivity should track number of claims "worked" per employee, as well as for the total billing area, and the number of re-billed claims. Such analysis allows determination of whether efficiency is negatively affected by excessive re-billing. If the re-bill rate exceeds industry standards, the cause should be queried. Quality assurance tracking will assess the registration error rate, which may indicate a need for front-end staff training.

Once the above data is collected, compare it not only to industry standards but also with regional practices. Each practice is different, with variations in state reimbursement requirements, staffing, payer mix, percent of up-front collection, and timing for account referral to collection. Moreover, differences in accounting functions can result in difficulty with comparisons. That said, certain health care standards have been proposed (see Box 9-4).[5]

After analyzing the data, look for recommendations for improvements. Some ideas to help reduce AR follow:

1. Offer incentives for signing dictations in the most timely fashion (see Chapter 14, "Voice Recognition Dictation").
2. Keep MDs informed of important changes in managed care contracts.
3. Review lost and late charges, which may allow for capture of significant revenue.
4. Conduct current and retrospective payment audits, which allow for recouping of underpayments thus maximizing AR.
5. Review on a regular basis internal and/or external CPT or ICD-9 coding, which should ensure that neither undercoding nor overcoding is practiced, thus maximizing potential revenue.
6. Have internal staff focus on AR less than 90 days old, which should increase cash.
7. Have one group of internal staff call and write to patients requesting payment, and have a second group call and write insurance companies after the patients have been contacted.
8. Verify primary and secondary insurance at time of encounter.
9. Collect charges in advance, based on an estimate of self-pay amounts.
10. Institute a minimum-payment schedule, scaled to the patients' income.
11. Develop an outreach program, stressing the importance of paying medical bills.
12. Accept credit card payments at the time of care delivery.

Scrubbers

Staying profitable requires keeping abreast with the numerous rules, policies, and guidelines established by the government and third-party payers, as reimbursement is the bulk, if not all, of practice revenue. Nonetheless, coding and policies constantly change, usually on an annual basis. One way to keep up to date is with a *scrubber*, which is a system that checks claims (prior to submission) against payer-specific coding compliance edits to ensure completion and absence of errors. This ensures a clean claim, which is less likely to be denied and leads to prompt payment thus decreasing AR. New systems are quite sophisticated, with payer-specific edits and quarterly coding updates, among other features. For example, the age-old question of whether a transabdominal and transvaginal ultrasound exam can be billed on the same day depends on local and national policy; a scrubber can be up to date with this issue, ensuring clean claim submission, maximizing the accuracy of billing, and minimizing rejections.

Many systems are Internet-based, with the capability of integrating with a practice's information system. Claims can be run individually or in batches. Problem claims are flagged and returned to the practice with an explanation, which enables the coding/billing staff to amend the claim prior to submission. This leads to decreased denials, reimbursement protection, recapture of missing charged revenue, compliance with Medicare requirements, and, ultimately, a reduction in AR. Scrubbers can tailor reports, as well as afford direct access to payer policies and coding compliance information. Ideal scrubbers are fast, processing 10 to 20 claims per second and providing real-time analysis. Granted, scrubbers entail an extra step in the billing process, but the potential of improved revenue likely outweighs having issue.

Moreover, the labor required for follow-up of rejected claims can be reduced as well.

Strategies in Dealing with Managed Care

If you are strategic in dealing with managed care, you can maximize potential collection and minimize AR days that are outstanding. Negotiating an ideal contract is clearly requisite, whereby payments are adequate, timely, and are collected without struggle. Unfortunately, obtaining such a contract can be challenging. A plan must be prepared before negotiations begin. Due diligence is naturally necessary, with knowledge of current and potential quantities of service for a payer's members. As this is a negotiation, and not an agreement by dictatorship, the contract goal is to serve both parties, providing a win-win result for both.

Key contractual elements include the following:

- Don't let the managed care plan dictate provision of services for certain patients, but not for others within the network; it should be all or nothing.
- Payment rates should reflect the number of services your practice provides, as well as how much the managed care plan needs your practice; an exclusive contract versus contracting with a large number of providers will alter the rate.
- The fee schedule should be concrete, not "to be determined by payer."
- Prepare for late payments by adding a late fee; thus fees for delays will hopefully offer incentive for prompt payment. A denial system based on mediation is necessary to prevent arbitrary denials.
- Ensure that modifications are made only by mutual agreement; allowing unilateral power to modify the contract is dictatorship in disguise. A clause permitting late claims—which will occur due to patients' failure to know who the primary payer is and administration's failure to obtain correct registration information—is necessary; otherwise, you can kiss a percentage of AR goodbye.
- Don't let hospital staff negotiate on behalf of radiology, as the interest of the practice may not be first and foremost in the minds of the hospital staff, which could lead to painful concessions.
- Collect data from the managed care plan to track actual payments, as they may be different from what the plan says they are; such information could be extremely useful in renegotiations.
- Follow-up of third-party payers is also integral to survival. AR should be worked starting with high value AR, AR greater than 120 days, then decreasing duration in AR. Know the five "W"s of dealing with payers:
  1. Who are you speaking with?
  2. What are they doing with the claim?
  3. When will the claim be paid?
  4. Where is the claim in their process, and where will the payment be sent?
  5. Why has the claim not been paid?
- Review files prior to calling payers to ensure that the discussion proceeds smoothly. It may be necessary to contact the patient and have him or her also contact the insurer to expedite payment. Payer meetings that allow many past-due claims to be addressed in one session also may provide increased efficiency.

DENIALS

Denials are a critical topic. Causes tend to fall into two groups: system denials, which result from an incomplete/improper claim, and payer denials, resulting from issues identified by the payer beyond the control of the practice. Denials should be interpreted as a means to identify problem areas that need addressing. Establishing a dialogue with payers can help to minimize denials, decreasing AR.

An ideal plan for handling denials would be to have all payers submit denials to a single address, where they are processed and resolved within five business days by a dedicated group of denial specialists. Denial categories would be standardized for each and every payer, to allow for proper tracking and reporting. Detailed denial reports, specifying denial volume and associated dollar values and broken down by denial type, payer, exam type, physician, and so on, could then be sent along to the appropriate individuals for timely resolution. Ultimately, such a process should reduce denials, improving AR. Other than auditing, referral to ACR communications guidelines and education on common coding problems may also reduce denials. In addition, credentialing should not be ignored, as failure to quickly acquire or renew physicians' credentials risks denials (see Chapter 25, "Credentialing and Certification").

NONPAYMENT AND PAYMENT DELAYS

While we're on the topic of managed care, living in an ideal world would be one in which there was a shared commitment to paying claims on time. However, this is not always the case. Disappointing behavior has included private insurance companies paying claims managers' escalating bonuses based on how long they could delay paying claims thus incentivizing delays and denials. Most plans promise payment within 30 days for clean claims, with some allowing up to 60 days. Prompt payment laws have been enacted in most states, albeit with quite a variation in the interpretation of the word "prompt": 15 days for Georgia versus 45 days for Pennsylvania. Note that the "cleanliness" of claims is up to interpretation as well.

BAD DEBT

The overall average private insurers' payment levels decreased from 1994 to 2001.[6] MedPAC attributes this trend to a shift of private enrollment out of indemnity plans into various managed care plans. In addition to decreases in collections, difficulties in successfully collecting also appear to have increased. It has been estimated that 40%[6] of the decline in the gross collections rate can be attributed to a reduction in net collections (i.e., secondary only to reduced ability to collect payments rightfully owed). The balance is due to decreases in allowed amounts or fee schedules relative to amounts billed.

A frequent cause of bad debt is inaccurate patient billing information and/or a relatively mobile patient population. One way to correct this issue is to use Internet-based search tools, which gather patient contact information from national databases. This represents a cost-effective,

labor-saving method to reduce bad debt, which decreases AR, thus improving the bottom line.

SELF-PAY PATIENTS

One primary source of bad debt is the self-pay patient, and how to effectively follow up with self-pay patients deserves separate attention. While there are special circumstances, such as screening programs for executive physicals and international health programs where payment is prompt and nearly complete, in general, self-pay—if not collected at the time of service—is closely linked to bad debt. In fact, the percentage of collections that go to bad debt will often be within a point or two of the unpaid self-pay percentage. Acknowledging that we became physicians to care for patients, we must seek appropriate fees for services if we are to sustain the patient care mission. Typically, payment is sought through a series of four or five letters sent to the patient. In a five-letter system, the first letter should serve as an immediate confirmation that the patient is indeed a self-pay client and state the summary of charges. The second letter should follow one week later in the form of a balance due statement and include payment options. If the balance due is not paid at this time by the patient, or a payment plan has not been laid out, a third letter should follow in approximately three weeks in the form of a past due notice. If still ignored by the patient, a fourth letter should follow as a delinquent past due notice. And finally, if the patient is still unresponsive, the fifth letter should serve as final notice, stating that the account will be turned over for collection. Letters should establish seriousness, urgency, state further action, and always provide payment options. Depending on practice policy, after the fifth letter, a collection call could be made. Legally, you may only speak with the patient or spouse. It is important to verify home and work telephone numbers and addresses (especially at initial registration). It is also important to ask for payment in full, ideally over the phone, by way of credit card. If the patient is unable to pay in full, offer other options, but maintain the sense of urgency. You must get a commitment from the patient and confirm agreements. Finally, documenting the call is critical.

If, after many letters and calls, patients fail to pay, options exist. Service to the patient can be legally suspended. The account can be turned over to collection. In the case of large dollar accounts, legal recourse could be a consideration, but this would prove expensive, given attorneys' fees. Small claims court, however, can be used without a lawyer. Make sure you do not provide future services unless it is a medical emergency.

WRITE-OFFS/CHARITY

Potential write-offs as uncompensated/unsponsored care include (1) the uninsured who are not expected to pay all or part of a bill, (2) the uninsured only able to pay part of a bill by way of a fee schedule based on income, (3) Medicaid or state/local patients who exceed coverage limits, (4) insured with catastrophic expenses in excess of a given percentage of annual family income, (5) Medicaid payments below the marginal cost, and (6) government program payments below cost.

Charity care allowances, arrangements to provide service at reduced rates, and provision for uncollectible accounts should be separately reported, not treated as AR. Services to a single patient can result in both charity care and bad debt. Concerning eligibility for charity care, consider the following: gross income with consideration to family size, geographic area, and so forth; net worth, to include both liquid and nonliquid assets less liabilities and claims against assets; employment status and future earning capacity; other financial obligations; amount and frequency of medical bills; and residual obligation after all other resources are applied, for example, Medicaid, welfare, and third-party payments.

COLLECTION AGENCIES[8]

While most people know that collection agencies are a valuable resource for recovering rightfully earned income, the criteria behind placing AR with an agency deserve review. Important points to consider are your radiology practice's credit policy and internal collection process. Credit policies should have a front end, detailing patient responsibilities and physician expectations, and a back end, stating the particulars of billing and collecting. With such a policy, the practice's business office can function with minimal input from physicians, only consulting them for unusual situations. In developing a policy, it must first be decided where the buck stops. Practice owners and/or physicians set rules, while business managers must grasp governmental and insurance regulations. Policy goals should establish that all AR is equal and all patients are billed the same. For example, if the collection agency has both surgical and radiology accounts, it might be inclined to pursue the surgical high-dollar value charges.

Statements must be accurate, readily understandable, and prompt. Statements should be regularly sent until fully paid, written off, or sent to an agency. Charges should not accumulate and patients should be informed of financial obligations. Slow billing encourages patient delinquency and tardiness by insurance companies; claims should be electronically filed daily.

Repeated statement billing is not without cost (not just Uncle Sam's stamp, you know). Accordingly, it must be determined how long unpaid balances will be carried. Most problems can be resolved within 90 days, with oldest AR approaching 120 to 150 days. Collecting accounts beyond 150 days is probably not cost effective, especially if billing is costing $3 per statement and you're trying to collect a $10 account.

Several points must be considered before AR is placed for collection. First, this will obviously alter the relationship between practice and patient. Perhaps this doesn't matter, especially in radiology, but it should be considered. Also, is the AR worth the collecting expense? Keeping an account open, either active or inactive, requires it to remain on the books, entailing internal or agency monitoring. All this leads to reports, letters, and phone calls. Can the account realistically be collected? If the patient is jobless and has no property, collection may be impossible. An elderly patient on Medicare may also not have resources. Unusual circumstances exist. A patient that frankly refuses to pay should be sent for collection after the practice's limit is reached. In contrast, a patient promising payment in 120 days, or when income is available, may result in an account kept longer than ideal, but at least with the assurance that payment will eventually be rendered. Be supportive when the patient is willing to assist in getting the balance paid.

In general, delinquent AR falls into three categories: AR that should never be sent for collection, AR that always should be sent to an agency, and AR that requires consideration.

Never send for collection: (1) AR entailing litigation, (2) worker's compensation cases, and (3) AR involving questioned quality of care. For litigation cases, lawyers often advise patients not to pay medical bills. Usually the attorney sends a letter of protection, which states the medical practice may get paid after the lawyer gets his or her percentage when the case is settled. If such an AR account goes for collection, the agency will increase the rate to legal level. Contingency fees for average AR at collection are one third the gross value, while the legal rate is greater than or equal to one half.

Worker's comp cases, if sent to collection, will be your bane. MDs will be called for depositions, practice staff will endlessly have to check the status, only to find out that the patient is going through the appellate process, which may take years. Of course a lawyer is involved, advising the patient to not pay the medical bill. After the lawyers get paid, don't expect much from that account, especially after the agency gets their percentage too.

Quality-of-care issues vary from dissatisfaction with the technologist or receptionist to accusations of malpractice. There may or may not be basis for complaint. Regardless, trying to get a disgruntled patient to pay is nearly impossible. If the practice business office cannot appease the unhappy patient, don't expect an agency to be able to, either. With a quality-of-care issue, an agency will shift the account back to the practice or close the account, stating that "efforts were exhausted" or some similar excuse.

In contrast, certain AR should *always* be sent for collection: (1) small balances (but not too small), (2) uncontested old accounts, (3) "skip" accounts (patient whereabouts unknown), and (4) patient fraud/abuse of services. The rule of thumb is, if internal billing costs exceed the balance, then send it to an agency. Better to pay the commission and collect a little, then to turn the account into a negative balance with internal billing costs. Moreover, this allows the practice staff to focus on more important, larger balances, which have a greater chance of collection. A limit for write-offs must also be established.

Skip accounts may not be the patient's fault, rather, a typo upon registration may have rendered the patient "lost." If simple Internet or telephone book searches prove unfruitful, agencies may have better luck.

In the case of fraud, such patients receive insurance benefit payments, which they spend, then refuse to pay the practice. This patient has no intention to pay. Aggressively pursue such an AR case. AR needing special consideration require MD involvement. Adhere to business principles to ensure equality of treatment. In the absence of a business reason to keep an account, send it for collection.

In selecting an agency, you should consider the following: medical specialization; a small, local, reputable agency; pleasant with practice staff; and a background that you have thoroughly researched. An agency familiar with medical issues will appreciate the doctor-patient relationship. Small local firms tend to achieve better results; they work hard as they need the business to stay afloat. Good firms belong to the American Collectors Association and participate in such organizations as the American Guild of Patient Account Managers or the Medical Group Managers Association. Always, always, always investigate the firm with the Better Business Bureau, the Chamber of Commerce, and the state attorney general. Negotiating a contract is important, as agencies will not state a lower limit to pursue AR, unless you negotiate one. The practice staffer appointed to deal with the agency should be watchful to ensure contract compliance. Moreover, it is important to verify that the accounts are being worked, not that the agency is merely collecting what the patient wants to pay. In addition, multiple collection agencies could be simultaneously used to compare performance. For example, 50% could go to one agency, 35% to another, and the remaining 15% to a third.

SELLING AR (FACTORING)

Selling or "factoring" of AR is a potential method to manage capital needs for a practice. Nonetheless, serious consideration must be exercised before entering into an agreement with creditors. Buyers could suddenly cease purchases, financing may be excessively complex and expensive, and the practice may (accidentally) not comply with the terms that lenders established. This may necessitate restitution or the practice may have to face fraud charges. So how does this help the practice?

Selling AR allows funds to become immediately available, rather than waiting until AR is collected. With such an accelerated cash flow, payables can be addressed sooner, sometimes resulting in a discount, or debts can be paid off sooner. Programs typically offer practices 50% of the expected AR value.

BORROWING AND LINES OF CREDIT

Borrowing against AR is another option to gain immediate cash. On one hand, borrowing does not improve the balance sheet, as debt is added equal to cash received. Moreover, the lender may impose restrictive covenants, limiting further incurrence of debt by the practice. Yet, on the other hand, operating lines of credit can provide cash on an ongoing basis. The cost of such a process is usually slightly higher than the prime interest rate and collateral may be required, for which AR could be used. Lines of credit can be obtained from commercial banks, vendors, savings and loans institutions, or savings banks.

AR SECURITIZATION

If selling AR, with all its warranties and discounts, seems too distasteful, AR securitization may be a more palatable alternative. A sponsor sells AR at a modest discount (10% to 20%) to a special-purpose vehicle (SPV), which is a corporation or trust legally related to the sponsor. The SPV borrows cash from a lender or issues securities (A1-rated commercial paper) to investors. As security for repayment, the SPV pledges the AR as collateral. When the AR is collected, the SPV pays principal and interest to the lender/investors or purchases additional AR. Similar to AR selling, the sponsor immediately collects cash, which can allow it to improve its debt-equity ratio, hence its credit rating. Even bankrupt sponsors stand to benefit, as the investment value depends on the AR value, not the sponsor's credit rating. The risk of nonpayment of the AR by a third-party payer or government agency is, relatively speaking, small.

CONCLUSION

As the largest asset of a practice, accounts receivable certainly deserves your utmost consideration. Savvy AR management can clearly enhance practice prosperity, while nonchalance will inevitably lead to doom and gloom. We hope that this chapter has been useful in giving you a better sense of AR and the management thereof. Lastly, remember that the most important aspect of a business-oriented approach to collecting AR from those able to pay is that we can continue our mission of service to all patients and also have adequate reserves to contribute to society's responsibility to the underserved.

Dos and Don'ts of Accounts Receivable	
Dos	**Don'ts**
1. Establish metrics of AR and review at least monthly. 2. Get the inputs correct for each patient. Gather appropriate demographic, insurance, payment history, and clinical information in advance of the visit.	1. Take your eye off the accounts receivable ball; it's a big one. 2. Forget that payers have no incentive to pay promptly. It is, however, your job to ensure that they do.

Dos	Don'ts
3. Focus on customer service and meeting needs and expectations.	3. Forget that the quality of collections is in part based on the quality of CPT and ICD-9 coding.
4. Develop an ongoing training program to keep staff up to date.	4. Let new regulations/codes pass you by.
5. Decrease AR by using a systematic approach.	5. Let yourself be wooed by quick-fix AR solutions.
6. Accept a moral obligation to assist those that are underinsured or uninsured.	6. Accept nonpayment without a fight.
7. Negotiate contracts wisely with clauses regarding issues of AR.	7. Accept a contract that does not address timely payments without penalty clauses.
8. Outsource if you cannot manage AR yourself.	8. Abrogate responsibility for AR lightly.
9. Consider incentivization plans for collections.	9. Offer only one way to pay (cash). Make other payment plans/options available.
10. Get what you deserve.	10. Leave money on the table.

REFERENCES

1. Mefford D: Four-square: Practice profitability stands on four foundations. MGMA Connex 3(8):44–48, 2003.
2. Gapenski LC: Understanding Healthcare Financial Management: Text, Cases, and Models, 2nd ed. Chicago, Health Administration Press, 1996, pp 651–693.
3. Office of Management and Budget, Final Rule, 5 CFR 1315, Sept. 29, 1999.
4. Sistrom C, McKay N: Costs, charges, and revenues for hospital diagnostic imaging procedures: Differences by modality and hospital characteristics. J Am Coll Radiol 2:511–519, 2005.
5. Nearhoff W: Adopting ideal standards to optimize PFS performance. Healthc Financ Manage 56(9):62–65, 2002.
6. Hogan C, Sunshine J: Financial ratios in diagnostic radiology practices: Variability and trends. Radiology 230:774–782, 2004.
7. Nordberg P: Beyond all measures: Criteria for the use and selection of a collection agency in a medical practice. J Fam Pract 38(5):514–520, 1994.

FURTHER READING

Cergnul J, Russell P, Sunshine J: Selected accounts receivable performance statistics for radiology practices: An analysis of the adjusted collection percentage and days charges in accounts receivable. J Am Coll Radiol 2:1019–1029, 2005.

DeGrote L: Internet-based search tools can help reduce bad debt. Healthc Financ Manage 56(6):34–36, 2002.

Kroken P, Carmody PW: The radiology reality show: Automating billing. Imaging Economics, November 2004, pp 61–64.

Ladewig T, Hecht B: Achieving excellence in the management of accounts receivable. Healthc Financ Manage 47(9):24–32, 1993.

McCormick E: The hidden costs of accounts receivable. Healthc Financ Manage 47(11):78–82, 1993.

Newton R: Measuring accounts receivable performance: A comprehensive method. Healthc Financ Manage 47(5):33–36, 1993.

Swayne L, et al: Unpaid radiology claims in New Jersey: Incidence and financial implications. Am J Roentgenol 183:3–7, 2004.

CHAPTER 10

Managing Expenses

David M. Yousem

INTRODUCTION

The ability to manage expenses and costs is equally important as managing assets and revenues in a good radiology practice. A group providing service at a lower cost than its competitor's can either reap greater profits in the setting of a fixed payment agreement, or compete more effectively to obtain greater volume or more lucrative contracts than the next group. Capitated contracts, a driving force in the analysis of expenses, assure that profit can be generated through lower-cost provision of services. Cost control may not be possible in, for example, the federal government, where spenders, often motivated in part by pork barrel politics, are not impacted by the residual of "profits minus expense"; but in private practice cost control has to be exercised. Without cost control, you cannot hope to maintain a sustainable radiology practice.

Controlling expenses begins with its characterization. A pretty straightforward characterization is an input/output, fixed and incremental cost model. The inputs are the costs for generating the outputs, which are purchasable to generate revenue. Inputs are what are required to produce an output, that is, a good or service.

Determining the magnitude or value of costs can be done in a couple of ways. One way of thinking about expense management is to define as inputs the goods and services your practice uses to produce its product, and to define opportunity cost as the value of each of those inputs in its best alternative use. Opportunity costs may also be thought of in terms of a required return on investment. Ask yourself, "How much money can I earn by using my money not for this expense, but in another way, for another vehicle, another investment?"

Incremental (Variable) Costs

Costs (or inputs) then need to be more closely defined. For the sake of discussion, assume you decide that investing in a new 64-detector CT scanner is the right opportunity. In determining what it will actually cost your imaging center, it should make sense that there will be some costs that can only be estimated as a function of the amount, or each increment, of a product or service that you generate. These are appropriately called incremental or variable costs. For example, there will be an incremental cost of providing a CD with each CT scan you perform. The more scans, the more CDs.

As in the CD example, this cost relationship may be linear or nonlinear to products or services generated. If you pay the same amount for each CD regardless of how many CDs you purchase, then this will be a linear relationship. However, if you get a volume discount—that is, 5% savings if you use over 100, 10% savings if you use over 1000—then it will be a nonlinear relationship. Technically speaking, nonlinear variable cost means that there is not a reproducible ratio of the added cost per unit product. This is because variable costs in some cases may actually accelerate or decline with increased use. A service contract that escalates with increasing use of a machine might be another "semivariable" nonlinear cost.

Other examples of variable costs might be contrast dye, laundry, and film costs. They increase with each study. Your electricity bill may even vary with the use of the imaging machine and hence might be considered a variable cost.

Fixed Costs

The CD burner itself, however, is considered a fixed cost. It is a one-time expense that does not increase with increasing study volume. Thus, fixed costs are seen as essentially independent of volume. Note that the "per-case fixed cost" decreases with increasing use. So purchasing a reliable system and running it efficiently is imperative. The CT scanner itself is another fixed cost if purchased, but can be converted to a less burdensome, partially variable cost if leased on a "per click" basis.

There is also what could be considered a combination of the variable and fixed costs, that is, a "step-function" cost. For example, when you started your business, you invested in your CD burners. If your volume grows and grows and you add CT scanners, there may come a time when your operations demand an additional CD burner. The volume drove up the

fixed and variable expenses, but not directly related to volume, as is seen with variable cost increments. Thus this step-function cost is one in which the costs increase by a fixed amount, as volume exceeds a given threshold. Another example of a step-function cost is the addition of another technologist to the team as the volume of studies increases, that is, adding another "shift" to accommodate increased volume.

Marginal Costs and Profit

The marginal cost of an action is the variable cost, as long as capacity has not been exceeded and a fixed cost has not been added with increasing volume. Thus it can be perceived as the change in total cost associated with an increase or decrease in volume. Marginal revenue is the change in total revenue associated with a similar increase or decrease in volume. As long as marginal (incremental) revenue exceeds marginal (incremental) cost, expanding a product line may be lucrative (marginal profit!). If marginal costs, because of the step-function addition of fixed costs associated with the increased volume, exceed marginal revenues, it is not worthwhile to expand the practice, unless it is a loss leader that generates revenue downstream in another aspect of your practice.

Sunk Costs

Sunk costs are costs that have already been paid out that cannot be reversed. Building an imaging center on a strip mall lot requires a lot of sunk cost (e.g., the cost of the land, development permits, etc.). Money used to pay for film processors 10 years ago in a new filmless environment can be considered sunk costs. Over the short term, most fixed costs are sunk costs. In general, the lower one's fixed costs are, the more likely one is able to make a profit—sometimes these fixed costs are referred to as "overhead," meaning costs of doing the business that can be readily changed but have to be met to make a profit.

Economies of Scale and Economies of Scope

Two concepts that are critical to understanding expense management are economies of scale and economies of scope. "Economies of scale" means bigger is often better, that is, a company achieves economies of scale when it lowers its cost per unit produced through increased production—its average fixed cost per product is less. Technically, from a revenue standpoint, economies of scale mean that increasing all inputs by X% will increase output by more than X%. For example, a large 90-member practice may be able to obtain lower interest loans, afford greater managerial sub-specialization (and thus increase efficiency), pursue bulk purchasing with associated cost savings, and afford equipment with greater throughput (thus increasing technical efficiency) than a 4-person practice. Consider Company A with two scanners in a building with similar expenses to Company B, which has only one scanner. The second scanner at Company A will enable a doubling of the ability to generate scans without a doubling of the costs (Company A would have the same marketing costs, bulk purchase savings on CDs, etc., as Company B).

This means that high-volume CT/MR/ultrasound practices may be able to get discounted rates on contrast dye, intravenous catheters, injectors, lubricants, oils, film, or even machinery, compared to groups with only modest volumes. This is another example of economy of scale. Imagine the improved profit you could achieve by increasing PET volume from three to six cases a day if the only fixed costs you were paying were the salaries of a technologist and a receptionist. Expenses are the same except for the isotope and CDs. Some insurers are so large that they can demand to be charged the minimum of your payer mix because they dominate the market with lives insured and can provide that coverage at a lower cost basis. Their size, as measured by members enrolled, affords them economies of scale "against" you—they pay you less.

The term "economy of scope" is exemplified by improved rates of payment by insurers for an imaging center that can provide full-service products to the patient, rather than only having a boutique practice specializing in one modality. For the payer it may mean one less contract to have to negotiate, and for the patient it means less parking, aggravation, and travel expense, by being able to drive to one site to have all of their imaging needs met. In fact, some payers are beginning to require a specific minimum of modality offerings as a tool to impede the growth of specialty imaging centers. "Full service providers" gain an advantage in contracting, hence economies of scale.

Operating Expenses

Operational expenses are those ongoing expenses required to keep the doors to your imaging center open every day. These expenses include the salaries and benefits of your employees (as always, the highest expense), rent/occupancy charges, maintenance costs for the facility (heat, electricity, insurance, janitorial, telephone, data lines, etc.), supply costs (usually a variable expense), and administrative costs (billing, collection, accounting, legal, financing, loans, leases, etc.). Marketing costs, particularly for start-up of a new practice or imaging center, may also be added to administrative costs. As an example, the average marketing costs for a new outpatient CT scanner site may be as high as $350,000.

Equipment Expenses

For radiology departments, another big expense is the equipment cost. While equipment costs may be an initial outlay, there are very few practices that can buy their equipment outright with "cash in hand." In many cases, the equipment is financed or leased at a specified interest rate, leading to an ongoing expense that is in part a capital expense, and in part an operating expense. In addition to the expense of equipment purchases, the expense of equipment maintainance (i.e., service contracts) must be considered a significant component of any budget of a radiology department. In some academic centers, the equipment costs and maintenance, and for that matter the personnel needed to run and support the equipment, are expenses sustained by the hospital rather than by the typical practice/university. For example, if one's practice is heavily weighted toward MRI scanning or PET-CT scanning, in which the equipment tends to run into the $4-million range, then these expenses must become competitive with how much can be allotted for employees' salaries (also often in the millions!). (See Chapter 11, "Purchasing Capital Equipment," for more information.)

Depreciation Expenses

Depreciation expenses refer to the declining value of a fixed asset as it ages over time. A fixed asset is something of value that cannot be easily converted into cash. Because of the limited flexibility of assets in this form, you are given a tax break for these fixed assets. Property, buildings, and equipment are examples of fixed assets. Given the average five-year lifespan of most of the equipment that imaging centers purchase, the value of that equipment decreases over time, but can be deducted as a noncash expense over that same time period. While this depreciation is recorded as an expense, the same amount may be recorded as a taxable deduction in the asset column, as a means of lowering income taxes. Straightline depreciation (reducing the value of the equipment equally each year over the projected lifespan of the machine) is the preferred pro forma method of accounting over taxable depreciation, which accelerates the loss of value of the equipment over the first few years of the economic life of the machine. By accelerating depreciation early on, you achieve a tax benefit that, in effect, provides improved cash flow.[1]

Accounts Payable

Under the current liabilities column on a balance sheet, you will find expenses of accounts payable, notes payable, accrued liabilities, salaries/wages/taxes, and accrued vacation. Long-term liabilities include loans/bonds payable and deferred pension liability. The difference between current and long-term liabilities is that the former is based on a payment schedule comprising the ensuing 12 months.

What are accounts payable? *Accounts payable* by and large are the expenses that occur within your practice and the monies owed to suppliers and vendors, due within 12 months of the transaction date (hence, they are current liabilities).

Notes payable denote money owed over the short term to banks or other creditors. Managing the source of revenue, as well as the expenses in a practice, is but one component of a successful radiology group. Some of the principles that have been discussed in Chapter 9, "Accounts Receivable," apply as well to accounts payable. Accounts payable (A/P) are the burden that the practice holds with respect to that balance of credit and debt. Accounts payable often refer to the ongoing expenses of the practice as opposed to its material

liability, which may be from items like imaging equipment and depreciation of such, or issues of bad faith.

Accrued Expenses

The term *accrued expenses,* or *accrued liabilities,* refers to obligations of payments that will have to be paid in the future, but payment has not yet been billed (e.g., wages or payments that are owed or taxes not yet paid). Accruals can be thought of in terms of the delays that occur in paying obligations. Even though an employee may work five days a week for four weeks, his or her salary may be accrued until it is an end-of-the-month payroll expense. In a similar fashion the payments for social security, Medicare, pensions, and other such benefits are considered accruals on a balance sheet. Generally, no interest is paid on these accruals (unless the business fails to adequately pay representative corporate taxes). Because of the "storage" of accruals until the end of the month, this money accumulated can be considered a free loan to the practice. From a payer's perspective, it would be best to pay employees once a year and accrue all the salary so that the payer can have that money at his disposal or in his account, earning interest during the year. Bimonthly or monthly payments, however, are the standard of practice nonetheless. If you have received supplies from a vendor and have inventoried those supplies into your asset list, but have not been billed by that vendor yet, that too is classified under accrued liabilities.

Salaries and Benefits

The vast majority of the money in accounts payable is tied up in salaries and benefits. In many cases, salary and benefit expenses account for over 60% of a practice's ongoing burden of expenses (Table 10-1). This should not be understated, as a company's employees are often some of the company's most valuable assets. Paying their salaries and benefits consumes a tremendous amount of money, as does creating the infrastructure for critical human resources. One of the worst things a company can do is to fail to make a salary payment to an employee. Trust by a company's employees is an intangible asset that is only appreciated when it is lost.

Table 10-1 Typical Annual Expenses, Medium-sized Academic Department of Radiology

Item	Cost	Percentage of Whole
Faculty salaries	5,810,206	38.1
Fringe benefits	2,867,417	18.8
Staff salaries	2,231,720	14.6
Student/postdoc salaries	1,336,166	8.8
Contractual services (including construction)	1,007,772	6.6
Faculty supplements	809,083	5.3
Other expenditures	544,520	3.6
Supplies and materials	349,130	2.0
Internal charges	301,653	2.0
Total	15,257,667	100

In most practices, the physicians and top administrators of the practice management team garner the highest salaries. The width of the spread between the highest salaries of the physicians and the practice management team, and the rank-and-file employees is a critical element to manage in a practice. In the best of all worlds, all components of the practice benefit from the success of the work product. Certainly, a patient's experience within a radiology department in large part depends on the front desk personnel, the schedulers, the technologists, and the accounting department members who collect the revenue. The provision of service in a radiology department requires a team approach in the best practices, and physicians who believe that it is largely *their* interpretation of a chest X-ray, head CT, or carotid ultrasound that is critical to the ongoing success of that practice are fooling themselves. All it takes is one bad front desk person and a significant proportion of patients will

not be returning to your practice whether you interpreted that ultrasound showing gallstones appropriately or not. Therefore, managing the incentive programs and benefit packages, and, yes, the salary spread from physicians to nonphysician members of the practice is critical.

Most potential employees look at the bottom-line salary when deciding whether to join a company. If the salary does not meet a certain minimum (set by the applicant or the "agent"), then the prospective employee will not even consider the job. Salaries must be competitive at a basic level to even open the door to discussion of the job and (also important) the benefits. The issue of benefits has become increasingly important because of the escalation of medical expenses for the working population. It is said that the average person spends approximately $7,000 per year for medical care and the average U.S. salary in 2004 was $44,695. Thus medical care expense represents approximately 16% of one's salary. Therefore, having a comprehensive medical care plan within a company as one of its benefits is essential. (It's also very expensive to the practice.) Having a variety of favorable medical care options from which to choose is also quite attractive, though again causes increased expenses. In our experience, medical and dental care options are key factors in an attractive employment option for prospective workers.

The other major expense that is also included in a benefits package is higher education reimbursement. This is one of the major advantages of academic practices versus private groups in that, in many institutions, the affiliation with the university leads to reduced rates for access to university facilities or for college tuition. This can sometimes be a factor in prospective employees of a certain age who have children approaching college. Usually there is a period of time that the employee must be on the team ("vetted") before he or she can obtain the college education employment benefit.

Other benefits that are often provided in a package for the employee include disability insurance, a small amount of life insurance, and a prescription drug plan, either included in the health care benefit insurance, or as part of a separate fund that may be used for co-pays, etc.

Defined benefit plans (i.e., pensions) and defined contribution plans, such as 401(k) and 403(b) plans, are attractive features to a recruitment package, but also tie up significant amounts of capital for long periods of time. Institutions may use second-party vendors to manage these options, with TIAA-CREF, Fidelity, and Vanguard leading the way with 403(b) and 401(k) plans. The amount of investment made by the employer is variable and may range from none at all to the maximum allowable. Providing annual IRA payments (currently up to $4,000 per year) versus using an employee matching program (e.g., one-for-one or a multiple thereof, whereby the employee puts in a certain amount toward a pension plan and the institution matches or doubles it), versus full funding of the annual pension expense by the employer, are all options that can be offered and can make a huge impact in a favorable employee recruitment decision if the salary is considered "borderline."

REDUCING EXPENSES

Managing one's A/P practice is as complex as managing the accounts receivable (AR) practice. With respect to AR, the main goal is to obtain the revenue from the various sources of your practice quickly so it can grow and be used by the practice. Employing effective strategies for collecting bills enhances the chances that you will receive as much of the money that you are owed as soon as possible (see Chapter 9, "Accounts Receivable"). Having a good corporate manager to oversee the A/P and AR is essential to a thriving practice.

However, with respect to accounts payable, the goal is to try to decrease the amount of money that is being paid out for the various services and to delay payment so that the required funds for these payments are earning interest or being put to work within your own practice as long as possible. Various strategies for delaying the payment of bills can be applied in the practice. Don't delay payment of your employees' salaries and benefits, though, unless you can accrue salary from weekly or bimonthly intervals to monthly paychecks.

What is the "cost of money" exactly? Accountants and finance managers know that in the financial markets, there is a certain amount and percentage of money that can be derived through financial investment. At the same time, there is a certain percentage amount that it would cost to obtain a loan for a given amount of money. The combination of these two factors is coined the "cost of money." The goal of your practice should be to earn more money as a percentage than the cost of money. For example, if you can earn 2% on your money in a bank account, but can earn 12% in an ultrasound venture, then you are exceeding by 10% the cost of money. If you pay 5% interest to the bank on a loan to purchase an ultrasound machine, but that ultrasound machine has a profit margin of 12%, you are still exceeding the cost of money by 7%.

Some of the strategies for managing the expenses of your practice include the use of incentive plans for paying debts off early. Today you often have the option of paying 95% of a bill within 30 days or the full amount within 30 to 60 days. A charge of an additional percentage is added if the account is paid after 60 days. In other words, you can sometimes save money by paying your bills early. On the other hand, if no discount is offered for early payment, you should wait as long as possible to pay the debts without incurring the wrath of the provider or without jeopardizing the relationship of the payer-payee pair. When dealing with the supplier of medical equipment that you need to have available reliably and on a regular basis—for example, catheters for a special procedure such as stenting—it's important to maintain a good relationship with the provider of that catheter so that you don't end up jeopardizing a patient's health on a delivery.

Just-in-time delivery is one means of controlling the A/P portion of the practice as well. Rather than having catheters or contrast agents that are on the shelf (having been paid for months in advance with the potential of expiring), just-in-time delivery allows you to pay as you go, obtaining the supplies needed at the time they are required. Once again, it is important to have reliable providers so that you can trust that you have the equipment when you need it. Providing this type of service has become, in this FedEx/Brown world, more commonplace for most companies. Again, you may be able to take advantage of a slight discount for early payment, or you may choose to keep your money in the bank and pay the bill when it is due.

Supply and Inventory Costs

As the volume of procedures increases, so will the list of supplies needed for those procedures; supply and inventory are considered a variable cost (Table 10-2). It is hard to predict at the beginning of the year how many procedures you will perform without historical data and without a barometer of what is happening in the field with respect to shifts from, for example, conventional arteriography to MRA and CTA. Properly adjusting to the requirements of the clinical load requires a ready supply of cash available at any given time. Therefore, supply costs are one of the principal components of the cash balance adjustments throughout the year. For instance, if you have an active interventional group, and there are a greater number of procedures, the variable cost may include the catheters, the coils, the stents, and the contrast dye.

Inventory costs include "carrying costs" and "ordering costs." Carrying costs are the costs of storage, maintenance, insurance, and handling of unused assets, as well as the interest on the money used to purchase the inventory. For example, if you are storing 10 platinum coils for aneurysm treatment at a total cost of $10,000 for one month, you are losing the interest from that $10,000 (in whatever investment vehicle you have at your disposal) for that month. If that yield is, say, 10% per annum, then theoretically you are losing (just in interest) $10,000 times 10% divided by 12, or $83.33 per month in carrying costs for the 10 coils.

Ordering costs include the time taken to order materials, the processing fees, postage, and/or delivery costs. In many cases, the benefits of ordering large quantities of materials may offset the carrying costs of keeping such items in inventory. If you have to pay just-in-time delivery fees to have an item at your immediate disposal, it may be more costly than the interest you lose in having the item on the shelf. So if FedEx charges you $12 to deliver one platinum coil, then the loss of $8.33 interest in a month on a single $1000 coil may be worth accepting to have it on the shelf. Of course, if a $1000 coil passes its expiration date while on the shelf and can no longer be used, then all benefits of this practice are negated. While this may be unlikely with items like platinum coils, there have been numerous occasions when we have had to discard old catheters because they were no longer in vogue or contrast dye that had been stockpiled at, unfortunately, a great price.

There's science (and art) to managing supplies and inventory. For example, mathematical models are available to determine the optimal amount of supplies to keep in inventory to minimize variable costs, known as the economic ordering quantity (EOQ). The EOQ equals the square root of 2, times the total sales in units, times the ordering cost for each order, divided by the carrying cost.

Start-up Costs for a Practice

What you start up your radiology practice, make sure you have all your start-up costs completely covered. These include the initial fixed costs of the equipment, rent or purchase of space, the employment of a receptionist, technologist, transcriptionist, as well as marketing and technology support staff, in addition to the radiologists and nurses. If you don't have all your start-up costs covered, you might find yourself in a deep financial quagmire. Once you hang up your shingle outside, and patients start to arrive, there will still be a substantial period of time prior to receipt of funds from your care of these patients. You will be in a relatively dangerous predicament for the accounts payable portion of the practice if the first payday arrives and you are without sufficient funds. Thus, it is

Table 10-2 Typical Unit Costs for MRI Services

Item	Cost	Percentage of Whole
Salaries and benefits	6.10	43.4
Supplies	2.46	17.5
Purchased services	1.97	14.0
Other	3.50	24.9
Total	14.03	100

important to do a cash flow analysis that accounts for required funding for operating, inventory, and financing, as well as expected revenue, to ensure that there will be cash in hand to cover the period of negative cash flow.

For this reason, starting a radiology practice by yourself is fraught with the difficulties of having enough cash assets at the outset to even support a practice as it grows. In most cases, assets will need to be borrowed to start your radiology practice: the cash flow analysis mentioned previously will help you to determine whether it is necessary to borrow and how much. It will also be needed to garner the support of lending agencies. In some cases, there are corporations that underwrite the expenses. Equipment manufacturers may even offer the radiologist the option of paying a "per click" fee for each study, rather than paying for the machinery outright. This per click arrangement means that for every patient who is imaged by the equipment, a set fee is sent to the equipment manufacturer. In some ways, this is an incentive for growth, and, if structured properly, can result in a reasonably pain-free means for obtaining radiology equipment. Many companies offer buy-out provisions and some will even use a lease-to-purchase agreement structure in which part of the per click fee is used to pay down the price of the machine.

Ongoing Practice Costs in the Real World

What does the literature say about practice costs? What is happening in the real world of running a radiology practice? A survey of practice costs in diagnostic radiology was performed and published by Sunshine et al in 2001.[2] Median total physician-related practice costs per FTE radiologist varied from a high of $61,000 in private nonacademic radiology groups to a low of $38,000 in hospital-based academic groups. Of these expenses, physician fringe benefits accounted for almost two thirds of the total physician costs in all settings. Of the nonfringe benefit expenses, malpractice insurance was the greatest contributor. The median total physician-related practice costs as a percentage of practice revenue ranged from 7% in private settings to 13% in academic ones.

Nonphysician-related practice costs included technical, administrative, and business support expenses. Median costs for technical expenses ranged from $33.90 to $36.60 per RVU across all types of practices. Most of these costs were related to technical personnel costs ($10.70 to $18.20 per RVU) and technical nonpersonnel costs ($18.10 to $23.60 per RVU). Administrative and business costs per RVU were in the $5.00 to $8.30 range, with the higher value limited to academic settings. Median total practice costs per FTE radiologist varied from $90,000 to $100,000 in hospital-only academic groups to $190,000 in nonacademic private groups at hospital and outpatient settings. Sunshine et al's data are comparable to the American Medical Association's (AMA's) report of total expenses, excluding professional liability insurance and physician payroll with an average of $148,000 per FTE physician, with a median value of $64,000.

Suggestions for Reducing Expenses

1. *Use VRD.* Convert to voice recognition dictation to reduce transcription costs (see Chapter 14, "Voice Recognition Dictation").

2. *Use extended disbursement floats.* Extended disbursement floats is the practice of slowing down payments to people to whom you owe money. By preserving the money in your bank accounts for as long as possible, you can earn interest on the money before you give it up.

3. *Pay bills electronically.* Like "floating" money, electronic payment of bills allows money to remain in your account for a longer period of time. Over the lifetime of a corporation that owes millions or billions of dollars, sending a check that arrives by U.S. mail two to three days early because it was mailed five days in advance of the due date versus transferring money electronically at the end of the business day on the last day that it is due can save thousands of dollars. Using electronic funds transfers also will reduce the relatively small expenses of postage, mailbox runs, and check printing. Once you are "automated," hours spent on sending out payments manually may also be reduced. Think of these procedures as extending the benefits of "direct deposit" to the payment scheme. When was the last time you

ran to the bank to deposit your paycheck? Think of the time saved in not having to fill out the forms and drive to the bank, wait in line, and so forth. That time savings can be applied to payments as well.

4. *Use information technology fully.* There was a time when couriers did a booming business in transporting films from one imaging center to another to be read by the radiologist. Teleradiology has revolutionized our field to the extent that new industries (e.g., nighthawk and dayhawk) have developed, which are reaping great profits through effective use of information technology. Get rid of films. Figure out a way of electronically sending images and reports to clinicians and/or patients in a fast, inexpensive, and secure manner.

5. *Increase efficiency.* Providing radiologists with a never-ending supply of cases to read on a workstation that is user-friendly is an effective way to improve the productivity of the physicians. For example, balancing the reduced efficiency of voice recognition dictation on the highest paid employee (the physician) with the cost of transcriptionist service must be made based on volumes and costs.

6. *Use economies of scale.* Paying less for high-volume items because of volume-based discounting is another way to reduce costs.

7. *Be a lean machine.* The administrative burden within an organization must be reduced to maximize profits. Having a large front office is only useful if it is scaled to the unit productivity. In many cases, the expenses of carrying salaries and paying benefits for some permanent administrative employees may be better applied to outsourcing work, or paying for interim consultants or temporary agency employees, to get past hurdles or projects that need the extra effort. Billing and collection agencies that specialize in these efforts may be more cost effective than the overhead of maintaining your own business office.

8. *Reduce unpaid claims.* Unpaid claims include revenue lost due to the care of uninsured patients, as well as those from managed care organizations that do not pay their bills. Prompt payment legislation

has not had the impact on the loss of revenue that occurs when payments by insurers or patients are delayed or not forthcoming. Billing costs for unpaid or late payment claims are significant and can eat away at a group's profit margin. In a three-month period, one 11-member radiology group in New Jersey had 2,808 unpaid claims and 10,658 late claims.[3] If one assumes five minutes of work time per problem claim, this would amount to over 1,000 hours of work applied to working these claims. The cost at a modest $12/hour salary would be over $12,000. Nonetheless, the revenue accrued for payment of these claims ($161,664) far outweighs the cost of pursuing the claims. Thus, hiring someone to pursue late or unpaid claims would be advisable if the burden of these claims is as high as those reported in New Jersey.

9. *Use electronic submissions to reduce storage/rental expenses.* Even the Centers for Medicare and Medicaid Services (CMS) has progressed from paper submission to electronic submission of claims. One of the advantages of electronic paper trails is the reduction in physical storage space required for housing copies of the paper submissions. Naturally, electronic submissions still require storage and redundant computer facilities at remote sites to prevent loss of critical data.

The electronic systems, when tied to the banking systems or accounts of some of your payees, eliminate the vagaries of the postal system, including mailing costs.

10. *Outsource accounts payable.* Many private companies now offer to electronically manage your accounts payable. This is particularly worthwhile for any benefits program that you offer the employees. It takes the blame and the burden off of the practice, since that is not the practice's core business, and it lets you choose a vendor whose core business is just this sort of thing. Another advantage is that these companies keep up to date on changes in regulations and requirements, something that a small radiology practice may not be able to do. Generally, these outsourcing agencies will save your staff time and, since they should

have insurance for disaster planning, they are held responsible to their clients at all hours of the day. When choosing a company, research its background and experience: most can provide excellent reports on use and expense histories.

Some other areas to think about would include the hiring of consultants to look at your expenses. Having a team expert in "best in practice" management may certainly be worthwhile if you find money leaving the business on a daily basis without a good explanation. Look at your competitors. If they seem to be making large profits and you are struggling to stay afloat, something is amiss. Consultants can help but only if they already understand the local environment and the corporate culture and are empowered to make the tough calls. Other effective strategies are to use benchmark data, readily obtainable from radiology management societies, to look at costs, such as cost of billing, or service contract. You can also explore the option of maintaining in-house physics/engineering equipment support to decrease service contract costs. Negotiate nonobsolescence contracts when there is maximum leverage so that upgrade

costs or unforeseen, state-of-the-art, "must have" software releases are at lowest cost. If you are a member, go to MD Buyline, and see if you are paying more than other customers. Demand the "best" pricing for the "best" equipment. Try going on the Internet and consulting the AuntMinnie.com website for peer advice.

CONCLUSION

Managing a group's expenses is nearly as important as managing revenues. In lean times, it will be the expenses that will dominate your stressors: How will I meet payroll? How much more money do I have to borrow? Understanding cash flow accounting will mitigate some of these anxieties and will allow for successful navigation through the perils of rising expenses. Juggling the unavoidable, high-fixed costs of imaging machinery and overhead—and salary and benefit expenses—with variable costs while still obtaining a healthy profit margin, requires the attention of the highest levels of the administrative team of a radiology practice.

Dos and Don'ts of Managing Expenses	
Dos	**Don'ts**
1. Pay bills electronically whenever possible.	1. Play games with or delay paying employees' salaries.
2. Recognize when additional volume will lead to new fixed costs and factor in these expenses.	2. Build volume in losing segments of the business unless collateral income is assured.
3. Provide benefit packages that attract good employees.	3. Forget that training expenses in the currency of your time sometimes "cost" more than money.
4. Grow/merge/accumulate to obtain economies of scale.	4. Monopolize.
5. Perform due diligence regarding return on investment and years to break even on capital equipment purchases.	5. Let your fleet of machines become a disadvantage to the group.
6. Understand your "cost of money."	6. Miss out on applying funds to other opportunities that have higher yields.
7. Use just-in-time delivery mechanisms for infrequently used supplies that can expire.	7. Carry heavy, unused, expirable inventory.
8. Use capital for morale building.	8. Rely on snail mail.
9. Outsource noncore functions.	9. Pay for long-term contractual services as opposed to hiring up.
10. Use IT to increase efficiency.	10. Be frivolous.

REFERENCES

1. Leibenhaut MH: Radiology applications of financial accounting. J Am Coll Radiol 2(March):241–253, 2005.
2. Sunshine JH, Burkhardt JH, Mabry MR: Practice costs in diagnostic radiology. Radiology 218(3):854–865, 2001.
3. Swayne LC, Fask A, Stelletell HD, Fanburg JD, et al: Unpaid radiology claims in New Jersey: Incidence and financial implications. AJR Am J Roentgenol 183(1):3–7, 2004.

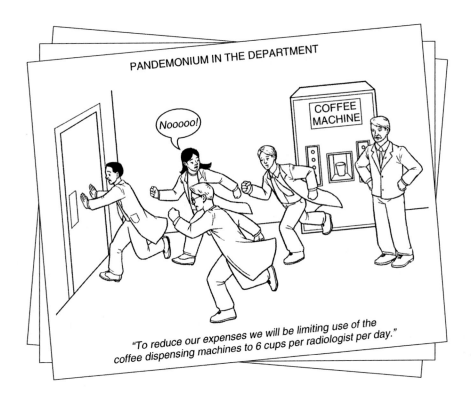

Purchasing Capital Equipment

Bob Gayler

The process of acquiring capital equipment has become more complex with the increasing sophistication of imaging equipment, and with the widespread dissemination of electronic image storage and retrieval. This chapter reviews a general approach to the purchase of capital equipment for a radiology imaging department. My experience is in hospital radiology departments, but most of the detail and approach are also applicable to outpatient imaging centers.

RADIOLOGY AS AN OVERALL HOSPITAL COMPONENT

In a hospital environment, radiology capital needs are typically very large compared to other departments. The endoscopy, information technology departments, as well as the operating rooms and bed and wheelchair replacements, are other relatively large consumers of capital. Since a majority of patients have imaging

procedures performed, there is usually support from other departments for radiology to have reliable, high-quality imaging devices. From the hospital administration standpoint, radiology operations usually are operated at a profit. However, the accounting details of payment by "diagnosis-related groups" has caused a reassessment of the "profitability" of imaging, so simply assuming that radiology is a profit center for the hospital will likely be erroneous. The details of this are beyond the scope of this chapter, but don't be surprised if hospital financial personnel are skeptical if you talk to them about financial return on equipment purchases, especially if the equipment is used primarily or even only for inpatients.

The purchase of capital equipment starts with a perceived need. The expression of this need may start at the user level, the administrative level, or may be related to a life cycle timetable. The replacement cycle should not be the same for all categories of equipment. Mature technologies, such as plain-film equipment, need not be replaced on a 10-year cycle, as they frequently last 12 or 15 years. MRI equipment, however, needs major upgrades for technical advance reasons at much shorter intervals.

PURCHASING STRATEGY

In a department equipment makeup, you should distinguish between profitable equipment, break-even equipment, and money-losing equipment. Hospitals require full-service imaging operations, while imaging centers may cherry-pick profitable operations. In the hospital it is essential to keep profitable equipment current so that revenue continues. Units that operate at a loss should be kept functional for as long as possible to minimize loss, as long as they are safe and meet regulatory requirements.

The three typical categories of equipment purchase are:

1. Current equipment in existing space
2. New equipment in existing space
3. New equipment in newly constructed space

The reasons for acquiring equipment include:

1. Age of the current equipment
2. Excessive downtime with current equipment
3. Regulatory issues with current equipment
4. Safety of current equipment
5. Important features on new equipment not available on current equipment (technological obsolescence); compatibility with information systems and electronic imaging system may also be a factor
6. Volumes greater than the current equipment can handle
7. Planned clinical or research expansion
8. Competition (to keep up with other hospitals or imaging centers)

It is important for management to keep an accurate inventory of current equipment, including age, use, maintenance costs, and service issues. These four components form the basis for any cost justification for replacement. Radiologist and technologist users, unless they are part of management, typically do not do a good job of forewarning management about performance issues, so management needs to anticipate problems. The simplest way of anticipating problems is replacement on a timetable, but this is frequently not possible in the cash-strapped health field. Management should also keep current on equipment development through trade shows, throw-away and technical journals, and the rumor mill. Peer-reviewed literature is a late indicator of technical advances in equipment.

CAPITAL BUDGET VERSUS OPERATING BUDGET

Many, perhaps most, organizations will separate the operating budget from the capital budget. This is logical and usually easy to understand, but there are some gray areas, into which capital and operating budgets fall and influence each other. Therefore, I will give a brief discussion and some examples of this overlap and mutual influence.

The capital budget is typically for discreet items that last for several years, typically six to ten years, occasionally longer. The organization will include an inventory list, detailing items that will usually need maintenance. Items that involve ionizing radiation will need state or federal registration, and frequently preapproval from some regulatory agency, before purchase or installation, depending on the state.

Capital budget items can be divided into major and minor, depending on the dollar value. This distinction is usually determined by the organization. The separation may be $5,000, $10,000, or $50,000. Thus, at a $50,000 cutoff, a mobile radiographic unit would be minor capital; a mobile fluoroscopic unit costing more than $100,000 would be major capital. A small ultrasound unit would be minor capital and a traditional ultrasound unit would be major capital. The distinction may be important considering the amount of lead time for budgeting, whether competitive bids are required, and whether a separate contract is required. There will be a certain dollar level, below which items that might look like capital equipment are actually supplies and are purchased from the operating budget. An example of a gray-area item would be an X-ray cassette, costing, for example, $1,200. This lasts more than one year, but usually is not tracked as a capital asset, and does not require outside maintenance but does require regular cleaning. If a group of cassettes is purchased as part of a computer radiography contract, it would be considered capital. Replacement computed radiography cassettes would ordinarily be purchased from operating dollars, however.

The operating budget is usually a one-year budget and includes salaries, supplies, rent, insurance, maintenance, and various contractual items, such as telephones. A merger area of overlap with the capital budget occurs with respect to maintenance. New capital items typically carry a one-year warranty. Therefore, the operating budget maintenance category would be decreased for one year each time a new piece of equipment is installed, and then either go back to the previous annual maintenance cost or increase if the new equipment is more complex. Putting together the operating budget therefore requires specific knowledge about when capital equipment items are coming off warranty and how much the service will cost when that happens. If the new capital items increase volume, supply cost will increase.

With the ubiquitous distribution of computers, a special category is required. Software is usually treated as an operating expense unless it is an integral component of a capital project. For example, you wouldn't buy a CT scanner with no software from capital dollars, and then buy all the software for the scanner out of operating dollars. However, *subsequent* purchase of software enhancements might well be considered an operating expense. This may be true, even if the software cost exceeds the traditional dollar cutoff points, such as $5,000, for distinguishing between operating expense and capital expense. It should also be noted that service contracts on computer equipment are typically more expensive as a percentage of cost than service contracts on traditional X-ray equipment.

When requesting new equipment, a cost and revenue analysis is usually required. This involves accounting input, since there are rules of financial operation to be followed. Categories for the user to be aware of include:

1. Equipment cost
2. Financing cost
3. Construction cost
4. Rent
5. Supplies
6. Labor
7. Overhead
8. Maintenance (including nonobsolescence agreements for certain types of equipment)
9. Additional PACS cost

These categories will be briefly discussed.

Equipment Cost

There will be additional comments on the purchase price later. At this prepurchase stage, there should be an estimated equipment price. It is important that this be the maximum *real* price (it is typically difficult to get additional money after the budget process is completed), but not *so* high that the proposal is denied. Intentionally overestimating is a ploy to be discouraged. Reasons for overestimating include not doing your homework in getting price estimates (so that there is no risk of having to ask for more money) and not having a reserve contingency, in case some other capital need arises. Consistently overestimating destroys one's credibility. Good estimates require discussion with two or more prospective vendors, who should know that these are "budgetary quotes," not best and final quotes. (See Appendix 11-1 for more information on return on investment.)

Financing Cost

This will vary from business to business. If the equipment is being purchased for cash, this does not apply. Vendors frequently have financing divisions and may offer lease arrangements, as well as financing the purchase price. Either borrowing the money to purchase the equipment or acquiring it through a lease involves complexities, which should be carefully reviewed by knowledgeable accounting personnel. However, the radiologist should be comfortable with all the language and conditions. Lease arrangements typically have a buyout provision at "fair market value" after five years. This buyout must be budgeted for, since most imaging equipment is kept longer than five years. Negotiating a fixed, low buyout value, such as one dollar, means that the buyer pays the full price in the 5-year period through the lease cost. The vendors are legally prohibited from "forgiving" a significant obligation remaining after a 5-year lease.

A special cautionary comment is appropriate: If a service contract is combined with a lease, be careful to separate out the purchase price before the service contract is added. The equipment should have a one-year warranty, so there should be no service cost the first year unless you are getting extended-hour coverage, or special glassware coverage, projected because of unusually heavy use (glassware coverage involves X-ray tubes and image intensifiers). After the first year and the service contract begins, payments are typically quarterly without interest for the service contract. If you want identical payments for the full term of the lease, you are in effect paying down principal early so your total interest should be reduced. In summary, compare financing options carefully and do not pay interest on the service contract.

Leases

Capital lease and operating lease are terms used by financial officers. You need to know the difference. A capital lease is paid by money designated for purchase, used for leasing instead. The reasons may have to do with capital markets. This is analogous to leasing a car when you have the resources to purchase it.

An operating lease is paid out of the operating budget as an additional category, like salaries and supplies. In the hospital setting this may be important, if radiology has a fixed operating budget with a separate capital budget. Will finance increase the operating budget to cover the lease expense? If not, you are unlikely to welcome an operating lease.

Example: Assume a $10 million operating budget annually with a $2 million average capital budget. Assume a lease of $1 million worth of this annual expenditure for $200,000 per year. If the operating budget does not increase, you will be spending $10,200,000, with a negative variance, therefore, of $200,000. The capital budget, underspent by $1 million, will look good for the hospital and your imaging administrator will be in hot water for failure to meet the budget.

Construction Costs

These are part of capital projects costs, so they form an important part of the "return on investment" calculation (see Appendix 11-1 for more information on return on investment). These are far more difficult to estimate than equipment costs. Working closely with an experienced facilities coordinator is the best general approach, but there are too many variables to come closer than ballpark numbers. The good news is that mobile radiographic units and c-arm fluoroscopic devices only need electrical outlets and alcoves and ultrasound units only need outlets, a sink, and floor space. Requirements for all other devices have significant construction features including:

Replacement in the Same Space

1. Electrical requirements may be different
2. HVAC (heating, ventilation, air conditioning) requirements may be different
3. Any ceiling-mounted equipment may be different
4. Floor conduits will likely be different
5. Floor weight will likely be different
6. There may be new picture archive and computer storage systems (PACS) requirements
7. Potential shielding requirement changes

New Equipment in Existing, Nonimaging Space

1. New electrical requirements
2. New HVAC requirements
3. New ceiling requirements
4. Floor conduit requirements
5. Floor weight issues
6. Plumbing issues for sinks
7. Lead lining when appropriate
8. Wall construction
9. Space for electrical cabinets
10. PACS connections
11. MRI (including magnetic shielding, acoustical shielding, radio frequency shielding, delivery route)
12. Plumbing (including restrooms and sinks)
13. Patient prep and holding areas

New Equipment in New Space

New equipment in a new space is the same as all of the items above under new equipment in existing, nonimaging space, but involves more complex planning.

You should be aware of infectious disease requirements concerning hand-washing, so sinks should be conveniently located in all exam rooms and in technologist work areas. You should also be aware that the Joint Commission of Accreditation of Healthcare Organizations (JCAHO) considers contrast media to be a drug and thus it must be kept locked in a cabinet or refrigerator and must have orders written for dispensing it.

Some vendors offer turnkey installations. In this situation, the vendor will hire the construction group. Vendors frequently have experience with contractors who are familiar with the imaging requirements. This can be attractive financially, but references should be thoroughly checked. The areas of potential misunderstanding with outside contractors include:

- Permissible hours of construction
- Impact on contiguous operations
- Length of project
- Staging area requirements
- Infection control
- Asbestos abatement
- Noise control
- Access routes for construction equipment
- Federal patient privacy regulations (HIPAA)
- Magnetic field issues on all sides

Rent

In commercial space, rent is on a square-foot basis. Imaging equipment has much different electrical requirements than office equipment, so discussion with the landlord must make clear how the utility cost will be handled. Hospitals typically roll imaging center space into their overhead. The formula for this is rather complex, since imaging overhead includes expensive construction space, high utility cost, as well as the more typical billing, security, parking, and general lobby and space cost. The overhead for imaging should not subsidize other functions of the hospital to the point where technical charges for imaging procedures are unrealistically high. Note that this "hospital overhead" is in addition to radiology department overhead.

Supplies

The best model to estimate supply use for new equipment is current supply cost on a per exam basis of the type of exam to be done with the new equipment. If volume growth is projected, obviously supply cost will go up.

Labor

Labor cost should be similar to the equipment being replaced, unless there are to be major increases in the number of exams, changes in the hours of operation, or changes in function.

Overhead

Imaging department overhead includes scheduling, billing, nursing support, purchase of non-imaging equipment, telephones, and department administration. This can be allocated to a piece of equipment based on a relative value unit basis. In other words, if a computed tomography scanner produces 10% of the relative value units for a department, the scanner would be responsible for covering 10% of the total department overhead.

Maintenance

Service contract costs can be used to indicate maintenance costs rather accurately. For the first year, equipment is typically under warranty. Warranties offered by the vendor cover standard hours and basic functions. If extended hours of coverage and extended component coverage are desired during the warranty period, there will be an extra charge. This charge will be part of the operating budget rather than the capital budget. Subsequent maintenance charges are also part of the operating budget. Be aware that as basic equipment is replaced with much more sophisticated equipment, the maintenance cost will go up, which increases the departmental operating cost. The difference between operating budget and capital budget was discussed previously.

Additional PACS Cost

This includes not only the networking costs but additional storage and display costs. Engineering to install and maintain the PACS applications will be a significant expense.

Once the allocation of the capital for the purchase of the equipment has been made, detailed planning begins. Preparation of the bid document, which sometimes is referred to as a Request for Proposal (RFP) can be drafted by one person and then modified on the basis of input from others. An ad hoc RFP team including major users—technologist, radiologist, physicist, and engineering—is suggested. Input from administration, the purchasing group, and the legal department will be needed at some point in the process as well. Components of the RFP include:

1. Overview of the function and location of the equipment
2. Component specifications
3. Options to be listed
4. Delivery parameters
5. Any special conditions (e.g., trade-in of current equipment)
6. Negotiation of maintenance contract

   The maintenance contract may be negotiated at the same time as the purchase sale agreement, or separately. If a service contract is intended for the equipment, you have no leverage in discussing service price, once the purchase price has been determined and the contract signed.
7. Negotiation of nonobsolescence terminology

   Any nonobsolescence terminology should be negotiated. You should be aware that this is a relatively new concept, and is not a term with universal meaning. Some dialogue will be necessary with respect to what each party understands are nonobsolescence agreements. If you want very broad coverage, you will pay significantly for this.
8. Electronic storage implications (including image transfer time and compatibility with existing archives)

When the bid document is completed, it is sent by the corporate office to selected vendors. A minimum of three vendors is recommended. The state and federal government facilities usually require invitations to more vendors depending on a variety of regulations. Of the bid document components outlined in the numbered list above, only Component Specifications" will be discussed in detail below. The others are intuitive.

Component Specifications

There are three levels of specification writing that may be used:

General Specifications

1. Advantages
   • It's fast to prepare for the buyer.
   • It's fast for the vendor to respond to.
   • There is maximum opportunity for the vendor to showcase a product.

2. Disadvantages
   • The buyer is open to salesmanship.
   • It requires spending the most time with the vendor.
   • Desirable details may be overlooked.
   • This is usually only suitable when the buyer has full decision authority.

Moderately Detailed Specifications

1. Advantages
   • It requires less time by the buyer than full-detail specifications.
   • Point-by-point vendor comparison is possible.
   • It ensures that the product is matched to the needs.
   • Good price comparisons are available.

2. Disadvantages
   • More preparation time is needed than for general specifications.
   • More vendor time is needed for response than for general specifications.
   • Desirable features may be omitted through simple oversight.
   • This level is appropriate when the user has a major voice in the decision process.

Full-detailed Specifications

1. Advantages
   • It enables a point-by-point comparison.
   • When the user has little or no input into the final decision, this is the most appropriate, and, since the vendor must meet specifications, a decision can be based on price.

2. Disadvantages
   • Preparation by the user takes the most amount of time.
   • The response time by the vendor is greatest.
   • Writing appropriate specifications requires thorough knowledge by the user.
   • Comparing quotes is time-consuming. Since more detail is stipulated in the RFP, the response will require that more items be compared.

See also Appendices 11-2, 11-3, and 11-4.

Purchasing Team

The department head and administration (hospital, imaging center) must have a strategy for acquiring capital equipment. The department head can directly participate in all phases, or delegate components of the process and retain either final decision authority or share the authority with the business side of the organization. In each situation, there will be variations, but input from direct users—radiologist and technologist, department management, physicist, and maintenance and construction personnel—are very helpful. For certain categories of equipment, such as mobile fluoroscopic devices, getting input from the surgeons familiar with the operating requirements can be extremely beneficial. Keeping these constituencies involved throughout the process will facilitate a smooth acquisition and installation process. The business side of the acquisition requires the engagement of legal, purchasing, and finance but they need not be involved in the early detail. The purchasing group may have access to comparison pricing information and access to user satisfaction surveys, which can be very helpful.

With any multimember group, face-to-face meetings are difficult to arrange, so group mailings sharing input, and a few two-to-three-member meetings can be used for decision making. It is essential that the major users be comfortable with the operational features of the equipment. Site visits, which will be discussed in more detail later, can be very helpful in gaining familiarity with the operational features.

Comments on Single Vendors

There are two basic ploys used by vendors to get around the bid process. These are both very seductive, so it is important to be alert to both of them. One is a long-term "demonstration" on loan, which can be done with ultrasound units, contrast injectors, mobile C-arms, and mobile radiographic units. Ultrasound and C-arm fluoroscopic devices are the most expensive, so these are the ones that the buyer is most susceptible to. The equipment will be new, there will be special pricing, the images will be better than what you are accustomed to, and the salespeople will bring donuts for the technologists, but you will not have looked at competitive equipment, and no competitive negotiations will have taken place. Management in charge of purchasing, in either the hospital setting or in the private practice arena, should rightly tell you "no deal" on arrangements of this type, even if you have the money. The other

vendor ploy is actually attractive and may be ethically and legally acceptable. This involves a major upgrade to existing equipment and works best if it is prebudgeted as such. Major upgrades should prolong the useful life to at least five additional years and cost no more than one third the price of new equipment. If it costs one half as much and adds one half of the expected 10-year life, there is no benefit over buying new. Also, an upgrade should require no construction. Upgrades at less than one third of the cost of replacement may be helpful in MRI, with respect to new applications or shortening exam times.

Single vendor purchasing may be justified when doing fleet purchases, such as mobile fluoroscopic devices and mobile radiographic units. In this situation, familiarity of operation is very important, prices are usually similar, and the vendor track record will be clear. Another special situation is with respect to computed radiography. Due to the complexity of this equipment and the importance of integration, it would probably be a disadvantage to have more than one CR vendor in a department.

Purchase Contracts

The vendor will have a standard contract. This will be included with a quotation, at the back, in fine print. For simple inexpensive equipment, this may be acceptable. It will be worded in favor of the vendor to a marked degree, however, so for expensive equipment, changes should be negotiated. There are several common areas of potential change:

1. Shipping costs, vendor or buyer
2. Rigging costs, vendor or buyer
3. Delivery to loading dock or place of installation. Liability is with the vendor to the delivery point with respect to any transportation damage
4. Warranty conditions
5. Terms of liability for patient or personnel injury
6. Performance guarantees during warranty
7. Payment schedule (down payment, delivery payment, turnover payment)
8. Collaboration regarding construction
9. Acceptance testing/turnover testing. Acceptance testing is a point of special emphasis. This should provide verification by a physicist

of the vendor specifications and include radiation output and electrical safety as well as all state regulations (federal regulations are typically delegated to the states for monitoring and enforcement). The vendor must file a compliance certificate with the state but this should not be relied on. The installation crew will frequently be independently contracted so details can be overlooked. Outsourcing happens at this point due to the sporadic nature of equipment installations. The rule "if anything can go wrong it will" applies. Installation of the correct grid, correct grid positioning, tube filtration, tube anode position, and all components are simple examples of easily overlooked issues.

10. Remedies for prolonged nonperformance
11. Integration with buyer's PACS systems

Service contracts will overlap with the purchase contract in areas of liability for injury and performance guarantees penalties. The usual remedy for uptime falling below a stipulated level is to receive "free days" of service. The formula is negotiable but should be based on logic. It should be recognized that the vendor and buyer both want a mutually beneficial relationship. Mutual fairness should be standard.

Whether to have a service contract with specific details depends on several circumstances. Some advocate multivendor service contracts. However, having service companies who are also serving competitors has its limitations. For example, while this may be appropriate for basic equipment, there are concerns about this type of arrangement for complex equipment, since it tends to result in longer downtime. The inconvenience of downtime is not felt in your administrative office, or in the administrative office of the vendor, but by the end user—you.

The value of the service contract to the vendor is that it provides a steady income stream, so the service manager can hire personnel and order equipment, in comparison to a "time and material" rate (in which time is billed at a high hourly rate and parts are billed at a high list price). The advantages to the buyer are that expenses are known and budgeted. The buyer should not have to pay a premium for this service and should end up paying less than the cost of time and material; there should be less downtime due to preventive maintenance. Therefore, a service contract can

be appropriate if the price is reasonable, compared to time and material. Special features of the maintenance contract include:

1. *Hours of coverage.* There is a premium for other than standard hours, that is, 40-hours-per-week coverage. Emergency department coverage should be extended, while individual circumstances should dictate whether extended coverage is appropriate for non-ED areas. (Most experienced service personnel do not routinely work nights or weekends, so extended hours of service will be done by less experienced service engineers.)
2. *Service contract.* Service contracts should include certain upgrades, usually including software upgrades.
3. *Glassware coverage.* Glassware coverage is the largest component of the service contract and includes the X-ray tube and image intensifier. Image intensifiers rarely fail, and X-ray tube life is determined largely by usage. Local experience should be reviewed to determine price appropriateness.
4. *Response time.* Response time includes telephone time and time for a service engineer to be onsite.

A few more rules of thumb regarding maintenance contracts:

- A basic X-ray equipment service contract should be 6% to 8% of the purchase price.
- For equipment with expensive tubes, the service contract should be 10% to 12% of the purchase price.
- Computer-based equipment should be about 15% of the purchase price, and software upgrades should always be included.

These rules of thumb presume average discount on purchase price, average hours of coverage, and average use. Coverage for PACS is a special situation, since hours of operation are conducted under the standard rule of 24-hour, 7-days-a-week, 365-days-a-year coverage.

Downtime Penalty

Vendor contracts typically indicate a guaranteed uptime percentage. The starting point in the negotiations may be 95%. We believe this is much too low since it is approximately one day per month downtime. Uptime should be at least 98%, or only three hours per month downtime. Most vendors will agree to this if preventive maintenance is not considered downtime. For downtime greater than this, penalties of increased service contract time without charge can be stipulated. The downtime can be averaged over a three-month period to avoid excessive bookkeeping. At first consideration, it may seem to be to the buyer's advantage to have downtime calculated on a 24-hour, 7 days-a-week basis. Except for ED equipment, this may not be true due to the size of the denominator.

If the service contract is not "24 by 7," there needs to be a provision for overtime rates in those circumstances when night or weekend service is essential to maintain operations. The rate should be substantially less than the standard time and material rate, typically about 50% of it.

An economic fact: You do not want to pay for overtime service if you have enough capacity to handle the volume with minor inconvenience. If you can handle planned downtime for preventive maintenance, do not insist on weekend preventive maintenance. However, if every Monday through Friday preventive maintenance costs you significant lost revenue, it can be good business to pay for weekend preventive maintenance.

Any contract is a compromise. Long drawn-out contract negotiations will delay equipment replacement and may create bitterness. It is helpful to have frank discussions with potential vendors at the RFP stage so that they are fully aware of your terms beforehand, in which case they may not wish to bid. The reality is that some equipment failures cause patient injury and the buyer must be protected in this event. Another reality is that some equipment does not perform as intended so the buyer also must be protected from this situation.

General Comments About Vendor Relations

Relationships between radiologists and vendors are based on ongoing use of modalities, so there is sustained contact after the equipment turnover. This usually means that there are periodic discussions about satisfaction or dissatisfaction with performance and service. These discussions can be helpful to the radiologist, in that problems are addressed, and helpful to the vendors since customer concerns may result in design changes in future models.

There is a danger in too much friendly contact between buyer and vendor in that congenialilty may lead to bias in the decision-making process. Socializing with vendors should be avoided. Many buyers unfortunately feel that vendors should provide perks as a thank you, but the buyer is legally and morally obligated to use objective criteria when spending government (Medicare and Medicaid) money. Consultantships, perks, and social contact have the potential to compromise objectivity.

Site visits are helpful and occasionally essential in evaluating equipment performance. When possible, these should be day trips to avoid the expense of hotel and dinner. If there are travel expenses, these are usually paid by the vendor and must be reported to the buyer's legal office, so that monitoring can be done. Money spent on equipment is ultimately patient's money or the taxpayer's money.

Most site visits are accompanied by a vendor representative. Bear in mind that these are artificial, as the vendor would not take you to see an unhappy customer. The customer, even if lukewarm about the product, will not admit to a mistake to a stranger. If you have a relationship with a radiologist at a site, a private telephone call may be more revealing than a visit.

Before you visit a site, study the brochure first. The more prepared you are, the more valuable the visit will be. If possible, have with you on the visit at least one other radiologist and a technologist. Depending on the specific situation, it can be very helpful to have an engineer or physicist with you as well, to raise questions that you as a radiologist may not think of. When at the site, mentally go through several exam situations for which the equipment will be used and move the equipment around. Put yourself in the position of the patient and have the technologist operate the equipment. Ask about interfaces to PACS. Make sure to see some images produced by the equipment. Get the names of the people at the site and write a thank-you note to them the next day.

EQUIPMENT ASSESSMENT

Networking is as important in equipment selection as it is in many aspects of professional life. Getting a user list from the vendor can be very helpful, in that you can call several users and talk to them without the vendor being present. You also may know someone at the site. The Klas Organization publishes a "best of" annual list, which can be helpful. There is an organization requiring a membership fee, MD Buyline, which gives pricing and user comments. The annual meeting of the Radiological Society of North America (RSNA) is very helpful in giving an overview but, in my opinion, you shouldn't make your decision there, unless you've done a lot of homework before the meeting. There are too many prospective customers present at a vendor booth to receive in-depth time from the rep, and as well, the trade-show atmosphere may give rise to emotional rather than reasoned decisions.

TIMEFRAME FOR CAPITAL EQUIPMENT

After the vendor receives the specifications for the RFP, they will need between two to three weeks to respond, depending on the complexity on the proposal. If it is unusually complex, they will need additional time.

Internal Decision Making

This is under the control of the user. At a minimum, the responses will need to be carefully read by all members of the decision-making team and a flowchart for comparison reviewed. If no site visits are needed, a minimum of two weeks should be set aside for this, however, it may take as long as several months. You should be aware that all of the RFP responses will have a time during which the quote is valid, so if the decision time is longer than the valid time with the quotation, you may need to get fresh quotations.

Paperwork Approvals

At our institution, paperwork approvals typically take four weeks for major capital equipment.

Legal Review

This typically takes from 4 to 12 weeks at our hospital. Once the order goes out, the time for

delivery from the point of view of the vendor is "after receipt of order," or ARO. This is when the vendor's clock starts. Delivery is usually between 60 and 90 days, which is appropriate when there is no construction. If there is construction, the following timetable is typical for us:

- Planning, 4 to 12 weeks
- Drawings, 4 to 8 weeks
- Engineering review, 2 weeks
- Permits, 2 weeks
- Bid, 2 weeks
- Construction, 1 to 6 months

Thus the total, if no construction is involved, will typically be 20 to 32 weeks from the time the specifications go to the vendor. If construction is involved, the schedule will be from 32 to 52 weeks from the time the vendor receives the specifications. Our experience is that angiographic labs typically take closer to two years. The delays in cathlabs are related to site visits, the number of people involved in the decision-making process, and the complexity of the construction planning.

BIGGEST MISTAKES IN PURCHASING CAPITAL EQUIPMENT

1. Confusing the salesperson with the product. It is obviously the goal of any company to have salespeople with good personalities, who are knowledgeable, dress well, and are attractive. The purpose of this is so that you will think that the product they represent will be of the same high quality as the salesperson. There may be some correlation between the quality of the salesperson and the quality of the product, but it is safest to assume that there is no correlation at all.

2. Failing to check out the local service operation. For this, there is no substitute for word of mouth and local reputation. The quality of service ultimately comes down to the individual service engineer. Service support back at the home office is important for certain essential things, but your uptime will depend more on local service people.

3. Believing surgeons. A few surgeons understand the economics of imaging equipment;

however, these are very few indeed. A few also are concerned about radiation safety. Our local examples of bad economic decisions based on surgeons' recommendations include:

- Fixed fluoroscopic units in the operating room (twice)
- Biplane mobile fluoro unit designed for hip surgery
- Lithotripsy device
- Cysto-table with fluoro

All had very low volumes.

4. Accepting a beta-level product in an area where you need reliability.
5. Buying a product near the end of its technical life; it will not be supported.
6. Getting a product from a company with a different primary focus. For instance, Pfizer, at one point, had an outstanding CT product. They discontinued development. Johnson and Johnson had an excellent MRI product. They sold it.
7. Assuming that a key feature is standard when it is an extra cost option.
8. Choosing equipment over the end-user's objection. Unless it is perfect, which is impossible, you will get endless complaints.

9. Buying a good product from an undercapitalized company. This can be a winner, but you have to have tolerance for high risk, because you might get stuck with an unsupported product.
10. Forgetting that more volume means more supplies, more PACs support, and thus higher overall expenses.

CONCLUSION

This chapter outlines a general approach to the purchase of capital equipment for a radiology imaging department. To summarize:

1. Maintain a detailed 5-year equipment replacement plan and a general 10-year equipment plan.
2. Retain current data on inventory of equipment, current exams, and current expenses.
3. Keep abreast of technical advances.
4. Treat the vendors professionally, not collegially.
5. Remember that money spent on equipment requires accountability by serious accountants.
6. Include the physicist and engineers as part of the purchasing team.

Dos and Don'ts of Purchasing Capital Equipment	
Dos	**Don'ts**
1. Keep the organization's needs uppermost on the list of priorities.	1. Assume that a large company does everything well.
2. Think of life-cycle costs, not just acquisition costs.	2. Believe that a nonimager can project volumes.
3. Learn construction requirements.	3. Buy a good product from an undercapitalized company.
4. Consult with other members of the imaging team—the technologist, physicist, engineer, nurse, and clerical and administrative staff. For equipment used by surgeons or endoscopist, involve the user.	4. Purchase a sideline product from a company whose main focus is elsewhere.
5. Make sure that the IT department is prepared for the equipment. They need to be on board from the time the specifications are prepared.	5. Acquire an early version of a product when you need high reliability.
6. Understand the sales contract. If the terms are confusing, ask your lawyer what they mean.	6. Forget that more volumes mean more supplies, more space, more infrastructure.
7. Attend the planning meetings. If you don't understand the symbols on the plans, ask.	7. Fail to remember that bottom-line finances ultimately must be respected.
8. Buy an architectural ruler and a 16-foot tape measure.	8. Forget that personal conflicts of interest are as seductive as financial conflicts of interest.

Dos	Don'ts
9. Understand the basics of the term "return on investment" (see Appendix 11-1). 10. Stick with the facts. Remember that you are a scientist. "More" is not a number.	

REFERENCES

1. Berlin JW, Lexa FJ: Finance for practicing radiologists. J Am Coll Radiol 2:254–262, 2005.
2. Berlin JW, Lexa FJ: An analysis of the buy-vs.-lease decision. J Am Coll Radiol 3:102–107, 2006.

APPENDIX 11-1. CAPITAL EQUIPMENT

Return on Investment

The concept of return on investment is reasonably straightforward. Specific institutional formulae may not be so clear, however. I will discuss the process used at our facility, since the general logic should be similar wherever you are.

1. The capital cost is determined, which includes equipment cost added to construction cost. Together, these are the initial expenses.
2. Annual expense is estimated for years one through five, or longer if desired. The same concept will work for the life of the equipment. Annual direct expenses for nonreplacement, new equipment include: salaries, supplies, maintenance after warranty, and any other expenses. Annual indirect expenses include: rent, utilities, building maintenance, billing cost, insurance, and are usually calculated as a percentage of direct cost rather than specifically determined. Our institution uses 25% of the direct cost, which is to be allocated to indirect cost.
   - Annual expense for replacement equipment may be calculated as incremental expense rather than total expense. Therefore, supplies and salaries, related to the increase rather than the total, are listed as annual incremental expense. Incremental, indirect expense is a percentage of the incremental direct expense.
3. Revenue for additional equipment is the number of procedures times the average collection per procedure. Revenue for replacement equipment is the number of incremental procedures times the average collection per procedure.
4. At this point you may be thinking, "That's unfair, why not use the total revenues?" The accounting theory is that the old equipment can be kept working indefinitely. If you can win the argument that it cannot, and the old equipment is fully amortized, you may convince your accounting staff to let you treat replacement equipment as if it is a new unit. If you do this, you must remember to pick up the total salaries and supplies rather than just the incremental salaries and supplies.
5. At this point, you have annual cost, direct and indirect, plus annual revenues. You can subtract the cost from the revenues to determine an annual profit. In very simple accounting terms, you would go year by year through the annual profit and figure when your profit exceeded the initial investment—that would be your payback period. Again, in accounting terms, this is what you actually do but with a correction for inflation. Your initial investment is worth less money each year but must be paid with then-current dollars. Your accounting department can tell you how much to factor in for inflation, and whether to increase salary and supply expenses in accordance with inflation. The following example, based on a CT scanner as a "new" rather than "replacement" device, may be helpful.

CT Scanner, New	Initial	Year 1	Year 2	Year 3	Year 4	Year 5	Total
CAPITAL							
Equipment	1,100,000	-	-	-	-	-	1,100,000
Construction	200,000	-	-	-	-	-	200,000
PACS connections	100,000	-	-	-	-	-	100,000
Total	*1,400,000*	*0*	*0*	*0*	*0*	*0*	*1,400,000*
REVENUE							
Procedures		5,000	5,500	6,000	6,500	7,000	30,000
Collections per case ($10 inc./yr)		250	260	270	280	290	1,350
Collections per year		1,250,000	1,430,000	1,620,000	1,820,000	2,030,000	8,150,000
Total		*1,255,250*	*1,435,760*	*1,626,270*	*1,826,780*	*2,037,290*	*8,181,350*
EXPENSES							
Direct @ $90/exam		450,000	495,000	540,000	585,000	630,000	2,700,000
Indirect at 25% (no inflation included)		112,500	123,700	135,000	146,200	157,500	674,900
Total expenses/year		*562,500*	*618,700*	*675,000*	*731,200*	*787,500*	*3,374,900*
Total margin/year		*692,750*	*817,060*	*951,270*	*1,095,580*	*1,249,790*	*4,806,450*

Revenues - Expenses (Operating Margin)			
		Present Value Factor 4%	Present Value
Year 1	692,750	0.96	665,040
Year 2	817,060	0.92	751,695
Year 3	951,270	0.88	837,118
Year 4	1,095,580	0.85	931,243
Year 5	1,249,790	0.81	1,012,330
Total	**4,806,450**		**4,197,426**

Average annual net present value = $4,197,426/5 = **$839,485**
Original cost = **$1,400,000**
Annual operating margin average $839,485/1,400,000 equals 60% = return on investment
1/.60 = 1.6 years return on investment
Note: Present value factor is artificially low.

Formula
1. Subtract annual expenses, direct and indirect, from annual revenues for years 1–5.
2. List by year.
3. Multiply each year by present value factor, giving a present value dollar amount for each year.
4. Add the 5 years present value dollar amount.
5. Divide #4 by 5.
6. Divide #5 by initial cost.
7. Divide 1 by #6. This is the payback period in years.

CT Scanner, Replacement	Initial	Year 1	Year 2	Year 3	Year 4	Year 5	Total
CAPITAL							
Equipment	1,100,000	-	-	-	-	-	1,100,000
Construction	50,000	-	-	-	-	-	50,000
PACS connections	100,000	-	-	-	-	-	100,000
Total	*1,250,000*	*0*	*0*	*0*	*0*	*0*	*1,250,000*
REVENUE							
Procedures above prior		1,000	1,500	2,000	2,500	2,500	9,500
Collections per case		250	250	250	250	250	1,250
Collections per year		250,000	375,000	500,000	625,000	625,000	2,375,000
Service contract saving		150,000					
Total		*401,250*	*376,750*	*502,250*	*627,750*	*627,750*	*2,385,750*
EXPENSES							
Incremental							
Direct @ $90/exam		90,000	135,000	180,000	225,000	225,000	855,000
Indirect @ 25% (no inflation included)		22,500	33,750	45,000	56,250	56,250	213,750
Total expenses/year		*112,500*	*168,750*	*225,000*	*281,250*	*281,250*	*1,068,750*
Total margin/year		*288,750*	*208,000*	*277,250*	*346,500*	*346,500*	*1,317,000*

Revenues - Expenses (Operating Margin)			
	Revenue - Expense	**Present Value Factor 4%**	**Present Value**
Year 1	288,750	0.96	277,200
Year 2	208,000	0.92	191,360
Year 3	277,250	0.88	243,980
Year 4	346,500	0.85	294,525
Year 5	346,500	0.81	280,665
Total	**1,467,000**		**1,287,730**

Average annual net present value = 1,287,730/5 = **$257,546**
Original cost = **$1,250,000**
Annual operating margin average = $257,546/1,250,000 = 21% = return on investment
1/.21 = 5 years return on investment

Formula
1. Subtract annual expenses, direct and indirect, from annual revenues for years 1–5.
2. List by year.
3. Multiply each year by present value factor, giving a present value dollar amount for each year.
4. Add the 5 years present value dollar amount.
5. Divide #4 by 5.
6. Divide #5 by initial cost.
7. Divide 1 by #6. This is the payback period in years.

APPENDIX 11-2. SPECIFICATIONS

As noted in the text, it is useful to think of specifications in three categories:

1. Short, general
2. Moderately detailed
3. Extensively detailed

We prefer to use Category 2—moderately detailed specifications—for most purchases. It should be remembered that for government contracts, or in any situation in which the final purchasing decision is not made by the user, Category 3 should be used.

Imaging can be thought of in seven categories of equipment:

1. Plain "film," mobile and fixed
2. Fluoroscopy, mobile and fixed
3. Angiography
4. Ultrasound
5. Computed tomography (CT)
6. Magnetic resonance imaging (MRI)
7. Nuclear medicine

There are related components, including physiological monitoring devices and contrast media injectors as well as PACS connectivity issues, storage, and workstation issues.

The imaging categories are sufficiently unique in that there are limited areas of overlap. Working familiarity with each is essential to writing the specifications. Therefore, users of the modality must be directly involved in writing specifications for their units.

For X-ray generating equipment, the basic components are:

- X-ray generator circuitry
- X-ray tube or tubes
- Tube support and collimator circuitry
- Patient table, wall-mounted film holder
- Image recording device, with any automatic detector circuits

For fluoroscopic equipment, the image intensifier and television chain are included. Dynamic image recording may be needed. For computed tomography, the gantry, image detector, and processor are the variables.

The basic X-ray system is a useful starting place for concept and comment. Current X-ray generators have a compact control unit, either wall-mounted or on a desktop, with the larger components included in a cabinet elsewhere in the room (older units had a large transformer box). Current transformers are smaller and less conspicuous and are typically included in cabinetry with other components. The operator control is by screen touch or push button. Many decisions formally made by the technologist regarding kilovoltage, milliamperes, and time are automatically selected based on exam type. However, equipment specifics still need to be stipulated concerning the operating range of kilovoltage peak, milliamperes, time, and automatic exposure response. X-ray tube characteristics of focal spot and milliamperage will be controlled at the generator and usually will be part of the exam parameters.

Tube mount travel is important. It is essential to have 40 inches above the table for full coverage and good geometry. For a wall-mounted film holder, vertical travel must be low enough to cover required standing extremities and high enough to cover standing cervical spine exams. Movement of the tube to cover the table, wall film holder, and stretcher must be considered. Orthopedic application must be provided for.

All vendors currently have elevator tables to accommodate easy transfer of patients from stretchers. Current table construction will usually be able to accommodate patients of up to 400 lbs. or more. A 4-way moveable tabletop greatly facilitates positioning. Tabletop movement controls should be both at the front and back part of the table so that cross-table lateral exams can be positioned without excess technologist movement.

Grid devices in the table and in the wall-mounted film holder should be high speed reciprocating. In a busy area, technologists will not have the time to change grids for different types of exams so that appropriate grid ratios and focal distances must be selected to reflect this.

The upright cassette holder or direct digital device should have adequate vertical travel for upright chest exams, cervical spine exams, and standing knee exams. The occasional skull examination may be done on either the wall-mounted film holder or on the table. Various cassette sizes should be accommodated. For the wall-mounted film holders, either right loading or left loading should be stipulated.

This can usually be deferred until fairly late in the ordering process so that room layout can be done before the side-loading characteristics of the film holder are stipulated.

Wall-mounted buckys may be close to the wall or may extend out. Consideration must be given as to whether space is required for the patient's knees under the cassette device. Some wall-mounted cassette holders can fold out so that they are horizontal. Whether this feature is ordered depends on the applications.

APPENDIX 11-3. EXAMPLE OF SPECIFICATIONS FOR RADIOGRAPHIC ROOM

The XYZ Hospital is requesting vendor proposals for replacing the radiographic equipment in Room 123, in the imaging department. The equipment will be used for standard radiographic examinations on adults and children. The equipment will be used primarily for inpatients. The quotation should include removal of the existing equipment. The vendor agrees to work with hospital facilities to indicate any required room modifications.

Generator

The power output rating is to be 80 kilowatts. The X-ray voltage should range from 50 KVP to 150 KVP. The equipment should be capable of supporting a high-speed rotating anode X-ray tube. One X-ray tube is to be supported. The unit should be capable of photo timing operations and able to support three detector chambers in the table device and three detector chambers in the wall-mounted film holder. The system should be capable of a full range of manually set nonphoto timed exposures. The equipment must be capable of carrying a series of standard techniques based on body part examinations. The equipment must have protective circuitry to prevent X-ray tube overheating.

X-ray Table

X-ray table should be elevator type. Tabletop must go as low as 22 inches above the finished floor and as high as 32 inches.

Four-way floating tabletop with electromagnetic locks: Tabletop locks must be at front edge and at back edge of table. Whether locks are foot controlled or hand controlled should be stipulated. The absorption characteristics of the tabletop should be no more than 0.6 mm of aluminum. The distance between the tabletop and the surface of the X-ray cassette should be no more than 4 inches. The tabletop should be capable of supporting a 350-lb. patient; a greater weight is desirable. The tabletop must be moveable with a 350-lb. patient on the table. The grid between the tabletop and the cassette should have a ratio of 10 to 1 or similar. The grid should be fine lined so that on ultra short exposures, the grid pattern will not be visible on the radiographs.

The upright film holder should be capable of going close to the floor for standing upright exams. Details should be stipulated. The grid and the upright film holder should be 10 to 1, and capable of use between 60 and 72 inches FFD. The absorption of material between the patient and the cassette should be no more than 0.6 mm aluminum.

The X-ray tube holder is to be ceiling mounted, of a general telescoping construction. The X-ray tube must be usable pointed toward the table, and in a cross-table orientation, angled in the long axis of the table, and used for horizontal beam radiography in the wall-mounted film holder.

X-ray tube holder must have mechanical safety devices in case of electrical lock failure. There must be automatic detents for the ceiling-mounted tube holder, for orientation to the center of the table and to the center of the wall-mounted cassette holder. Standard radiographic distances should be indicated visually and by detents.

X-ray Tube

X-ray tube should be focal spot 0.6 mm small, 1.0 mm or similar large. Stipulate the heat unit and anode storage capacity. Stipulate the X-ray tube heat unit storage capacity. X-ray tube should have high-speed rotor circuitry.

X-ray collimator must be of high quality to minimize radiation outside the selected field of radiation.

Delivery to be within 90 days after vendor receives order.

Equipment must meet all state radiation safety requirements and pass inspecting physicist's evaluation.

Applications training to be provided onsite for two days.

Equipment is to come with one-year warranty including glassware. Details of warranty to be included with the vendor response.

Vendor to submit service contract proposals for years two through five based on 40-hour per week, Monday through Friday service with stipulation of additional charges for off-prime service cost.

This room is to be a completely functional room. Any omissions from the specifications above are to be brought to the attention of the purchaser prior to the completion of an order.

APPENDIX 11-4. INTERVENTIONAL RADIOLOGY RFP

The XYZ Hospital is currently requesting bids for the IR room 10 in IGIL (Image Guided Interventional Lab), CMSC 5 to be addressed. The following is a list of technical, service, and warranty items that we would like addressed.

A: Generator

A01—List power requirements needed to support equipment being quoted.

A02—High voltage output: High frequency.

A03—Power output rating: 100 KW is preferred.

A04—High voltage output range: 50–150 K.

A05—Tube current output range: 10–1000 mA.

A06—mAs output range: 1–1000 mAs.

A07—Pulsed fluoroscopy: Please indicate steps available.

A08—Manual independent selection of KV, mA, time, and focal spot size.

A09—Automatic Exposure Control (AEC) shall be included with the capabilities of selecting separate dominant fields.

A10—In Automatic Exposure Control the mA can be programmed at any value less than maximum.

A11—Anatomical programming shall be included.

A12—Tableside generator control, as well as control booth generator control, shall be provided with the unit.

A13—An in-room status display shall indicate generator parameters to the operator.

A14—Unit shall be equipped with Dose Monitoring Equipment to provide indication to operator of the amount of radiation that the patient is receiving in real-time and collectively.

A15—Unit shall indicate X-ray tube heating and alarm or notify operator if limits are being approached.

A16—Unit shall be capable of setting acquisition technique from the previous fluoro exposure (no trial acquisition exposures). Unit shall indicate how much fluoro time is needed to accomplish this task.

B: X-Ray Tube

B01—High-speed rotating anode 150 PkV. 0.3 mm small, 0.6 mm medium, and 1.0 mm large focus. Micro focal spot in addition to the three above for pediatric needs. Tube shall be a hand-selected tube to ensure true focal spot specifications.

B02—Minimum 1.5 mHU anode capacity and 2 mHU housing heat unit capacity. Tube shall also have an external circulation cooler.

B03—Over temperature heat sensor mounted to X-ray tube interfaced to inhibit exposure if activated.

B04—Warranty for X-ray tube will be a minimum of one year of full coverage for initial X-ray tube. Standard tube warranty will apply on subsequent tubes.

B05—Provide current cost of X-ray tube being quoted.

B06—Vendor agrees to install, calibrate, service, and perform preventative maintenance service on any and all pieces of vendor's equipment installed in room regardless of where replacement X-ray tube is purchased.

C: Collimator

C01—Collimator shall be automatic sizing to receptor.

C02—Collimator shall be capable of both automatic and manually controlled rotational movement.

C03—Collimator shall have iris collimation as well as independent shutter collimation. It shall also have semitransparent shutters as well as a finger filter. If finger filter is not available, optional products (e.g., bolus bags) shall be provided to accomplish said task.

C04—Power requirements: No external power provided. If additional power is required please state.

D: Multidirectional C-Arm, TABLE

D01—Table shall have the following motions: (please complete list by filling in the amount of travel and the speed of movement)

Movement	Amount	Speed
1. Table tilt		
2. Table vertical motion		
3. Table longitudinal movement		
4. Table transverse movement		
5. AP C-arm LAO/RAO		
6. AP C-arm Cran./Caud.		
7. AP C-arm longitudinal movement		
8. AP C-arm transverse movement		
9. AP II vertical motion		
10. PA/AP imaging		

D02—Collision protection shall be provided to protect patient operator and equipment.

D03—Emergency shutoffs shall be easily accessible in the event of mechanical or electrical failure.

D04—Tabletop shall be capable of withstanding 400 lbs. or more with table fully extended for CPR. Please list your specs.

D05—Accessories: Detachable hand grips, shoulder rest, patient step, table side rails, alternate wide tabletop, and two premium table pads shall be included in purchase.

D06—Power requirements: No external power provided other than stated in the generator section. If additional power is required please state.

D07—System to be capable of "Rotational Angiography."

E: Radiation Control

E01—Two radiation shields (Mavig 6290/Z-60/110–80/80-UL) shall be provided including installation.

E02—Tableside mounted radiation shields to be included.

E03—List any other radiation control devices available for unit as an option with pricing.

F: Imaging Components

F01—Flat Panel Detection System. Describe your methodology, detection process (direct, indirect, etc.), and image acquisition performance expectation.

F02—A monitor suspension shall be provided to attach to the ceiling that will provide space for two 21 in. (54 cm) Active-Matrix Liquid Crystal Display, plus space for the two hemodynamic LCD.

F03—Vendor agrees to run cables for the monitoring equipment at time of installation.

F04—Four high-quality Active-Matrix Liquid Crystal Displays will be provided, capable of both 1K and 2K display. Two Active-Matrix Liquid Crystal Displays will be in the control area and the other two mounted in the suspension, one for live AP, the other for Roadmapping. Also list LCD manufacturer and replacement price of LCD.

F05—Provide specifications that provide high contrast resolution and low contrast resolution numbers for the liquid crystal display/digital image detector combination for each of the modes available. Describe measurement method and tool being used. Comment: Interested in magnification abilities to adjust for neonates/infants.

F06—Digital shall be capable of doing road-mapping with landmarking and peak opacification.

F07—Digital fluoro should be capable of doing last image hold with the capability of storing selective holds to disk. Unit should also be capable of fluoro cine loop.

F08—Digital fluoro shall work in conjunction with X-ray generator to provide pulsed operation. List pulse fluoro modes that are available.

F09—List minimum and maximum storage capabilities of disk. Also indicate if image is compressed to disk and what type of compression is used.

F10—Unit shall be capable of doing online, real-time subtraction.

F11—List analysis packages that are available for the digital, along with pricing.

F12—Unit shall be capable of image reversal from left/right and top/bottom.

F13—Unit shall be capable of variable frame rate acquisitions in fluoro, DA, and DSA. List available frame rates and modes.

F14—Describe the manufacturer's intention for pulsed fluoro, whether for image improvement, or patient dose reduction. Describe what level of patient dose reduction we can expect when using pulsed fluoro mode over continuous fluoro mode.

F15—Provide pricing for options such as DVD, thermal paper printer, DICOM output, and so forth.

F16—Provide DICOM conformance statement. Must be integrated with current archive. This may be referenced online.

F17—Must be compatible with the current work list provider.

F18—State all DICOM compatible options included with the basic system. Quote all additional DICOM compatible options separately.

F19—Describe your network transfer speed from image processor to a compatible network archive in images/second for all DICOM display formats.

F20—Describe manufacturer's configuration adjustments for neonates, infants, and children.

F21—Provide information, including pricing on integrated ultrasound unit for localization.

F22—Quote contrast media power injector, Med Rad.

F23—Provide option physiological monitors compatible with system. Display shall be LCD type.

F24—Quote OR light, ceiling mounted.

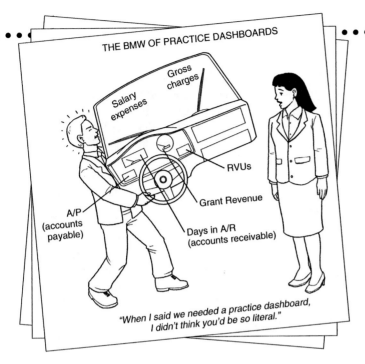

CHAPTER 12

THE BMW OF PRACTICE DASHBOARDS

Gross charges

Salary expenses

RVUs

A/P (accounts payable)

Grant Revenue

Days in A/R (accounts receivable)

"When I said we needed a practice dashboard, I didn't think you'd be so literal."

Making Cents of Metrics

F. A. Mann, Peter Ghavami,
Joseph Marotta, Michelle Bittle,
and Joel A. Gross

INTRODUCTION

Metrics serve as one of many useful communication tools, which help team members focus on those enterprise functions that most closely predict success (drivers). When people are aligned along values, goals, and milestones, they tend to work well together. That said, "Making Cents of Metrics" is a synthesis of our personal experience of managing, by trial and error, in various workplace settings (e.g., industrial linen industry, private practice in internal medicine, and university-based academic radiology practices) over the past 35 years. While we are decidedly not management experts or academicians of management science, we have collectively produced and successfully applied a set of metrics and frameworks that has made significant improvements in practice. This chapter is an overview of how we did it

and how you can apply the same techniques to achieve more from your radiology practice.

GOALS

You can create very powerful links between your group's missions and the metrics you use to assess your organization's success in achieving those missions. In a sense, thoughtfully developed metrics should capture the "drivers of achievement" for your group. Of course, metrics are just tools used to illuminate the path you are on, and cannot represent or replace the capabilities or the will of your organization to really attain its stated missions. Getting the "right metrics" takes time and experimentation, and then additional reflection to refine them. To start the process of metric development and implementation, however, we advocate three simple rules:

1. If you can, measure what is important.
2. If you cannot measure what you believe is important, do not abandon the idea (leave it as an unfinished milestone), but audit a surrogate process.
3. Where you can find no reasonably measured events, survey important stakeholders.

METRICS AT A GLANCE

The collation of selected metrics into a single management report is like an automobile dashboard or an instrument panel of an airplane. By having a look at the dashboard, we can see, at a glance, "how we are doing." The dashboard conveys "as is" data (e.g., altitude, speed, direction, residual fuel capacity, etc.), "to be" or future data (e.g., time and distance to go, etc.), "environmental stability" data (e.g., engine temperature, oil pressure, local traffic, etc.), and "target versus actual" data (e.g., actual fuel consumption vs. predicted fuel consumption, actual vs. predicted waypoint times, etc.).

ASSUMPTIONS

If you expect metrics to be your guide, your organization should have a mission and a hunger for achievement. In our experience, motivated, mission-driven groups know (or have strong suspicions about) what the drivers of achievement are for their organizations, and these drivers are typically relatively few in number ($n \leq 20$). Metrics are typically most beneficial when complexity complicates processes ("it's a mess"), and not when tasks are simple and isolated ("this is easy as pie"). We use qualitative judgments about complexity and scalability in the selection and development of metrics. For example, the difference between net collections and net expenses (i.e., profit vs. loss) at the organizational level does not, in itself, point to specific opportunities for improved performance. However, analyzing the same metric for each of the market segments (or for each radiologist) in which your organization competes will almost certainly show meaningful variations that will

suggest opportunities for increased or decreased effort. Importantly, routine use of enterprise-spanning metrics requires the infrastructure for collecting and analyzing such subunit data to be designed into your systems up front.

But, there are caveats: While it is generally true that "you cannot manage what you cannot measure," not everything that can be measured can or should be managed. Einstein is alleged to have said, "Not everything that counts is measurable and not everything that is measurable counts." Moreover, very often it is not possible to effectively measure all of the key motivators of your organization's success, even if you know what they are. If you do not have the information systems from which to collate relevant data, as well as the information technology (IT) staff who know how to extract the data that feeds your "dashboards," what we propose—if maintained entirely by hand—might well become an exercise in futility. Finally, times and circumstances change, and so should your metrics. Challenging the appropriateness of your metrics should be part of your regular business or strategic planning.

METRIC TYPES

We track four distinct but interrelated types of metrics:

1. Qualitative
2. Quantitative
3. Budgeting
4. Trending

Qualitative and quantitative metrics are primary data sources from which budgeting and trending information is synthesized.

Qualitative measurements can be taken from carefully constructed surveys (e.g., stakeholder comments related to their expectations and satisfaction), process verification audits (e.g., protocol compliance, credentialing, etc.), and environmental assessments (e.g., benchmarking, best practices, demographics, regulatory assessments, etc.). Although numeric, we personally treat audits and most environmental assessments as qualitative metrics, because they do not directly measure the outcomes for which we hope they are surrogates (e.g., audits for compliance with performance of a documented preprocedure verification [PPV] as a surrogate for one dimension of patient safety, or maintenance of subspecialty certification as a proxy for provider skill).

Quantitative measurements include directly measurable and often technical events. Since there can be "no margin, no mission," we track the various subroutines of our revenue cycle (e.g., procedural volumes performed and coded, relative value units [RVUs], denials by type and resolution status, gross and net revenues, profit/loss, Fig. 12-1A–C). As well, we directly measured various cycle times (e.g., resource utilization, time to develop and implement new services, etc., Table 12-1) and, where applicable, market share. We calculated measures of central tendency (e.g., mean,

Table 12-1 Drivers and Metrics

# Objectives	Measure	Source Data (Frequency)
1. Compassionate Care	1. Surveys — patients/family	1. Community relations (quarterly)
	2. Letters — patients/family	2. Collated through modality and site-of-practice centered cross-functional teams (monthly) (Fig. 12-2)
	3. Incident reports	3. Patient Safety Net (monthly) (UHC®, Chicago, IL)
2. Safe Care	1. Letters — patients/family	1. Collated through modality and site-of-practice centered cross-functional teams (monthly)
	2. Reports — incidents	2. Patient Safety Net (monthly) (UHC®, Chicago, IL) (Fig. 12-3)
	3. Reports — complications	3. Ibid; and, Morbidity and Mortality Conferences (monthly)
	4. Reports — deaths	4. Ibid.
	5. Patient-safety protocols compliance	5. Audits of policy-driven practices (e.g., "Pre-Procedure Verifications"; syringe labeling; documented communication of emergent and urgent diagnostic findings) (quarterly)
	6. S-number analysis to guide minimization of radiation exposure (ALARA)	6. Analysis of S-number data from CR header information routinely taken from the IIP (Fig. 12-4)
3. Timely Care	1. Wait times — schedule	1. Spot checks against RIS (manual; monthly) (Fig. 12-5)
	2. Wait times — start	2. RIS "ABCD" (Arrival, Begin, Complete, Depart) tracking points reworked into "Resource Utilization" report by resource (monthly) (Fig. 12-6)
	3. Report availability	3. RIS "Unsigned Reports" and "Outstanding Reports Display" showing real-time numbers of preliminary reports awaiting provider signature; PACS-based script showing real-time number of unreported cases in each clinical worklist; "Milestones" reworked into "Report Turnaround" report by individual provider showing summary of timeliness of reporting and report finalization for the prior month (Fig. 12-7)

Continued

Table 12-1   Drivers and Metrics—Cont'd

# Objectives	Measure	Source Data (Frequency)
	4. Unreported cases	4. Departmental Web page access of extracted PACS-based, hourly update of totals of unreported studies by specified worklists (e.g., unread orthopaedic examinations, unread trauma center examinations, etc.)
4. Highly Valued Care	1. Surveys — patient/family	1. Community relations (monthly)
	2. Surveys — internal staff/ providers	2. Department and community relations (annually)
	3. Letters — patients/family	3. Collated through modality and site-of-practice centered cross-functional teams (monthly)
5. Accessible Care	1. 1st and 3rd available appointments	1. Spot checks against RIS (manual; monthly) (see Fig. 12-5)
	2. No. of rings to answer telephone	2. Automated...
	3. Elapsed time from request to consultant availability	3. Survey — referring providers, and comments extracted from cross-functional team meetings
	4. Report turnaround times	4. "Milestones" reworked into "Report Turnaround" report by individual provider showing summary of timeliness of reporting and report finalization for the prior month (see Fig. 12-7)
	5. Residual resource capacity	5. RIS "ABCD" tracking points reworked into "Resource Utilization" report by resource (see Fig. 12-6) (monthly)
	6. "Secret Shopper"	6. Blind calls to department, reported at cross-functional team meetings
6. Cost-effective Care	1. Use of validated clinical prediction rules	1. QA audits of councils-approved institutional practice guidelines[5]
	2. Ratio of revenue/cost	2. Calculated from departmental balance sheets (Fig. 12-8)
	3. Surveys — patient/family	3. Community relations performs regular surveys and results are reported to departments by point-of-service
7. Accurate Diagnoses	1. Peer review	1. RadPeer™ (ACR, Reston, VA) and user-reported discordant cases (Fig. 12-9)
	2. Risk management reports	2. HMC risk management consults with department on all potential legal cases that involve radiology
	3. Discordant diagnoses: radiology-pathology; radiology-surgery	3. QA review of cases in which radiology diagnoses differ from pathology or surgery findings
8. Education Regarding Optimal Practices	1. Surveys — patient/family	1. Community Relations (monthly)

Continued

Table 12-1 Drivers and Metrics—Cont'd

# Objectives	Measure	Source Data (Frequency)
	2. Interpretative services participation	2. PSN (Patient Safety Net™, UHC Chicago, IL) reports where interpreters are absent or late (quarterly)
	3. Written and oral education materials	3. Review of patient/family procedure explanation materials at cross-functional team meetings (annual)
	4. CME presentations	4. Self-report from practice partners (annual)
	5. Educational exhibits	5. Self-report from practice partners (annual)
	6. Quality control feedback to radiology technologists	6. Summary and trending of PACS-based QC folders with direct feedback to responsible radiology technologist (Fig. 12-10)
9. New Knowledge	1. Enumeration of strategic clinical needs and related clinical partners	1. Solicitation and collation of clinical service chiefs about clinical and management "challenges" amenable to collaborative improvements
	2. Peer-reviewed publications	2. "Community of Science" biographies linked through departmental Web page and maintained at regular "green book" reviews (e.g., quarterly to annually) (Fig. 12-11)
	3. Grants and contracts	3. Self-report from practice partners (annual)
10. Mutual Respect	1. Survey — faculty, staff, and trainees	1 & 2: Under development
	2. 360° evaluations of leadership	
11. Teamwork	1. Team training	1. Percent of target individuals completed formal training (annual) (Box 12-3)
	2. Team projects	2. Under development
12. Individual and Collective Growth	1. Documentation of additional training for all personnel, including: management skills, relevant CME or CEU	1. Personnel review (annual)
	2. Peer-to-peer training	2. Mentorship listing as part of personnel review (annual) (Box 12-4)
13. Quality Assurance	1. Documentation showing routine practice changes arising from QA data	1. Cross-functional team milestone management of TASKS arising from collated data from PSN, PACS-based QA folder (Fig. 12-12)
	2. Documentation scalable from individual provider to department	2. Standardized reporting matrix and definitions used throughout institution (quarterly) (Fig. 12-13)
14. Operational Efficiency	1. Trend data showing increasing value (output/ cost or output/resource)	1. Calculated from financial balance sheets, and resource utilization data (Fig. 12-14)

Continued

Table 12-1   Drivers and Metrics—Cont'd

# Objectives	Measure	Source Data (Frequency)
15. Outcomes	1. Milestone management showing interval changes in metrics, especially against budget	1. The "dashboards"
16. Fiscal Responsibility	1. Profit and loss	1. Departmental balance sheet (Fig. 12-15) and Clinical Summary Reports (Fig. 12-16)
	2. Revenues as $/FTE; $/RVU	2. Calculated in balance sheet (see Fig. 12-8)
	3. Costs as $/FTE; $/RVU	3. Calculated in balance sheet (see Fig. 12-8)
	4. Performance against budget	4. Calculated in balance sheet (Fig. 12-17)
	5. Revenue cycle data performance against benchmarks, against budget	5. Standard and ad hoc reports detailing gross and net collections, adjustments, bad debt, etc.; unworked denial inventories; patterns of first-time denials by faculty, payer, examination type; etc. (Figs. 12-18 and 12-19)

median) and, especially, variance (e.g., standard deviation, standard error), in which we tried to guide group performance to targets (e.g., using sensitivity number as a metric of radiation dosage for computed radiography to minimize individual and population radiation exposure). Often, to consolidate or arrive at a single indicator, we created compound variables, or ratios to reflect system efficiencies (Box 12-1).

These metrics can be used for benchmarking your organization's performance against others, or to just measure your own performance. Certain techniques, such as Data Envelope Analysis (a linear programming technique for assessing relative efficiency of operational units that can incorporate multiple inputs and outputs),[1] can determine if subunits within your organization are on the leading edge (envelope margin) or among the trailing performers. A variety of commercial programs are available to support such analyses, and there are even some free online syllabi with freeware.[2]

Budgeting metrics are the foundation of milestone management, and are simply an exercise of analysis and resultant actions arising from the comparison of actual and expected performances. We believe each of these metrics must reflect critical waypoints or performance specifications necessary for the achievement of desired goals, and should have a priori thresholds that trigger an organization's introspection and action (Box 12-2).

Although trending of metrics is a common planning tool, we often use trending of metrics when we incrementally budget for changes in specific processes (e.g., reducing report turnaround times by 10% per month). Depending on the primary data, we may use various regression or hazard models to "predict" future performance (e.g., possible volume growth over the next 36 months, likely time until an MR resource reaches saturation, etc.). Trending of

---

BOX 12-1

Return on investment (ROI)
Return on equity (ROE)
Volumes/full-time-equivalent (FTE) employee
RVU/case (Fig. 12-6)
RVU/FTE (Fig. 12-16, by individual radiologist)
Revenue and cost per FTE (Fig. 12-8)

BOX 12-2

Targets for Budgeting Metrics

Maximum patient waiting times
Report turnaround times
First-time denials for medical necessity from a given payer
Profit (loss)/RVU

BOX 12-3

HMC "Green Book" Reviews Regarding ACLS, ATLS, BCLS Certifications*

Faculty member: XX
Track: TA
Academic rank: TA
Date of review: 5/9/06
Approximate date for next review: 10/06

Follow-up Items

1. Teaching: Focus on teaching residents to "run the facility."
   a. Incorporated into orientations.
2. Administration: If there is sufficient time, would be very helpful for XX to assist in ad hoc projects. FAM will talk with LG and JM to list possible assignments and review these with XX.
   a. Extensive efforts around credentialing of PAs, compensation for Teaching Associates, compliance with CMS and CIA billings, and initial efforts in development of career pathway for TAs in Radiology.
3. XX update CV in COS, will meet with EH.
   a. Completed.
4. Consider greater involvement in academic products, such as educational exhibits. Staging of solid organ injuries, examples of contrast extravasation. Range of pathology for appendicitis, etc.
   a. Not undertaken.
5. Increase TG's involvement in QA.
   a. Completed.

Clinical Performance

Self-evaluation: Assumed the primary role in providing coverage for cardiac stress testing. Focuses on providing clinicians clear and timely imaging advice, especially with outside examination reviews in polytrauma cases. Remains very efficient, increases the efficiency of attending radiologists by triaging consults, providing clinical coverage that allows for on-service teaching by faculty, resident, and fellow attendance at noon conferences, and facilitates triage of work through the facility (especially, CT).
Life-support certification (BLS, ACLS, ATLS): ACLS, re-certified PA boards (98th percentile).
Based on Departmental and HMC MSQA QA data: No issues.
Based on Compliance data:
  HMC HIPPA: No complaints.
  Billings: < 0.5% header mismatches, no pattern.
Report turnaround times: 100% < 24 hr.

*"Green Books" are folders maintained on all HMC-based faculty and contain faculty-specific metrics and the documentation of regular reviews in which "contracts" for future performances are made by both the reviewer and the reviewee.

select variables against time (growth velocity and acceleration), volumes (e.g., marginal costs), and revenue/cost (e.g., financial efficiency) helps inform group leadership about future risks and promising opportunities. For example, if your group's strategy for its "commodities business" is to grow through superior cost control, trending cost/RVU compared to your competition will allow your leadership to better assess the strategic risk, and to appropriately price your "product."

KNOW AND BELIEVE IN YOUR BUSINESS

Success does not derive from wishful thinking in the boardroom, but from the right strategy, reinforced by habitual and proper execution of critical tasks at the many and varied "points of service" (i.e., "in the trenches"). Organizations are well served when they understand the what's and how's of those critical tasks on which future

---

BOX 12-4

HMC "Green Book" Reviews

Peer-to-Peer Contracts

1. HC: Life support certification: HC will contact BT for information.
2. FAM/HC: Define career pathway.
   a. HC: Focus area that HMC has sufficient volumes to support clinical research.
3. FAM/HC: For unrestricted Washington State Medical license, HC requires 2 years of ACGME training. For ABR eligibility, HC needs to apply for a waiver based on 4 consecutive years at one ACGME-approved institution as faculty member.
   a. What HC would like to be doing in 5 years: Interested in diagnostic radiology, and finds ERad more interesting than, for example, pure body imaging.
   b. ACGME: When and what? Between 2007 and 2009. Preferable Body Imaging and MSK (if MSK is ACGME); otherwise, pediatrics or nuclear radiology.
      i. FAM will discuss with MB and TD this week as to availability for AY07 or AY08.
         1. 01/06/06: FAM spoke with MB, re: CH interest in body imaging fellowship in either 2007 or 2008. MB requested that HC contact her directly.
      ii. FAM will assess whether or not MSK plans to become ACGME-certified fellowship.
         1. 01/06/06: FAM e-mailed FC requesting FC consider having fellowship ACGME accredited.
      iii. FAM will query EE re: pediatric fellowship availability for AY07 or AY08.
         1. 01/06/06: FAM left request for EF to call.
   c. ABR:
      i. Current CV.
      ii. Verification of: medical school; foreign clinical year training; foreign radiology residency; foreign radiology board certification (HC to check with ABR for advice on resolution of these criteria); radiology training in an institution that has an ACGME-approved diagnostic radiology residency *or* full-time faculty appointment in an institution that has an ACGME-approved diagnostic radiology residency appointment.
      iii. Outline of the 4-year plan to meet the guidelines, which needs to include a letter of support from the departmental chair and program director.
         1. FAM draft letters for NB and SS, after discussions with them and JN.

---

performance rests, and can measure them. For example, in answering the telephone, optimal friendliness and timeliness demonstrated by the support staff will improve customer satisfaction. If the phone is not answered properly, encourage the staff to improve those skills; if answering the phone is well executed, acknowledge it as a competitive advantage. Another example is the accuracy of billing and coding. Your practice can use metrics, such as the number of rejects and denials, to determine its effectiveness in generating revenues. Just as "economy of scale" arises from a theoretical competitive advantage, which allows an organization to capture larger market share, our attractiveness as providers of choice often rests on perceived value, and value added relative to the "market" (i.e., our competitors). Obviously, objects of perceived value differ by industry and market segment (e.g., safety: extreme sports vs. commercial airlines;

cost: commodity goods, such as paper napkins vs. specialty goods, such as tailored suits). It follows that thoughtful introspection precedes the development, modification, and interpretation of metrics you believe are important to guiding mission achievement.

USING YOUR ORGANIZATION'S MISSION TO SELECT ACHIEVEMENT DRIVERS AND RELEVANT METRICS

In this section, we briefly recapitulate the extraction of achievement drivers and derivative metrics from the Mission and Values statements for our department. Parenthetically, our mission statement was developed to reflect the missions and values of the University of

Washington School of Medicine and Harborview Medical Center (HMC), as written in their statements of mission and values. Some organizations have a formal system of missions, visions, and objectives. These statements are hierarchically defined and link the mission to yearly objectives for each department.

Our first step was to review our Mission and Values statements and extract mission-derived objectives. The following is our mission statement and enumeration of the explicit organizational objectives:

"We are an academic healthcare service whose primary mission within the bounds of fiscally responsible practices is to provide:

1. Compassionate, safe, and timely performance of diagnostic and therapeutic radiological procedures that are highly valued by both patients and referring care providers;
2. Easily accessible, cost-effective, and accurate radiological services and consultations;
3. Education about the optimal practice of radiology for our patients, staff, trainees, other healthcare providers both internal and external to the institution, and the public; and,
4. New knowledge through research directed at strategic clinical needs defined in collaboration with our clinical and administrative colleagues."

Values derived from vision and goal statements were also included in enumerating the 16 mission- and values-derived objectives that follow:

1. Provide compassionate care
2. Provide safe care
3. Provide timely care
4. Provide highly valued care
5. Provide easily accessible care
6. Provide cost-effective care
7. Provide accurate diagnoses and consultations
8. Provide education about optimal practice of radiology
9. Provide new knowledge through research
10. Promote mutual respect
11. Promote teamwork
12. Promote and improve individual and collective growth
13. Emphasize quality assurance
14. Emphasize operation efficiencies
15. Emphasize outcomes
16. Be fiscally responsible

How can we measure where we stand and whether we are making progress relative to these objectives? Table 12-1 shows three columns: Objectives, Measure, and Source Data. References to all figures (except Fig. 12-1) are in the Source Data column, and illustrate some of the formats in which we portray collected data. The figures suggest how we synthesize decision capable information from their regular aggregation and review.

Creation and maintenance of "virtuous cycles"[3] of improvement using these collated data require administrative structure appropriate to your organizational strategy and good management habits. As noted above, these strategies and structures necessarily vary by locality and market focus across radiology practices.

At HMC, we rely on cross-functional teams organized by modality (e.g., angiography, CT, MRI, nuclear radiology, ultrasound, etc.), site of practice (e.g., trauma center, OR, main radiology, etc.), and function (e.g., billings, IT), which meet at least monthly to oversee appropriate "resourcing" of tasks. We also assess and then guide necessary individual (Boxes 12-3 and 12-4) and system performances pertinent to mission achievements. A broad representation by relevant stakeholders (e.g., hospital administrators, nursing, radiology technologists, radiologists, physician practice administrators, medical physicists, etc.) populates these cross-functional teams, and the teams are accountable to senior leadership for task execution.

How often do we survey our data? As noted above, most performance data are reviewed in cross-functional groups monthly, against either target or budget. Accountable individuals, however, track critical functions daily (such as billings postings, patient safety events, etc.). Although our strategic planning process is said to be "annual," for us it is a continual process that seeks regular assessments of business environment change, alterations in our internal capacities (human and technological), and community expectations.

Of course, collecting and reviewing data is meaningless *unless* decisions and actions ensue. We practice "thresholding," that is, we use thresholds (targets or limits) based on statistical process management practices for those processes that lend themselves to quantitative assessments (such as average age of accounts receivable [AR], report turn-around times, extravasation of intravenous contrast at CT, etc.) to determine when ad hoc in-depth reviews are indicated. We base our "need to respond" on how critical the function is in its particular market segment, and our historical wisdom. For example, inability to accommodate elective outpatient studies within 48 hours receives an escalation of audit frequency from monthly to daily, once a threshold is passed and remains outside acceptable parameters. In-depth review and correction will be implemented at the next month's cross-functional group meeting. Using trending to anticipate future needs (when significant lead time is necessary to garner resources necessary to adequately respond, e.g., purchasing new MRI scanners), we incorporate reviews into our capital assessments as part of our strategic planning.

These cross-functional teams, in conjunction with weekly HMC radiology faculty and hospital departmental managers meetings, are the "spinal cord" of our systemic communications practice. The teams use a standard agenda format that is tailored to their areas of focus. These cross-functional teams are the effectors of change for our organization, the translators of thoughts from departmental leadership to the willful action of the organization, whether the issue is development of new business or how to make improvements in examination scheduling. One important underlying theme in all of our meetings is use of "root cause" analysis[4] structure to analyze performance variations and shortfalls. In the end, however, organizations must show the will to act on data at variance with their goals, visions, and missions.[5]

DIFFERENCES BETWEEN PRIVATE AND ACADEMIC PRACTICES

After the conclusion of this chapter, you'll find a list of dos and don'ts of metrics. Do they depend on your practice setting? Not really. We believe there are few, if any, important differences between private and academic practices. The perceived differences are just that—perceived, since the concepts we espouse here are universal. We politely observe that some academic practices outperform many private practices on all financial metrics, and that some private practice groups have more grant and contract funding than many so-called academic ones. "Successful" organizations, whether private or academic, manage to stay in business and continue to achieve their missions while living up to their values.

CONCLUSION

We live in interesting and complex times. And, in complex systems, "the devil is in the details." Myriad factors influence the success of organizations, most importantly, the quality of their people, especially if they work well together. The quality of communication is most essential in determining the ability of groups to work together, to form highly reliable organizations. The regular dissemination and collective review of and response to thoughtfully and doggedly collated data and derived metrics on determinant performance drivers should form one of the most important corridors with which to align the "hearts and souls" of your organization.

Dos and Don'ts of Minding Your Metrics	
Dos	**Don'ts**
1. Recognize the profit margin. Remember, "no margin, no mission." For the organization as a whole and for every elective product line, measure how much income exceeds expense. For nonelective product lines, how much does actual metric exceed budget?	1. Get caught up in the glory of merely having data to admire. Don't collect it if you don't have the courage to act on what you find. 2. Misuse the data you've collected. Collecting data but failing to use it effectively is costly.

Dos	Don'ts
2. Emphasize innovation by building better mousetraps.	3. Just stand there; do something. Show energy. Stagnation in this market is a killer.
3. Develop name recognition—"Who *are* those guys?" To stay in the lead, organizations must have continuous improvement of product lines and personnel.	4. Allow emotions to completely override logic. It may be your "pet" metric, but if it's misleading the team, abandon it.
4. Be efficient. Want to change habits? Measure the timeliness and execution of campaigns, programs, processes, and acquisition of new habits.	5. Miss your systematic and periodic reviews. They help to realign metrics with changes in organizational strategy and structure.
5. Demonstrate passion. If your organization lacks passion, it won't be a good place to work, so why measure at all?	6. Use metrics that under- or misrepresent the "drivers" for your organization's achievement. Be certain to measure what matters to your customers and stakeholders.
6. Review and realign metrics with changes in organizational strategy and structure.	7. Forget that complexity can confound judgments: "How long will it take you to learn that we do not use data to make decisions around here?"
7. Develop "scalable" metrics that can be rolled up from the smallest unit to the largest (such as $/RVU as both expense and revenue, which can be applied to individual CPTs, radiologists, market segments, referring clinicians, and the organization as a whole).	8. Underestimate and underinvest in informatics infrastructure and skilled IT personnel.
8. Include, discuss, and attempt to track important and desired metrics that are not currently measurable.	9. Exclude the naysayers. They are often the keys to innovation and self-analysis.
9. Establish organizational purpose and alignment. No metric can lead you to where you are not going.	10. Violate process fairness. For the sake of the "hearts and souls" of team members, and to prevent those members from disengaging or having low morale, leaders must be respectful of dissent and differing opinions and accountable for their own mistakes and errors in judgment.
10. Implement and practice effective systemic communications through the use of highly autonomous cross-functional teams.	

REFERENCES

1. Emrouznejad A: Data envelopment analysis home page, available at: http://www.DEAzone.com/.
2. Beasley J: Operations Research Notes, available at http://people.brunel.ac.uk/~mastjjb/jeb/or/dea.html/.
3. Senge PM: The Fifth Discipline: The Art and Practice of the Learning Organization. New York, Doubleday, 1990.
4. Liker J: The Toyota Way. New York, McGraw-Hill, 2004.
5. Hanson JA, Deliganis AV, Baxter AB, Cohen WA, et al: Radiologic and clinical spectrum of occipital condyle fractures: Retrospective review of 107 consecutive fractures in 95 patients. AJR Am J Roentgenol 178:1261–1268, 2002.

SUGGESTED READINGS

Chandler AD: The Visible Hand: Managerial Revolution in American Business. Cambridge. Mass, Harvard University Press, 1977.
Davemport TH: Competing on analytics. Harvard Business Review (January 2006), pp 99–107.
Kaplan RS, Norton DP: The Balanced Scorecard. Boston, Harvard Business School Press, 1996.
Pfeffer J, Sutton RI:: Evidence-based management. Harvard Business Review 84(1):63–74, 2006.
Sirkin HL, Keenan P, Jackson A: The hard side of change management. Harvard Business Review (October 2005), 109–118.
Tuchman BW: The March of Folly: From Troy to Vietnam. New York, Alfred A. Knopf, 1984.

Figure 12-1 Billing cycle. **A,** Coding production and "header" mismatches (discordant description given by radiologist and examination scheduled).

	Jul-03	Aug-03	Sep-03	Oct-03	Nov-03	Dec-03	Jan-04	Feb-04	Mar-04	Apr-04	May-04	Jun-04		
Exams:														
Hospital	16702	16323	17091	15900	13900	18200	16000	18409	20346	20438	20405	21503	203776	
pro-fee								18175	18931	18825	13060	19769		
Header Mismatches:														
Hospital "B" status	57	99	52	43	32	22 n/a	44	58	53	100	103			
MD/PA	143	102	150	127	65	119 n/a	223	204	338	336	308			
%	3.24%	2.62%	3.57%	3.31%	3.67%	3.26%	1.65%	1.39%	2.07%	2.40%	2.09%			

	Jul-04	Aug-04	Sep-04	Oct-04	Nov-04	Dec-04	Jan-05	Feb-05	Mar-05	Apr-05	May-05	Jun-05	
Exams:													
pro-fee	19855	19487	18906	17234	16228	17422	17959	15849	19770	17396	18348	19379	217830
Header Mismatches:													
Hospital "B" status	63	121	74	134	92	72	12	15	8	9	16	31	
MD/PA	303	246	308	269	297	274	318	251	317	307	373	410	
%	2.15%	1.86%	2.02%	2.34%	2.39%	1.96%	1.84%	1.67%	1.64%	1.61%	2.12%	2.23%	

	Jul-05	Aug-05	Sep-05	Oct-05	Nov-05	Dec-05	Jan-06	Feb-06	Mar-06	Apr-06	May-06	Jun-06	YTD
Exams:													
Hospital	22138	21906	20464	19984	17570	19001	20454	18646	20679	21050	21806	21789	2003
pro-fee	18884	20794	18606	17785	16467	17073	17821	16159	18115	16749	19129	19073	2004
Header Mismatches:													
Hospital "B" status	29	28	9	17	13	16	24	26	26	22	35	38	2005
MD/PA	414	375	341	330	313	255	266	327	407	400	434	352	2006
									-35				
									1.77				
%	2.34%	1.93%	1.86%	1.95%	1.97%	1.53%	1.64%	1.97%	2.39%	2.13%	2.45%	2.04%	

YTD: 2006 43343; 2007 46949

	Jul-06	Aug-06
Exams:		
Hospital	22506	23743
pro-fee	20221	21246
Header Mismatches:		
Hospital "B" status	20	27
MD/PA	427	421
%	2.21%	2.10%

YTD: 2006 39676; 2007 41467

N/O yearly totals: 2003 174008; 2004 203776; 2005 217830; 2006 219258

A

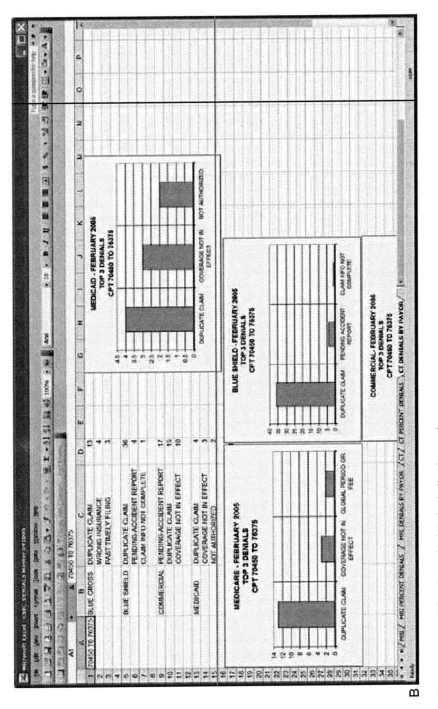

Figure continued on next page

Figure 12-1, cont'd   **B,** CT denials by indication and payer.

Figure 12-1, cont'd C, Denials for allegedly inappropriate medical necessity.

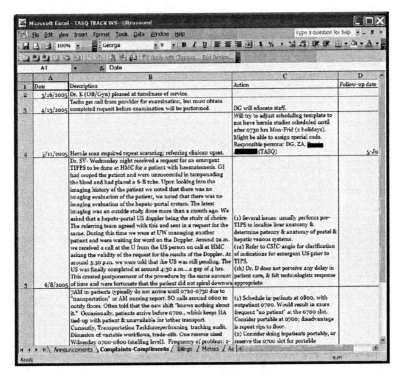

Figure 12-2   CSIS-US compliments and complaints.

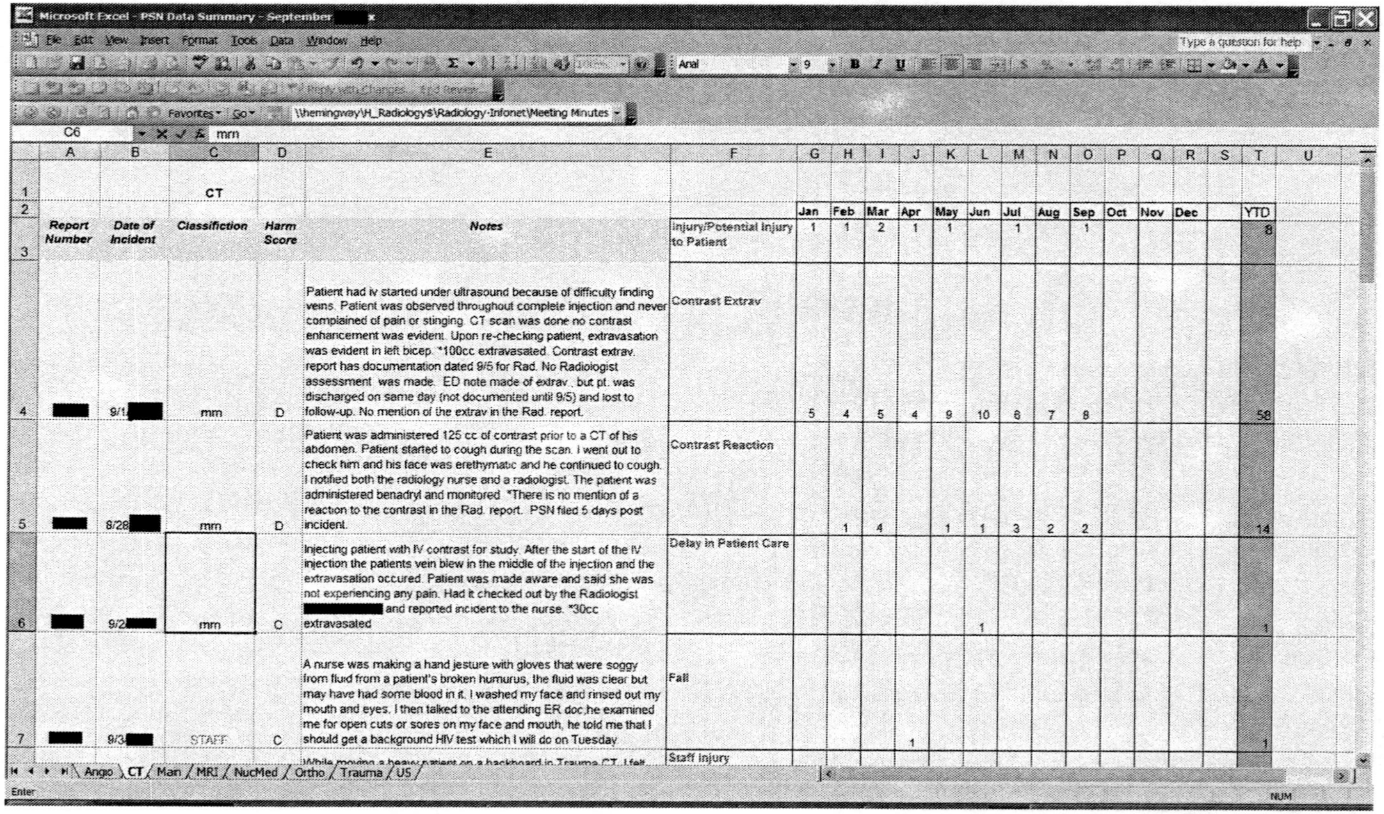

Figure 12-3   CT PSN summary.

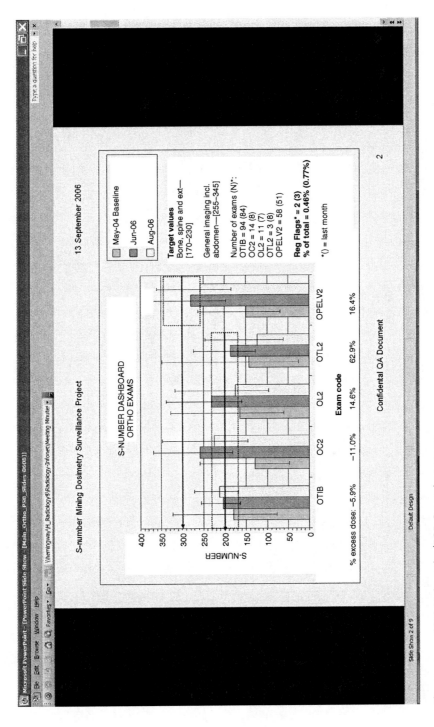

Figure 12-4 CSIC-Main ortho/PSB S-number report.

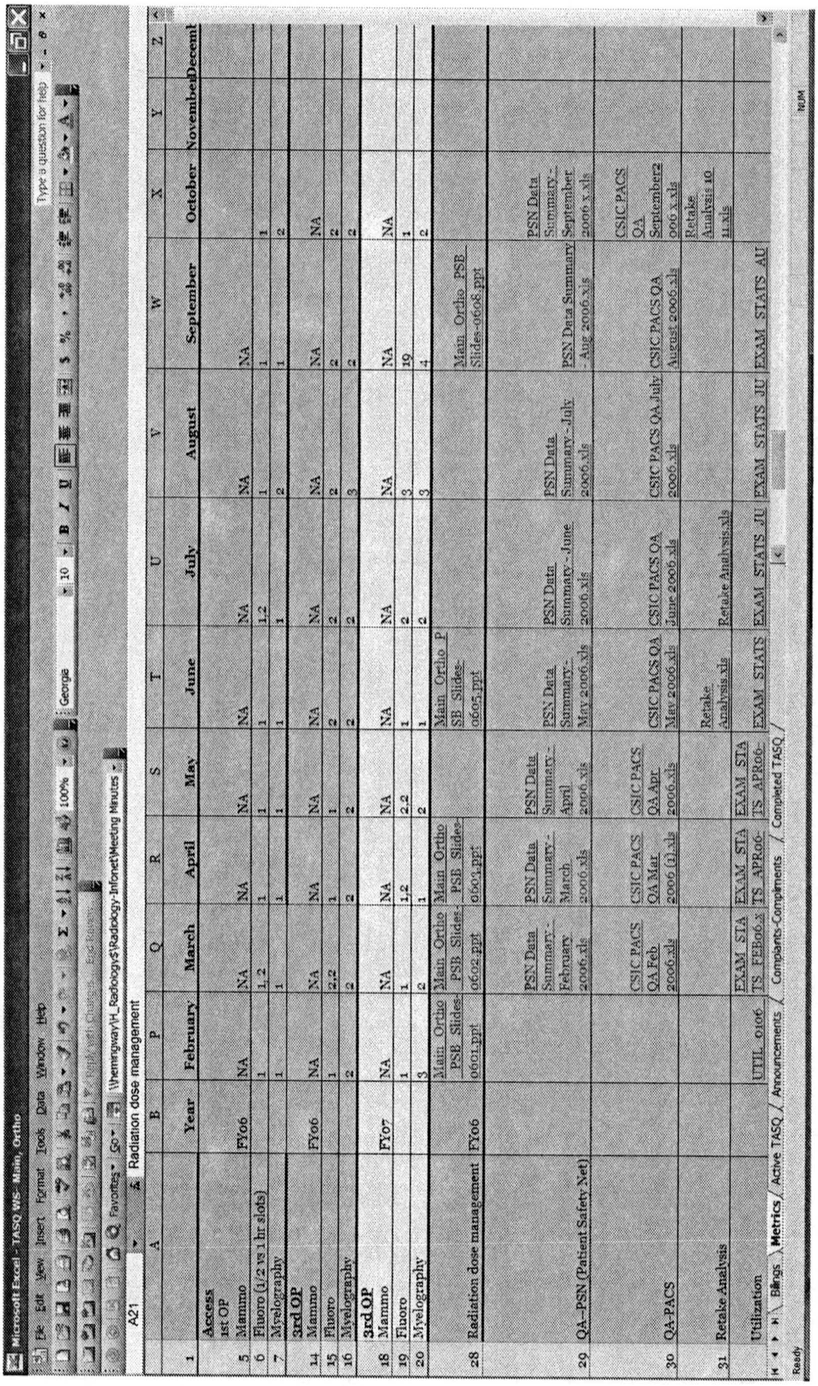

Figure 12-5 CSIC-Main 1st and 3rd OP appointment availability.

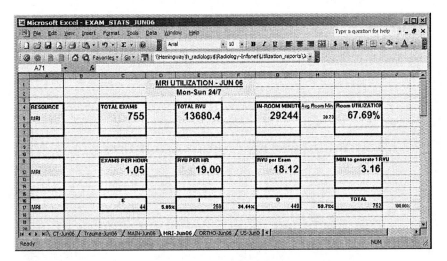

Figure 12-6 CSIC-MRI resource utilization reports.

Radiologist	Completed to Finalized			Completed to Preliminary				Preliminary to Finalized		
	Average Time	Daily Average Within 24 Hours (Exams)	Within 24 Hours (%)	Average Time	Daily Average Within 12 Hours (Exams)	Within 12 Hours (%)	After 2 Days (%)	Average Time	Daily Average Within 8 Hours (Exams)	Within 8 Hours (%)
	< 2h	50.9	99.2%	< 2h	50.8	99.1%	0.3%	< 2h	48.0	93.6%
	4-6h	49.5	99.5%	< 2h	49.2	99.0%	0.3%	4-6h	35.5	71.4%
	10-12h	43.6	77.0%	8-10h	38.7	68.2%	0.6%	4-6h	48.3	85.1%
	2-4h	39.2	98.9%	< 2h	38.3	96.7%	0.3%	< 2h	36.8	92.8%
	2-4h	39.5	97.6%	< 2h	37.1	91.7%	0.9%	< 2h	37.9	93.6%
	2-4h	31.6	99.6%	< 2h	30.4	95.8%	0.2%	< 2h	30.2	95.2%
	4-6h	28.7	91.2%	< 2h	29.1	92.5%	0.4%	2-4h	27.0	85.8%
	10-12h	19.3	72.9%	2-4h	23.0	86.6%	1.1%	8-10h	15.4	58.0%
	4-6h	22.4	97.2%	< 2h	22.1	95.8%	0.3%	2-4h	17.2	74.8%
	6-8h	14.5	91.5%	4-6h	13.7	86.2%	1.2%	2-4h	11.9	74.8%
	10-12h	16.6	79.6%	8-10h	13.0	62.4%	2.2%	2-4h	19.1	91.6%
	6-8h	13.7	91.8%	4-6h	12.5	83.2%	1.1%	< 2h	13.9	92.9%
	2-4h	12.4	98.2%	2-4h	11.3	89.0%	0.0%	< 2h	12.6	99.5%
	28-32h	7.3	36.6%	10-12h	9.3	46.8%	6.3%	12-16h	8.8	44.2%
	< 2h	8.8	100.0%	< 2h	8.8	100.0%	0.0%	< 2h	8.8	100.0%
	6-8h	12.3	96.7%	6-8h	8.6	67.6%	0.5%	< 2h	12.7	100.0%
	20-24h	7.5	54.1%	8-10h	7.1	50.8%	3.5%	8-10h	7.6	55.0%
	16-20h	10.7	74.4%	8-10h	6.6	46.0%	1.1%	4-6h	11.3	78.7%
	4-6h	6.8	92.5%	2-4h	6.5	88.1%	0.4%	2-4h	6.5	89.0%
	8-10h	7.3	90.4%	4-6h	6.4	79.2%	1.2%	4-6h	6.1	75.6%
	16-20h	7.0	62.1%	8-10h	6.4	56.4%	1.4%	6-8h	5.8	51.6%
	8-10h	6.6	82.3%	4-6h	6.4	79.1%	4.8%	4-6h	6.2	77.1%
	10-12h	10.2	89.0%	8-10h	5.9	51.4%	2.5%	< 2h	11.3	98.3%
	6-8h	5.7	94.1%	2-4h	5.8	96.8%	1.1%	4-6h	3.8	63.1%
	10-12h	7.3	89.7%	8-10h	4.0	48.6%	0.4%	< 2h	7.6	92.9%
	4-6h	2.7	90.4%	2-4h	2.7	89.4%	4.3%	< 2h	2.9	94.7%
	6-8h	2.0	92.4%	2-4h	2.0	93.9%	3.0%	2-4h	1.6	77.3%
	2d	0.0	0.6%	12-16h	1.6	30.9%	3.0%	36-40h	0.1	1.2%
	6-8h	1.4	86.3%	< 2h	1.6	98.0%	0.0%	4-6h	1.4	86.3%
	10-12h	1.0	71.4%	2-4h	1.2	85.7%	2.4%	10-12h	0.7	50.0%
	8-10h	0.7	80.8%	2-4h	0.8	96.2%	3.8%	6-8h	0.5	61.5%
	40-44h	0.2	20.0%	6-8h	0.8	71.4%	5.7%	36-40h	0.3	22.9%
	28-32h	0.5	45.7%	8-10h	0.7	62.9%	8.6%	20-24h	0.5	45.7%
	6-8h	0.5	73.9%	4-6h	0.6	78.3%	0.0%	2-4h	0.7	91.3%
	24-28h	0.7	50.0%	12-16h	0.5	32.6%	4.3%	8-10h	0.8	54.3%
	16-20h	0.4	57.9%	4-6h	0.5	73.7%	0.0%	10-12h	0.2	36.8%
	24-28h	0.2	23.1%	10-12h	0.5	53.8%	11.5%	10-12h	0.2	26.9%
	10-12h	0.3	75.0%	2-4h	0.4	91.7%	0.0%	8-10h	0.2	58.3%
	< 2h	0.5	100.0%	6-8h	0.3	56.3%	0.0%	< 2h	0.5	100.0%
	8-10h	0.3	66.7%	8-10h	0.3	66.7%	8.3%	< 2h	0.4	100.0%
	40-44h	0.0	5.9%	8-10h	0.3	47.1%	0.0%	32-36h	0.0	0.0%
	32-36h	0.1	19.0%	10-12h	0.2	33.3%	0.0%	28-32h	0.1	14.3%
	4d	0.0	11.1%	6-8h	0.2	66.7%	0.0%	4d	0.0	11.1%
	32-36h	0.0	0.0%	8-10h	0.1	66.7%	0.0%	24-28h	0.0	0.0%
	16-20h	0.4	72.2%	12-16h	0.1	22.2%	0.0%	2-4h	0.6	100.0%
	10-12h	0.1	66.7%	12-16h	0.1	66.7%	33.3%	10-12h	0.0	33.3%
ALL RADIOLOGISTS	6-8h	491.7	86.4%	4-6h	466.2	81.9%	1.1%	2-4h	462.1	81.2%

Figure 12-7 Report dictation turnaround times: Summary for December 2006.

YTD wRVU/MD-FTE	YTD Expense/wRVU	YTD Expense/tRVU
8,634	$55.04	$39.63
ANNUALIZED wRVU/MD-FTE	YTD Net Revenue/wRVU	YTD Net Revenue/tRVU
25,902	$54.20	$39.02
	MARGIN:	-1.53%

Figure 12-8 HMC radiology balance sheet, indices quadrant.

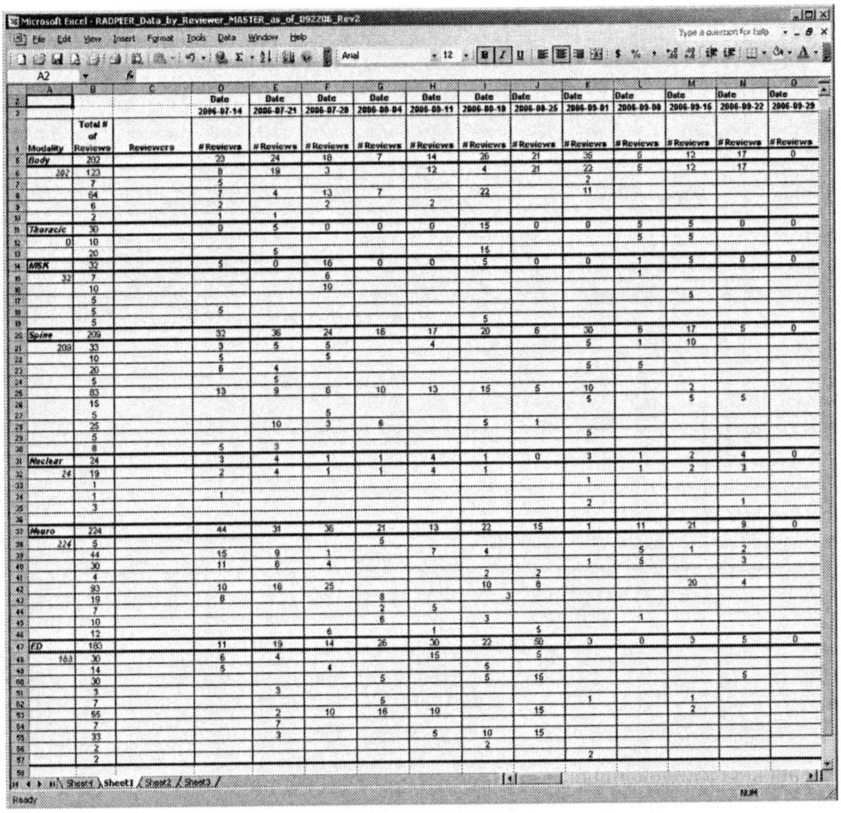

Figure 12-9 Compliance with RadPeer™ by section.

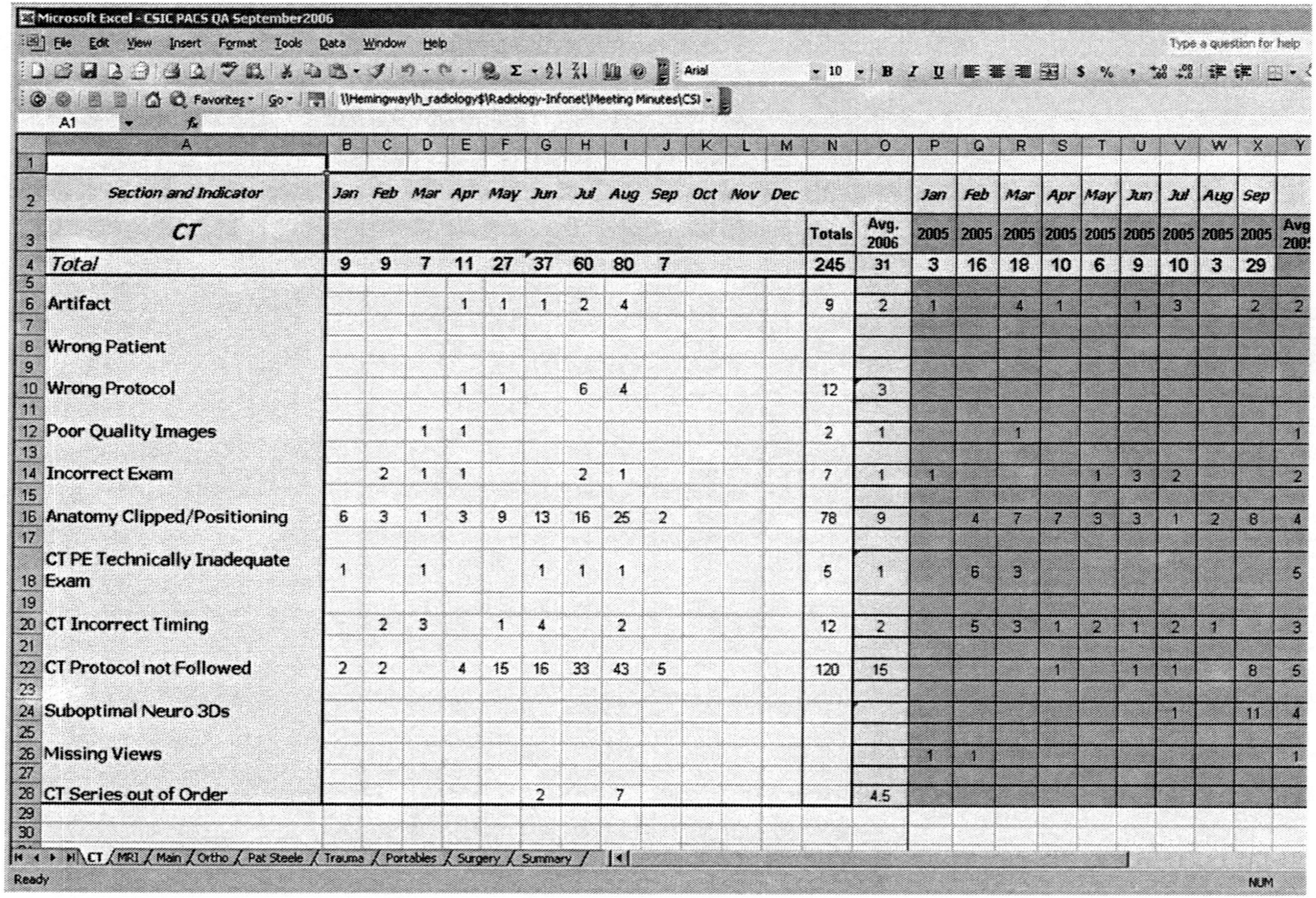

Section and Indicator	Jan	Feb	Mar	Apr	May	Jun	Jul	Aug	Sep	Oct	Nov	Dec	Totals	Avg. 2006	Jan 2005	Feb 2005	Mar 2005	Apr 2005	May 2005	Jun 2005	Jul 2005	Aug 2005	Sep 2005	Avg 2005
CT																								
Total	9	9	7	11	27	37	60	80	7				245	31	3	16	18	10	6	9	10	3	29	
Artifact				1	1	1	2	4					9	2	1		4	1		1	3		2	2
Wrong Patient																								
Wrong Protocol				1	1		6	4					12	3										
Poor Quality Images			1	1									2	1			1							1
Incorrect Exam		2	1	1			2	1					7	1	1				1	3	2			2
Anatomy Clipped/Positioning	6	3	1	3	9	13	16	25	2				78	9		4	7	7	3	3	1	2	8	4
CT PE Technically Inadequate Exam	1		1			1	1	1					5	1		6	3							5
CT Incorrect Timing		2	3		1	4		2					12	2		5	3	1	2	1	2	1		3
CT Protocol not Followed	2	2		4	15	16	33	43	5				120	15				1		1	1		8	5
Suboptimal Neuro 3Ds																					1		11	4
Missing Views															1	1								1
CT Series out of Order						2		7						4.5										

Figure 12-10 CSIC-CT PACS QA folder review.

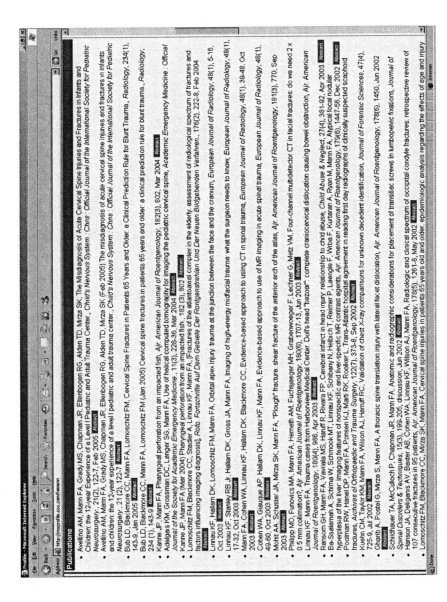

Figure 12-11 HMC radiology department faculty publications.

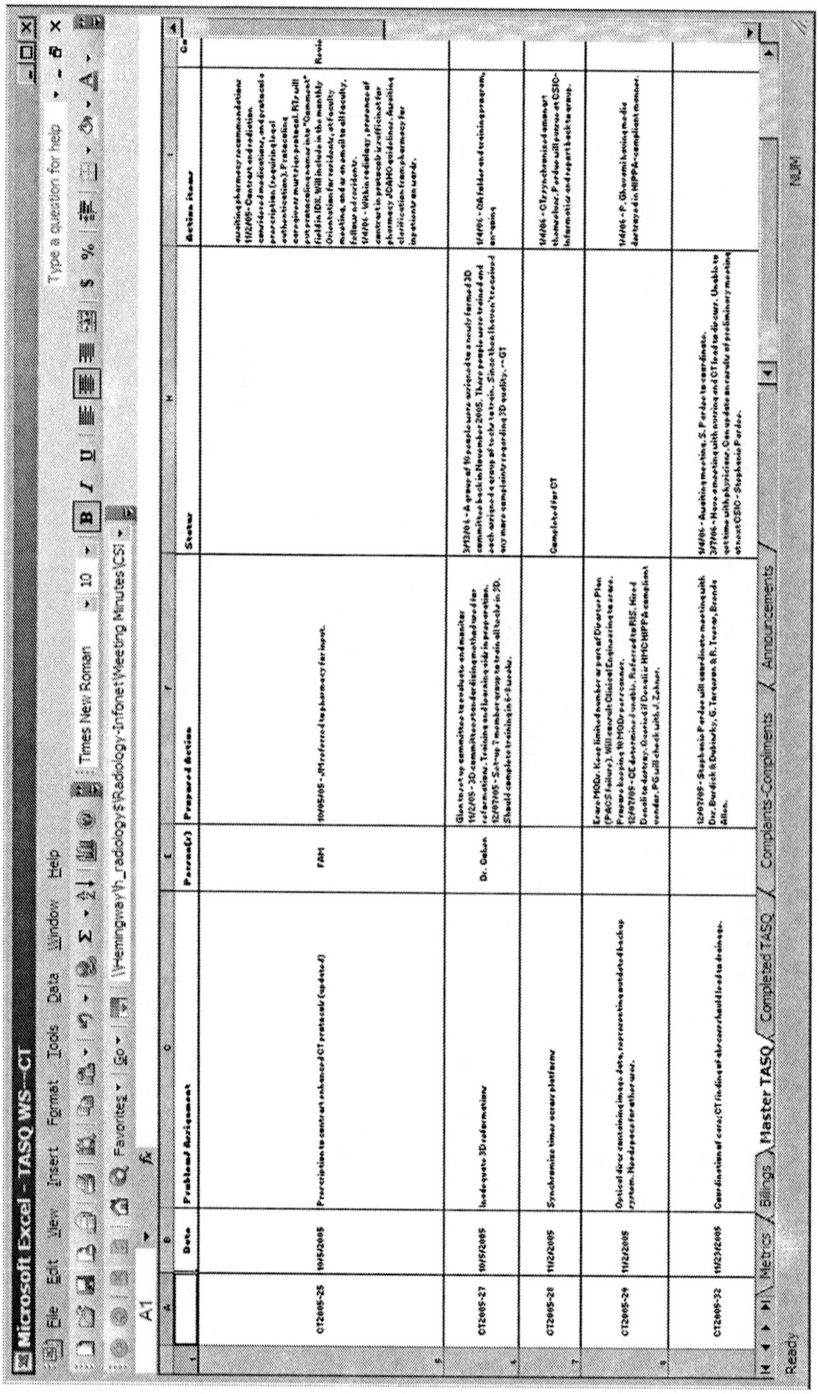

Figure 12-12 CSIC-CT TASQ worksheet.

9/26/05-1/15/06	total	agree with	discordant	A1	A2	A3	A4	B1	B2	B3	B4	C1	C2	C3	II	Total Acute % (A1+A2+B1+B2)	Acute intracranial % (A1 + B1)	Acute extracranial % (A2 - B2)	total %
	8	8														0.00%	0.00%	0.00%	0.00%
	316	300	16	2	3	3		1	1		1	1			4	1.90%	0.95%	0.95%	5.06%
	97	91	6				2				1				3	0.00%	0.00%	0.00%	6.19%
	5	4	1		1											20.00%	0.00%	20.00%	20.00%
	79	75	4	2			1								1	3.80%	3.80%	0.00%	5.06%
	1	1	0													0.00%	0.00%	0.00%	0.00%
	10	10	0													0.00%	0.00%	0.00%	0.00%
	1	1	0													0.00%	0.00%	0.00%	0.00%
	124	118	6	2	1		1								2	2.42%	1.61%	0.81%	4.84%
	8	4	4	2		2										25.00%	25.00%	0.00%	50.00%
	292	271	21	2	3	2	6				2	1	1		4	1.71%	0.68%	1.03%	7.19%
	65	64	1	1												1.54%	1.54%	0.00%	1.54%
	27	27	0													0.00%	0.00%	0.00%	0.00%
	260	250	10	1	2	2	1						1		3	1.15%	0.38%	0.77%	3.85%
	83	81	2				1								1	0.00%	0.00%	0.00%	2.41%
	3	1	2		1									1		33.33%	0.00%	33.33%	66.67%
	309	301	8		1		2						1		4	0.32%	0.00%	0.32%	2.59%
	152	143	9	1	1		1	1			1				4	1.97%	1.32%	0.66%	5.92%
	1	1	0													0.00%	0.00%	0.00%	0.00%
	91	89	2			1									1	0.00%	0.00%	0.00%	2.20%
	3	3	0													0.00%	0.00%	0.00%	0.00%
	3	2	1												1	0.00%	0.00%	0.00%	33.33%
	64	61	3	1											2	1.56%	1.56%	0.00%	4.69%
	9	9	0													0.00%	0.00%	0.00%	0.00%
	3	3	0													0.00%	0.00%	0.00%	0.00%
	2	2	0													0.00%	0.00%	0.00%	0.00%
	18	18	0													0.00%	0.00%	0.00%	0.00%
Totals (res)	2025	1920	105	14	13	10	15	3	0	1	2	3	2	7	26	1.48%	0.84%	0.64%	5.19%
Totals (res+fellow)	2043	1938	105	14	13	10	15	3	0	1	2	3	2	7	26	1.47%	0.83%	0.64%	5.14%

A - Missed	B - Misinterpreted	C - Overcall	C - Overcall
1. Acute Intracranial	1. Acute Intracranial	1. Old called new	1. Old called new
2. Acute Extracranial	2. Acute Extracranial	2. Normal variant	2. Normal variant
3. Non-Acute	3. Non-Acute	3. Not present	3. Not present
4. Possible/uncertain	4. Possible/uncertain		

Figure 12-13 Resident discordant cases.

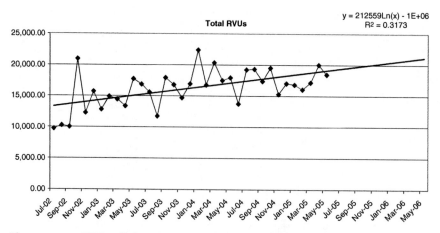

Figure 12-14 HMC radiology balance sheet, RVU regression models.

Microsoft Excel - HMC Radiology Pro Strategic Planning_Balance Sheet thru May 2006

| | Research overhead% | 12.83% |
| | Administration overhead % | 12.83% |

Harborview Medical Center UW-M Department of Radiology FY06 Projected RVUs & Cash	Actual Faculty Clinical Salary & Benefits	Faculty HMC Admin Salary & Benefits	HMC Director's & Christie Library Fund	HMC Operational Expenses	(NET from OPERATIONS) PRE HOSPITAL FUNDING RADIOLOGY NET REVENUE	HOSPITAL FUNDED FACULTY SUPPORT	POST HOSPITAL FUNDING RADIOLOGY NET REVENUE	YTD POST HOSPITAL FUNDING RADIOLOGY NET REVENUE	Budgeted DEPT RESEARCH TAX	Budgeted CENTRAL DEPT BUDGET NON-RESEARCH OVERHEAD	RESERVES
		1.4	97,500.0			#########			700,000.00	700,000.00	
Jul-05	$442,804	$35,700	$8,125	$755,949	$2,637	$283,333	$285,970	$285,970	$58,333	$58,333	$169,303
Aug-05	$442,804	$35,700	$8,125	$754,286	($1,531)	$283,333	$281,803	$567,773	$58,333	$58,333	$165,136
Sep-05	$442,804	$35,700	$8,125	$780,681	$64,582	$283,333	$347,915	$915,688	$58,333	$58,333	$231,249
Oct-05	$442,804	$35,700	$8,125	$757,559	$9,787	$283,333	$293,121	$1,208,809	$58,333	$58,333	$176,454
Nov-05	$442,804	$35,700	$8,125	$752,370	($6,326)	$283,333	$277,005	$1,485,814	$58,333	$58,333	$160,339
Dec-05	$442,804	$35,700	$8,125	$748,687	($15,552)	$283,333	$267,781	$1,753,595	$58,333	$58,333	$151,114
Jan-06	$442,804	$35,700	$8,125	$743,196	($29,300)	$283,333	$254,026	$2,007,621	$58,333	$58,333	$137,359
Feb-06	$442,804	$35,700	$8,125	$709,463	($113,797)	$283,333	$169,536	$2,177,157	$58,333	$58,333	$52,869
Mar-06	$442,804	$35,700	$8,125	$772,872	$45,022	$283,333	$328,356	$2,505,512	$58,333	$58,333	$211,689
Apr-06	$442,804	$35,700	$8,125	$735,929	($47,609)	$283,333	$235,824	$2,741,337	$58,333	$58,333	$119,158
May-06	$442,804	$35,700	$8,125	$741,250	($34,180)	$283,333	$249,153	$2,990,490	$58,333	$58,333	$132,486
Jun-06	$442,804	$35,700	$8,125			$283,333			$58,333	$58,333	
Projected FY06 totals		$428,400	$97,500	$8,252,242	($126,177)	$3,400,000	$2,990,490		$700,000	$700,000	$1,707,157

Income Statement / FY06 Projected RVUs & Cash / urReg RVUs and $ per RVU /

Figure 12-15 HMC balance sheet, P&L.

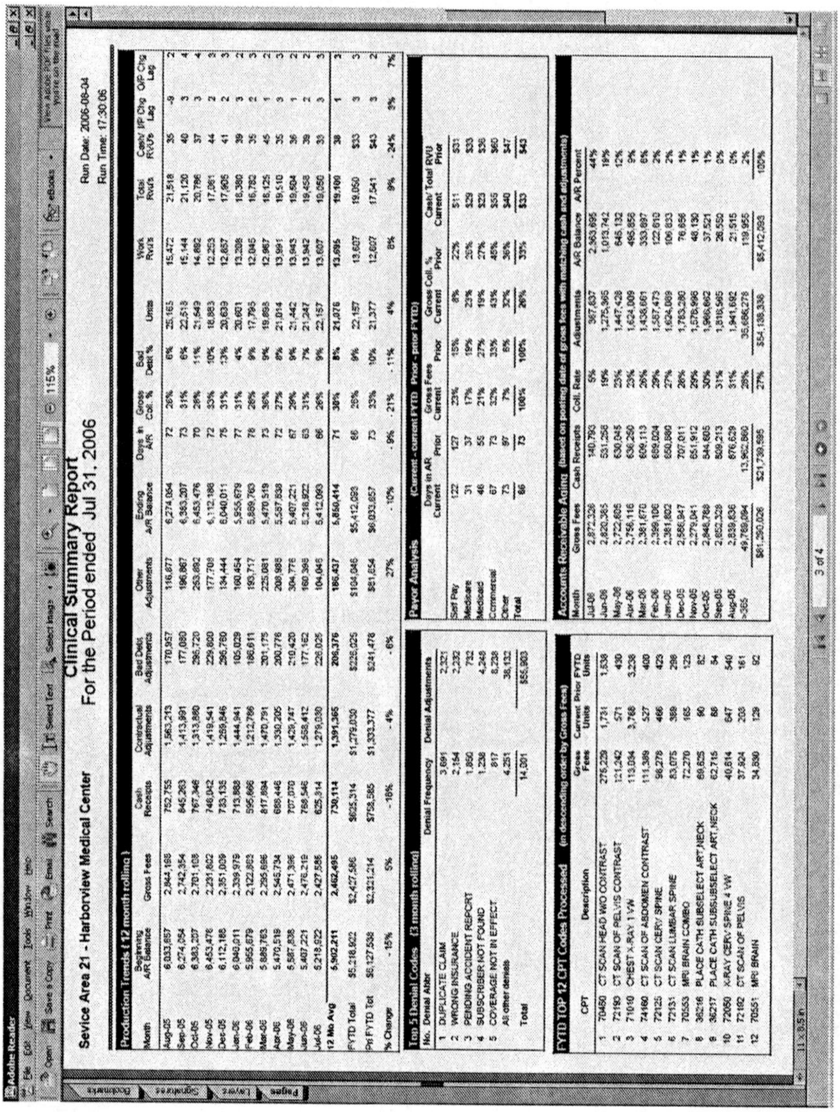

Figure 12-16 Clinical summary reports.

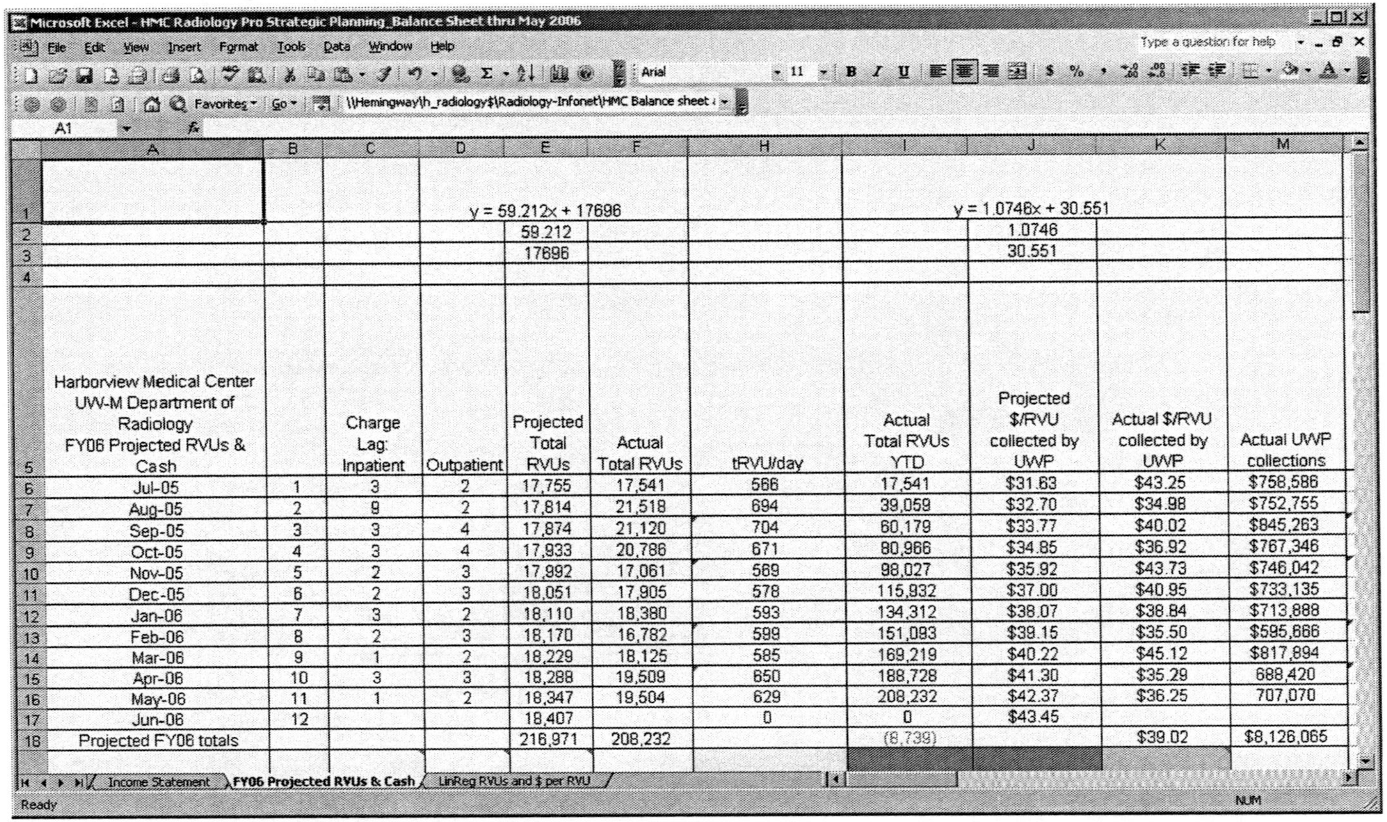

	A	B	C	D	E	F	H	I	J	K	M
1				y = 59.212x + 17696					y = 1.0746x + 30.551		
2					59.212				1.0746		
3					17696				30.551		
4											
5	Harborview Medical Center UW-M Department of Radiology FY06 Projected RVUs & Cash		Charge Lag: Inpatient	Outpatient	Projected Total RVUs	Actual Total RVUs	tRVU/day	Actual Total RVUs YTD	Projected $/RVU collected by UWP	Actual $/RVU collected by UWP	Actual UWP collections
6	Jul-05	1	3	2	17,755	17,541	566	17,541	$31.63	$43.25	$758,586
7	Aug-05	2	9	2	17,814	21,518	694	39,059	$32.70	$34.98	$752,755
8	Sep-05	3	3	4	17,874	21,120	704	60,179	$33.77	$40.02	$845,263
9	Oct-05	4	3	4	17,933	20,786	671	80,966	$34.85	$36.92	$767,346
10	Nov-05	5	2	3	17,992	17,061	569	98,027	$35.92	$43.73	$746,042
11	Dec-05	6	2	3	18,051	17,905	578	115,932	$37.00	$40.95	$733,135
12	Jan-06	7	3	2	18,110	18,380	593	134,312	$38.07	$38.84	$713,888
13	Feb-06	8	2	3	18,170	16,782	599	151,093	$39.15	$35.50	$595,666
14	Mar-06	9	1	2	18,229	18,125	585	169,219	$40.22	$45.12	$817,894
15	Apr-06	10	3	3	18,288	19,509	650	188,728	$41.30	$35.29	688,420
16	May-06	11	1	2	18,347	19,504	629	208,232	$42.37	$36.25	707,070
17	Jun-06	12			18,407		0	0	$43.45		
18	Projected FY06 totals				216,971	208,232		(8,739)		$39.02	$8,126,065

Figure 12-17 HMC balance sheet, revenues, actual vs. budget.

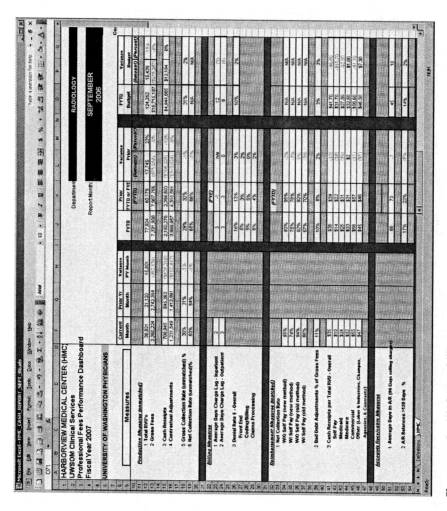

Figure 12-18 HMC UWP billings report.

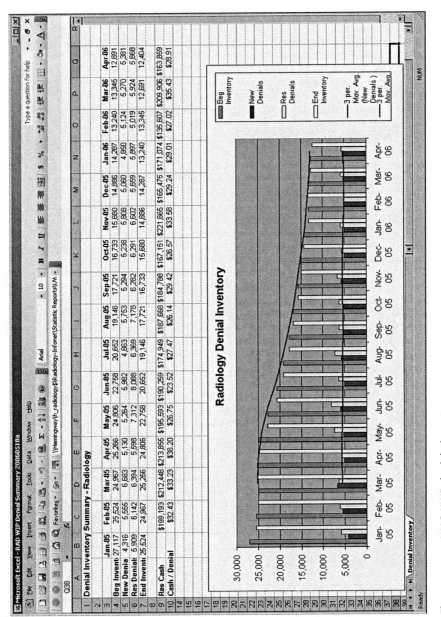

Figure 12-19 HMC UWP denials inventory.

PART 3A

BUILDING AND MANAGING
A PRACTICE: NUTS AND BOLTS

CHAPTER 13

Information Technology Systems

Peter A. Janick

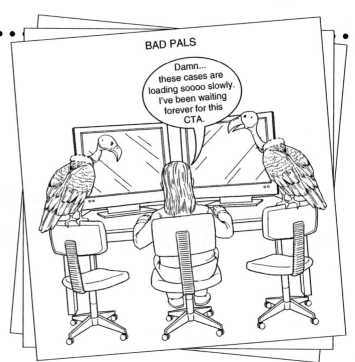

INTRODUCTION

In the beginning...there was the film jacket. Well, not really. My first day on the job as a practicing radiologist was at the Baltimore Children's Hospital, a former polio hospital converted into a sports medicine mecca. As I plowed through the stack of film jackets, I noticed five or six tall file cabinets along one end of the room. Many months later I summoned up my courage and opened up one of the drawers. Inside were hundreds of glass plate radiographs from which I randomly picked up an unbelievable image of Potts disease, just like in the textbooks. Handling those fragile pieces of glass, I immediately understood the importance of the development of cellulose film (even if it could spontaneously combust), and finally acetate, in advancing the management of X-rays. The film jacket was the crowning glory. The jacket organized and held the radiographs. Some institutions would even compartmentalize studies into subfolders within

the film jacket to improve organization. The front of the jacket provided the patient name, labels based on the medical record number to help organize the jackets within the film library, and a list of the studies contained within the jacket. Radiologists would often adorn the outside of the jacket with helpful synopses of the interpretations for previous studies and pithy comments concerning the patient's history. A clever pocket or envelope within the jacket held the old reports and worksheets. A plastic jacket would hold the new study, the requisition, any reports or worksheets, as well as the film archive. The movement of the film jacket defined work flow. First images were obtained and placed into the plastic jacket. If it was an ED case, the images were whisked to the ED and then retrieved later, usually well after the patient departed the ED. The new films were returned to the film library where they were matched with the film jacket containing the old studies. From there, the study was hung on an alternator for the radiologist to interpret. When

I was a resident at Duke, this model was pushed to the limit and each patient not only had a film jacket but a board on the alternator based on the hospital service—to find the films, you just had to go to that service's alternator. Radiologists would move from alternator to alternator to read the newly hung films.

Unfortunately, this approach was severely limited by virtue of the reality that the film jacket could be in only one place at a time. Matching the new films with the old jacket was tedious and often problematic. If a jacket was misplaced, or worse, sequestered in the trunk of the bone attending's Mercedes because it was a great case, it might never be found. It was all too easy to put one patient's films in another patient's jacket, or to totally scramble the contents of one patient's film jacket, forcing the next radiologist to spend 10 minutes reordering the jacket or, even worse, assume that the film was lost, and not bother to make the comparison. If the radiology specialist was in a different building or work area, he or she could not be consulted unless the jacket was physically brought to the physician. Most institutions (including Duke, before an enormous reading room was constructed) had a window in the film library—often covered in chicken wire or glass for the physical protection of the film clerk from the long line of often surly supplicants queued up to get their films for rounds. As a medical student on my surgery rotation, I once was banished to accompany one of the surgical interns on his day-long quest to round up all the surgery patients' X-ray jackets for afternoon surgical rounds. Hours elapsed trying to locate all the cases. Due to inefficiencies in moving films from one department to another, the radiologists typically would never read the ED films while the patient was still in the ED. If a department didn't have enough alternators, the radiologists would read the alternators and then flee the hospital (especially on the weekends) in "blissful" ignorance, assuming that everything had been read knowing the cases wouldn't be hung again until morning. When I first got to Lansing, Michigan, this meant that it could take until Tuesday afternoon to clean up weekend plain films from the ED.

Before the days of word processors and fax machines, the radiology report was typed on a multisheet carbon form by a transcriptionist working on a typewriter. Once signed by the reading radiologist, a copy would go into the film jacket, a copy into the departmental file, and a copy into the permanent paper chart. Like the film jacket, the patient's paper chart can only reside in one location at a time—if the chart is gone, the radiology report too is gone. With the development of the mainframe and mini computer, database systems were developed to hold the pertinent information. Radiology information systems (RIS) were created to better manage the report information contained within the film jacket, as well as to better manage the tracking of the film jacket and its contents. Bar codes on the film jacket and a bar code reader attached to the RIS terminal simplified the process of signing out and tracking the film jacket. Orders could be generated within the RIS or received from the hospital information system (HIS). A paper requisition could be printed out for each study, which could be annotated with history, study comments, contrast doses, or used as a face sheet for a detailed tech worksheet. Once a study was dictated, the transcriptionist could type the report on a computer terminal rather than a typewriter, entering the text directly into an electronic record within the RIS. The report could then be accessed directly by the reading radiologist and signed electronically. Corrections could be made to the typewritten report rather than scrawled in longhand between the lines of the report. Copies of the report could be automatically printed or printed on demand, as well as viewed electronically.

RADIOLOGY WORK FLOW

Radiology studies begin as orders from referring physicians for their patients—outpatients, inpatients, and ED patients (Fig. 13-1). The clinical context and medical necessity of the test needs to be established and transmitted with the order to the radiology department. The study needs to be placed into the schedule for the appropriate modality. If the patient is an outpatient, the time and location of the test, as well as any pretest instructions, need to be communicated to the patient. Any special preparation for the study needs to be initiated at the appropriate interval before the study. Patients need to be registered if they are outpatients and their insurance/payment information needs to be recorded. If the patient is an ED denizen

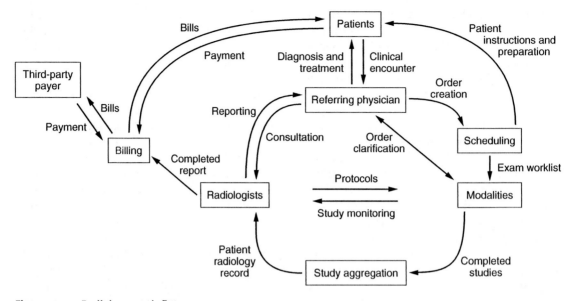

Figure 13-1 Radiology work flow.

or inpatient, transport needs to be summoned to bring the patient to the appropriate imaging device at the scheduled time. The technologist needs to interview the patient or review the clinical chart to supplement the clinical history in the order, and confirm that there is no contraindication to performing the study. The technologist also needs to confirm that the patient is the correct patient, that the procedure is the correct procedure, and that it is performed on the appropriate location/side.

The technologist performs the study and prepares the images for the radiologist, who may need to be consulted before or during the procedure to direct the imaging protocol. The study needs to be completed by the technologist and disposables, such as contrast or catheters, may need to be inventoried. The images are viewed by the radiologist and interpreted within the clinical context of the patient history. Any prior comparison or complementary exams need to be compared to the current exam and a report is prepared. For certain procedures (e.g., mammography), the study may need to be categorized. If the findings are critical or the clinical situation requires it, the radiologist may need to transmit a preliminary interpretation in advance of either the final interpretation or transcription of the dictated report. The final report needs to be reviewed and signed by the interpreting radiologist. If there are unexpected findings of clinical significance, this needs to be conveyed directly to the referring physician. There also needs to be confirmation that the referring physician received these results. That report needs to be transmitted to the referring physician and possibly other physicians (e.g., the primary care physician, a consulting specialist, etc). Once the final report has been completed and signed, the study needs to be billed. The images may need to be reviewed by the referring physician or a consulting physician who may also wish to review them with the radiologist or with the patient. A copy of the images might need to be prepared for the patient to take to a physician outside of the institution. Finally, the study needs to be available for comparison with future studies or for review at clinical conferences.

This work flow is standard for any department, whether it is paper/film–based or digital. However, as the number of studies per day climbs beyond 50 or 100, computerizing the process greatly increases its efficiency and accuracy.

ROLE OF THE RIS AND THE HIS

The RIS manages and stores the textual information for the patients, the studies, and the study reports (Box 13-1A and B). The RIS can stand alone or be integrated with the HIS. With a stand-alone RIS, the imaging-

BOX 13-1

A. RIS Functions	B. HIS Functionality

A. RIS Functions

Patient Information
    Patient Name
    Medical Record Number
    (See Box 13-2)

Study Orders
    Procedure Requested
    Exam Indication
    Physician
        Ordering
        Attending
        Primary Care
        Consulting

Modality Scheduling

Study Information
    Accession Number
    Patient Questionnaires
    Patient Interview
    Study Protocol
        Protocol Details
        Protocol Deviations
        Reason for Deviation (e.g., Patient
          Condition, Machine Malfunction)
    Contrast, Dose Record (Nuclear Medicine)
    Contrast Reactions
    Study Complications
    Study Worksheets (Nuclear Medicine,
      Ultrasound, Vascular Ultrasound)
    Mammography Categories
    Film/View/Series/Pulse Sequence Information
    Sedation Record
    Catheters, Filters, Coils, Stents, Supplies

Study Reports
    Prelim Reports
    Final Reports
    Report Transcription and Approval

Film Tracking
    Location
    Sign-out Record

Billing Information
    Insurance Information
    Study Precertification
    Advanced Beneficiary Notice
    Coding

Departmental Quality Assurance

Interventional Complication Record

Departmental Activity Tracking

Departmental Statistical Reporting

B. HIS Functionality

Admission Discharge Transfer (ADT) Information
    Patient Name
    Medical Record Number
    (See Box 13-2)

Medical Alerts and Allergies

Responsible Physician
    Attending Physician
    Referring Physician
    Primary Care Physician
    Consulting Physician(s)
    Resident Physician(s)

Order Entry
    Laboratory, Microbiology, Anatomic Pathology
    Diagnostic Testing (Cardiology, EEG, EMG)
    Nursing, Respiratory Therapy, Physical Therapy
    Medications

Diagnostic Testing Schedule

Pharmacy
    Medication Administration Record
    Medication List

Nursing Record

Clinical Data Repository
    Clinical Laboratory
    Anatomic Pathology
    Microbiology
    Hematology and Coagulation
    Cardiology
    Neurology
    Pulmonary Function

Transcribed Reports
    Admission History and Physicals
    Discharge Summaries
    Operative Notes
    ED Visit Notes

Patient Problem List

Bed Control

Transportation Management

Scheduling
    Diagnostic Testing
    Surgery
    Physical Therapy, Rehabilitation

Billing Information
    Insurance Information
    Advanced Beneficiary Notice
    Coding

related HIS functions are taken up by the RIS itself. Specifically, in most hospital environments, the HIS either contains or is closely integrated with a master patient index (MPI), which stores the name and medical record number of the patients in the information system. Additional demographic information (Box 13-2) is stored and is important for verifying if, for example, "Ann Smith" in one hospital system is the same "Ann Smith" in a different hospital system. Automated systems

are now available that will match multiple criteria, providing a level of confidence that entries in the different systems match. Maintaining the integrity of this index is essential. If a single patient has several entries within the MPI, that patient's studies will be treated as belonging to different patients and comparison studies can get lost. Insurance information is entered into the HIS and must be kept current and accurate to assure reimbursement. (That's why you're always asked to show your insurance card and it gets copied over and over!). The HIS should provide access to laboratory, anatomic pathology, and cardiology studies and may also hold transcribed reports such as ED notes, surgical notes, admission history and physicals, and discharge summaries. The HIS may also hold the medication administration record and nursing care documentation.

BOX 13-2

Patient Information

Name

Maiden Name

Medical Record Number

Account Number

Date of Birth

Place of Birth

Sex

Marital Status

Address

Phone

Employer

Work Phone

Next of Kin
  Name
  Address
  Phone

Social Security Number

Insurance Company
  Plan Number
  Individual Number
  Name of Covered Individual

Secondary Insurance Information

Race

Nationality

Religion

ORDER ENTRY

Order entry may occur directly through the RIS or through the HIS. The order entry process is crucial for obtaining the appropriate clinical history for interpreting radiographic studies and to prove medical necessity for billing purposes, especially for negative studies where the exam can only be coded based on the clinical indication. In larger academic institutions or organizations with employed physicians, the importance of billing may seem secondary, but the old adage, "No margin, no mission" rings true. In the private practice setting, failed billing means no salary. The referring physician has little incentive to provide a detailed description of the clinical scenario—both because of the effort it requires and the high likelihood that the information is going to get lost anyway in traditional paper-based systems. Lastly, some referring clinicians feel it is better to get a radiologist interpretation that is unbiased by clinical history, and then with that interpretation, try to integrate the clinical history with the "findings" themselves. This approach fails to recognize that most radiologists count on the clinical history to constrain what might otherwise be an exhaustive list of differential possibilities and, more importantly, does not enable a directed optimized search, given the vast number of

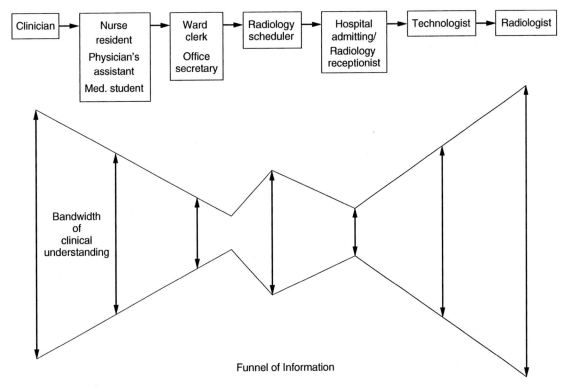

Figure 13-2 Order entry process.

images/anatomy that must be surveyed in a modern day imaging study (e.g., a 64 slice CT).

The order entry process in most institutions consists of a dysfunctional game of telephone tag (Fig. 13-2). Information gets passed down a funnel through personnel with decreasing medical understanding. By the time the requisition gets to the radiologist, the indication may bear little relationship to the original order, or morph into a twisted homonym like bad voice recognition. Unfortunately, a significant amount of information needs to be passed along to optimize scheduling and study interpretation (Table 13-1). The patient name needs to be reconciled with the MPI for the new study to be viewed in the context of all their prior studies. The ordering physician as well as primary care or consulting physicians must be recorded so that the report can find its way back to the appropriate physician. Also, there should be contact information in case more information is required. Finally, the ordering system needs to be sophisticated enough to encompass multiple studies or panels of studies, where it becomes arbitrary when one portion of the

study ends and the next begins, such as a chest, abdomen and pelvis CT or cervical, thoracic, and lumber spine MR. While such studies may be interpreted by different sets of radiologists in an academic center, they are usually interpreted in the private practice setting by a single radiologist generating a single report. The indication for the one segment of the examination may need to be different from that for the other segments (i.e., abdominal pain will not work for the chest component of a chest abdomen pelvis CT). The order also needs to allow for the addition of specific instructions, such as the type of protocol for the exam (e.g., Hi Res or PE CT of the chest), requests for certain readers, special attention to specific areas or special instructions for how the study is acquired (e.g., thin cuts through a certain region, not to use a certain arm for IV access, contrast restrictions, etc). The order entry process must have fields to hold the appropriate information; by virtue of their presence, it is more likely that the appropriate information will be acquired before the patient reaches the imaging facility.

Table 13-1 Order Entry Information	
Incoming Information	**Outgoing Information**
Name	Time and location of exam
Age	Diet instructions
Sex	Medication instructions
Medical record number	Preparation for exam
Contact information	Requirement for another driver
Insurance type and precertification	Post-op care requirements
Study requested	
Special study instructions	
Clinical indication	
Underlying conditions	
Prior surgery, implanted devices	
Allergies	
Medications (certain procedures)	
Expected findings	
Priority of exam	
Physician name	
Other physicians to receive report	

As the interaction between the office secretary and the radiology scheduler is often time-consuming and frustrating, many institutions have instituted Web-based ordering forms to allow clinicians to order directly. The system lets the secretary choose among the openings for the time of the procedure, or simply indicates that a radiology scheduler will contact the patient directly to schedule an appointment. Preparation information and directions to the facility are also available for printing. The advantage of a forms-based system is the ability to control the pick list of indications by procedure and to make certain fields mandatory. While it is not legal to only list the actual International Classification of Diseases, 9th revision (ICD-9) codes that are payable, it is considered acceptable to use descriptive phrases, which can be later mapped back to the proper ICD-9 codes. Innovative institutions, such as Massachusetts General Hospital, have built computerized entry systems to screen the submitted indications and return a color-coded appropriateness score (green, yellow, red) back to the user, based on the American College of Radiology (ACR) appropriateness criteria. If the appropriateness score is marginal or very low, a more appropriate study is suggested, based on the ACR criteria. Physicians can still override the suggestions and order the study, regardless of the low score, but they do so infrequently. The scheduling systems may compare study indications to local medical review policies (LMRP) and prevent scheduling of studies that fail to meet the criteria. Unfortunately, LMRPs are not available for all studies and apply only to certain carriers. The reality is that virtually all insurers have strict criteria for which indications are acceptable, but very few choose to publish those policies.

SCHEDULING PROGRAM

The scheduling program may be embedded directly in the RIS or HIS, or it may be a stand-alone radiology specific or enterprise-wide product. If order entry information is populated within the system, it is important that this information flows back to the RIS and appears on the study requisition. Interfaces between products from different vendors may be problematic so don't assume that this will occur seamlessly, as it may require significant effort or expense.

The scheduling program can be tailored to the departmental resources and integrated to the radiologist work schedule to ensure that the appropriate imaging device, ancillary equipment, appropriate personnel, and a qualified reader are all available at the designated time and place. Based on the schedule, patients can be contacted in advance by support personnel to confirm that preprocedural instructions, preparations, medication changes, and so forth, are properly carried out. Patient notification can also decrease the no-show rate by providing a reminder to the patient of an upcoming scheduled appointment. This helps to maximize the chances that the study can be successfully and efficiently performed. The system should also alert the clerical staff as to which procedures will require precertification from the insurance carrier. The scheduling system should balance patient preferences for imaging location, or time of procedure, with efficient use of the imaging location devices and personnel. Obviously, it is imperative that the information in the order and the procedure requested be as accurate as possible so that studies don't have to be delayed, rescheduled, or reassigned to alternative locations because they are inappropriate for the designated time slot.

Schedules need to be accessible to the technologist and department coordinators so that appointment for inpatients, ED patients, or add-on patients can be inserted appropriately into the schedule. Also, review of the schedule by the radiologist at the beginning of the day may help identify cases that require a call to the referring physician for more information or that would benefit from an alteration in the standard imaging protocols. Carrying out these tasks before the patient makes it to the scanner table prevents indecision and delays, while the patient is lying, uncomfortably in the missile tube.

PATIENT INTERVIEW

Due to the uncertainties of the order entry procedure detailed above, it is of vital importance for the technologist to interview the patient, or to have the patient complete a study questionnaire. Contraindications to procedures—such as allergies, medications, implanted devices, or underlying medical conditions—need to be noted as they may require modifications to study protocols or impact study interpretation. The ability to store "alert" information within the RIS can prove invaluable when the patient returns and is unable to communicate due to their condition, or just forgets to mention an allergy or condition. Information gleaned by the technologist regarding prior surgeries, smoking history, underlying diseases (e.g., cancer, diabetes, asthma, collagen vascular disease or trauma), as well as prior radiation therapy or chemotherapy often proves pivotal for interpreting the study. If the patient has a palpable

mass, area of tenderness, skin discoloration, swelling, deformity, mole, sinus tract, or other pertinent physical finding, the details need to be recorded for the interpreting radiologist and markers should be placed appropriately. The acquired information needs to be typed into the RIS, annotated on the requisition, or entered into a worksheet.

DICOM WORK LISTS

Keeping track of patients in a busy hospital setting is of utmost concern to prevent patients from receiving the wrong study or having the images stored under the wrong patient name. In modern systems, the schedule within the RIS can be exposed to the computer controlling the specific modalities by way of structured work lists, conforming to the Digital Imaging and Communication in Medicine, or DICOM, standard. This allows the technologist to simply select the patient name and study directly from the DICOM work list and have that patient's data (name, patient number, study number, date of birth, study description, etc.) directly entered into the console of the modality. Some systems support bar coding the patient armband to ensure the correct patient identification. While modality compliance with DICOM work lists is widespread, most modalities and RISs do not support transfer of corrected information back from the modality to the RIS if there has been a change in the study performed. Instead, the technologist must open the RIS independently, usually on a second computer to enter the required information.

STUDY INFORMATION

Details regarding the study performed need to be stored in the RIS for a variety of reasons. The type and volume of contrast (or dose and activity of radiopharmaceuticals) and the method of administration need to be documented for billing purposes. Some insurers require including contrast doses in the body of the radiology report, so the information must be readily available for the radiologist at the time of dictation. Contrast reactions need to be recorded. Many institutions will record consumables for billing and/or inventory control. Certain study information needs to be available for the radiologist at the time of interpretation, be it within fields of the RIS or recorded on the requisition or a worksheet. This includes significant deviations from the procedure, such as an inability of the patient to achieve or maintain a certain position, inability of the patient to follow instructions or comply with the requirements of the exam, unwillingness of the patient to allow contrast administration, inability to complete the exam due to patient claustrophobia, infiltration of contrast, machine malfunction, or delay of a portion of the exam to a later time. If this information is missing, the radiologist will have to expend extra effort to call the technologist to find out why the study is incomplete or improperly performed. Worse, if repeats or extra imaging are to be completed at a later time, the radiologist may dictate the study before it has actually been completed. Certain modalities, particularly ultrasound and nuclear medicine, generate numerous measurements that are most efficiently presented in worksheet format. Pictorial representations within a worksheet are also important for vascular ultrasound and mammography.

Ideally, information is entered directly into the RIS and is available electronically at the time of interpretation. However, most RIS systems are not robust enough to eliminate paper requisitions. Few systems exist for populating worksheets electronically except for narrow applications, such as ultrasound. Most institutions still transfer paper requisitions or employ document-scanning systems to archive paper requisitions and/or worksheets.

RADIOLOGIST REPORT GENERATION AND REVIEW

At the time of study interpretation, all the acquired information regarding the patient, the study, and the patient's past radiology history needs to be available at the radiologists' fingertips to facilitate interpretation. Ideally, the information is filtered and arranged in an optimum order and style for maximum efficiency (see the "RIS-PACS Interface" section later). The

radiologist dictates the study either into a voice recorder for subsequent transcription or directly into a voice recognition program (see Chapter 14). The advantage of the voice recognition program is that the report is immediately available to the radiologist to correct and approve directly within the dictation application; the disadvantage of it is that since the report is immediately available to the radiologist, he or she may be tempted to correct the report immediately (which improves report turnaround time) at a potential cost of disrupting work flow and image analysis concentration. The dilemma—review and sign, or save for later to edit?—reflects a shift of effort from a lower expense resource (the transcription) to a higher one (the physician). Caution should always be exercised when this "effort-shifting" occurs in that there must be a demonstrable gain in quality, efficiency, or customer satisfaction to offset the cost.

With conventional transcription, the transcribed report needs to be imported into the RIS and made available to the radiologist for approval. There needs to be a mechanism for the radiologist to know that reports are awaiting approval. Next, the radiologist must open the reports within a viewing application and cycle through the reports. Editing may be possible directly within the application or may require opening the report in an external word processing application. In a busy practice where each radiologist is interpreting 100 to 200 exams per day, the efficiency of the report approval process is crucial, especially when the transcription service is poor. Also, unless transcription is very quick, the radiologist must be able to remotely approve their reports either from home, from another facility, or from their vacation hotel room. Most systems will not send the report to the referring physician or initiate billing until the report has been finalized. Once approved, the report needs to be locked for legal purposes and any further modification must be made in the form of an addendum. Last of all, there should be an administrative tool that alerts the "boss" to unsigned reports; this produces the sometimes needed "loving" reminder that all reports must be signed. It is also useful if the system can generate standard reports to show report turnaround and sign-off times. This should be a motivator and a generator of important measures of quality.

REPORTS

Once produced, reports must be transmitted to the ordering physician. While this sounds easy, it is by no means trivial. First, the report needs to be transported either by fax, mail, or courier. Many physicians work at multiple locations so the report must be transmitted to the correct location within the physician's practice. The practice support staff must then take the report and place it with the patient chart. Physician practices will call for overdue reports and need to either directly access the report or want to know why the study has yet to be completed or interpreted. Remote computer access to the report is desirable but most practices will still want a printed copy for their chart. As physician practices adopt ambulatory electronic medical records (AEMR), there will be increased pressure to develop direct electronic interfaces to automatically populate the report within the AEMR. Creation of these interfaces is currently an arduous and expensive endeavor. Communities are starting to look at development of the Region Health Information Organization (RHIO) to facilitate results distribution. However, RHIOs are years to decades away for the vast majority of the country. Reports also need to be transmitted to the primary care physicians and other consulting specialist physicians, as well as the attending physician. Although the same report distribution mechanisms can be employed, they can only be triggered if the system knows on the front end which physicians also need to receive a report. Reports also must be readily available to the radiologist consulted on a case and for the ED or hospital physicians admitting new patients.

BILLING AND CODING

Once the report is finalized, billing of the study needs to be triggered. In many hospital systems, the signing of the report pushes the study to the billing system. ICD-9 codes obtained during the order entry process may be automatically submitted along with the current procedural terminology (CPT) code for the study description in the RIS. The system must know the correct billing information so the bill gets routed to the appropriate third-party payer and only for studies that are appropriate to bill (i.e., not diagnostic-related group [DRG] inpatients). Unfortunately, automated billing often is not accurate. Review of the final report is often required to determine what CPT code(s) are supported by the actual study procedure performed. Also, the most appropriate ICD-9 codes for the study may come from the study findings, rather than from the clinical indication, especially if little care is taken to ensure appropriate indications before the study is performed.

Certain studies, primarily mammography, have strict requirements for characterization based on the findings. Once the studies are coded, that information needs to be maintained in the RIS, or in a dedicated mammography RIS, so that the appropriate analysis, quality assurance, and follow-up can be performed. With mammography, there are statutory requirements for patient notification letters and biopsy results tracking that are greatly facilitated by computerization within the RIS. Interventional radiology programs have also been created to facilitate direct physician coding of procedures. These systems also are useful for maintaining procedure logs, following patients, documenting QA, tracking complications, and managing inventory supply.

BIRTH OF PACS

Picture archiving and communication systems (PACS) began to take form in the late 1980s and early 1990s. The PC revolution had just begun, and, after the introduction of the Macintosh computer in 1984, relatively inexpensive computers were suddenly capable of displaying grayscale pictures and not just pixilated text (assuming that you don't count the goofy images created from typed text!). Two compelling needs in radiology pushed forward the development of PACS: (1) bringing portable chest X-rays to the ICU, and (2) interpretating CT, ultrasound, and nuclear medicine images from home. In my first private practice job in 1990 at Sinai Hospital in Baltimore, Maryland, ICU chest studies were hung on their own alternator in a small room just outside the ICU. This provided rapid and convenient viewing of the images for the clinical staff. The disadvantage, however, particularly for the radiologists, was that those portable chest and abdominal radiographs were separated from the rest of the film jacket, which also contained the old studies from other modalities, such as CT. Furthermore, it distanced the films from the radiologist: the practical implication was that the radiologist would only trek upstairs once a day in the late morning to read out all the films for the past 24 hours.

For years, the ED physicians would interpret plain films after hours. In many institutions, other physicians might bring chest x-rays performed on their house patients to the ED physician, or to the ICU pulmonologist for a "curbside" consultation. This by and large freed up radiologists from most after-hours duties—except for coming in early on the weekends to read out the accumulated piles of films or returning to perform the occasional after-hours procedure. This became problematic with the advent of CT and MR—studies interpretable only by the radiologist—which meant he or she had to come in to evaluate emergent studies at night.

The initial efforts at solving this challenge were difficult in that networks lacked bandwidth and there was not an accepted image transfer standard. Thus, even before the proliferation of Ethernet networks and DICOM-based image transfer, enterprising companies devised means to frame grab images from the video screens of the CT scanners, or to use a video camera to generate computer images from sheets of film. Because the images were captured from video, they were only 8-bit images, which precluded significant windowing and leveling. Bone windows and soft tissue windows had to be transmitting separately. The images were then highly compressed and sent over phone lines by modem to the radiologist at home. However, the images were of sufficient quality to keep the radiologist from having to come in to the hospital, making the systems extremely popular. The most difficult task was transferring the home reading console from radiologist to radiologist, as they were too expensive for all but the richest partner to purchase one of their own.

Crucial to the development of PACS was the development of high-quality, digitally acquired plain radiographs. Conventional X-ray film has a photographic emulsion layered onto a medium, first glass, then cellulose, and later acetate. The silver grains in the emulsion are exposed by direct interaction with the X-ray photon. This yielded extremely detailed films but at the price of high radiation doses. Thus the next step was the development of phosphor screens, which interacted with the X-rays to yield a flash of light that exposed the photographic emulsion, rather than the X-ray beam itself. The screens increased efficiency of exposure by the incident X-rays, which allowed for a decrease in X-ray dose, but with a narrow band of acceptable exposure. With CR (computer radiography), a photostimulatable plate is placed within the X-ray cassette. When exposed with X-rays, the plate captures a latent image. Unlike the film screen combination, the CR plate has a much more linear relationship between intensity and exposure, which allows for much wider latitude in appropriate exposure. The plate is removed from the film cassette, and a laser scans the plate line by line. When an exposed area of the plate is struck by the laser, a flash of light is produced and measured by a photomultiplier device. The position and intensity is recorded to create the digital image.

Digital radiography (DR) is similar to CR except that the CR plate is replaced with a solid-state detector, which directly captures the image. The advantage is that the image is obtained instantaneously and potentially at a higher contrast resolution. However, the expense of the detector makes a DR room similar in price to a conventional room plus a high-volume CR reader. Since this must be duplicated in each room, DR is substantially more expensive than CR for multiple rooms. Initially, the digitally acquired images were simply printed with laser film printers. The advantage of the digital image is that a greater dynamic range is acquired than can be viewed on a sheet of film (even with a hot light!). The image can be windowed and leveled to bring out contrast in different parts of the image, that is, the lungs versus the retrocardiac region, or to standardize the grayscale appearance of the images. Images from initial CR systems were still printed and reviewed on film. The ability to generate consistent windowing and leveling, as well as the decreased need to repeat over- or underexposed images, was deemed important and valuable enough to justify the more complicated system, despite the continued expense of printing film. CT, MRI, nuclear medicine, and ultrasound are

206

all digital modalities but initially were all interpreted on film. Images could be viewed on the modality console but getting the images out of the machine to view on a computer was difficult.

Through the forethought of the RSNA (Radiological Society of North America) and the ACR, a standard file format and image transfer scheme called DICOM (digital imaging and communication in medicine) was not only developed but successfully adopted by the entire medical imaging industry. While rigorous compliance to DICOM standards has occasionally been elusive, particularly for nuclear medicine, it has allowed images to be sent by any modality from any manufacturer to be successfully aggregated by any PACS system. DICOM is a wide-ranging standard, which places a standard header on each image file containing patient, study, series, and image-specific information. Proprietary information can be placed into the header, which can, unfortunately, lead to some incompatibilities between different PACS and modality vendors. The standard is broad enough so that different types of compression schedules (LZW, RLE, JPEG, JPEG-2000) can be employed. DICOM contains methods for displaying lists of available images for transfer or viewing, and mechanisms for the actual transfer of images to and from a storage device, printing, and displaying work lists of pending studies so that demographic information can be directly imported into the modalities. A standardized method for transfer of patient and study information had been developed by the HIS industry—HL-7 (Health Level 7)—allowing transfer of RIS data to PACS.

By the early 1990s, the PC revolution had produced desktop computers capable of displaying and manipulating high-resolution grayscale images. High-resolution monitors capable of displaying up to $2,500 \times 2,000$ pixels were also developed with the high luminescence levels required for image interpretation. Computer networks—first, proprietary systems developed by military contractors, such as Loral but later Ethernet, ATM (asynchronous transfer mode), and Gigabit Ethernet networking schemes—allowed sufficient bandwidth to move the large imaging data files. This

culminated in the Baltimore Veteran's Administration Hospital radiology department, which opened in 1993 as the first truly filmless hospital. Whereas much of the system was proprietary, it nevertheless demonstrated that imaging could be interpreted efficiently and effectively on computers. Over the next 10 years, PACS was commercialized and commoditized. Systems were developed by Agfa, Siemens, and Kodak. Loral was purchased by GE Medical Systems, which enhanced a commercial product. Many of the Loral engineers who did not join GE developed the Fuji Synapse Product. Dominator Radiology and ALI (later purchased by McKesson) also produced systems. Web-based systems were developed for remote viewing at the University of Pittsburgh and Massachusetts General Hospital and later commercialized, respectively, as Stentor (now owned by Philips) and Amicas. A number of other systems have been developed over the years, including Cedara, IDX, Cerner, Emageon, and dozens of small companies.

CURRENT PACS

While the various PACS systems all have their points of differences, they all share similar fundamental functionality (Fig. 13-3).

RIS-PACS INTERFACE

There needs to be an interface between the PACS system and RIS. Unless the two systems are directly integrated by a single vendor, information is sent from the RIS to the PACS system using an HL-7 interface. HL-7 is a message format in which information is encoded into simple text streams with a standardized order of the discrete information items. Standard message structures are available for ADT (admission discharge transfer) patient information (i.e., name, number, insurance, diagnosis, etc.) as well as order information (ORM) and report information (ORU). An interface is required to translate the incoming information (25,000 messages a day at my 550-bed hospital). If the RIS does not have the capability to generate the DICOM work

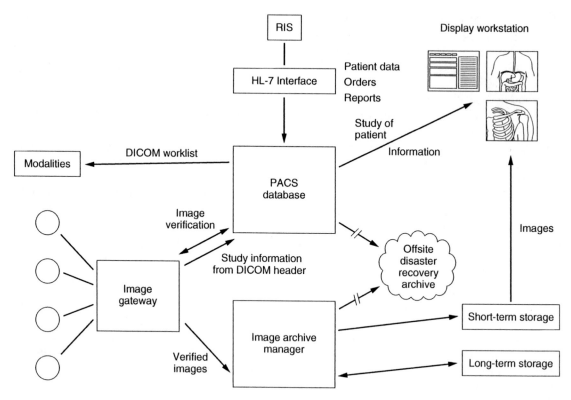

Figure 13-3 Basic PACS functionality.

list described above, which is common, the PACS system will have to generate the DICOM work list containing the outstanding orders for studies that the individual modalities can access. Once an item on the list is selected by the technologist, typically all the patient information and the study accession numbers are automatically retrieved and entered into the appropriate fields directly on the modality. This minimizes typographic errors and information reconciliation after the study is sent to the PACS system.

IMAGE TRANSFER FROM THE MODALITIES

The PACS system needs to accept images sent by the various imaging modalities. The DICOM specification allows the modalities to send images in a standard fashion for all PACS systems. A process within the PACS system needs to parse out the study and image data contained in the DICOM header, which is verified against the study and patient data transferred from the RIS

to ensure that the correct images are matched to the correct study and patient. Studies that fail to verify are exiled to a "dump" file to await repair, hidden from the users. The study, series, and image numbers need to be aggregated and stored in the PACS database; each study, series, and image is assigned a unique identification number (UID) so that the image files can be later easily retrieved for display. Slice- or image-specific information, such as projection, table location, series description, and so forth, is stored in a database for later display on the image overlay. A quality control (QC) functionality is present within PACS systems to allow the arbitrary division of studies—for example, splitting off the chest portion of a CT scan from the abdominal portion so that the portions can be interpreted under separate accession numbers by different radiologists. Also, images can be moved from study to study when they are inappropriately attached to the wrong study (e.g., putting the lateral lumbar spine with the PA and lateral chest). Finally, incorrect patient or study information can be corrected within the PACS database.

IMAGE STORAGE

The images themselves need to be stored in an efficient and cost-effective manner. Most systems have a short-term cache, a long-term storage device, and a second (and sometimes third) copy for disaster recovery, in case the primary storage device is destroyed for whatever reason. Typically, the short-term cache is a redundant array of inexpensive or independent devices (RAID), or a number of hard disks aggregated into a single functional unit. The data are spread over several disks to speed the rate of data storage/retrieval, as well as redundantly store the information. If one of the component hard disks fails, it can be replaced and the information regenerated from the information stored on the other disks. Depending on the architecture, RAID can be directly attached to the server by an SCSI (small computer system interface) interface, be available from a storage area network (SAN) attached by fiber channel (a very fast storage network interface), or be accessed by way of a standard Ethernet connection, such as network attached storage (NAS).

A single enterprise-wide SAN can service multiple storage needs within a health care system thereby consolidating maintenance and administrative functions. For longer-term archival storage, digital linear tape (DLT) or magneto-optical disk (MOD) systems have been employed. MOD is near the end of its life cycle and may be replaced by DVD for small systems, or ultra-density optical (UDO) or Blu-Ray for larger systems. The density of data storage has been doubling every two to three years, greatly reducing the cost of storage. Unfortunately, many of the new systems are not backward-compatible with old systems. Migrating from an old archive system to a new system for a large archive may take months to years, depending on the speed of the media readers. Typically, a device would have a rack full of the media, several reader drives, and a robotic arm to move the disks back and forth from storage to the drives for reading. While the information can be retrieved from the RAID hard disks within seconds, it takes 10 to 30 minutes to retrieve the files from the long-term storage, depending on where the information is on the tape and how many other retrieval tasks are ahead in the queue. In the last few years,

the cost of spinning disk has declined precipitously to the point where it is often cheaper to just expand the SAN to accommodate the long-term storage, rather than to purchase the DLT, MOD, or other media. Finally, a copy of the images and data needs to be maintained for the worst-case scenario—a catastrophic failure due to explosion, fire, flood, and so on.

For disaster recovery, the data need to be saved to a remote location so that the entire system can be reconstructed from scratch, if necessary. Because such a retrieval can be exceedingly slow (imagine restoring 100 terabytes of data from 25,000 DVDs!), some determined organizations have even considered having redundant systems to allow for a "hot" switch between the separate systems to keep downtime to an absolute minimum. Other large hospital systems are building central data centers with independent energy sources in hardened bunkers to service multiple hospitals. One chain in Florida stored the PACS systems for seven hospitals in a single central data center. When the hurricanes of 2004 ravaged the state, the hospitals individually all lost power but the data center and PACS systems never stopped running.

In 2006, high-speed, backed-up RAID cost less than $3,000 a terabyte. This means a 4,000 slice CT containing 1 gigabyte (GB) of lossless compressed data costs $3 to store—compare that to the $1.50 per sheet price of film. Furthermore, the cost of hard disk space continues to drop precipitously. There used to be a science in balancing RAID and long-term storage with intelligent prefetching rules for pulling in the most critical prior exam and dropping studies not recently viewed. This functionality was really important when we only had enough cache to hold five days' worth of studies. But now it is typical to hold at least a year's worth of studies in cache and some institutions talk of replacing DLT libraries with low-cost spinning disk archives, or eliminating a separate long-term archive all together and keeping everything short-term RAID. Also, as the cost of storage continues to plummet, interest in long-term lossy image compression for archival purposes is waning, despite the proliferation of multidetector CT. (It is important to note here that offsite storage and redundancy of patients' protected health information are not optional: HIPAA requires the maintenance of offsite data backup.)

STUDY SELECTION

PACS systems must allow users to rapidly and efficiently find and display studies. Searching for studies individually by patient name or medical record number is effective but highly inefficient, particularly for volume reading. Organization of studies by location, modality, dictation status, or date all have their place. For clinicians, organization of study by patient location facilitates rounds. However, displaying lists of patients based on location may violate HIPAA regulations. The ability to sort patients and studies by referring and/or consulting physicians or by service would get around the HIPAA regulations and make X-ray rounds highly efficient for the clinicians. However, this would require scrupulous efforts to correctly attach physicians to patients within the RIS. For the radiologist, sorting lists by modality, body part, dictation status, age, and study acuity, and placing them into work lists is essential for enhancing radiologist productivity. Flexibility in setting up the work lists is also critical, as radiology practices often evolve highly customized work flows.

IMAGE DISPLAY

The radiologist or clinician needs the appropriate tools to visualize and maneuver through the images for the selected studies. The images need to be organized in an efficient and effective manner to speed viewing and facilitate comparison with prior studies. Prior to PACS, radiologists read from banks of viewboxes or alternators, providing four over four, or six over six or more viewboxes. Initial image display systems tried to mimic viewboxes with four or eight monitor systems. Over time, however, it has become standard to have two image display monitors at most sites, due to the degradation of system speed with large numbers of monitors, the difficulty in visualizing the additional monitors, and the high cost of high-resolution monitors. A third color monitor is now standard at most PACS workstations for viewing RIS information. Most radiologists realized that it was much faster and took less effort to cycle through the images on a single monitor with the mouse than to shift their eyes from monitor to monitor.

For plain films, the current study can be displayed on the left monitor, while the comparison study is displayed on the right. The entire screen can be filled with a single image or divided into any number of individual viewports containing an image from within the same series (tile mode) or different series (stack mode). As different readers and different modalities have different optimal viewing paradigms, the display software must be highly flexible. Many systems provide for custom "hanging protocols" to order and display studies in a consistent manner, facilitating comparison. In the film era, it was most efficient to display CT and MR images with a tiled set of images, 15 or 20 to a page. When PACS systems were first developed, the screen was divided and images displayed on the monitor to mirror the typical film display. Most radiologists found it more efficient to display different series in a single viewport and to track through the images with a drag of the mouse, much as we used to preview images on the CT or MR scanner by spinning the track ball. Computer systems can now scroll through hundreds of images within seconds. The advantage is that the eye can perceive subtle changes in intensity and shape, and distinguish between tubes (vessels) and balls (masses).

With the explosion of MDCT (multidetector computed tomography) images, stack mode begins to break down. Scrolling through thousands of images is tedious without an extremely fast computer and a highly athletic index finger. Developments in 3-D workstations have resulted in an MPR (multiplanar reconstruction) paradigm, in which the individual axial slices are reconstructed into a volume and displayed in three orthogonal planes. As the entire volume is fed into memory, the user can navigate extremely rapidly through the entire volume in any plane with smooth transitions. Any off-axis plane or even a curved plane can be rapidly generated. With the 64-slice scanners, the volume data is truly isotropic and reconstructed images have the same resolution in all planes. Over the next few years, look for these tools to be embedded directly within the PACS viewing software—either directly or through integration with third-party software. Volume rendering and maximum (and minimum) intensity projection options will also migrate from dedicated 3-D workstations to standard PACS reading stations. Current systems tend to have only rudimentary tools for ultrasound and nuclear medicine. Look for future systems to seamlessly handle ultrasound cine loops or "clips." Now that PET (positron emission tomography) is widespread, multiplanar PET/SPECT (single photon emission computed tomography) views and fusion capabilities should move from dedicated workstations to the standard PACS viewers. With the addition of extra memory and a more capable video card, high-end PACS stations can also meet the specifications for dedicated 3-D and modality workstations. Color images can be viewed on the third monitor of the PACS system.

The eye can only perceive up to 256 different shades of gray or eight bits of data. CR, CT, and MR images all contain 12 bits or more of intensity information, which are reduced to 8 bits by window and leveling of the data. PACS systems make it very easy to adjust the window and level, either manually or, particularly for CT, using preset window/level combinations. Inverting images between white on black and black on white becomes very useful, particularly for plain films, for viewing lines, pneumothoraces, and ribs on chest X-rays. Most systems allow for a particular series to be cloned to additional viewports. This is most useful for CT, allowing an image to be simultaneously viewed in soft tissue, lung, and bone windows. Most systems have correlation tools that allow the user to click on a location with an image and display that particular point on other CT or MR series, regardless of the series orientation or plane of section. Series in the same plane can be linked and correlation lines displayed on orthogonal or oblique images. Images can be linked based on table position so that series with different slice thicknesses can still be synched. Such tools are also useful synchronizing comparison studies of the same modality or for comparing CTs and MRs.

Image magnification is useful and most systems will have a variety of different tools for either magnifying the entire image (or a portion of the image), as well as displaying the image at life size or at a 1-to-1 pixel representation. Images can be rotated in any direction, or flipped around a horizontal or vertical axis.

The order of series within a study or the order of images within a series can be rearranged. Images can be viewed statically or in a cine mode. Images usually can be exported both as DICOM images as well as standard JPEG images with or without annotations for use in educational presentations.

IMAGE ANNOTATION

In the film era, most radiologists felt naked without their grease pencils for annotation. PACS workstations allow textual annotations as well as arrows in a variety of styles. Standard snippets of text (i.e., spine levels) can be saved in a list and picked from a drop-down menu. Different vendors have semiautomated tools for facilitating spine labeling. Measurement tools for region of interest density/intensity measurements, distance measurements, and simple angle and Cobb angle measurements are present on all systems and are typically very easy to use. Images can be aggregated into special summary "key images" series, either automatically based on the presence of annotations or manually based on user selection. Keywords can be added to individual images, series, or studies for teaching purposes, to facilitate finding images or studies by user-defined criteria, or for identifying cases for clinical conferences. Most systems have calibration systems for refining measurements based on external markers, due to inherent magnification or for modalities such as ultrasound and digitized films.

IMAGE EXPORT

Much of the cost savings of PACS is its ability to eliminate the need for film. At $1.50 or more for a sheet of film, not to mention the time required to film studies and the decreasing margins for imaging, a low-cost medium is needed for transporting imaging studies to referring physicians, particularly those beyond the reach of the facilities-wide area network. Indeed, with 1000 slice CTs, filming studies is cost prohibitive. Image distribution on CD is now standard, due to its low cost and the ubiquity of CD-ROM drives on physicians' computers. Robotic systems, which will burn the CDs and print your logo and patient identification information on the back of the CD, are available and affordable. Many vendors have devised simple viewers that are burned onto the CD and can be run on the target PC without formal installation. Other vendors have devised Web-based front ends to remotely control CD creation at a high-volume, central CD burner. Image CDs are a very handy transport mechanism but the CD-based viewers are hobbled by the low data access speed from the CD and the limited capabilities of the embedded viewer.

The image viewers are all different, which can stress out computer software–challenged physicians. For instance, removing the CD before closing some viewing programs can lock up the physician's computer. Also, some vendors store the images in a non-DICOM proprietary standard which precludes importing the images into other PACS systems. Ideally, the CD would be used to simply transport the images and the office staff of the receiving physician would simply import the images into a workstation at their office, much like ripping music CDs into iTunes. The physician could then view the images at hard disc speeds, employing a full-featured viewer with a user interface with which the physician is familiar and facile regardless of where the images were acquired. It is preferable for all studies of a patient to be burned to the same CD. This negates the need to be shuffling CDs back and forth through the CD drive to try to make comparisons on serial studies. Many of the programs burned onto CDs do not allow simultaneous viewing of multiple studies from different dates, which is problematic. A widely used program, eFilm from Merge Healthcare, has many of the required functionalities listed above and is widely available at affordable pricing for both individual and enterprise-wide use.

MONITORS

Just as CR development was crucial to the ability to digitally acquire plain radiographs, the development of high-resolution monitors was essential to the efficient interpretation of images. The native resolution of CR is 2500×2000 pixels, giving a pixel size of approximately 0.068×0.07 mm.

Viewing such images on a standard 1024×768 monitor entails either loss of special resolution or the need to magnify the images and pan the entire radiograph. Cathode-ray tube (CRT) monitors were developed, capable of displaying 2500×2000 pixels, and allowing a radiograph to be displayed at native resolution in its entirety on a single monitor. These monitors, however, were very expensive ($10,000 to $15,000 each) and, due to the high brightness, were subject to degradation, limiting their effective lifetime to two to three years. Arguments raged over what resolution was truly required for effective plain film interpretation.

Over the last three years, liquid crystal display (LCD) flat panel displays have revolutionized the consumer and PACS monitor marketplace. The LCD monitors are sharper, brighter, and slower to degrade than the old CRT monitors. This has significantly improved the contrast resolution of PACS monitors and studies have convincingly shown that plain films can be effectively read on 2000×1500 (3 megapixel) LCD monitors with equal or greater success than on 2500×2000 (5 megapixel) monitors. Grayscale, 3-megapixel monitors are now widely available for approximately $5,000 each. Monitor brightness is a key attribute for successful PACS usage. DVD viewing is a key driver for consumer acceptance of LCD monitors in the home marketplace. This has lead to the development of large 1900×1200 pixel, 24-inch-color monitors (e.g., Dell 2407 WFP), now under $900, with brightness levels at the lower end of medical grade. These function superbly for clinician and home use. Some institutions use these monitors for reading, including plain films. However, they are color monitors and I find that the 3-megapixel, grayscale monitors are much better suited for high-volume interpretation. I also greatly prefer 3-megapixel monitors over lower resolution color monitors for MR—especially MR mildly degraded by motion artifact or poor signal to noise.

WORKSTATIONS CONFIGURATION

Most systems allow for different workstation configurations. Most radiologists prefer a three-monitor configuration: two 3-megapixel gray-scale monitors for image viewing, and a third 1600 × 1200 pixel color monitor for RIS functionality. The color monitor also allows color visualization of ultrasound, nuclear medicine, functional MRI, perfusion, and 3-D images. A dedicated ultrasound or nuclear medicine workstation may benefit from two or three all-color monitor configurations. The technologists need access to the images, particularly in CT and MR, to review prior studies to help define the appropriate area of interest and ensure that similar protocols are performed for follow-up studies as well as to guarantee that all images from the current studies have actually made it to PACS. Typically a single 1600 × 1200 pixel color monitor system will be adequate. High-volume ED and ICU clinical review systems benefit from two or three monitor setups. Depending on how carefully the clinicians actually view plain films, 3 MP monitors may be required. For CT and MR viewing (by neurosurgeons, neurologists, orthopedists, etc.), a two-monitor setup with large 1900 × 1200 pixel monitors (i.e., 24-inch) works very well and is surprisingly cost effective.

Similar setups or single monitor setups work well at home. High-end laptops (i.e., those costing $2,000 to $3,000) will support 1900 × 1200 pixel resolution on their screens and will typically also have two video ports, allowing them to be attached to dual external 1900 × 1200 pixel monitors (at home or in the office). Many new monitors have integrated USB connections, so a mouse and keyboard can be attached to the monitor. The laptop is then plugged into the monitors and a USB port, effectively allowing it to be used as a desktop computer for image viewing. Hardware requirements will vary but dual processor workstations will provide outstanding speed of use for high-volume reading stations. Load up your workstations with 2 GB of memory, or 4 GB if you have integrated 3-D capability. Once your operating system and PACS supports 64-bit processing, you can increase the memory beyond 4 megabytes (MB). Hard disk space is now so cheap and plentiful that it is rarely an issue (expect at least 200 GB). For home or clinician use, expect at least a mid-range system and 1 to 2 GB of RAM memory. Dual monitor systems are advised if you plan frequent access. Video cards should have at least 128 MB of RAM for

standard monitors. The 3-megapixel, grayscale monitors will require dedicated high-resolution video cards.

INTEGRATING RIS AND PACS

Traditional RIS and HIS systems evolve very slowly. Part of the reason is that extreme care must be taken to assure data integrity, rock solid stability, and backward compatibility with prior versions. The market is not that large and once tied to a specific vendor, it is an extremely arduous process to switch to an alternative product. Migration of data from one system to another is a nightmare. These systems tend to be based on fixed database structures so adding new fields can be problematic or serve as an excuse for the vendor to charge outrageous professional service fees. Furthermore, in many legacy systems, the size of the data fields may be constrained to 24 or 36 or 64 characters, which limits the complexity of information that they can hold. As a result, the functionality of most RIS systems has not kept up with the rapid evolution of radiology.

As a result, most radiology departments have looked to the PACS system to solve their most pressing information transfer and work flow issues. To meet the challenge, PACS systems have evolved surrogate RIS systems that duplicate the reports as well as patient and study metadata within the PACS database. The radiologists interact almost exclusively with the PACS system, both for images and old reports. In many departments, the radiologists only use the RIS to approve reports if they don't have an independent transcription system. While image storage and display are straightforward, information transfer and work flow management are much more problematic and idiosyncratic. Successful PACS implementation is less dependent on the vendor than on the ability of the radiology department to successfully integrate their disparate systems.

RIS systems typically don't have the capability to handle study worksheet information. Newer systems will allow lengthy comments to be attached to study records but rarely provide modality-specific customizable data entry fields. As a result, many departments rely on paper-based worksheets or add written annotations to a paper requisition. Document imaging is a mature technology for many industries outside of medicine. Low-cost, high-speed, double-sided scanners are readily available commercially. Ideally, the PACS system will have an embedded scanned document viewer displayed on the third monitor of the PACS workstation. This allows the radiologist to view the clinician-completed request/order sheet and try to decipher the handwritten, sometimes cryptic clinical indication. The data may reside in a separate application also available for viewing on the third monitor. However, to enhance productivity, there must be an easy method to synchronize the study in the image display window with the document in the third-party viewer.

The most common, but least attractive, solution is to save the scanned image as an additional series in the study and display it in a viewport on the image display monitors. Although this requires the least effort, it does place the worksheet information with the study permanently, accessible to all viewers of the images, including the clinicians, the patients, and the patient's lawyers, even when the study is exported from the system. This is particularly problematic when the worksheets contain tech diagnoses that may or may not be correct. Similarly, problems can arise if comments about patient behavior are included. It's like hanging your dirty linen in front of the picture window in your living room! The advantages and disadvantages of paper-based systems are summarized in Table 13-2.

Many PACS systems have built-in application programming interfaces (API) to allow integration with external processes such as a browser, a dictation system, 3-D reconstruction software, or in-house custom applications. The interface can pass contextual information, such as the user name, and study information, such as the medical record number and study accession number. Some systems also allow for two-way communication with an external application able to open the PACS system to a particular patient or study. This allows an enterprising radiology IT department to build its own custom RIS, reporting system, or digital requisitioning application. Though this requires considerable expense and in-house programming expertise, the advantage is the ability to create a highly customized and

Table 13-2 Scanning Paper

Advantages	Disadvantages
Limits changes to pre-PACS workflow	Writing must be legible
Existing forms can be used	Data cannot be corrected nor can additional information be added without scanning another sheet of paper
Little or no programming or customization required	
Computer access not required to add data	No error checking or mandatory completion of fields
Allows external documents, such as H&Ps, outside reports to be added to the system	Data cannot be repurposed or rearranged
	Cannot query the data without first keying information into the computer
Scanning equipment is low cost	
	Information cannot flow directly to the reporting system
	Finding information becomes problematic as the number of pages of scanned information increases
	If scanned into the Image Display space, all viewers see all the information

efficient system. Custom forms can be created for each task, be it order entry, tech patient interview, study worksheets, radiology preliminary or final structured reports, QA reports for problem cases, and custom work lists based on site-specific criteria or urgency of interpretation. Entering the data on the computer instead of digitizing paper means that the data are accessible in database format and can be searched. Users can be authenticated, and every step is time/date stamped. Information can be repurposed and fields can be rearranged depending on the context. Requisitioning information (Box 13-3)

BOX 13-3

Requisition Information

Patient Name
Study Accession Number
Patient Medical Record Number
Sex
Age
Patient Location/Patient Type
Facility
Priority
Study Description
Reason for Study (Signs and Symptoms)
Clinician's Expectations
Ordering and Attending Physician
Underlying Conditions
Prior Surgery
Relevant Medications
Summary of the Patient Interview
Summary of the Study Worksheet

Modern Times, the radiologist never stops talking while the studies and relevant clinical information flash by in rapid succession. The advantages and disadvantages of this approach are summarized in Table 13-3.

Structured report systems have proven popular for certain modalities, particularly mammography and ultrasound. Some ultrasound systems will directly pull measurements from the ultrasound machine into the report. Many 3-D workstations will create semiautomated reports for cardiac scoring, cardiac function, and stent graft planning measurements.

Unfortunately, most interfaces between the RIS and either the modalities or the PACS are one way, only flowing outward from the RIS. Thus, if an exam changes at the time of data acquisition, changing the entry in the modality will not migrate back to the RIS without the tech logging on to the RIS application and making the change. IHE (Integrating the Healthcare Enterprise) is an initiative begun by the Healthcare Information and Management Systems Society (HIMSS) and RSNA to provide an advanced framework based on DICOM and HL-7 to facilitate the two-way migration of information between medical information systems and devices. Look for improvements in integration between future systems in the next 5 to 10 years and lobby for your PACS vendor to implement IHE support.

can be listed in the order that it is dictated and salient information can be abstracted and summarized from the order entry and tech worksheets (Fig. 13-4) and not left to the radiologist to glean from a complex form. Integration of the PACS system with the digital dictation system allows the accession number to be directly entered into the dictation station. Much like Charlie Chaplin tightening widgets in the film

Links to EMR, QA, Stat cases, Teaching file, Schedule

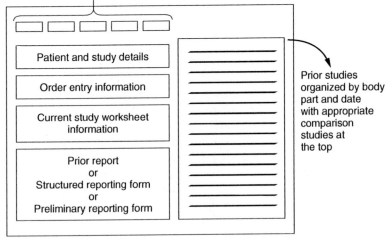

Patient and study details

Order entry information

Current study worksheet information

Prior report
or
Structured reporting form
or
Preliminary reporting form

Prior studies organized by body part and date with appropriate comparison studies at the top

Third monitor

Figure 13-4 Requisitioning information tech sheets.

Table 13-3 Computerized Requisitioning

Advantages	Disadvantages
Computerized forms creation allows structured data acquisition with check boxes, radio buttons, and dropdown lists	Initial expense of developing system as functionality is not readily available commercially
Forms easily customized	Usually requires in-house support and programming capability
Can make certain fields mandatory	Requires using a computer for data entry
Functionality only limited by creativity of designers	
Entries at every step are user, date, and time stamped	
Information can be presented, rearranged, or repurposed, based on the user context	
Information can be prepopulated into reports, decreasing what needs to be dictated	
Acquired data is computer searchable for whatever purpose	
Data from prior tests can be summarized and displayed with current data	

PRACTICE CONSEQUENCES OF PACS

PACS has greatly increased the efficiency and effectiveness of the radiologist. However, like most disruptive technologies, there is a price to be paid for these advances and unintended changes are forced on radiology practices.

"Just in Time" Reading

With PACS, the images truly are available anywhere in the enterprise immediately at the completion of the study. Once a clinician sees a study appear on the PACS system, she or he expects to click on the report button and see at least a preliminary report. The trauma surgeons now walk from the CT scanner to the reading room as their patient rolls back to the ER, expecting an immediate interpretation. The radiologist can no longer hide behind "the case hasn't been filmed and hung yet" and cannot claim that the comparison films are not available when someone comes by and requests to view a study. Pressure is high to keep up with the flood of studies, so radiology staffing has to match the ebb and flow of production. It is important to maximize the efficient information exchange on the radiology requisition. When it only takes 60 seconds or less to read a chest radiograph, an extra 10 to 20 seconds spent searching for the clinical indication or the results of a prior exam has severe consequences for productivity.

Disruption in Radiologist/Technologist Communication

In the film era, the radiologist had to be physically located close to the film processor and therefore was close to the modalities themselves. It was easy for the technologists to walk over and discuss issues with the radiologists. With PACS, the interpreting radiologist may be in an entirely different location so communication becomes more difficult. With subspecialization, several radiologists may be responsible for the interpretations of different studies performed on a single CT scanner. Clear work flow patterns are required so the technologists know which radiologist to call for consultation.

In the past, the radiologist knew a study was completed when the films were delivered. With a paper-based requisitioning system, the delivery of the paperwork by the technologists also indicates that the study is ready to read. As PACS allowed studies acquired in one location to be read in another, it made moving the paperwork around even more difficult. Also delays in transporting paper down the hall became a bottleneck for reading cases. Moving to a paperless system allows work to be shared by local and remote readers. It heightens the need for a computerized communication system to facilitate flow of protocol information to the technologist, study request information from the referring physicians, and historical/worksheet information from the technologist back to the radiologist. Without a paperless solution, most viewing areas must be armed with multiple fax machines to receive paper requisitions from multiple modalities and multiple imaging sites.

Unfortunately, it is problematic knowing when a study is actually completed, particularly for CT with delayed imaging and postprocessing times. It becomes very important for the technologist to document deviations from the standard protocol so the radiologist knows a study is completed, even when all the requisite series/images are not present. Regrettably, most PACS systems do not have an "in progress" status and once any images are present in PACS, the study is given a "new" status. Since two-way communication between the modalities and the RIS is rare, completing the exam on the modality does not automatically tell the RIS that the study is completed. That becomes an extra step for an overworked tech on a separate computer and may not be performed until much later. Ideally, closing a study in the RIS would trigger a change in the PACS study status from "in progress" to "new," or "completed but not dictated," but most systems don't have this capability. With some systems, sending an additional image or reconstruction to a study marked "dictated" may change the status back to "new," triggering the study to be interpreted a second time by a different radiologist (it's particularly embarrassing when the dictations don't match!). Ideally, the technologists have a mechanism to complete a study and have it register as such within the PACS system. It also would be helpful if the modality could send a message to the PACS system regarding the total number of images to be sent, so that the PACS system "knows" when all the images have been received.

As the number of radiologists covering a given location increases and the number of scanners covered by each radiologist increases, the understanding and familiarity between the radiologists and technologists become much weaker. Clearly articulated protocols and greater attention to documenting the details of the exam become more important as the likelihood decreases that the technologist knows exactly what the reading radiologist wants.

Disruption of Radiologist/Clinician Communication

Since the clinicians can easily review images, either directly from the wards or from their offices, there is less need for the clinicians to visit the reading room. Challenging cases will still bring the clinicians to the reading room for consultation but more and more conversations occur over the phone with both physicians viewing the images simultaneously. Radiologists still call clinicians with critical findings or to seek more historical information regarding difficult cases or procedures. Exchange of information in the order entry process and the reporting process becomes more important as the casual information exchange in the reading room becomes more infrequent. Interpretation may be "outsourced" to a radiologist in a different location within the practice or, at night, perhaps to an entirely different country by a different set of radiologists. There needs to be an effective communication system between the radiologist and the referring physician—particularly when real-time transcription or voice recognition systems are not employed.

As the distance between the radiologist and technologist, as well as the radiologist and the referring physician, increases there is, alas, a loss in the substance and tenor of communication exchanged between the different parties. Collegial conversations over coffee while waiting for the films to drop out of the film processor are gone. As with the technologists, it becomes harder for the radiologists to know all the clinicians when cases come from increasingly greater distances. The camaraderie and sense of pulling together is lost, especially as everyone tries to enhance their "productivity" and "efficiency." Interruptions become annoyances rather than opportunities for exchange and improvement of the study or interpretation.

COMPLEX WORK FLOW AND WORK LIST STRATEGIES

As practices enlarge, PACS enhances the ability of the practice to divide the workload along subspecialty lines, regardless of where the study was performed. However, the ideal work flow within the institution may be more complex. If nobody wants to be the plain film specialist, the practice must force someone to take that role each day or devise a more complex work flow to share the burden. The pediatric radiology reader would like to search by age-specific criteria but would still like to search by location-specific criteria to capture older patients with pediatric-specific problems on pediatric wards or clinics. The ED reader may prefer a single point of contact rather than strict subspecialty coverage, which may necessitate altering work flow. The PACS system needs to allow each radiologist to access her or his specific work list with a single mouse click. The art is in constructing the appropriate queries to choose the appropriate patients. It is often too tedious to select the appropriate studies individually from a more general work list. If this is not possible, work flow may be dictated more by the search capabilities of the PACS system rather than by the desires of the radiology practice. New studies may be added to the end of the work list as they are completed, so that the radiologists can move from study to study without having to return to the study search page (thus avoiding time spent in locating the unread studies and reloading the visualization software). Ideally, the system should have some capability to sort high-priority cases to the top of the work list: as new urgent cases are added to the list, or preliminary reads are requested on unread cases, those need to move to the top of the list.

AGGREGATE STUDIES AND APPROPRIATE COMPARISONS

With multidetector CT scans, the speed of image acquisition has made it easy to obtain optimal chest, abdomen, and pelvic CTs in a single acquisition. Most PACS systems have difficulty in dealing with multiple studies with a single accession number, since they are incapable of placing the study into more than one category. They also present an order entry challenge as the different parts of a multilocation study may require separate indications to ensure medical necessity (i.e., "abdominal pain" doesn't justify the chest CT). It is important that the appropriate prior comparison films are automatically fetched and displayed as well. The prefetching algorithm must be sophisticated enough to bring over the appropriate comparison across different modalities. It must also know what views are within combined studies so that comparisons are made between, say, a chest X-ray and the chest view in an acute abdomen series (e.g., four-view abdomen) or a rib film or the chest X-ray in a metastatic bone survey, or even the AP thoracic spine view. Sorting the list of prior exams by anatomic location in patients with long lists of prior examinations can facilitate identification of appropriate comparisons as well. This becomes especially important in institutions where location prefixes may be added to study descriptions, so sorting a study list alphabetically will not group similar studies together. The radiologist must feel so confident in the PACS system that when a comparison film is not displayed, he or she knows it does not exist and will not have to spend time searching for possible comparisons in a long, complex study list.

REMOTE ACCESS AND REMOTE READING

For the PACS workstation to display images at the speeds required by the radiologists for volume reading, the workstation needs a very fast network connection to the PACS image server. For most general reading, a 100 MB or faster Ethernet connection is minimally required for volume reading, although Gigabit Ethernet (GbE) is clearly preferred. Fortunately, GbE connections are now cost effective for hospital LANs, and new PC workstations typically have a GbE adapter built in. This allows near instantaneous retrieval of even 1000 to 2000 slice CT studies. Modality vendors, however, may only ship computers with 10 or 100 MB network cards. For high-volume CT and MR systems, it is important to force the vendor to supply a Gigabit network card if your network will support it. Otherwise, image transfer will be bottlenecked at the modality before hitting the GbE network. Hospital systems have become more complex with multiple campuses and satellite clinics. However, the telecommunication industry has invested heavily in optical fiber connectivity in many metropolitan centers, allowing high-speed connections even in geographically dispersed hospital systems.

However, for remote viewing outside the comfort of the hospital LAN, the realities of bandwidth requirements stress the user's ability to rapidly review images. Image compression can greatly facilitate remote viewing. An uncompressed CT image is approximately 0.5 MB, a standard 256×256 MR image is 0.125 MB, and a standard plain film image is 10 MB. DICOM images can be losslessly compressed by a ratio of approximately 2:1. Lossy compression can be applied to images with very little loss in image fidelity—certainly 6:1 for CT and MR and 15:1 for plain radiographs. Further image compression can also be applied to plain radiographs up to 30:1, with more loss of image fidelity (yet still acceptable to tell if the fracture is angulated or distracted, or if the lung base is opacified or clear). Furthermore, for plain films, the native image resolution is 2500×2000, which is significantly higher than most home or physician office monitors. If the plain film resolution is decreased to match the resolution of the screen, for example, 1280×1028, an additional 4:1 compression is possible. Also, even if you wish to review the present study at full resolution, there is no reason the comparison can't be highly compressed.

The proliferation of broadband access and hospital systems' adoption of high-speed Internet connections makes review of images from home or from clinician's offices practical. Time must be spent working with IS to ensure facile virtual private network (VPN) access, but soon you too will be viewing images from Starbucks on your laptop and you will have no excuse not to sign your reports while you are on vacation!

Different strategies have been employed to achieve efficient remote viewing. Unfortunately, there is a dichotomy in physician requirements for remote image review. On one hand, primary care physicians and general surgeons just want a quick look at a limited number of images to either plan their course of action or to demonstrate abnormal findings to their patients. On the other hand, there are the consulting radiologists, neurosurgeons, vascular surgeons, orthopedists, and neurologists who need to see *all* the images and require the same complete diagnostic tool set as the interpreting radiologist.

Early PACS workstation clients were not well suited for remote access and the workstation pricing model also precluded deploying the clients remotely. Several vendors (e.g., Agfa Web 1000, GE Web Viewer, AMICAS, Siemens MagicView) developed Web-based simplified systems for remote access. The crux of this strategy was to provide a lightweight simplified viewer with only modest hardware and software requirements. Such systems worked admirably with plain films. However, the simplicity of these viewers was also their downfall as they allowed only limited functionality and performed poorly with large MR and CT datasets. Typically, these systems maintained a second separate image library and employed a separate server, which was an advantage as it kept the main server from getting bogged down responding to the needs of scores of users throughout the institution. Yet this was also a disadvantage for two main reasons: having to store images in more than one place and creating synchronization issues for annotations, measurements, dictation status, and window and level values. Many systems were based on Java and at least a few had conflicting requirements regarding the installed Java version, forcing clinicians to choose between installing the viewer from one institution or the viewer from another.

Subsequently, more advanced Web-based systems (Fuji, Stentor) allowed for a more robust client for remote viewing but a not-quite-so-rich client for in-house reading. Such systems also moved the software sales models away from a per-seat hardware/software workstation model to software-only, concurrent-user licensing models, in which an unlimited number of clients could be deployed. However, as the client becomes more sophisticated, there is a commensurate increase in the size of the client download, as well as increases in the memory and processor speed for optimal performance, making deployment more difficult—particularly outside of the hospital.

While this may not be practical for hundreds of casual viewers, it has been a godsend for the hard-core remote users who demand full functionality. With improvements in computer and network speed, improved storage access, and higher performing database servers, systems using a single unified image database are now much more practical. Look for vendors in the future to develop a second, easy-to-use, simplified client for casual viewing that will supplement the full-featured client, both pulling images from the same server.

Whether the viewer is Web-based or a stand-alone application, the image data are transferred to the remote computer and manipulated within the application on that computer. An alternative approach to actually moving image data is to use a screen-sharing application, most commonly a Citrix server. The PACS application runs on a central server local to the PACS server so image transfer is not rate limiting. Instead, the pixels on the screen are transmitted to the remote computer. As those pixels change, the screen data is retransmitted. Think of it as having a very long (and somewhat slow) monitor cable between your monitor and the thin client server back in the main department. The speed of thin client access is still very dependent on network bandwidth. This is exacerbated by the relatively high-screen resolution required (between 1280 × 1024 to 1600 × 1200 pixels) and the pixel color depth (true 24-bit color) typically required to allow true grayscale representation. Citrix servers are designed to allow multiple users to connect simultaneously. While this works in settings in which the users employ low-screen resolution and color depth, multiple PACS users will bring a Citrix server to its knees. If each active PACS user has his own dedicated server, performance is satisfactory. However, it is expensive for the host institution to implement multiple Citrix servers if the number of concurrent users will be high. A similar approach has also been employed for 3-D reconstruction by TeraRecon, in which a proprietary board on the central server rapidly performs reconstructions so that screen data are transferred to a remote computer to view the images. This works quite well for network speeds above 100 MB but becomes excruciatingly slow at network speeds below 10 MB.

It is important to distinguish remote access from remote reading. Accessing a PA and lateral chest radiograph or a 30 slice head CT over a fast cable connection with a modest amount of compression can occur in under a minute, while a 500 slice MR or a 150 slice abdominal CT may take three to five minutes and a 1200 slice CT angiogram may take 10 to 15 minutes. These times are acceptable for reviewing an emergent case from home and obviate the need to return to the hospital. However, such performance is far too slow to support productive reading for a remote facility or from home. A caching mechanism or automated query and retrieval (subscription) system is important, as physicians don't mind waiting up to 10 to 15 minutes to download a study, as long as they can do something else in the interim. Volume reading requires a faster connection such as dual point-to-point T1 lines or a caching mechanism to allow images from a remote facility to dribble into the workstation at T1 speeds (1.5 MB) over time. This allows the radiologist to sit down at the workstation for 10 minutes and read the images accumulated on the hard disk over the last hour at full speed.

SELECTING AND IMPLEMENTING A PACS SYSTEM

A successful PACS implementation requires extensive planning and organization. It is important to define a team of individuals to understand the existing work flow in the organization and develop a vision for optimizing functionality and productivity for the future. The vendor needs to be selected and a contract negotiated. Finally, the system must be implemented and the users trained. It is also essential to have a long-range IT (5-year) plan that involves a capital and operating cost projection. As opposed to the more predictable standard depreciation cycle of an image acquisition device, IT costs accumulate in the form of transmission, display, personnel, and storage costs.

PACS PROJECT TEAM

Select champions from all aspects of the department and hospital to push the project forward. A strong radiologist champion is required to set the direction and scope of the project as well as to ensure that the requisite clinical functionality is present in the system. A strong lead technologist is required to bring understanding of the patient flow and technologist work flow. The department manager brings a clear understanding of the outside demands on the department, as well as skill in navigating the budgetary hurdles in the organization. A savvy IT project manager is needed to efficiently plan the requisite computer systems and networking solution. IT must also be involved in the planning of the interfaces to the HIS/RIS, electronic medical record (EMR), dictation systems, and any other clinical systems. It is important to involve clinician power users to ensure their PACS access requirements are met. Their help will become invaluable following implementation to help "evangelize" the system to their less-computer-secure brethren. Also, involve your departmental VP or CIO to help negotiate the deal—they usually have a wealth of experience brokering difficult contracts. If you don't have capable personnel eager to put in the effort to carefully evaluate your requirements, consider hiring a PACS consultant to help you out. Remember that the PACS is an enterprise-wide endeavor; include hospital and outpatient center IT personnel in the mix, not just your departmental support people.

DEFINE THE VISION FOR YOUR PROJECT

It is vital to understand the actual flow of information in and out of your department. Moreover, you need to have a vision for how you wish information to flow: Do you want to continue with paper, employ a document scanning process, or implement a fully digital order entry/requisitioning system? Get a crash course in PACS at the annual Society for Imaging Informatics in Medicine (SIIM; formerly SCAR, Society for Computer Applications in Radiology) meeting. Take a few field trips to luminary sites to understand how they organize their work flow.

It is important to learn what the full capabilities are of your HIS, RIS, and EMR, and to understand the long-term vision for the EMR.

Make sure your PACS has the tool set and integration capabilities to deliver on that vision and to facilitate seamless integration and adoption. Look at the wider role your institution plays with affiliated hospitals and the patient referral patterns both in and out of your institution to ensure that studies can easily flow in and out of your facility.

Take a close look at your current clinical practice to understand the display issues for the various modalities. Box 13-4 illustrates studies that most PACS workstations do not handle well. Where will this image display functionality reside? Within the PACS system, on third-party viewers integrated on the PACS workstation, or on a separate dedicated workstation?

Assess your current hospital remote network access capabilities and evaluate whether they will suffice for PACS access. Determine if clinicians will access images directly with a PACS client installed on their computers or by way of a Citrix solution. How will images be integrated into the EMR—by a hyperlink to the PACS system, by a context-sharing link in the EMR directly to the PACS client, or through a separate embedded client within the EMR? Finally, will your PACS system integrate with an RHIO, either directly or by passing all the studies to a separate system?

BOX 13-4

Challenging Exams for PACS Workstations

Real-time Multiplanar Reconstruction and 3-D Rendering
CT and MR Angiography
CT and MR Perfusion
PET and SPECT Viewers
Nuclear Medicine Cardiac Studies
Nuclear Medicine Renal Studies
Ultrasound Cine Loops (Clips)
3-D Ultrasound
MR Spectroscopy
Functional MRI
Angiography Image Subtraction and Pixel Shifting

WHO WILL RUN THE SYSTEM?

When hospitals first started implementing PACS systems, they typically were radiology initiatives run by radiology personnel, often to make up for deficiencies in the IT-run HIS and RIS. As PACS has matured, the huge increase in the volume of image data coupled with increased user expectations for performance and access has made systems more complex to operate and manage. The computer expertise to maintain servers and SANs may be more efficiently provided by the Enterprise IT department as they can use the same personnel that manage the other hospital systems. With advances in hierarchical storage managers, it is quite feasible to host the PACS data on an Enterprise-wide SAN, along with the other hospital data.

Determine if your IT department truly has the ability to run this sort of system. If so, you can purchase a software-only solution and save a considerable amount of money. Otherwise, you will need to consider a turnkey system or application service provider (ASP) model with the PACS vendor responsible for maintaining the core systems. Alternatively, if you are a small system, you could partner with a neighboring, large health system on PACS, rather than trying to go it on your own. As hospitals aggregate into integrated health delivery organizations, it makes sense to aggregate PACS within a multi-facility Enterprise PACS system rather then multiple independent stand-alone systems. This allows the smaller institution to have a more robust, better-supported PACS system as well as potential access to all the studies from all the institutions within the PACS system.

The telecommunication boom of the past 5 to 10 years has greatly increased the availability of optical fiber connections between institutions, providing superb network performance. The smaller institutions need only purchase the CR equipment, display workstations, and gateways. Not having to duplicate the servers and SAN or personnel to maintain them can drastically decrease the size of investment for the smaller hospital. Instead, the smaller institution will typically pay the hosting organization a one-time-per-study charge to store the cases. This is an advantage for the larger host institution because it provides an income stream to defray the cost of its own PACS system, since the incremental burden on the PACS servers and the cost of the storage is minimal. It also provides revenue to finance redundant servers or storage, consolidate disaster recovery, and hire additional support staff. PACS administrators, like radiologists, have to be on call 24/7, so increasing the number of PACS administrators lessens the call burden on each support individual.

The PACS administrator or an associate IT administrator needs to have an in-depth understanding of the technical requirements of the servers, databases, and network requirements for the system, as well as training in trouble-shooting and maintaining the PACS and RIS applications. It is important to have a PACS administrator with strong ties to radiology—who has technical experience in image acquisition, a clear understanding of radiology work flow and technologists' needs, and experience with patient care issue. These are all qualifications that might be overwhelming for someone coming into the job straight out of a nonradiology IT background. The PACS administrative team needs great interpersonal skills and the patience of Job to interface with the technologists, the radiologists, and especially the clinical users throughout the institution.

VENDOR SELECTION

Having crafted a cogent vision for your PACS future, you need to find the appropriate PACS partner to actualize your dream. Traditionally, this means crafting a request for proposal (RFP) document, sending it to a preliminary set of vendors, narrowing the field to a manageable number of vendors, going on site visits to evaluate the products, and then negotiating a final contract. A number of national consulting firms generate "white paper reports," comparing the different PACS solutions, while others conduct customer satisfaction surveys and publish the results online (e.g., http://healthcare. knowl edgestorm.com, www.healthcareitnews. com, www. himssanalytics.org, www.healthcomputing.com). Your hospital likely participates in a Hospital Purchasing Consortium, which may also provide surveys for their member organizations. These provide a good source for generating the long list of PACS vendors. Google may work just as well, too.

Your PACS vision must be clearly described in your RFP document. Sample RFPs are available on the Internet and for $5,000 to $10,000, you can contract with a PACS consulting firm to help you construct the RFP. I would not get too obsessive about the details of the RFP, as the vendors will send you pretty much the same information, regardless of what you say you are looking for. The major vendors have dedicated RFP writers who can turn around a 200-page RFP in a week or two and are highly skilled at casting their product as your perfect solution regardless of the product's true capability.

Make sure you get reference sites from each vendor that share your same RIS/HIS and closely parallel your size and type of institution. Rather than accepting the ones that they select, who will likely be effusively pleased with their product, ask to have a list of the installations from one to two years ago (in chronologic order) and then interview five consecutive customers to get a more unbiased view. Once you narrow the field down to three or four realistic contenders, go on site visits, concentrating on similar-sized institutions that also use your RIS/HIS products. Try to get a feel for how the users are actually using the software—you may need to watch from the other side of the reading room out of the corner of your eye as people hate to work while someone is watching. Finally, go to a SIIM meeting (or an RSNA annual meeting, although it is much more hectic) to check out the different systems. Allow time (particularly at the end of the show, when the booths are not that crowded) to sit and play with each of the vendor's user interfaces to see what is most comfortable. Take notes about the features in each and compare how the different systems handle frequently used tasks. Most PACS vendors have user group meetings the day before the SIIM show. If you have a front-runner, go to the user group meeting to find out other users' concerns and talk with system administrators from around the country. Most vendors' user groups also have e-mail list servers, which may be another venue to see what issues other users are experiencing. Again, more important than the issues is the responsiveness of

the vendors to the issues and the degree of satisfaction of the users with the vendors' product support. Remember that you will be using this system for the next 10 years, at least (you hope), so you'd better be really comfortable with how the user interface works and confident that the product will allow you to work most efficiently.

Carefully research the financial stability of your vendor. If your vendor is gone, you could be left with an orphan system and have to replace the entire system. If the vendor is absorbed by another company, will the product be maintained or is the purchaser just looking for market share and will then force you to migrate to the new owner's system? Is the current product offered up to date? Does the company have a clear development pathway and sufficient financial resources to ensure that the offering will remain state of the art? Don't assume that functionality promised in the next upgrade will happen in the time frame touted by the vendor. Are nonobsolescence packages offered at affordable prices?

FINANCING PACS

Know the financial and accounting strategies that your institution prefers to use for equipment purchases. Specifically, does your institution prefer to buy or lease? Does your institution expect some risk sharing and cost savings guarantees from the vendor? Which portions of the contract should fall under the capital budget and which should fall under the operating budget? There is no right answer, so go with what is most comfortable for those paying the bills. The vendors just want to sell the equipment so they will be extremely flexible on how the system will be financed. They will be happy to finance the deal, shift the service contract to the capital cost of the equipment, or work out a leasing structure. Your administration usually won't be nearly as flexible.

You will be asked to provide a cost justification for your PACS. The falling price of computer equipment and PACS software makes this easier but it is still difficult to arrive at cost justification based on hard costs alone. Film savings and decreasing costs for film storage are a large component of the cost justification. Space is saved as large film rooms are no longer necessary. Litigation is potentially avoided, given the increased availability of comparison films and the decreased frequency of unread or lost films. Again, it is important to not underestimate current and future film usage (the 64-channel CT really helps here!) as this will negatively impact your estimated cost savings after PACS. The caveat is that you have to work hard to deliver on keeping down filming costs for referring physicians. Money is also saved by not having to repeat lost or misplaced exams, as well as not having to repeat exams because of improper exposure, as CR and DR are more forgiving.

Although you have to hire a PACS administrator, employee costs will still decrease, particularly in the film room and libraries. Transcriptionist costs will be less if you incorporate voice recognition. For small institutions, decreasing employee costs becomes harder as it is much easier to eliminate the second, third, or fourth film room employee, but not the *only* film room employee on a shift, as they may have vital functions elsewhere in the department. Promising improved turnaround times for ED and inpatients can be translated into institutional savings but is also a double-edged sword, as you will have to adjust radiology staff appropriately to keep that promise (bean-counting administrators won't forget!). Depending on the size of your organization, recognize that a sizable portion of a full-time employee's time will be needed to ensure that the clinician users are comfortable and capable of reviewing images online. Not doing this could well result in a backlash that will lead to duplication of costs, resulting from a clinician being mandated to print and store images on an ongoing basis.

The most significant cost reductions arise from greatly increased radiologist productivity and referring physician time savings. Unfortunately, in the eyes of the administration, unless the radiologists and/or clinicians are hospital employees, those savings don't count! Yet, luckily, even the smallest hospitals now understand the inevitability of implementing PACS, although administrators may still try to get budgetary concessions out of radiology in return. If all else fails, it is better medicine. Last, "pay for performance" is upon us and attaining quality metrics will be very difficult without PACS.

PACS CONTRACT

Negotiating the PACS contract is an arduous process and should be left to individuals in the organization with proven experience in negotiating large contracts. The radiologist may need to intercede to help the vendor understand how their institution works, or to aid the hospital in understanding the relative importance of different aspects of the project, especially which portions of the project cannot be cut.

Make sure the software licensing scheme will allow you to add the appropriate number of workstations throughout your organization. Try to obtain an enterprise-wide licensing scheme that allows you to provide—both efficiently and cost effectively—the appropriate client software to all your current and future clinical users. You may have to accept a concurrent user limit or a usage- or volume-based charge. Per seat charges should be avoided, as that limits the number of places that a radiologist can sit, which is particularly onerous if your institution has sites that are staffed for only part of the day.

Plan for upgrades and enhancements either by placing them in the contracts or keeping money available in future budgets, depending on what works best in your organization. You can choose to pay for upgrades by purchasing an "Evergreen" service contract that keeps your software current. This is particularly valuable if you have a software-only contract. If you are dependent on your vendor for hardware, be vigilant because free software upgrades may lead to expensive hardware upgrades (and professional services to install the hardware) that effectively negate the value of the free software upgrade. Try to lock in the service contract costs so you don't get hit with unexpected service rate increases. It is imperative to get uptime guarantees with a financial penalty if these are not met. Also beware of your administration trying to stretch out the depreciation schedule for the PACS system to 7 or 10 years, to make their budgetary numbers more appealing to their board. Given the seemingly unstoppable increase in computer speed, your system is likely to be outdated in 5 years. You don't want to deal with the added burden of incomplete depreciation when you have to financially justify your next upgrade. A nonobsolescence clause can be beneficial if the vendor is about to upgrade to a new platform at the time of initial contracting.

Find out what others have paid for the same product, either by talking with colleagues or by using a buying guide consultant company, so you can be certain you are getting the best deal. Don't announce your final selection until you have a contract you can live with. Don't feel bad about playing the vendors against each other—they expect it and won't give you their best price unless you play the game. Scrutinize your contracts very closely—especially at the end with last-minute cost reductions. Portions of the product may be unexpectedly eliminated to achieve those cost reductions, which will end up costing you much more to restore (than the actual savings) if you don't discover them until after the contract is signed. Also, make sure that the system functionality is appropriate for the size of your institution now, as well as in the next 5 to 10 years. Estimate growth liberally. If you go with a product for small institutions, don't assume that the products will be usable if your institution doubles in size.

It is extremely important to expend all necessary effort to get a truly accurate picture of your current volume and a realistic prediction of your future volume. If you are about to add a 64-channel CT, you must account for the dramatic increase in image volume. Once you have selected a vendor, all the pressure on the vendor is off and whatever additions you need to make to the project come at list price, rather than the highly discounted, initial purchase price.

While it is hard to think of divorce while you are getting married, provision must be made in the contract for what happens if you choose to switch to another PACS vendor. Issues concerning the ownership of the images, guaranteed access to images, and agreements for support during future PACS migrations need to be addressed in the initial contract.

IMPLEMENTING PACS

Having installed hundreds of systems, the PACS vendors have become very proficient at system installation. The vendors will be very helpful in guiding you through the installation process and customizing it to meet your institution's particular needs. Typically, CR will be installed a few weeks prior to the official PACS "go live" day. Images are printed in the interim but can be stored and added to the PACS system. The RIS HL-7 interface needs to be built and tested in advance of installing the PACS servers. Once the PACS servers and image storage devices are installed, image transfer from the CR can begin, as well as the routing and testing of CT, MR, nuclear medicine, ultrasound, and fluoroscopy images. This gives time for radiologists who have never used PACS to become familiar with soft copy reading. Images should be populated in the PACS server for a week or two to both test the system and to build up a small archive of images. Radiologist and technologist training on the display stations can begin. On the go live date, all operations are switched to the PACS systems and film production is halted (hopefully). If the radiologists don't have prior experience reading on PACS stations, different modalities can be brought online sequentially. Try to keep the schedule light, and increase staffing bit by bit for the first couple of days after going live. Initially, continue the preexisting flow of paper while everyone acclimates to the new system. Clinicians who access a high volume of studies—such as the ED and ICU physicians—need to be trained just prior to the go live date, and a concerted effort needs to be made to train the remainder of the clinical staff thereafter.

Training contracts can be obtained at the time of purchase. The PACS administrators need to attend the vendor's administrator course in advance of the system installation. System training for anyone else more than a day or two before going live is usually not useful because users will very rapidly forget everything if they are not continually using the system. It is essential to have trainers available for a few days before and after the go live date. The trainers also need to be available for the afterhours shifts. The trainers will also train in-house trainers, who in turn will be responsible for training nonradiology personnel after the initial start-up. Local expertise is a must. It is also very helpful for the vendor's trainer (or trainers) to schedule a return visit after a month, and again in six months, to answer questions and consolidate learning. Also at that time, once the users are comfortable with the basic system, they will be able to learn more advanced techniques from the trainers, who can be helpful in sharing strategies to increase efficiency.

After going live, comparison films can be digitized into the PACS system. Remarkably, an archive of only a couple of weeks substantially cuts down the number of comparison films requiring digitization. After everyone is comfortable with reading studies on PACS, changes can be made to adjust to the flow of information/paper throughout the department. A scanning process or digital requisitioning system can be implemented. Outside studies on CDs can be imported to the growing archive. Remarkably, within a month after going live, the department will no longer understand how they managed to live without PACS.

Eliminating film within the department is very easy and can occur immediately after going live with PACS, provided you have buy-in from the clinicians. Usually the last people to accept filmless imaging are the orthopedic surgeons—who love the feel of plain X-rays—and the busy surgeons who have to get used to filmless viewing in the ORs and the technique of "sterilely" scrolling and holding selected images. The computer screens must remain active and not "fall asleep" during four- to six-hour operations. So be sure to provide the ED and ICUs with fast, dual screen workstations and make certain that you have at least a simple PACS viewing station on every ward. This will satisfy your internal users and will get the referring physicians hooked on reading studies digitally.

Weaning the referring physicians off of film outside the boundaries of the hospital LAN requires planning and education. Audit your film sign-out process to determine which physicians most want to view their images on film. As you approach the go live date, make sure that you have worked out the networking and VPN issues so that these high-volume users can view their images digitally. You may even have to "loan" them a workstation for viewing and make sure to provide them with a PACS client with enough functionality to meet their needs. If they reside in a professional building next to the hospital, get IT to wire that building and connect it to the LAN. Eliminating network bottlenecks will give you the most bang for your buck for improving remote access. CDs work well for physicians who only rarely want to see images, or for patients traveling to distant specialists who for the most part are accustomed to using them.

PACS AND HEALTH INFORMATION EXCHANGE (HIE) IN THE FUTURE

Increasingly, clinicians are adopting AEMR in their office practices. Though lagging behind AEMR adoption, hospital EMRs will also become common in the future. The entire medical record will be stored digitally in the EMR, and more and more clinical information will be entered in structured format. While many clinicians still dictate their notes, it is easy to visualize a not-too-distant future in which all clinical information—that is, the patient problem lists, the clinical history, the patient physical exams, the drug lists, the nursing record, the clinical laboratory results, and the anatomic pathology reports—will be digitally accessible within the EMR.

Clinicians need to bill just like radiologists and use the same ICD-9 codes to justify their charges. Clinicians are motivated to use their AEMR products to automate their billing processes though they are not willing to expend much energy to facilitate radiology billing. Hopefully, soon, clinicians will be able to order studies directly within their AEMR using an interface they are comfortable with. Their system will search through the AEMR for the ICD-9s that would support the ordered test. If the ICD-9 codes are missing, the physician would be prompted to choose a more appropriate test or provide a justification for the ordered test. If the patient has had a similar recent study, the clinician would be alerted and given the option to review those reports and images. If the prior study is very recent, the clinician would be prompted to explain why a repeat study is needed so soon.

The ICD-9 codes will automatically be attached to the order and automatically transferred by HL-7 to the preferred radiology provider, along with the appropriate supporting portions of the record. These ICD-9 codes will be hyperlinked directly back to the textual portions of the note, allowing the radiologist to access the clinical narrative and place the study in the proper clinical context directly from the third monitor on the PACS workstation. Furthermore, the radiologist could link to the community's RHIO to access prior reports and studies from any of the other radiology providers in the community.

With time, RIS systems will leapfrog PACS. PACS will be relegated to image storage and image retrieval while work list, worksheet, and reporting functions will all reside in the RIS. Study requisitions will be accessed as computer forms. Pertinent clinical information such as creatinine levels, known medical alerts, medications, prior surgeries, and underlying conditions would be automatically pulled from the EMR and displayed for the technologist. Modality workstations will directly access the RIS and changes to the study made on the modality would be reflected back in the RIS. While performing the study, the technologist will complete the form on the computer to enter the additional clinical information gleaned from talking with the patient. Details regarding irregularities in the procedure could be entered on the form and contrast or supplies used during the study will be logged. When the technologist has finished working through the form, the study will be marked as closed and all the data will be transferred to the appropriate location, be it the modality, PACS, RIS, or the reporting system. The modality would confirm when all the images are resident within PACS and the study would be marked as ready for interpretation.

The radiologist will work from a customized work list within the RIS based on her or his work assignment for the day. STAT cases, or studies requiring expedited interpretation, would be clearly identified or promoted to the top of the work list. When the study is opened for interpretation, the requisition will be displayed with the clinical indication, procedural description, volume, and type of contrast all added to the standardized report template so the radiologist need only dictate the body and conclusion of the report. Simple/negative reports could be handled by clicking a normal button or by voice command, using a simple structured report, obviating dictation. Comparison studies will be sorted by body region with the most appropriate comparison listed at the top. Positive findings will be abstracted from the prior reports and summarized. Previous clinical indications will also be summarized if a patient problem list is not available. The patient's record in the EMR will be easily summoned in context for review of operative notes, discharge summaries, or clinical notes if more detailed clinical history is required. Images from anatomic pathology as well as from endoscopy or arthroscopy will be available to facilitate clinical correlation or quality assurance. When a critical finding is found, clicking one link will automatically page the ordering physician or the after-hours on-call physician. A record will be opened so the communication with the appropriate clinician can be documented and receipt confirmed.

The radiologist will generate a report, marking pertinent findings with arrows or measurements. These positive findings in the report would be hyperlinked directly to the markup on the pertinent images. The clinicians will then receive the report at their AEMR or hospital EMR by way of an HL-7 interface. When the clinician reviews the completed report, clicking on the links would open the hyperlinked images in the PACS client on the clinician's workstation. Conversely, clinicians reviewing the images could also click on the markup to view the appropriate portion of the radiology report detailing the findings.

CONCLUSION

PACS has greatly increased radiology productivity and efficiency. Improved information transfer will increase clinical accuracy and effectiveness. The future will be hyperlinked and integrated!

Dos and Don'ts for Implementing PACS	
Dos	**Don'ts**
1. Go to a SIIM meeting or a PACS course and learn from the pros before you start your search.	1. Assume that your equipment vendor's or RIS vendor's offering will make the best PACS for you and skip an exhaustive evaluation.
2. Set up a strong interdisciplinary team to evaluate your needs and define your vision.	2. Think the radiology department can handle PACS without strong IT support.
3. Take the time to really understand your current work flow and determine how you want it to change after PACS.	3. Underestimate your future imaging volume and undersize your system.
4. Visit luminary sites, especially those that are institutions that use the same RIS as you. Learn how they make the system hum and take the time to really assess the workstation functionality.	4. Take for granted that all systems will handle PET, nuclear medicine, angiography, MPR, or ultrasound well.
5. Listen to your techs and make sure the system will enhance their productivity.	5. Presume the next version of the software will fix all current issues or be delivered on time.
6. Work hard on developing a truly paperless work flow.	6. Believe that integration of all your different systems will be inexpensive to implement, or that all your other applications will work on your PACS workstation.
7. Negotiate for future upgrades and unlimited PACS clients in your contract.	7. Assume the vendor will see to it that work flow with their product will match your vision.
8. Invest in the fastest network you can afford and a big pipe to the outside.	8. Underestimate the number of workstations you need and cut corners on memory or processor speed.
9. Make sure your dictation or voice recognition system integrates flawlessly with your PACS workstation.	9. Suppose you will be filmless without proactively working with your high-volume film requestors.
10. Hire a very talented PACS administrator and provide him or her with sufficient support staff.	10. Skimp on the number, size, or screen resolution of your monitors.

LIST OF ABBREVIATIONS AND GLOSSARY

ACR—American College of Radiology

ADT—Admission Discharge Transfer, or patient information. Also an HL-7 message type for transferring patient information.

AEMR—Ambulatory Electronic Medical Record

API—Application Programming Interface. Built-in method for integrating different computer programs.

ASP—Application Service Provider. Scheme in which you don't own the software or hardware but pay a volume-based fee to the provider.

ATM—Asynchronous Transfer Mode. Networking scheme to enhance networking efficiency.

BLU-RAY—Next generation optical disk holding 25 GB on a single-layer disk or 50 GB on a double-layer disk.

CD—Compact Disk. Optical disk holding 650 to 700 MB of data.

CPOE—Computerized Physician Order Entry

CPT—Current Procedural Terminology. Coding system for medical procedures developed by the American Medical Association.

CR—Computed Radiology

CT—Computed Tomography

DICOM—Digital Imaging and Communications in Medicine

DLT—Digital Linear Tape

DR—Digital Radiography

DRG—Diagnostic-Related Group

DVD—Digital Video Disc. Optical disk holding 4.7 GB on a single-layer disk, or 9.4 GB on a double-layer disk.

EHR—Electronic Health Record

EMPI—Enterprise Master Patient Index

EMR—Electronic Medical Record

GB—Gigabyte. 1000 bytes or 8000 bits.

HIE—Health Information Exchange. The process of exchange of medical information.

HIMSS—Healthcare Information and Management Systems Society

HIS—Health Information System

HIT—Health Information Technology. Computer-based technology to manage health information and HIE.

HL-7—Health Level 7. A standard specification for sending health care messages.

ICD-9—International Classification of Diseases, 9th revision

IHE—Integrating the Healthcare Enterprise. Initiative of RSNA and HIMSS to use DICOM and HL-7 to improve transfer of health care information.

IS—Information Systems

IT—Information Technology

JPEG—Joint Photographic Experts Group. Standardized image compression scheme.

JPEG 2000—Joint Photographic Experts Group 2000. Image compression schedule using wavelet compression.

LAN—Local Area Network

LCD—Liquid Crystal Display

LMRP—Local Medical Review Policy

LZW—Limpel-Ziv-Welsh. Lossless data compression algorithm.

MBS—Megabit Per Second

MDCT—Multidetector Computed Tomography

MOD—Magneto-optical Disk

MPI—Master Patient Index

MPR—Multiplanar Reconstruction

MR—Magnetic Resonance

ORM—Order Request Message. HL-7 message type for transferring order information.

ORU—Observation Result Unsolicited Message. HL-7 message type for transferring test result information.

PACS—Picture Archiving and Communication System

PET—Positron Emission Tomography

RAM—Random Access Memory

RSNA—Radiological Society of North America

SAN—Storage Area Network

SCAR—Society for Computer Applications in Radiology (now SIIM)

SCSI—Small Computer System Interface. Standard interface and command set for transferring data between devices, especially hard disks, used in high-performance systems.

SIIM—Society for Imaging Informatics in Medicine

SPECT—Single-Photon Emission Computed Tomography

QA—Quality Assurance. Oversight responsibilities.

QC—Quality Control. Testing activities to assure that specifications are adhered to.

RAID—Redundant Array of Inexpensive Devices (now also Redundant Array of Independent Devices)

RHIO—Regional Health Information Organization

RIS—Radiology Information System

RLE—Run Length Encoding. A lossless data compression algorithm.

UDO—Ultra-density Optical. Successor to MOD containing 30 GB of data (future generations to hold 60 and 120 GB).

UID—Unique Identifiers. In DICOM, unique strings of numbers to describe studies, series, and images.

VPN—Virtual Private Network

WAN—Wide Area Network

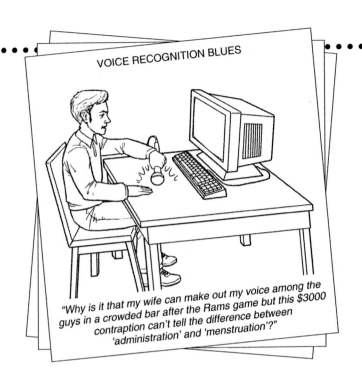

CHAPTER 14

VOICE RECOGNITION BLUES

"Why is it that my wife can make out my voice among the guys in a crowded bar after the Rams game but this $3000 contraption can't tell the difference between 'administration' and 'menstruation'?"

Voice Recognition Dictation

David M. Yousem

INTRODUCTION

The use of voice recognition dictation (VRD) for on-time delivery of radiology reports is a great source of both pride and frustration for radiologists. At the same time, it has special appeal for business administrators and information technology specialists in radiology groups for different reasons. This chapter discusses the issues related to VRD, including the marked growth of this aspect of radiology practice, for better or for worse.

DEFINITION OF VRD

While some refer to "voice recognition" as the ability to identify a person by his or her voice, and "speech recognition" as the process of converting speech to text, for the purposes of this chapter both features will be referred to as "voice recognition dictation," or VRD.

THE IMPORTANCE OF THE RADIOLOGIST'S REPORT

What is the end product of a radiologist's work? The official finalized report. That is our contribution to patient care. A radiologist's report should be concise, complete, timely, accurate, and helpful to patient management. When clinicians evaluate radiologists' reports, some of their most common complaints relate to the availability of the reports (Box 14-1). When clinicians are asked to rank their demands for a high-quality radiology report, the items of priority, from high to low, are: (1) accuracy, (2) timeliness, clarity, completeness, and (3) text that is well organized (and mentions pertinent negatives).[1]

USE OF VRD

The use of voice/speech recognition systems for reporting cases should help to achieve these goals, not thwart them. In particular, with its immediate provision of a report and its widespread availability throughout the radiology information system (RIS) or electronic patient record (EPR), it should address the top three complaints listed in Box 14-1. However, there are several requirements that must be met by a VRD system, which will make the product readily acceptable as noted in Box 14-2.

VRD is a means of improving report turnaround times (RTT) in a radiology practice. When functioning well, it may also reduce transcription expenses and delays in bill submission (see subsequent sections in this chapter), which can significantly impact the revenue and expense equation in a radiology practice. As of 2003, 13% of radiology departments at hospitals with more than 100 beds were using VRD. That number has probably swelled to 40% in the four years since (personal communication, James Philbin).

The primary driver of this growth has been customer service—not radiologist convenience—particularly during the phase of adapting the work flow modifications that can occur with real-time report review and editing. As such, the level of clinical patient enthusiasm may be matched by the lack of enthusiasm by the radiology department. The "cost" of the implementation is often felt in the gastric mucosa of the "dictator."

THE NUTS AND BOLTS OF VRD

The technology underlying VRD is a highly sensitive speech microphone combined with a computer processor that subtly discriminates between a variety of voice inflections and tones. The technology of this module is also able to detect probabilities that certain words will appear in proximity to each other: for example, it is able to predict that there is a greater likelihood that the word "reflux" (rather than "reflex") will follow "gastroesophageal," even though these two words may sound very similar, given a person's particular speech pattern.

An individual's speech pattern, voice volume, and certain inflections must be initially registered in a "voice print" (personal phoneme-allophone library), created when first using a VRD system. In the past, this was a 20- to 30-minute process, which required reading several passages of text provided by the computer software so that the module could distinguish the consonant and vowel sounds pronounced by the individual speaker. This is particularly necessary in a society where individuals may hail from anywhere in the world and pronounce words with marked variability. That this process can be accomplished at all is phenomenal, given the ethnic diversity across a radiology department. Yet the technology has now advanced to the point that within just five minutes of first sitting down with a VRD system, you're able to start dictating official radiology reports. (For some, however, reading through a greater number of text passages to gain higher accuracy rates is beneficial, if not essential.) This "streamlining" of the voice registration process has led to wider acceptance of VRD.

It might seem intuitive that the text passages on which the voice print is constructed should be composed of medical terms when applied for use in a radiology department. Although this is true to an extent, the ability to capture the widest array of consonant combinations and vowel patterns is probably just as critical to obtaining the most useful voice print. In some cases, when starting out with a VRD system, reading a lengthy passage from a Walt Disney story may be more useful than reading through esophagography reports by a mammographer.

The contextual piece is another critical component of the VRD software. How does a computer system know how to handle homonyms such as "red" and "read," or "build" and "billed"? Once again, the VRD module assesses the probability of the combinations of adjacent words when choosing the "best fit." As an aside, most VRD systems also have a spell-checker function that, before sending a report out in its final stage, will prompt you for misspelled words with options for insertion. As opposed to the Microsoft Word function in which my spelling of "oposed" is auto-corrected to "opposed," whether appropriate or not, the VRD systems are more likely to highlight the word as misspelled for you and provide you with options. You may choose to leave it as is or to replace the word with a similar-sounding one, such as "apposed" or "posed."

To improve the VRD system's accuracy, make sure it has a specialty-specific lexicon of words to choose from. It makes sense that with fewer words to choose from the likelihood that the correct word in context will be applied to the dictation by the radiologist will increase. Hence, some vendors of VRD provide a medical lexicon, specific for physicians, rather than offering a universal lexicon. Of course, this means that some words may need to be added to the vocabulary list if they are not typically associated with a medical context, and many radiology groups benefit by adding and subtracting words that are frequently used in their unique environment (e.g., referring physicians' last names) or rarely encountered (e.g., the word "duodenum" for a dedicated full-time neuroradiologist). You can also, while maintaining the overall vocabulary, manually elevate or demote the probability of certain words, making the list an even more effective medical dictionary.

One colleague recounted the story of how frustrated he became because his pronunciation of the word "marked" (i.e., as two syllables, "mar-kid," rather than "markt") returned the VRD transcription of "market." Since "marked" was a word that, as a chest radiographer, he used several times a day, his frustration level was quite high. Unfortunately, in the universal lexicon that was employed in his version of VRD software, the word "market" was deemed a vital word that could not be deleted. The work-around for this type of situation is exasperating but can be effective nonetheless. He had to trick the VRD program by pronouncing the individual word "market" as "mar-keeeet" so that the overlap with his "mar-kid" would be reduced.

As a neuroradiologist I dictate a lot of lumbar spine studies. Hence the combination of "L" with the numbers "4" and "5" occur at a high rate in my speech pattern voice print. This led to an unusual phenomenon when the calendar clicked over into the years 2003 to 2005 because my pattern is to dictate dates for comparison studies using the pattern of slashed numbers such as 8/10/05. Unfortunately, after six years of "L5"s, when I pronounced the year as "oh-five," the VRD transcription repetitively would list the date as "8/10/L5." Since I frequently combine "L" with "3" and "4" and "5," it transcribed L3, L4, and L5 as 03, 04, and 05. Several times a day I would have to make this correction before the computer trained me: either I had to exaggerate and round my "OHHHs"; pause after saying "oh" (allowing it to transcribe that number) before adding 3, 4, or 5; or I had to say "zero-five" rather than "oh-five." It is examples like these, in which both terms are used very frequently, that you realize, alas, the computer module is not a human transcriptionist. Humans, it is hoped, would never make such an obvious mistake on a daily basis.

After the voice print has been made, you can begin to use VRD for radiology reporting across the department. Usually the voice print is stored in a central VRD server so that with each log-in to a new computer with VRD installed, that same voice print can be retrieved from the server, rather than having to repeat the process on each computer across the dictating environment. In a similar fashion, the edited lexicon for the individual (with his/her deletions and additions) can be retrieved from the same central storage device.

Because the environments in which the VRD computers are located may vary in their acoustics and background noise, most VRD programs will require an initial volume and microphone quality check for that unique environment. This usually requires a one-time-only reading of a single paragraph of text in which the microphone adjusts to the optimal settings for that person's voice and ambient noise. A second paragraph to assess the microphone's quality for discrimination is read, also generally just a few sentences of basic text. This also is done just once, for each software upgrade. When the VRD module is integrated into the radiology information system, the headers for the individual case are displayed on the VRD screen when the case to be dictated is selected. At this point, there are several options for using VRD.

OPTIONS FOR USE OF VRD

Digital Dictation with Remote Transcription

In the absence of a voice recognition system, a radiologist reports his findings into a recording device prior to this voice file being manually converted into text. This has become more efficient with the use of digital dictation: the voice dictation is then sent to a human transcriptionist, bypassing the computer module

that does the immediate translation on the screen. This effectively replaces the use of mini-tapes and tape recorders that were the previous generation of transcription devices. With digital dictation, a remote transcriptionist can log into the overall system and hear the radiologist's voice, transcribe the text, and return the completed report to the radiologists' signature queue for electronic signature. Whereas this is probably the fastest and most user-friendly means of dictating a case, it incurs the "cost" of the delays of transcription—the going back and forth of transcribing and signing—and depends on a reliable and potentially costly pool of transcriptionists, who can provide 24/7 coverage. Nonetheless, in a high-volume setting in which the cost of extra time spent by the physician by using the *complete* package for VRD is prohibitive, this option is beneficial to keep in reserve.

Initial VRD with Transcriptionist Correction

Using this option, the radiologist uses the full VRD module for transcription and produces an immediate report. However, rather than correcting one's own report, the radiologist defers that duty to a transcriptionist who listens to the report while reading the VRD transcription and makes the contextual corrections in the report for the limited number of words or phrases that the computer incorrectly chose. Depending on the typists' speed in keeping up with the dictating radiologist's rapidity of speech, this may or may not gain a time advantage over just sending the case to digital dictation. In some cases, a radiology department may provide the unedited preliminary VRD report to the clinicians by way of an EPR for viewing. That way, colleagues from the clinical side can log into a patient's report to listen to the same dictation before transcription, if necessary. The danger here is that neither the radiologist nor the transcriptionist has reviewed this report that is now accessible to the clinicians, and the inaccuracies of missed words ("there are *no* masses seen in the right lower lobe" vs. "there are masses seen in the right lower lobe") or misspelled words may lead to poor patient care. Once again, using the transcriptionists as proofreaders will decrease the physician time in correcting his or her reports but will incur the "time" cost of reports going back and forth between transcriptionists and radiologists for finalizing after review, signing electronically, and sending the completed report on to the patient record.

A slight modification that can shorten the time to final report yet avoid the frustration that can occur when a voice file is inadequately recognized is to reserve the "send to transcriptionist" option for when a report is particularly complex, there is not an adequate template, or the voice recognition accuracy is lower than usual in the report and requires editing. In instances in which an accurate report is generated by voice recognition, an immediate sign-off could occur without the transcriptionist as an intermediary.

Complete VRD (No Transcriptionist)

Using VRD to create final reports, and bypassing the use of a transcriptionist, obviously uses the module to its fullest advantage. In this scenario, the case is completely dictated and transcribed locally on the radiologist's host computer, reviewed at the same time (or later) by a radiologist, and sent to the patient record without the use of a transcriptionist. The specifics of how to implement this interface are at the discretion of the dictating radiologist. With some modules, the text appears as the radiologist dictates each phrase so that he or she can see how the computer is translating his or her voice in real time. Another option is that the completed text appears only at the end of the report's completed dictation.

The advantage to the former methodology is that you can detect if there is a gross problem with the VRD system after only a sentence or two, rather than finding out after a 5000-word dictation that the system was not on, or, because of interference, was translating the abdominal CT scan into the Gettysburg Address in Pig Latin. In addition, immediate viewing of the text as you dictate allows you to efficiently use "tabbing" functions for preordained templates (macros, see subsequent section) of reports to reduce the number of words needing to be translated into text. Concurrent translation also lets you pick up the repetitive errors being made by the VRD and adjust the speech accordingly (round the "ohs" or shorten the "mar-keeeeets"), if those words are being used many times in the same report. Otherwise you'll be making the same corrections again and again throughout the report.

The disadvantage of immediate translation is that the appearance of the text can be distracting—with the dictation showing, your eyes stray from the images on the screen quite frequently. While this may lead to more accurate interpretation of the voice, the cost of not focusing on the images at hand may lead to less accurate interpretation of the images. So, viewing the text only at the end of the dictation when it "magically appears" from the cue provided by the microphone, prevents these distractions and allows you to turn from the singular important task of interpreting the case to the next task, that is, reviewing and correcting the report.

If VRD attained the six sigma levels (i.e., 3.4 errors per 1 million opportunities) that our vendor colleagues ascribe to it, it'd be more popular than sliced bread. In reality, if a VRD system is 95% to 98% accurate in its capture of a person's voice into translated, transcribed text—this is the industry standard, and it has done a very good job. Yet what does 95% to 98% accuracy mean to the radiologist? For those who read screening chest radiographs in which reports may be 10 to 20 words at most, it means that there may be a single correction in every four to five reports. However, for those that read combined chest, abdominal, and pelvic CT scans of patients in a cancer center it often means that, in your 300-word report, there will be 6 to 15 corrections to make, some of which may be totally out of context, frankly embarrassing or, at worst, potentially dangerous to the patient's health. Once again, these are often mistakes that a human transcriptionist can correct and identify with ease, but in the VRD environment require constant vigilance by the VRD radiologist.

Of note, picking up a VRD error can be more difficult that detecting a transcription error. The previously cited error between "opposed" and "apposed" would not be an error a good transcriptionist would make. However, errors such as this, which are phonemically similar, can defy the radiologist's ability to detect them. The days of briefly looking at a report, trusting your 30-year-veteran departmental typist, and quickly scribbling your signature on a paper report are long gone with the VRD system. You must review the report carefully and make the corrections yourself for the maximal *potential* benefit of the patient and your clinical colleagues.

Clearly, the degree to which VRD is accepted by radiologists will vary by practice patterns, voice clarity of the individual radiologist, and his or her experience with it. There are compelling reasons why VRD should be adopted and used with its full capacity function.

Use of Templates/Macros

Obviously, the solution to reducing the number of words that need correcting is to reduce the number of words that are transcribed. I believe that in some circles the reports have become more cryptic as radiologists attempt to decrease the potential word errors by shortening their reports. Is a "Normal" report really any less informative than a report that reads "No evidence of infiltrates. Normal cardiothoracic ratio and mediastinal structures. The costophrenic angles are sharp with no evidence of effusions or pulmonary Kerley B lines to suggest congestive heart failure"? As long as the specific clinical question asked is also answered, perhaps the former is not less meaningful in terms of conveying adequate medical information. It can also not be diminished that our third-party payer friends are putting great emphasis on documentation, so a more verbose report can convey to the coders that a comprehensive review was not only well done but also well documented.

More often than not, however, radiologists instead resort to the construction of personalized templates. With the use of templates, the radiologist can be expansive in the detail of what he or she did *not* see while limiting the number of words translated. Thus, for a normal chest radiograph, the radiologist merely has to insert, either by voice command or by mouse clicks, the "Normal Chest" template and the entire report can be produced without a single word dictated and finalized without review. Also, insertion points can be created for providing the individual patient history or to insert a data point that may be patient specific (e.g., the patient's cardiothoracic ratio with minimal/moderate/marked degenerative changes in the thoracic spine).

These templates (also called macros) are particularly useful in settings in which: (1) there are a lot of normal studies, such as for the emergency department or screening studies; (2) the technique used for the study is stereotypical and must be provided as part of the report (e.g., the pulse sequences for a routine lumbar spine MRI scan); (3) serial measurements are made as part of a standard report (e.g., fetal measurements for dating gestational age using ultrasound); and (4) the report prompts a radiologist to look at specific areas for pathology, as in a carotid angiogram in which the common carotid origin and bifurcation are observed for narrowing, followed by a vessel-by-vessel analysis of anterior circulation branches for stenosis. If the radiologist in the latter case can reduce his or her report to the six words "no," "minimal," "moderate," "60," "minimal," and "no" for a report that states, "There is NO evidence of stenosis at the common carotid origin from the aorta. The external carotid artery shows MINIMAL atherosclerotic change at the common carotid bifurcation. The internal carotid artery shows MODERATE 60% stenosis at the common carotid artery bifurcation. There is MINIMAL carotid siphon narrowing and NO narrowings of anterior and middle cerebral artery branches," he or she will be using templates advantageously while the tabbed prompts force him or her to look at all the critical sites of the anatomy as a check-off list.

This use of a template is also a very good teaching tool for trainees, since it also directs them to look for specific locations and types of pathology and forces them to make measurements for relevant data points. One could argue that the speed gains in tabbing through reports in this fashion compensate for the loss of time spent correcting the 3% to 5% of words in reports that require a more freestyle type of textual dictation, but, unfortunately, this has not been our experience. These templates are stored centrally on the server so that they are available at each VRD-containing computer and are not lost in local crashes. Templates can also be shared among users for more uniform reporting. These will be helpful in maintaining compliance with and implementing "pay for performance" initiatives.

Trainees as Transcriptionists

In academic settings, the trainees often become pseudotranscriptionists in a variety of potential scenarios. In one situation, the attending radiologist will dictate the case using VRD and ask that the trainee do the correcting and proofreading before the attending finalizes the report. In other words, on completion of the report, while the attending is calling a clinician about the case, or pulling up the next case on the PACS (picture archiving and communication systems), the trainee is reviewing the report for any errors before pushing the case to the EPR in its final form. In another context, the attending arrives at the VRD station with a preliminary report having already been transcribed by way of VRD by the trainee and edited appropriately so that all the attending radiologist has to do is to review the case, check that this previously dictated report is accurate, and push it to the patient record. This type of prereporting might actually be well used in fetal ultrasound settings, in which the ultrasonologist provides all of the data points for the fetal sizes and the radiologist merely has to verify the numbers, check for congenital anomalies, and send a finalized report to the EPR. (Whether the clinical team can see the preliminary report by the trainee or the sonologist will vary according to departmental policy.)

Avoid "forcing" implementation of VRD. In some departments, in order to overcome resistance to adopting VRD, the alternative systems—tape recorders—have been removed from the reading station. If VRD is subsequently not well implemented, the radiologist or trainee will end up typing the majority of the report, and efficiencies will be lost.

BENEFITS OF VRD

Reduction in Report Turnaround Times (RTT)

Clearly, the ability to produce a finalized report within a matter of seconds that appears in the EPR, where any physician can access it almost contemporaneously, is a tremendous improvement in the quality of patient care. The impact of VRD in our practice setting is best demonstrated with emergency department (ED) cases in which the immediate access and reduced turnaround time of the reports can significantly reduce the length of ED visits and also the traffic of telephone interruptions from the ED clinicians to obtain verbal reports. In fact, there are good arguments to prioritize the ED cases from the work lists over the less urgent outpatient studies so that immediate, appropriate care can be given to the ED patients.

Across the board, using VRD definitely leads to reduced report turnaround times (RTT), since the going back and forth with transcriptionists is eliminated (this assumes that the radiologist is dictating and finalizing as he or she goes). There is the option of just sending the reports as "preliminary" in the VRD-transcribed state and then, at a later date, running through all of the batched reports in one setting and correcting them as one would the delivered paper reports from the transcription pool. In such a case, there still is likely to be a reduction in RTT but not as dramatic as the immediate "dictate and finalize" practice pattern. The full use of VRD also allows for relatively easy attainment of the JCAHO (Joint Commission of Accreditation of Healthcare Organizations) standards, from study completion to finalized report in most practices. And, since the RTT is often one parameter tied to practice-based incentive plans, the radiologist who uses VRD to its full potential has a financial motivation to implement the program as well. This is often the focus of practice quality improvement projects for maintenance of certification.

Reduction in Delayed Bill Submission (see Chapter 9)

In the practice pattern of yesteryear, the typing pool may have been a source of delays in preliminary reports being provided to the radiologist, depending on the volume of studies and the pool's capacity to handle those studies. Let's imagine a CT scan that is performed at 3 PM on a Monday. It is then read and dictated on a microphone tape at 4:45 PM. The transcriptionists have already made their last rounds to pick up tapes for the day. The case gets transcribed the next day by 10 AM and is delivered to the radiologist in paper form by noon. He revises the report and signs the paper version at 3 PM and that paper copy is returned to the typist or billing people by 5 PM that day. In most cases, the bill will go out the next day since it is the finalized signed report that usually enables the submission of the Medicare Part B bill to the payer. This situation is not uncommon in many radiologist practices, let alone practices in which that same radiologist is at another facility (or on vacation or weekend break) the next day. Thus the bill may take an extra one to two days to be sent out, as opposed to the scenario in which the radiologist uses VRD with no transcriptionist and the report is sent out in finalized form at 4:48 PM the same day as the case was performed. It also enables electronic automatic submission of the bill, again faster than the paper copy being the prompt to the billing department to send out the bill for the professional component of the study.

While one might think that the "cost" of one or two days of delay in submission of a bill would have little impact, this plays out at a much larger level when one has a busy practice. Imagine a healthy practice of $30 million in net revenues and a "cost of money" of 10% (for more on "cost of money," see Chapter 10, "Managing Expenses"). If one can cut two days from the time of procedure performed to the time the bill is submitted, what would the potential impact be? If the cost of money is 10%, then over a year that potential revenue could be reduced (or accrued) by $3 million. Dividing that $3 million by 365 days yields a daily cost of money of $8219. For a two-day delay this is $16,438, which would be a nice annual bonus to pay out to the radiologist who fully uses VRD. While the numbers may seem relatively small, it will vary depending on the efficiency of the system, the billing practices of the group, and the typical delays in the group's transcription service. For each day saved, that's $8219, merely in the cost of capital benefit.

Reduction in Cost of the Transcription Pool

Yes, you can completely eliminate transcriptionists if you're using VRD fully. Within my neuroradiology division of nine radiologists billing over $36 million in charges each year, we went from a transcription expense attributable to our work of $80,000 per year to $0. We do not use transcriptionists at all. We can create addendums or revise reports or finalize all of our work without the use of one hour of transcription expense, despite a volume that generally runs over 80 to 100 CT scans a day and over 50 to 70 MRI studies a day. Obviously, it is appropriate to have backup available in the event of system outages, but these temporary employees may be hired with the use of third-party vendors on an as-needed basis, rather than retaining full-time, in-house employees. Our former transcriptionists, long-standing employees of our department, have been retrained to be patient service coordinators within our department, or digital file managers. Many of the transcriptionists' positions were eliminated through attrition as more and more sections within the department moved to VRD: some left to type for less "advanced" radiology groups. One thing to consider, of course, is that we have shifted work from a lower-expense staff member to our most expensive employee. For a time, while learning the VRD system, the cost benefit is lost in the decreased efficiency of the doctor.

Improved Header and Clinical Information

Since VRD is linked to the RIS, header information is readily transferable from one system to the next. Instead of, say, scrambling to find the correct medical record number from the spelling of a patient's name to link the dictation to the correct patient, the VRD system does this for you (or for the typist). It may employ a strobe light to bar code the patient data, or it may have a pull-down menu of patient names to choose from. In its most effective implementation, the VRD system will also transfer the clinical information and ICD-9 code from the electronic physician order entry into the "Indication" field of your dictation. Wouldn't it be nice not to have to guess at what the clinician's scribble on the request slip was and to have this transferred without even dictating it into the correct history field? These are the goals of the "smart" VRD system.

Other Benefits

Other VRD benefits include:

1. Expediting patient care.
2. Reducing the work of practice managers and physicians who must field calls for reports on cases that are still in the "waiting to be transcribed" pool.
3. Eliminating the need for radiologists to re-review cases that they have become unfamiliar with by the time the transcribed report makes it back for signature.
4. Eliminating the need for runners who bring transcribed reports back and forth to the radiologists for signature.
5. Reducing the risk of having proxy signature of cases when a radiologist leaves for vacation or goes to another facility the next day—all the cases are signed and sent as they are dictated with no leftover cases. In fact, proxy sign-off should never be done for billing compliance reasons, particularly in an academic setting in which the attending will not be able to attest that he or she actually reviewed the images, not just the resident.

The realization of these benefits, particularly number 2 above, requires change management for the clinicians. It will not be atypical that they will come seeking a verbal report, even though a VRD report is awaiting them in the EPR.

Modifying reports following a prior read by a trainee can also be improved with VRD because you'll have a clearer picture of the likely interpretation conveyed to the clinician at the time that the resident made the preliminary read. This certainly will be an improvement over mere recollection or the jottings on the requisition by the trainee.

Other recent advances in VRD have allowed dictation to be performed over telephone lines while preserving an adequate and accurate voice print. The microphones for VRD have also become more specialized, allowing the hand-held microphone to become the substitute for a mouse on the VRD computer. Still other systems enable the use of a headset, which allows the radiologist to maintain optimal positioning of the microphone to the mouth, thus freeing the hands to manipulate the images being interpreted. (Sharing of headsets is discouraged due to health reasons.)

DOWNSTREAM EFFECTS

Downstream effects of VRD are predictable. Because of the need for relative silence while dictating, and the propensity of most radiologists to leave the microphone on while pausing to review the images (a behavior that is actually detrimental to speech recognition over the long run), the usual banter between an academic radiologist and the trainee is reduced. The resident or fellow is less likely to interrupt the reporting radiologist with questions while the attending is in the process of VRD. The modest reduction in efficiency—because of the radiologist using the VRD system—also leads to a greater strain on the system to get the reports read within the workday. When residents were surveyed as to the impact of VRD on their training, 81% reported that VRD led to an increase in the amount of time it took to dictate a case and that the reliability was less than that of traditional transcription.[2,3] This led to a negative impact on the available time for teaching during the workday. This negative impact on resident education was of a greater magnitude at higher volume centers. Some residents and attendings voiced concern that having a third monitor to deal with is distracting and time-consuming, and detracts from "face time" with the trainee. However, the reduced number of phone calls because of immediate reporting increases mentor-mentee communication time. Also, the increased dictation time with VRD may be mitigated by the attending and trainee working in parallel on two independent workstations, yet this also impedes the learning experience, since the trainee working alone on a worksation sees fewer cases.

Feedback when readings are checked remotely tends to decrease. If the radiologist is reviewing cases from home that the trainee has input by way of VRD earlier in the day, he is less likely to call the trainee to provide feedback over simple misses like old lamina papyracea fractures, lens implants, mastoiditis, or old lacunar infarctions, than if he were sitting next to the fellow. It's unfortunate because this type of critique is essential for removing "blind spots" from a trainee's technique of image review. So VRD allows for easy remote reviewing and editing, but the feedback loop suffers.[3] (Many VRD programs are advanced enough that they can be used over the phone for dictation. This is not widely employed, however, since the command system using telephone keys is often awkward.)

Nonetheless, there are beneficial aspects to resident education that may not be immediately apparent. Because most residency programs using transcriptionists have the residents wait to enter reports until the attending radiologists have reviewed the cases with them, the attendings aren't able to assess the knowledge base of the residents as well as when the resident is predictating with VRD. In the latter case, the resident is more likely to commit fully to an impression of the case and to look at it in greater detail, rather than a perfunctory review "until the attending shows up to give the answers" or a cursory scribble on a request slip. As a faculty member, one is much more

able to get a sense of holes in the trainee's scan-and-review technique, or blind spots, when the trainee uses VRD in advance of review. One can also assess the maturity/accuracy of their differential diagnoses when you can see how they would have dictated the case on their own. This assumes a work flow in which trainees put in preliminary VRD reports while the attending is away from the reading station. Furthermore, if the attending reports the cases on his or her own at the end of the day, it means that both the professors and the trainees get to leave at the same time, having completed the day's work, rather than the pattern in which the attending reviews the case with the trainee and leaves the dictating to the resident or fellow afterward. Of course, this can also be said to be possible at the end of the day with transcriptionists. With transcriptionists, next-day signage of the reports often leads to re-review of at least a small percentage of cases to make sure the rights and lefts were correct or that the corrections for gaps in transcription were accurately addressed. "Was that case really Mr. Smith? I thought it was Miss Jones. Better check." When one leaves the workstation after VRD, all the cases are dictated, up-to-date, reviewed, and available to the clinicians.

Deitte reports that, in her experience, it takes longer to review and edit a trainee's report than it does to report it herself, even with VRD.[3] I agree. The residents' reads then actually serve to *decrease* the time available for teaching. The temptation is to pick up the speech mike and just do it yourself. Alternatively, Deitte advocates group reading sessions in which everyone is looking at the case but the attending is doing the VRD. The negative to this approach is that the resident fails to learn (actively) the technique of report generation.

The resident can generate the report and keep track of what needs to be changed and then change it after readout: in a multi-PACS station environment, this does not have to be less efficient for the attending, but it will be for the trainee.

Another downstream effect of VRD is to raise the expectations of clinical colleagues as to the RTT. As stated previously, by prioritizing ED cases, you can reduce the overall

240

time from study performance to finalized report to less than 30 minutes. This is very desirable and beneficial to patient care until it becomes a 24/7 expectation. In our current VRD environment, the clinicians become irritable if an ED report into the EPR is delayed by as much as two hours. This means that taking a 90-minute lunch break with the trainee to discuss life's little mysteries outside of the department of radiology is verboten. It also means that the only time one gets calls from the ED are when they are demanding the report on a case that is delayed to the PACS. In exams where multiplanar reconstructions are required, 3-D volumetric studies need to be reviewed (CT angiograms), or in difficult cases in which reference material must be consulted, a 30-minute turnaround time becomes an expectation that is very difficult to meet. In short order what was once a delight to the ED clinicians (finalized reports on screen within an hour) quickly become an expectation, placing a large burden on the radiology team.

Clinician-radiologist communication on cases also has suffered because of VRD. Since reports are available so quickly into the EPR, the surgeons and clinicians no longer call the radiologists as frequently to find out what the case showed (during the natural delay between dictation and human transcription). There is less verbal exchange of patient data. Fortunately, the EPR has improved the written data exchanged between the departments. Therefore, just as the referring physician may no longer call the radiologist to find out the results from that day's study—referring instead to the VRD report on the EPR for the final result—the radiologist is more likely to refer to a clinic or discharge note to gain further insight into the patient's history, rather than paging the referring physician. The communication that occurs is richer in detail and formality using the EPR, but does create a more pervasive sense of the radiologist as the "shadow doctor"—unseen and now unheard—just a producer of timely, accurate readings into the EPR.

In its stead, because of the efficiency of the PACS, more interdisciplinary conferences can be scheduled with the clinicians, since the cases are read (but not dictated) more quickly by the radiologists. The importance of multidisciplinary conferences cannot be understated in the era of VRD. This is the main feedback loop with the clinicians and gets the radiologists front and center in a patient care environment in which we can thrive.

VENDORS OF CORE SPEECH ENGINE TECHNOLOGY

Two of the vendors' products of VRD in radiology reporting are Dragon System's Naturally Speaking PowerScribe and IBM's VoiceType Medspeak-Talk Technology. Unfortunately, these products have been bought and sold so many times that it will be difficult to predict who will own what at the time of this book's publication. Nonetheless, the two *dominant* products of the core speech engine technology are first, as already mentioned, Naturally Speaking PowerScribe (Nuance Communications) and SpeechMagic (Philips). The previously mentioned IBM product—VoiceType Medspeak-Talk Technology—is also still supported. These engines, however, are not truly usable without a supporting product that incorporates radiologist work flow and integrates with other departmental systems. For a comparison of the two core speech engine technologies, based on their own literature, see the Appendix. Some basic requirements of the systems are summarized in Boxes 14-3 and 14-4.

VENDORS OF COMMERCIAL SOFTWARE PACKAGES

With many similarities between the two leading speech engines, the noticeable differences for the end user come from the commercialized software applications that drive the work flow and present additional tools for the radiologist. The three leading suppliers of this technology are Commissure, Dictaphone, and MedQuist. Aside from using different core speech engines (both Commissure Rad Where and Dictaphone PowerScribe use Dragon, and MedQuist SpeechQ uses SpeechMagic), there is a substantial differentiation between each

BOX 14-3

Technical Needs Critical to Easy Implementation of VRD

1. Make sure that the operating system is appropriate for the VRD function; use vendor's preferred platform configured as recommended. This may mean limiting the other applications that can be accessed on this PC.
2. Ensure that the VRD file server has the correct memory, disk space, and processor speed and can receive messages from the RIS.
3. Ensure that the VRD module can speak to the RIS by way of Health Level 7 (HL-7). This is almost assumed today, although some RIS systems will require the use of a file drop or other communication methods. The VRD platform should support the easy mapping of interface fields both into and out of the system to allow for local RIS configuration differences.
4. Ensure that structured query language (SQL) data storage of a report can be converted to an HL-7 message to the RIS and EPR.
5. Have adequate initial and follow-up training. Mandatory one-on-one training is needed before a user can be productive on a VRD system. Instruct trainers, since each year new residents, fellows, faculty, and employees will enter the group.
6. Optimize the microphone for the environment.
7. Have the PC configured to auto restart during off-hours. VRD systems place heavy demands on the computer; daily reboots will minimize the problem.
8. Ensure that a full test environment is available. This will require a test server and PCs to allow all upgrades to be fully tested in a simulated production environment. Final testing should be done by actual users of the system prior to deployment.

BOX 14-4

Nontechnical Issues to Be Addressed for VRD Implementation

1. Financial analysis
2. Build consensus with leaders
   - Radiologists and nonradiologist physicians
   - Administration and technical staff
3. Choose vendor with experience in type and size of your practice
4. Appropriate staffing for implementation, training, and maintenance
5. Effective training and retraining strategies
6. Defer payments until 30 days after full acceptable implementation

the application beyond just the speech component. The best systems should incorporate other various additions that improve productivity and enhance work flow above and beyond just transcription. It is also critical to look for an application that provides benefits not only to the radiologists, but also to the patients, the trainees, the administration, the IT personnel, and the referring clinician base as well. All else aside, it is these "extras" that will differentiate a superior system (Box 14-5).

The following are critical to quality factors from an IT director's standpoint:

1. Interface (accuracy, reliability of information interfacing with HIS or RIS).
2. Work flow (true two-way results—clinical information available to reader and reports available to clinicians, accurate and maintainable work lists).
3. User interface ("intuitiveness" of bells and whistles and buttons and clicks).
4. Voice recognition quality (important, especially if the above items in number 3 don't work well, you won't notice that this one does).
5. General reliability (ease and quality of vendor and in-house support—it's going to break, how quickly it's fixed is critical).

of the leading market players. Table 14-1 illustrates a breakdown of product features.

When selecting a VRD system, it is important to explore all the tools that make up

Table 14-1   Comparison of Vendors*

	Commissure RadWhere	Dictaphone PowerScribe	Agfa TalkStation	MedQuist SpeechQ
Dragon NaturallySpeaking 8.1	×	×	×	
SpeechMagic 6.0				×
Integrates with most major RIS/PACS	×	×	×	×
Ability to merge data in macro fields	×		×	×
Supports resident workflow* dependent on RIS interface	×	×	×	×
Fax, print, and e-mail from application	×	Print only	×	×
Telephone access		×	×	×
Integrated critical communication tools	×			
Integrated access to clinical knowledge	×			
View previous reports	×	Limited	Limited	×
Microphone options	Nonproprietary	Proprietary	Nonproprietary	Nonproprietary
Electronically sign reports	×	×	×	×
Image capture capability	×			
Radiology-specific language models	×	×	×	×
System automated macro population	×			
Audio file playback	×	×	×	×
Voice command navigation support	×	×	×	×
ICD-9 coding capability dependent on RIS interface and billing work flow	×	×	×	

*Data current as of January 2007.

BOX 14-5

Wish List for VRD Systems

1. Maintains 100% accuracy.
2. Uses spelling and grammar checking.
3. Enables access to and inputs patient information including ICD-9 coding, old reports, problem lists.
4. Performs ACR teaching file coding automatically.
5. Has easy template usage and scrolling that can be prepopulated.
6. Detects errors in left and right incongruity in the reports.
7. Knows clinicians' preferences for report delivery (fax, email, paper, electronic, pager) and verifies receipt of the report. Reliably notifies physicians of critical findings.
8. Allows flagging of teaching file cases, morbidity and mortality conference cases, trainee error cases.
9. Permits flagging of cases for determination of diagnosis in the future with link to pathology reports that notify radiologist when histology has been determined.
10. Gets the diagnosis correct every time!

Dos and Don'ts for VRD Systems

Dos	Don'ts
1. Include radiologists, IT support people, technologists, nurses, and administrators in vendor decisions.	1. Skimp on VRD systems. A bad one will infuriate the physicians.
2. Allow the radiologist to make the final decision.	2. Constrict individual customization.
3. Emphasize accuracy in the selection process.	3. Buy a product that does not have a limited medical lexicon.
4. Have full integration with RIS/PACS.	4. Rely entirely on VRD without an emergency backup system, including one that does not require electricity (e.g., battery-powered handheld dictaphones).
5. Provide multiple options for use by physicians.	
6. Minimize needs for frequent upgrades.	
7. Store voice prints on servers with redundant architecture.	5. Have VRD on a single system server.
8. Have multiple trainers available, especially at peak, new-employee times.	6. Be cursory in system implementation.
9. Allow conferences for users to exchange secrets (and hints) to success.	7. Allow the frustration of the first week or two with the system to cloud judgments.
10. Distribute widely and have spare units.	8. Buy a product that requires multiple commands/clicks to get the job done.
11. Maintain a close vendor relationship.	9. Blame the physician for the wrong VRD system.
	10. Undertrain.
	11. Be inflexible to change.

CONCLUSION

Voice recognition dictation comes at a cost: the ease of picking up a dictaphone and letting a professional medical typist do the rest in a reliable manner is lost. However, the benefits far outweigh the minor inconvenience and, by using templates, one can regain that lost efficiency. From the standpoint of the ultimate health care parameter—patient care—there can be no doubt that VRD, by speeding up the communication of radiology reports, has improved the radiology service. Given the advances in the technology of VRD over the past two to three years, the future is even more rosy for those radiology groups who make the commitment to VRD programs.

REFERENCES

1. Johnson AJ, Ying J, Swan JS, Williams LS, et al: Improving the quality of radiology reporting: A physician survey to define the target. J Am Coll Radiol 1(July):497–505, 2004.
2. Gutierrez AJ, Mullins ME, Novelline RA: Impact of PACS and voice-recognition reporting on the education of radiology residents. J Digit Imaging 18(2):100–108, 2005.
3. Deitte L: Challenges to radiology education in the new era. J Am Coll Radiol 3(July):528–533, 2006.

APPENDIX

For more information on the major products/vendors that support VRD systems, please see the websites below:

http://www.commissure.com
http://www.dictaphone.com
http://www.medquist.com
http://www.agfa.com/en/he/products_services/all_products/talkstation_radiology.-jsp?p=2

Quality Improvement Programs

John A. Bonavita

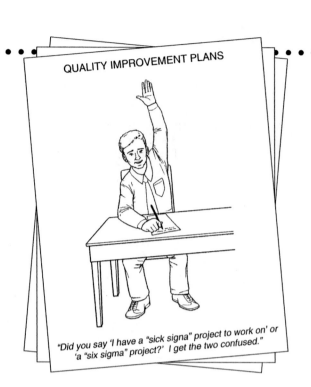

QUALITY IMPROVEMENT PLANS

"Did you say 'I have a "sick signa" project to work on' or 'a "six sigma" project?' I get the two confused."

Maria Gonzalez, a third-year student at the NYU School of Law, is older than most of the other students in her class. Her younger son has finished high school. Her husband used to work at Port Authority, but since 9/11 she has been alone. The end of what seemed like an endless road is just ahead of her. It's been tough to pick up the pieces; she's just begun to date again.

While sitting in a tax law class, she begins to feel slight discomfort in her side, not anything awful, but something that registers in the back of her mind. A week passes, it returns, but this time, it's more like a toothache; she can no longer sit comfortably in class. She calls her sister's internist at NYU, Dr. Luong, and is given an appointment for the next day.

The next morning, she is the first patient of the day. Before she even has any time to collect her thoughts, she is in with the internist and exchanging the usual pleasantries. From the moment they meet, she notices his attention to detail throughout the examination. She's impressed, thinking, "He's actually taking time to listen to me!" Even though the exam goes by quickly, it seems like it was thorough. Maria remembers, "Boy, did that hurt when he pressed on my left side!" As she returns to the front desk, the office staff schedules an abdominal ultrasound at the NYU Faculty Practice Radiology for the next morning.

Maria arrives at the radiology office on First Avenue at 9:00 AM for her 9:15 scheduled examination, waits in a line of ten people, and is shown into ultrasound at 9:30. "Not as fast as yesterday," she thinks. She's beginning to get nervous, worrying that she shouldn't have kept that appointment with her adviser downtown at 11:00. A tall thin woman with an Eastern European accent greets Maria at the door of the ultrasound department. On the way to the exam room, they talk about why Maria is here for the exam. Maria explains that her pain has moved to the left side of her abdomen, but is somewhat lower than yesterday. The tech disappears to talk to the radiologist. Maria begins to think how strange it is that the woman never bothered to introduce herself.

After about five minutes, the technologist comes back to tell her that her doctor has decided that a pelvic ultrasound, rather than an abdominal ultrasound, would be better suited to her condition. "Ok, whatever they think is right. What's the difference? But now I have to drink water? Oh brother, I'm really going to be late."

After drinking what seems like gallons of water, Maria waits outside, beginning to get a little impatient at this point ... and her bladder is full to the bursting point. She crosses her legs, she's not sure she will make it. Finally, another young woman brings her back to the ultrasound room. The pelvic ultrasound is done but she is told that an endovaginal scan is necessary. She is told to go and empty her bladder. "Now I'm supposed to empty my bladder?" The technologist performs the exam more quickly than Maria had anticipated, exits to speak to the doctor, who, believe it or not, comes into the room and repeats the whole endovaginal scan, and soon leaves the room.

Maria is soon told she can go home and that Dr. Luong would be calling her. It's an uncomfortable night; worrying about the results, she hardly sleeps.

Early the next morning, Dr. Luong's office calls. "Now I have to go back and get a CAT scan today," Maria muses. "It's probably easier to go to the place nearby in Brooklyn. It's got to be easier than yesterday!"

INTRODUCTION

At first glance, this narrative seems only slightly germane to a discussion of quality in radiology. Nonetheless, let's take a look at it. Every organization thinks that it offers a quality product to their consumer. In the automobile industry, it may be a hot convertible; in Silicon Valley, the "latest and greatest" computer chip. For radiology, the product is somewhat more nebulous but still very much a product. Our product, in its simplest form, is the radiology report—but not just the report, rather the entire experience of the examination. The consumer in radiology is the patient, the doctor, the insurer, the employer who pays the insurer. Is it all of the above? Last, as the customer varies, do the relevant measures of quality vary or stay fixed? The analysis of these issues in Maria's story can serve as an instructive example of the

developments in the conceptualization of "quality" over time.

HOW QUALITY MANAGEMENT BEGAN

The formalized quest for quality is a relatively new innovation. Until recently, the search for quality has been a largely informal, self-initiated, and self-monitored process, with variable results. The transition to the modern concept of "quality management" arose, not out of a sense of altruism, but rather through competitive market forces.

By the end of World War II, the United States was in a position, by virtue of its size, wealth, location, and status as victor, to rule the world economically. The losers of the war were forced to compete, either by virtue of perceived superior workmanship (Germany) or superior price (Japan), for their smaller share of the market. To meet the challenge of American economic hegemony, Japan, in particular, decided that it needed to evolve from the cheapest provider, which would only last so long, to the highest-quality provider.

Quality management was introduced as a formalized concept by an American engineer, G. S. Radford, in 1922.[1] In the 1930s, a Bell Labs statistical engineer, W. A. Shewhart, began to concentrate on manufacturing errors by codifying the incidence of specific recurring errors so as to prevent their reoccurrence.[2] More significantly, Shewhart maintained that price without an understanding of quality is meaningless and that concentration on low price alone will lead to additional expense. During World War II, another statistician, W. Edwards Deming, began to develop expertise in "quality" issues, while working for the U.S. government to improve the efficiency, or "kill ratio," of war materials.[3]

The time, nonetheless, was not right for acceptance of quality management concepts. With its seemingly limitless future, American business largely rejected them as superfluous. Deming's "PDSA" cycle (discussed below) did not take hold until he traveled to Japan, where it was embraced enthusiastically. At the same time, an associate of Deming's, J. M. Juran,

BOX 15-1

Deming's "14 Steps"

1. Constancy of purpose
2. Adopt cooperation
3. Stop mass inspection
4. Stop concentrating on price alone
5. Constantly improve
6. Training
7. Multifaceted leadership
8. Fear out; trust in
9. Break down internal barriers and competition
10. No slogans
11. Manage by objectives
12. Remove barriers to joy at work
13. Education and self-improvement
14. Everyone is responsible

From Deming, W. Edwards, *Out of the Crisis,* pages 23–24, adapted; ©2000 W. Edwards Deming Institute, by permission of The MIT Press.

also in Japan with Bell Labs, was occupied translating Shewhart's innovations into a customer-centric approach to quality.[4,5] Their combined success in teaching and facilitating "statistical process control" in the realm of communications infrastructure soon spilled into other businesses in Japan, most notably automobile manufacturing. The resurgent Japanese economy began to adopt these concepts as the only means of evening the economic playing field.

Deming returned to the U.S., where his work went unnoticed until the publication of his book *Out of the Crisis* in 1982. In it he described a "system of profound knowledge" of how complex organizations work and introduced a plan of necessary steps—his "14 points"—for the transformation of American industry (Box 15-1).

Quality Control, Assurance, and Management

Three distinct and evolutionary concepts of quality management evolved over the next decades: quality control, quality assurance, and total quality management (Table 15-1). These will be discussed briefly here and will be elaborated on subsequently in the discussion of their applications in radiology.

In the first concept, quality control (QC), the mechanics of production are evaluated in an informal (i.e., usually internal) and sometimes sporadic manner with the aim of correcting errors (rather than preventing them, which

Table 15-1   Quality Initiatives, Comparison

	QC	QA	TQM
Object	Technical issues	Clinical issues only	All activities
Subject	Equipment	Individual focus	Each step of work process
Reviewers	Radiologist and chief technologist	External reviewer and radiologist	Internal team
Review style	Informal	Formal	Formal
Focus	Measurement outside range	Errors anticipated	Continuous optimization of process
Goal	Correction of errors	Prevention of errors	Stay ahead of customer expectations
Creates	Defensiveness	Defensiveness	Team spirit
Action	None	Correct error	Correct cause of error
Efficiency and effectiveness	Not covered	Not covered	Key issue

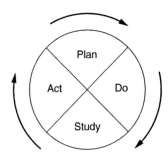

Figure 15-1 Shewhart cycle for learning and improvement. (From Deming, W. Edwards, *The New Economics for Industry, Government, Education,* second edition, Shewhart Cycle figure, page 132; ©2000 W. Edwards Deming Institute, by permission of The MIT Press.)

is a later development; see QA below).[3] Specific data measurement points were established for which ranges of acceptability were defined. Under QC, action is retrospective and is taken when a measurement falls outside a predefined range of acceptability. The only real innovation in this step is the quasi-formalization of the process of review and the use of statistical analysis.

The next step in the evolution of the quality cycle tackles the prevention of errors before they occur, rather than after. More comprehensive than QC, quality assurance (QA) is still retrospective but becomes more anticipatory in its prevention of errors, which is done by establishing a predetermined set of standards, the adoption of which will hopefully anticipate and prevent repetitive problems. The adherence to these standards is not just monitored internally, but also formally by external agents. In QA, standards are established first and the process of production is designed to fit those standards.

The third stage in the development of "quality" was revolutionary. Total quality management (TQM), the result of the innovations of Shewhart, Deming, and Juran, is the overarching philosophical (rather than merely operational) approach, whereby customers' expectations are not just met but continually exceeded. Deming's genius was the incorporation of multiple feedback loops throughout the entire process of manufacturing, Juran's the "discovery" of the consumer, and Shewhart's the introduction of a formalized set of guidelines for learning and improvement, known as the Shewhart cycle, or the PDSA cycle.[2] This cycle—Plan, Do, Study, Act

(Fig. 15-1)—has subsequently been expanded to the FOCUS-PDSA cycle—Find (a process to improve), Organize (to improve that process), Clarify (a current knowledge of the process), Understand (the sources of process variation), and Select (the process to improve).[6]

TQM as an overall philosophy is implemented by an operational approach known as continuous quality improvement (CQI). In TQM, each step in the making of a product is continually broken down, analyzed, and upgraded. Quality management, while monitored passively by outside agencies, is actively embraced by each member of an organization. Each individual is incorporated into the improvement process, so that there is universal "ownership" of responsibility. This emphasis on individual members each contributing to the team was born of necessity in impoverished postwar Japan. For example, sparse instruction manuals had to be shared by all members of the team, from the lowest paid worker to the highest manager.[5] CQI does not replace QC and QA but, rather, pushes them to a higher conceptual plane by focusing on the entire system, not just the end product. Problems are predicted and anticipated, not just corrected. The organization and all of its members become pro-active rather than re-active. Process, rather than product, becomes the key determinant in this dynamic approach.

QUALITY INITIATIVES IN MEDICINE

In the 1970s, there were forays into bringing the tools of "quality" to the practice of medicine. For example, in 1975, the Joint Commission of Accreditation of Healthcare Organizations (JCAHO), issued a 10-step monitoring and evaluation program of professional services standards called the 10-Step Quality Assurance Process (Box 15-2).[7]

Under these standards, steps taken to assure quality of care were to be documented and supplied to JCAHO on demand. This initial experiment in QC was voluntary—it was not under market pressures and was largely unmonitored—and so, as one might expect, it soon failed. (There was no financial penalty for not taking the program seriously.)

BOX 15-2

JCAHO 10-Step Quality Assurance Process

1. Assign responsibility for monitoring and evaluation activities.
2. Delineate the scope of care.
3. Identify the most important aspects of care.
4. Identify indicators for monitoring.
5. Establish thresholds for the indicators that trigger evaluation.
6. Collect and organize data for each indicator.
7. Evaluate care when thresholds are reached to identify opportunities to improve care.
8. Take action to improve care.
9. Assess effectiveness of the action.
10. Communicate results.

The concept of quality management was introduced into health care by Berwick and Laffel in seminal papers published in 1989.[8,9] Their basic points were that (1) the traditional medical quality paradigm of performance measured against standards with subsequent modification of outliers would not allow health care organizations to operate in a manner commensurate with that used by industry, and (2) these quality principles and techniques used by industry would have to be adopted by medicine.

In 1991, the JCAHO presented a new program that was quality management–focused and was more ambitious and comprehensive than the previous programs.[10,11] The JCAHO's *Principles of Organization and Management Effectiveness*[11] mirrored the then-evolving concepts of TQM, namely:

It is important to have the commitment and direct involvement of both clinical and management leadership.

- "Quality" must be defined for the organization and this definition communicated to its members.
- Key processes and systems should be examined scientifically and continuously improved.
- Information gathering, specifically customer satisfaction, should be identified as a key priority.
- Education, employee empowerment, and teamwork should be intrinsic to the improvement process.

This JCAHO initiative gradually evolved, over the next decade, into the National Committee for Quality Assurance (NCQA). In its 2005 publication, "The State of Health Care Quality," the NCQA introduced the concept of pay-for-performance incentivization of physicians: "Why should we pay the same amount—or worse, pay *more*—for low-quality care than we do for the nation's best? Paying for performance just makes sense."[12] In their conclusions, the NCQA recommended the following:

- Measurement and public reporting do indeed work to enhance quality.
- Payment for physicians, institutions, and health plans should be tied to quality and thus rewarded.
- Consumers should be supplied information.[12]

The early areas of adoption of quality management techniques were largely confined to administrative areas: specifically, scheduling, billing, report turnaround times, and patient records.[13] With increasing demands of the payers (insurers) as impetus, attention over the last decade has shifted to more critical-to-care issues, such as quality of care, appropriateness of procedures, and patient safety, specifically drug therapy.[14]

The impetus for change, however, has not been merely external. Internal inefficiencies also decrease revenue. According to the Juran Institute, "the costs of poor quality (COPQ) are the costs of unplanned, unnecessary waste. Studies have shown costs of poor quality to run as high as 15 to 29% of sales revenue, an extraordinary sum of money lost. The total cost of poor quality in the United States health care system is 30% of the $1.3 trillion spent annually on health care."[15]

Quality Initiatives in Radiology

Radiology has substantially lagged behind the other fields of medicine, primarily because of its immunity to the financial pressures of primary care in the face of the seemingly ever-expanding future provided by burgeoning technology. Let us review the three stages of quality management as they have been adopted in radiology (see Table 15-1).

Quality Control (QC)

Quality control (QC), while informal and self-regulated, has been a part of radiology from its inception. A look at follow-up conferences in academic and nonacademic practices from the 1950s until now provides some clues. These meetings generally concern clinical issues only, are self-monitored, and are accompanied by a fair amount of defensiveness, naturally. Other than embarrassment there have been few motivators for preventing errors. A few conscientious persons might try to figure out where and when they made an error in judgment. For example, you're asked at a follow-up conference to determine whether an error is a minor or major discrepancy. Needless to say, if I were to monitor my own errors, I could always find an excuse to make my discrepancy minor. (As early as 1992, the JCAHO began evaluating radiology practices in earnest and deemed that informal interdepartmental review was no longer acceptable. "JCAHO [was] interested in real peer review with opportunities for education and improvement."[11])

To a large degree, institutionalized QC in radiology has meant monitoring imaging techniques and radiation exposure (usually an annoying afterthought, taken care of internally by the chief technologist).[16,17] Imaging equipment has been tested for years on a periodic basis to ensure conformity to regulations. Reparative steps are performed only when and if these data points fall outside of the prescribed limits.[18] Examples include analysis of film quality, including technical factors such as development chemicals, pH, contrast, artifacts, and verification of adequate radiation safety (including room and building shielding). Even an admirable effort made by the American College of Radiology (ACR) Program for Site Accreditation for MRI is not quite up to snuff: although its QC program emphasizes machinery calibration, safety, and standardization of exams, there is to date virtually no analysis of professional capability (Table 15-2).

Quality Assurance (QA)

There has been some transition from QC to QA (quality assurance, also referred to as "conformance quality"). The evolution of breast imaging is a good example of this migration. Up until the early 1990s, quality in breast imaging meant a shockingly informal—at least by today's standards—approach to accuracy, patient notification, and image optimization. With the onset of the Mammography Quality Standards Act (MQSA), the approach to accuracy has become a more serious endeavor with real and formalized plans of improvement. Patient notification is no longer informal and is legislated. The correction of errors in the mammographic image, its interpretation, and patient notification become less important than the prevention of errors in these areas (Table 15-3).

Table 15-2 Quality Control in Radiology

Object	Technical issues
Subject	Equipment
Reviewers	Radiologist and chief technologist
Review style	Informal
Focus	Measurement outside range
Goal	Correction of errors
Creates	Defensiveness
Action	None
Efficiency and effectiveness	Not covered

Table 15-3 Quality Assurance in Radiology

Object	Clinical issues only
Subject	Individual focus
Reviewers	External reviewer and radiologist
Review style	Formal
Focus	Errors anticipated
Goal	Prevention of errors
Creates	Defensiveness
Action	Correct error
Efficiency and effectiveness	Not covered

Total Quality Management (TQM)

The shifts from QC and QA to total quality management (TQM) in radiology have been both internally (the ACR, individual practices) and externally (JCAHO) driven. Economic necessity, as in postwar Japan, has been the real driving force behind these shifts. During the 1990s, with an increase in the number of insurers in certain U.S. markets, came greater competition for employers' business. The insurers were forced to compete with each other regarding quality of services, and not only just concerning their *own* services—such as ease of use and number of services provided—but also those of their member providers (us). We (i.e., the providers) were judged on the basis of availability, timeliness, customer satisfaction, and "quality." What had heretofore been a nebulous topic, "quality" was now an issue that demanded our attention. Specifically, in radiology, "quality" has come to mean exam appropriateness criteria, surgical and pathological confirmation of results, timeliness of scheduling and reporting (including notification of important results or discrepancies), and film repeat rates. In successful practices, quality of care has emerged as a leading factor in competition for payers' dollars.

As noted previously, TQM attempts to look at every step in the manufacture of the organization's "product"—in the case of radiology, the radiology report—by encouraging members from every part of the organization (radiologist, technologist, secretary, front desk) to exceed the customer's (i.e., patient, insurer, employer) expectations. To empower each of its members, the radiology practice looks beyond the individual radiologist, technologist, or worker (as just a scapegoat for failure) and to the intrinsic *institutional* causes of an individual's poor performance. The democratization of the process makes seemingly equal players, if not partners, of the radiologist and front desk person. This may sound like a fantasy, but for TQM to work, the inevitable social barriers that develop between the "boss" and the "employee" must be broken down. In theory, at least, the technologist, for example, freed from the "big brother" mentality of the radiology factory, takes ownership of the entire process of TQM

and the end product. (Paradoxically, after World War II, Japan benefited from a ruined economy, which minimized wage differences between entry-level employees and CEOs. However, this took place in a country in which the *social* unit, rather than the *individual*, was paramount.) The underlying assumption, rather than an altruistic or political fantasy, is pragmatic—that is, increased efficiency equals increased quality—which equals increased customer satisfaction (purchasing), which leads to increased profit.[19] Although the social structure in the United States is quite different from that of Japan, the demands for TQM are the same. And so too in the radiology practice (Table 15-4).

In the evolution of TQM, the ACR, in 2005, formally defined quality of care as "the degree to which health services for individuals and populations increase the likelihood of desired health outcomes and are consistent with current professional knowledge."[3] This was a crucial shift, which had started with just technical factors (QC), then moved from interpretative accuracy (QA) finally to outcomes measurement (TQM).

"Specifically, with regard to diagnostic imaging and image-guided treatment, quality is the extent to which the right procedure is done the right way, at the right time, and the correct interpretation is accurately and quickly

Table 15-4 Total Quality Management in Radiology	
Object	All activities
Subject	Each step of work process
Reviewers	Internal team
Review style	Formal
Focus	Continuous optimization with process
Goal	Stay ahead of customer expectations
Creates	Team spirit
Action	Correct cause of error
Efficiency and effectiveness	Key issue

communicated to the patient and the referring clinician."[3]

Remember Maria? All the things that we did wrong!

"The goals are to maximize the likelihood of desired health outcomes and to satisfy the patient."[3,20]

Here it is, at last: "... to satisfy the patient." After one hundred years of radiology, we have finally arrived, formally, at this rather obvious point.

Accurate diagnostic information is to be gathered at the lowest risk of exposure (dose, contrast, danger) at a minimal but realistic cost. The quality product becomes not just an accurate report but rather the answer to the clinician's problem, given in a timely fashion and in a manner that satisfies the patient.

Continuous Quality Management

With the concept of customer-centric outcomes measurement, continuous quality managment (CQM) in radiology had begun in earnest.[21-24] The consumer's expectations are not only to be met but exceeded.[25] However, Deming noted several common impediments to progress, which he called the "7 Deadly Diseases"[7] (Box 15-3).

These seven points are essential to keep in mind in the pursuit of exceeding customers' expectations. CQM, in radiology as elsewhere, requires commitment, both financial and manpower, and is not a short-term solution. It may require 6 to 12 months to get staff knowledgeable enough to begin training them, then 6 to 12 months to complete the first stage of training, and up to a decade for implementation.[7]

BOX 15-3

Deming's "7 Deadly Diseases"

1. Lack of constancy of purpose
2. Short-term profits and thinking
3. Performance merit rating
4. Management mobility
5. Use of known figures only
6. Excessive medical costs
7. Excessive liability costs

From Deming, W. Edwards, *Out of the Crisis*, pages 97–98, adapted; ©2000 W. Edwards Deming Institute, by permission of The MIT Press.

Conventional organization behavior, such as performance rating and fixed roles within organizational management, must be jettisoned. This point, performance merit rating (which is Deming's third "deadly disease") is of utmost importance but is also a bit counterintuitive because CQM does not benefit from a supervisor providing a performance appraisal. The rationale is that such a performance appraisal will shift the employee's focus to pleasing his or her boss, rather than the customer. Finally, CQM initiatives are not yet universally successful. The main reason for failure is the lack of proper training. Other reasons include insufficient incentivization or recognition, lack of urgency, or absence of a champion for the project. It is invariably a slow process.

Summary of QC, QA, and TQM

Remember Maria's arrival at our office on First Avenue? Where did we go wrong? To find the most glaring transgression, you don't need to look any further than the issue of social rudeness, or ineptitude, as Maria wasn't even given the common courtesy of an introduction. More than anything, this conveys the all-too-real feeling that she is looked on as a commodity. It is bad enough that Maria is forced to wait, even longer than at her own doctor's office, but, more egregiously, her preparatory directions were confused and, in reality, incorrect. She was given little explanation why her initial request was wrong, why an endovaginal scan was needed and performed, and what the result of her exam was. The radiologist came and went with an air of indifference.

Through the use of QC, we would have perhaps analyzed the radiologist's interpretation, which would have been top rate, done in a great department. With QA, in this instance, we would have analyzed the technical quality of the ultrasound machine, also top rate. But with TQM we would have looked at the whole unfortunate interaction, analyzed it, and determined how to prevent it from ever happening again (Table 15-5).

In effect, TQM is the only approach that illuminates the obvious. The *total* experience was anything but top rate. NYU's FPO (Faculty Practice Office) Radiology, with its CQI (continuous quality improvement, another term for

Table 15-5 QA, QC, TQM, and Maria Gonzalez

	QC	QA	TQM
Review	Chief of staff	QA nurse	TQM team
Subject	Reprimand of tech	Review of results of ultrasound	Each step of Maria's experience
Object	Correction of "rude" interaction	Ultrasound accuracy	Make Maria's (and all patients') interactions pleasant, efficient
Action	If Maria complains	QA "event"	Plan to make techs part of "team," take more personal responsibility

TQM) team, would confront its deficiencies by analyzing all the major activities in the imaging center, including scheduling, the patient visit itself, the examination, the interpretation, and the transmittal of results. The team would not "blame" the scheduler, the technologist, or even the radiologist, but would instead look internally and determine the philosophical and procedural defects that guaranteed this bad result.

According to G. E. Hanks, these points in the experience concern structure, process, outcome, and functionality.[26] Every activity in the imaging facility would be identified, not just those that failed in Maria's case. Standards would be analyzed and then established by representatives of the entire team, with an emphasis on customer needs, in a process that would allow for continuous improvement. Proactively, CQI would not only identify the problems but also would anticipate them, and in doing so would improve the entire system.[27] This process comprises several steps, according to the PDSA cycle (Fig. 15-2).

THE PDSA CYCLE

In the **PLAN** stage of TQM, the quality team is established. Ideally, the team should be comprised of a small number of people representing every process of production, with complementary skills and a common purpose.

In the **DO** stage, the specific issues are identified. Goals are defined, operating procedures are established, information is shared, and specialized/technical information is provided. According to Juran, quality goals must be specifically worded such that their achievement can be measured.[4] Vague statements such as "No patient will leave the center dissatisfied" or "We strive for quality" are meaningless.

A major innovation in CQI in this phase is the use of scientific and statistical methods to identify intrinsic systemic flaws, rather than mere periodic examination of the end product and subsequent repair of defects. These scientific methods include the use of flowcharts, cause-and-effect diagrams, Pareto charts, fishbone charts, and multivoting.

Flowcharts isolate the steps in a process to identify the "weak link." The Pareto chart, a histogram that displays the decreasing order of frequency of causes of errors or missteps, helps identify which issues need to be dealt with first (Fig. 15-3). The Pareto "principle" states that whenever there are multiple causes of a problem in quality, just a few of those causes account for the majority of the problem, hence the adage that 80% of problems are attributable to 20% of the employees.[7] A conventional histogram is a bar chart that represents the frequency of causes of errors without a specific order (Fig. 15-4), and a fishbone chart is a multifactorial diagram that can evaluate multiple causes of a problem (Fig. 15-5).

The **STUDY** phase is made up of the statistical evaluation of the data collected, the identification of the problem, and the generation of alternatives.

In the final, or **DO** phase, group solutions are posited, and the revision to the plan (the "change") is implemented.

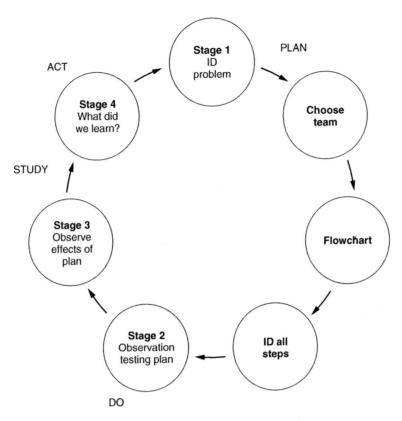

Figure 15-2 Flowchart for imaging center issues.

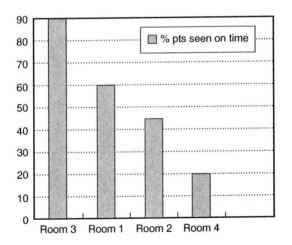

Figure 15-3 Pareto chart.

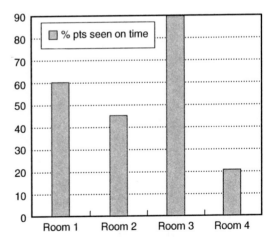

Figure 15-4 Conventional histogram.

CQI AT NYU RADIOLOGY

The first step in the development of a quality program at NYU was the articulation of a vision. Quite simply, we decided that we wanted our FPO to be the best radiology practice in the world and, if not the entire world, at least New York. This was not a flippant decision. Each radiologist, technologist, administrator, and secretary would start her or his day with this first thought: "Will what I do today, with this specific patient, that will enable us to be the best practice in the world?"

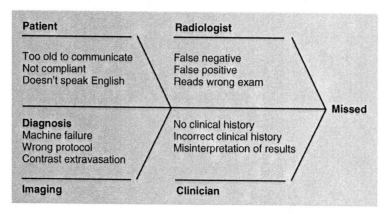

Figure 15-5 Fishbone chart.

It is not an insignificant thought. For each of us, there is a responsibility not only to each other but to the whole enterprise. With this sense of empowerment comes a profound sense of duty: for example, I have a 12 o'clock meeting in one minute. Do I read this seemingly insignificant stat chest x-ray, which will take five minutes, and be a little late or do I hope they can get someone else to read it instead?

Naturally, the success or failure of FPO radiology rests on this sense of responsibility. We are all responsible for knowing and implementing the vision, mission, and principles of the organization. Our *vision statement* describes our desired future, how we wish others to view the organization, and defines an appropriate target. Our *mission statement* is the concrete definition of the product, the scope of each individual's responsibility, and our goals toward optimal efficiency.

Step 1 (PLAN)—The Team

Before embarking on the implementation of a Total Quality Improvement (TQI) Program at Faculty Practice Radiology, a team had to be established. The team comprises representative members of all branches of the office: radiologist, management, front desk, secretarial staff, patient ombudsman, CT technologist, general technologist, ultrasound technologist, business office, housekeeping. The leader is not the highest-ranking member of the team but rather the person most suited to motivate the team toward its final goal or mission.

As noted by Weinreb, several factors must be kept in mind when forming this team.[28] The number of members should not be unwieldy, perhaps no more than 10 to 12 people. Failure or struggle by the team or by its individual members is a good thing, and should not be discouraged. Communication and flexibility are paramount for all members.

Step 2 (DO)—The Cause of Suboptimal Performance Identified

After the establishment of a mission statement and the "quality" team, the customer must be identified. In manufacturing, this is easy: the customer is the consumer. However, in radiology, there are multiple layers of customers: the patient (Maria), the referring clinician (Dr. Luong), the insurer (the payer), and the employer (in Maria's case, the City of New York). All have different needs; some are internal and some external customers. "Internal customers ... are the beneficiaries of [the] departments' tasks and activities [specifically Maria]. External customers are those entities ... outside the organization who receive services and/or provide revenue."[29] A major issue to be recognized is the conflicting needs of the internal (Maria) and external customers (the insurer), best exemplified in the registration process. Maria would like to get through the registration process as quickly and as painlessly as possible. The painlessness of the patient's experience can be antithetical to the billing, utilization, and quality needs of the radiologist, the insurer, and the payer.

Step 3 (STUDY/CHECK)—Systematic Collection and Analysis of Data

Once the mission has been established, the customer has been identified, and the CQI team has been chosen, the component steps in the customer experience can be identified and analyzed. The team will then identify the process issues that need to be addressed by a process of multivoting and rank ordering. In multivoting, each member of the team votes on which one third of the total ideas or events are the most important; in rank ordering, these ideas or events are ranked in order of importance, with "1" being the lowest rank. The issues with the highest component are addressed. At NYU, these processes have been (and are) evaluated on an ongoing basis by the quality committee, using a Radiology Report Card (Box 15-4).

Once again, let us return to Maria and her less-than-ideal experience at our office.

BOX 15-4

NYU Radiology QA/QI Report Card

Group 1: (vs. National Benchmark)

- Percent of studies dictated within 24 hours of study completion
- Percent of unreported studies (completed and never dictated)
- CECT extravasation and contrast material reaction rates
- Post-chest CT biopsy PTX rate
- Percent of randomly audited studies with major variance identified (Section QA tracker initiative)
- Percent of MR/CT studies that need to be repeated because of poor quality of initial exams; measure percent of incomplete studies
- Physician recall rate for diagnostic screening mammography
- Technical repeat rate for screening mammography
- Breast procedure complication rates incidence of post-neuron interventional procedure neurologic events
- Incidence of post IR or NIR procedure hemorrhage requiring patient transfusion or transfer to monitored setting
- Pediatric CT dosage compliance
- Misadministration rate of radiopharmaceuticals

Group 2: Measure

- Patient satisfaction
- Percent of resident and/or ED reports with major variance
- Percent of successful amniocentesis

Group 3: Measure

- Bellevue Hospital ED resident major variance
- Percent of incorrectly interpreted CT PE exams
- Percent of reports containing dictation typos and mistakes
- Percent of reports not containing appropriate measurements or comparison to priors
- Percent of studies ordered inappropriately
- Wait times (OB ultrasound, mammography)
- Percent of resident ultrasound reports with major variances
- Repeat examination rate
- Number of sentinel events
- Percent of cases where "time out" procedure not recorded in medical record
- Reports with inappropriate content (indications, procedure, findings, impression)
- Usage of macro templates in reports

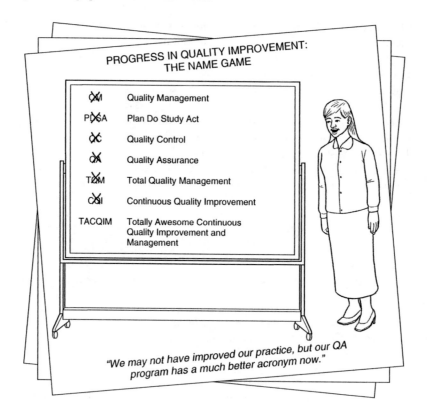

PROGRESS IN QUALITY IMPROVEMENT:
THE NAME GAME

QM — Quality Management
PDSA — Plan Do Study Act
QC — Quality Control
QA — Quality Assurance
TQM — Total Quality Management
CQI — Continuous Quality Improvement
TACQIM — Totally Awesome Continuous Quality Improvement and Management

"We may not have improved our practice, but our QA program has a much better acronym now."

It is not the individual mishaps that are important for us in Maria's case. What the team first needs to do is to conceptualize what would have been her ideal experience, simply and then in detail. By analyzing Maria's story, as she navigates her way through our system, we can anticipate the myriad of problem issues that could arise and take proactive steps to prevent them from happening, well before they occur.

Swensen and Johnson trace such a theoretical patient path through the diagnostic imaging process in their Radiology Quality Map (Fig. 15-6). Several key interaction points are identified in Swensen and Johnson's schema, which I would like to characterize as "opportunities" that either disappoint the patient or, more constructively, of course, delight the patient (Fig. 15-7). It is instructive here to examine the opportunities for excellence by following Maria's experience.

Opportunity 1: Study Ordered

Maria Gonzalez, a third-year student at the NYU School of Law, is older than most of the other students in her class.... It's been tough to pick up the pieces; she's just begun to date again.

Maria, although fictitious, has a real and complex life. She is more than just a "case," or a "consumer." Just as important as our vision statement is the realization that every patient that we see is a complex, scared, sometimes impatient, sometimes confused person, who has come to see us for an answer to a problem. You don't go to the radiologist on a lark; you go because there's a problem that you're nervous about. This sense of anxiety is present in all patients, no matter how placid they appear on the surface. If we're going to make NYU Radiology the best practice in the world, we have to be mindful that Maria, and all our patients, might be visiting us feeling scared, or even with a sense of dread, and rightfully so, considering the number of horrible things we see.

As she returns to the front desk, the office staff schedules an abdominal ultrasound at the NYU Faculty Practice Radiology for the next morning.

The first step in Maria's journey is the ordering of the exam by the office staff. Remember, in almost all instances, it is the staff and not the physician who orders the study. They can't always be expected to know exactly the right

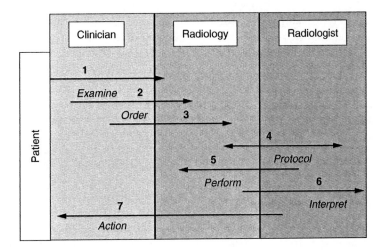

Figure 15-6   Patient pathway.

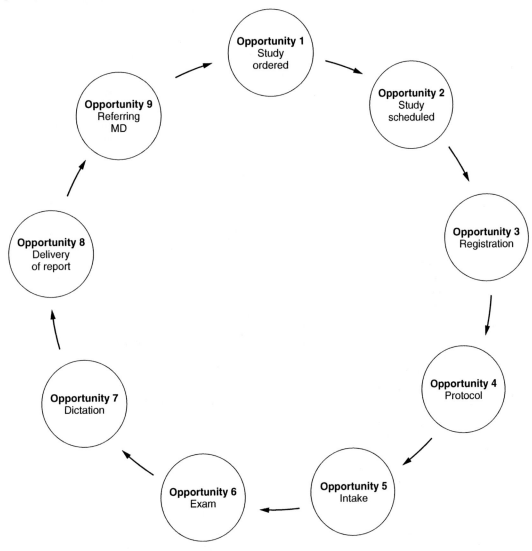

Figure 15-7   NYU "Opportunity to Excel" map.

study to order and the rationale for the study. Even the physician won't know the intricacies of changing radiology procedures. So some guidance is needed.

Hsi Li Han, a 45-year-old, high-powered Manhattan lawyer, is scheduled for a CT scan of the chest at FPO Radiology to evaluate chest pain. The scan is performed uneventfully. After the scan, as the radiologist reviews the results with him, he asks, "What about my coronary arteries?" The radiologist then looks at the patient's prescription, which requests a coronary artery CTA. "Hmmm.... How do I fix this mess?"

In this case, I was the radiologist. With a program of QC or QA, we would file an incident report, documenting who was at fault in this miscommunication. A formal reprimand would be issued with the hope that this would prevent such errors in the future. In TQM, conversely, we would sit down as a team, try to find where the system went wrong, and decide that perhaps an e-based order entry system might better assure that the clinician's requests will be carried out.

The ACR has "Appropriateness Criteria," a set of guidelines developed by radiologists to aid physicians looking for answers to specific clinical problems.[30] There are substantive issues with these criteria, however. On a concrete level, they don't take into account the severity of the patient's clinical status or the timeliness required in addressing the specific clinical issue. On a more abstract level, the criteria have been developed by radiologists themselves for other physicians who are the users.[31] (Unfortunately, these criteria have been developed in enough of a vacuum that these "other physicians," for whom these criteria would be important, haven't really been notified of their existence.)

The only way to implement such criteria, then, is to make them an integral part of the ordering process itself. Up-to-date radiology information systems (RIS) have just begun to make inroads into this area but to date, in most places, this is still a dream. Physician order entry (POE) systems are being implemented to guide the scheduling process to the appropriate examination electronically. This is also a useful first step (see Chapter 13, "Information Technology Systems" for more information on this subject).

There are innovative examples throughout the country. An interesting approach to the ordering process has been put into practice at the Massachusetts General Hospital in its radiology order entry (ROE) system.[32] This is similar to a proposed NYU e-ordering system that has not yet been implemented.

A system of homegrown appropriateness criteria has been incorporated into the ordering process itself, helping the clinician determine the best way to answer the specific clinical question. This process does not offer a series of billable histories for a specific test, which could be of questionable legality. Rather, it starts with the clinical dilemma and guides the clinician to the appropriate study. Just as important, the system, by design, is not punitive or overarching, but helpful. For example, if there is a special circumstance, the clinician can, in effect, bypass the system or ask for assistance.

At the NYU Faculty Practice, we have not yet been so innovative. A more rudimentary, albeit effective, system has evolved. CT and MRI examinations at NYU are tailored to very specific indications, in effect forcing clinicians to provide a detailed history to schedule particular examinations. Every afternoon, the next day's requests are previewed and modified to the tailored exams by radiology house officers. In this manner, questionable indications can be referred back to the chief technologists, who can make more complete inquiries. After intake, on the day of the examination, the patient is given a detailed form to complete and is interviewed by the CT team, while the patient is being prepared for the scan. While three and four layers of safeguarding have been incorporated into the system to ascertain that the correct study is performed, none of the individual steps are particularly burdensome to the patient.

Opportunity 2: Study Scheduled

Ordering and scheduling is usually a single process. Scheduling is composed of several factors: the exact time and location of the examination, patient preparation, basic insurance information, directions to the office, and the answering of specific questions.

In its publication To Err Is Human, the Institute in Medicine discusses the factors that lead to patient error and establishes a set of five principles, which can be usefully applied to the design of safe health care, whether in a small group practice, a hospital, or a large health care system[33] (Box 15-5).

One of these principles is the timeliness of delivery of care. Enough flexible time must be built into the schedule to accommodate emergencies. Other indications, however, are quasi-emergencies, such as the screening mammography callback patient, who needs to be seen in a timely fashion. A screening program should not be contemplated without the assurance that these patients can be scheduled for follow-up studies within a week's time.

In an attempt to speed up the scheduling process, an open e-book format or "patient portal" can be instituted, whereby the referring office or patient may be able to book a time slot, to be subsequently reviewed by the scheduling department.

After about five minutes, the technologist comes back to tell her that her doctor has decided that a pelvic ultrasound, rather than an abdominal ultrasound, would be better suited to her condition. "Ok, whatever they think is right. What's the difference? But now I have to drink water? Oh brother, I'm really going to be late."

BOX 15-5

Institute in Medicine Principles for the Design of Safe Health Care

Principle 1. Provide Leadership

- Make patient safety a priority corporate objective.
- Make patient safety everyone's responsibility.
- Make clear assignments for and expectation of safety oversight.
- Provide human and financial resources for error analysis and systems redesign.
- Develop effective mechanisms for identifying and dealing with unsafe practitioners.

Principle 2. Respect Human Limits in Process Design

- Design jobs for safety.
- Avoid reliance on memory.
- Use constraints and forcing functions.
- Avoid reliance on vigilance.
- Simplify key processes.
- Standardize work processes.

Principle 3. Promote Effective Team Functioning

- Train in teams those who are expected to work in teams.
- Include the patient in safety design and the process of care.

Principle 4. Anticipate the Unexpected

- Adopt a proactive approach: Examine processes of care for threats to safety and redesign them before accidents occur.
- Design for recovery.
- Improve access to accurate, timely information.

Principle 5. Create a Learning Environment

- Use simulations whenever possible.
- Encourage reporting of errors and hazardous conditions.
- Ensure no reprisals for reporting of errors.
- Develop a working culture in which communication flows freely regardless of authority gradient.
- Implement mechanisms of feedback and learning from error.

Patient preparation, as in Maria's case, can become a real embarrassment. Certainly, detailed instructions are needed at registration, but also directions to download instructions, if available to the patient, have proven to be quite effective. Referring patients to patient preparation documents on a website may be useful, especially for the more tech-savvy consumers of the 21st century, but not all patients have easy access to computers. (All website documents for patients should be geared to a high elementary/middle school educational level to effect maximal compliance.)

Opportunity 3: Registration

Maria arrives at the radiology office on First Avenue at 9:00 AM for her 9:15 scheduled examination, waits in a line of 10 people, and is shown into ultrasound at 9:30. "Not as fast as yesterday," she thinks. She's beginning to get nervous, worrying that she shouldn't have kept that appointment with her adviser downtown at 11:00.

Registration lines have been the major impediment to patient satisfaction.

E-registration is a concept that has been successfully adopted at several medical offices at NYU Medical Center. This program is being planned at the present time for FPO Radiology. E-registration lets the patient choose the time and location for a study, gives directions and appropriate instructions, and allows for entering insurance information. The motivation for e-registration is being built into the real-time registration process itself. Rather than having these patients stand in the same intake lines as the other patients in the waiting room, e-registrants will be fast-tracked to the correct clinical area. This process also helps ensure HIPAA compliance by helping to keep patient scheduling information confidential.

Genevieve Briarly, the wife of a trustee of New York University, has flown into New York from her home in Palm Beach to have a CT scan of the chest to evaluate a questionable pulmonary nodule, which was seen on a virtual colonoscopy performed in Florida. She is, as everyone in the city knows, a charmer who never expects special treatment, even though she and her husband are major donors to the medical school. She steps off the second-floor elevator and is immediately greeted by the pandemonium

of FPO registration. After a couple of minutes waiting on line, she decides to leave. Somewhat out of character, she grumbles to her assistant, "I thought they had arranged everything for me!"

For all registrants, whether e-registrants, real-time registrants, or walk-ins, a "patient representative" or "schmoozer" system has been implemented. The most outgoing member of our registration staff has been freed of all responsibilities other than meeting and greeting. She meets people as they walk off the elevator into a long corridor, which, because of its design, looks confusing and formidable. She guides people to the appropriate line in registration. She saunters up and down the waiting corridor, talking to everyone, joking, playing with kids. She is equally at home talking about the most mundane things with patients, as well as the fear or confusion they feel, while waiting for their studies. If there is a potential mix-up in ordering or some other problem, she will go "backstage" to see if the radiologist can solve the problem. If the patient is waiting too long, she will, in a very gentle way, move things along. In every outpatient office I have been associated with, this has been the most effective waiting area/registration improvement we have implemented. The patient has an ombudsman, a friend, in the department. They don't feel like a complete stranger.

Opportunity 4: Protocol

A series of detailed standardized protocols, which are established by each section, are tailored to particular, organ-specific clinical indications. This "best practice" approach to standardization of examinations is reviewed weekly in conferences and meetings.[34] Failure to establish and follow standardized protocols will cause difficulty in patient follow-up. (Adherence to standardized protocols is a key feature in ACR accreditation.)

Opportunity 5: Intake

A ... woman ... greets Maria at the door of the ultrasound department. On the way to the exam room, they talk about why Maria is here for the exam. Maria explains that her pain has moved to the left side of her abdomen, but is somewhat lower than yesterday. The tech disappears to talk to the radiologist. Maria begins to think how strange it is that the woman never bothered to introduce herself.

As noted above, intake offers an appropriate time to establish that the correct study is being performed and to determine whether there are any contraindications or significant dangers of the study. This is the first real one-on-one social interaction, the "make-or-break" site of the patient's experience. The patient can tell very quickly whether the people in the office really care about her or regard her as "just a patient, a case, a body." Especially in the situations of patients who, because of specific illnesses, are frequent visitors, this one-on-one time can afford the opportunity to ask whether the patient would like to speak to the radiologist concerning the results of the exam. In our practice, more than 90% of the offhand comments on the patient satisfaction questionnaire are based on this interaction.

Opportunity 6: The Exam

The pelvic ultrasound is done but she is told that an endovaginal scan is necessary. . . . The technologist performs the exam more quickly than Maria had anticipated, exits to speak to the doctor, who . . . comes into the room and repeats the whole endovaginal scan, and soon leaves the room.

The issues of CQI during the examination are largely the issues encompassed in the ACR accreditation standards. For example, in CT, they include:

- Specific examination reviews
- Examination identification and labeling
- Documentation of clinical protocols
- Physicist survey and phantom images

Opportunity 7: Dictation

I get a note in my mailbox from Dr. Giovanetti, complaining that she had sent her patient Mrs. D'Elia to FPO to follow up on a mass seen in the liver on a prior CT scan. Somehow, I made no comparison to the previous examination!

Not an unreasonable report at first glance. However, let us examine it for a moment. We never answered the clinician's question (Box 15-6A and B).

In QC or QA, it's my error, I'm embarrassed, defensive. In CQI, however, the questions are, "Why did I not see the old films? Was it that the patient had two separate accession numbers, making the old studies 'invisible'? Was I rushed by having to read a series of stat chest X-rays that morning? Was there no notification of old studies by the technologist?" The team will need to look at all of these factors and figure out a way to remedy them, rather than simply blaming me, the technologist, or the IT department for our roles in this error.

The radiology report, as a legal and medical document, should stand independent of the individual interpreting radiologist.[35] Standardization of reports has been one of the most contentious issues in the practice. Reporting styles are a mirror of a radiologist's training and experience, combining local culture, prior mentoring, previous mistakes, and his or her own individual way of thinking. In its systematic approach, standardization can reduce variation and liability risk and may significantly reduce misunderstanding on the part of the clinician.[36] As advocated by several authors,[34,37] a proposed format for the radiology report copies the format used in reports in scientific journals (Table 15-6).

This format is familiar in style to most physicians' reports and follows the general outline recommended by the ACR.[38] Wilcox also offers several grammatical suggestions for reporting, which are quite useful.[34] They include the following:

1. Keep the intended reader in mind . . . the referring physician, patient, lawyer.
2. Use the active rather than passive voice (makes you sound more sure of yourself).
3. Separate ideas by paragraphs (easier to read).
4. Use complete sentences and definite or indefinite articles.
5. The impression should not be longer than the findings.
6. Number and rank by importance the conclusions.
7. *Never* say "Clinical correlation is recommended." (Say what you mean. Do you think they're not going to correlate clinically?)

Rather than propose a single standard of reporting, it may be helpful to establish guidelines for reporting, as noted below (Box 15-7).[38a]

BOX 15-6

A. Clinician's Nightmare Report

CT ABDOMEN AND PELVIS

CLINICAL INDICATION: Carcinoma of the breast
Axial CT of the abdomen and pelvis was performed from the level of the diaphragm to the symphysis pubis, using 4 mm nonoverlapping sections.

PERTINENT FINDINGS:
A single 3 mm left axillary lymph node is seen. The patient has had a previous left mastectomy. A 0.9 by 0.5 cm right pretracheal node is seen, as is a 4 mm subcarinal node. Subpleural parenchymal scarring is noted anterior on the left, felt to be related to prior radiation.
A 2 mm low-density mass is seen in segment 7 of the liver, which is too small to characterize. There is a high-density area of sclerosis seen in the body of T12, which may represent a bone island and is unchanged from prior examinations. There are several pulmonary nodules. A 2 mm nodule is seen in the right upper lobe, which is unchanged from the examination of November 2005. Three small nodules, measuring 1, 2, and 2 mm are seen in the lingula. Calcification is seen in the right coronary artery. A cluster of small nodules with a "tree-in-bud" configuration is seen in the right middle lobe, consistent with infectious bronchiolitis, unchanged from the previous exam.

IMPRESSION:
1. Four small pulmonary nodules are seen, which are unchanged since November 2005. Further CT follow-up recommended to establish stability.
2. Too small to characterize liver mass. Recommend MRI for further evaluation.
3. Probable bone island T12. Recommend bone scan.
4. Coronary artery calcification.
5. Infectious bronchiolitis right middle lobe.

B. Clinician's Nightmare Report

CT ABDOMEN AND PELVIS

CLINICAL INDICATION: Carcinoma of the breast

Axial CT of the abdomen and pelvis was performed from the level of the diaphragm to the symphysis pubis, using 4 mm nonoverlapping sections. [NO MENTION OF CONTRAST . . . PROBLEM WITH BILLING!!!]

[NO MENTION OLD FILMS COMPARED!!!]

PERTINENT FINDINGS:

[ALL ONE PARAGRAPH . . . HARD TO READ . . . IMPORTANT FINDINGS MIXED IN RANDOMLY WITH OTHER NONIMPORTANT FINDINGS!!!]
A single 3 mm left axillary lymph node is seen. [PLEASE!!! IS THIS IMPORTANT???] The patient has had a previous left mastectomy. A 0.9 by 0.5 cm right pretracheal node is seen, as is a 4 mm subcarinal node. Subpleural parenchymal scarring is noted anterior on the left, felt to be related to prior radiation. A 2 mm low-density mass is seen in segment 7 of the liver, which is too small to characterize. [THIS WAS EVALUATED A YEAR AGO AND SHOWN TO BE A CYST!!!] There is a high-density area of sclerosis seen in the body of T12, which may represent a bone island and is unchanged from prior examinations. A bone scan is recommended for further evaluation. [THIS WAS PRESENT A YEAR AGO. DO YOU REALLY THINK THIS IS A MET?!!!] There are several pulmonary nodules. A 2 mm nodule is seen in the right upper lobe, which is unchanged from the examination of November 2005. [THESE WERE PRESENT A YEAR AGO. THEY'RE NOT METS?!!!] Three small nodules, measuring 1, 2, and 2 mm are seen in the lingula. Calcification is seen in the right coronary artery. A cluster of small nodules with a "tree-in-bud" configuration is seen in the right middle lobe, consistent with infectious bronchiolitis, unchanged from the previous exam.
IMPRESSION: [THE IMPRESSION *SHOULD* READ]:

No evidence of metastatic disease and no change from the prior examination.

[THIS IS WHAT THE CLINICIAN NEEDS TO KNOW—IS CHEMO WORKING?]

Table 15-6 Journal Style Format for Radiology Report

Journal Article	Radiology Report
Title	Title
Abstract	—
Introduction	Indication
Method	Procedure
Results and Discussion	Findings
Conclusion	Impression

Reprinted with permission of Anderson Publishing Ltd. from Wilcox, JR, The written radiology report. Applied Radiology Online. July 2006; 35(7). © Anderson Publishing Ltd.

The first of these guidelines is that the report should make some attempt to address the clinical issue. In published reviews, radiologists have been noted not to answer the clinical concern of the referring clinician in nearly 50% of cases.[39] In this same review, clinicians were confused by the radiologist's dictations in nearly the same percentage of cases. The clinical history should be mentioned at the introduction to the report, certainly for billing purposes. The ACR standards incorporate this billing requirement and recommend including the corresponding ICD-9 (international classification of diseases) diagnosis code in the indication, to aid in billing.[37] Within the body of the report, a statement should be made as to whether the clinical findings explain the clinician's question.

The second guideline is that the procedure be described. This description is not only required for billing purposes; it also gives

---

BOX 15-7

Guidelines for Reporting

Guidelines for Resident Dictations

Step 1. Address the clinical issue
Step 2. Description of study
Step 3. Comparison to prior exams
Step 4. Where to describe key findings
Step 5. Organs evaluated
Step 6. Impression or diagnosis
Step 7. Lexicon
Step 8. Typographical errors

---

the next radiologist who sees the patient a frame of reference, so that specific issues may be addressed in a standardized fashion. Mention should be made of the type of examination performed, the use or nonuse and amount of contrast, and imaging planes performed. Since insurers occasionally require justification for other imaging planes, 3-D reformatting, or the performance of more examinations, such as an endovaginal scan in a pelvic ultrasound, a mention of the reason for these extra steps may be required to justify billing. Examples are that the coronal reconstruction was performed at the referring clinician's request or that the endovaginal examination was deemed necessary because the ovary could not be seen on the conventional transabdominal study.

The third guideline states that there must be a comparison to older examinations. A summary of the findings of older examinations may be a helpful starting point in the discussion of findings. This could serve as the springboard for the discussion of findings on the new examination. If the prior examination is an outside study, a description of the location and date of the study should be made if a question arises in the future.

The fourth guideline concerns the most important findings in the specific patient being studied. If a very structured, organ-specific or checklist report is used, the clinician will know where to look for findings in a specific location.[40,41] However, if the reporting style is more casual, the most important findings should be discussed first, so that they will not be buried in the body of the report, amid a discussion of sometimes meaningless trivia. The clinician does not want to read a PhD thesis and probably is not interested in the "findings" part of the exam; consequently, brevity is key.[42]

The fifth guideline addresses ACR guidelines for reports. For example, the ACR guidelines for review of ultrasound examinations require that mention be made of specific structures and findings. Examples include mention of visualization of the cervix on pelvic ultrasounds and Doppler wave form in the aorta on ultrasounds of the aorta. A brief mention of the normal organs seen on an examination is certainly helpful. This would also answer the clinician's concern as to whether a specific organ was evaluated in an examination. As noted by Wilcox, the use of the journal or scientific format of reporting assumes a "null hypothesis."[34] With such a hypothesis, only findings outside the expected range of normal—that is, positive findings—require inclusion in the body of the report. The specific negatives that address the clinical indication may be included if useful. Hence, the use of the term, "PERTINENT FINDINGS."

The sixth guideline requires the impression, diagnosis, or conclusion. This part of the exam is the product. It has been noted in some series to be the only portion of the report read by nearly 50% of clinicians.[41] Here, the radiologist gives the clinical answer to the question posed. This should be a clinical diagnosis, not a rehashing or description of radiographic findings. In certain instances, such as simple extremity fractures, it may suffice, without a discussion of findings, since they tend to be the same. A differential diagnosis in order of likelihood is expected and there may be a suggestion as to the next imaging study to be performed to narrow that differential diagnosis. The following are useful templates for reporting, not to be used as absolutes but as reminders of what issues should be addressed in each report (Boxes 15-8 and 15-9). Notice that the ultrasound report is much more descriptive of structures; specifically, since the issues mentioned in the body of the report are specifically addressed in ACR guidelines.[43]

The seventh guideline deals with the attempt at standardization of terminology within a specific department. Sobel et al found, for example, in a review of thousands of Medicare patient examinations, 14 different ways of describing congestive heart failure.[44] Within our own practice, there is no agreement on the meaning of terms as basic as "cephalization." An attempt at standardization of basic terminology should be a first step. This may include terms such as:

- "Congestive heart failure" (What are the criteria used to make this diagnosis? Should any attempt at its description be made on portable chest X-rays?)
- "Infiltrate versus pneumonia"[45]
- "Pulmonary nodule" (Should 1 to 2 mm nodules be described? What is the specific departmental guideline for their follow-up?)

BOX 15-8

Template for CT Abdomen and Pelvis

CT ABDOMEN AND PELVIS
CLINICAL INDICATION: _____
EXAMINATION PERFORMED: Axial CT of the abdomen and pelvis (with/without) IV contrast from the level of the diaphragm to the symphysis pubis. (Positive oral contrast was used.) (Coronal reconstructed images were performed at the referring clinician's request.)

CONTRAST: 97 cc of . . .
(No significant technical limitations are present.)
(There are no prior examinations available for comparison/This examination is compared to the prior CT of the abdomen and pelvis performed on . . .)

PERTINENT FINDINGS:
On the previous examination, the patient was described as having (summary of prior impression).
The KEY FINDINGS in this patient are as follows: (. . .)
(This could explain the patient's clinical presentation/findings.)

The OTHER FINDINGS include:
(. . .)
The LIVER; BILIARY SYSTEM and GALLBLADDER; SPLEEN; PANCREAS; KIDNEYS, URETERS, and BLADDER; RETROPERITONEUM, AORTA, and LYMPH NODES; PERITONEAL CAVITY; BOWEL; PELVIC ORGANS; VISUALIZED LOWER THORAX; and BONES are within normal limits.
There has been no change from prior examinations.

IMPRESSION:
(No significant abnormalities.)

- "Fatty replacement of the liver on ultrasound" (Does increased echogenicity mean fatty replacement? How to decide it is not due to technique?)
- "Abnormally thickened endometrium" (Whether to use 5, 7, 8 mm in a postmenopausal patient may not be as important as internal consistency.)
- "Criteria for percent stenosis on carotid ultrasound" (Internal inconsistency from standard

BOX 15-9

Template for US of the Pelvis

US of PELVIS
CLINICAL INDICATION: _____
The patient's LMP was (...).
EXAMINATION PERFORMED: (Transabdominal
and endovaginal) ultrasound of the pelvis.
No significant technical limitations are
present. (The endovaginal examination was
performed at the referring clinician's
request.)
(This examination is compared to the prior ...
performed on ....)/(There are no prior
examinations available for comparison.)

FINDINGS:
On the previous examination, the patient
was described as having (summary of
prior study).
(Discussion of KEY FINDINGS ....) MAKE SURE
TO TALK ABOUT THE MOST IMPORTANT
FINDINGS FIRST!!!
YOU MAY WANT TO ADD ...
(These findings may/do not explain the
patient's clinical question.) (Include only
if pertinent.)
(Generalized review of normals ... erase areas
discussed above.) IN THIS AREA, YOU CAN BE
AS BRIEF AS YOU WANT AND CAN USE YOUR
OWN WORDING.
The UTERUS is normal in size and appearance. It
measures ... × ... × ... cm. No myometrial
masses are noted.
No definite CERVICAL abnormalities are seen.
The ENDOMETRIUM is normal in size and
appearance for the patient's menstrual
status. It measures ... × mm in diameter. No
masses are noted.
The RIGHT OVARY is normal in size and
appearance for the patient's menstrual
status. It measures ... × ... × ... cm. No
significant masses are noted.
The LEFT OVARY is normal in size and
appearance for the patient's menstrual
status. It measures ... × ... × ... cm. No
significant masses are noted.
No significant fluid is seen in the CUL-DE-SAC.
(There has been no change from prior
examinations.)

IMPRESSION:
(MAKE SURE YOU GIVE A DIAGNOSIS AND NOT
A DESCRIPTION OF RADIOGRAPHIC FINDINGS,
i.e., RADIOLOGY SPEAK).

characterization is a major red flag in ACR accreditation.)

This has lead to an initial attempt by the ACR to standardize the radiology lexicon.[46] The result of external legislation, the ACR Breast Imaging Reporting and Data System (BI-RADSTM),[47] has evolved into an essential component of breast imaging and, as a result of uniformity of reporting patterns, has aided significantly in the overall improvement in the quality of breast imaging interpretations.

Complaints from referring physicians regarding highly variable reporting styles have led some practices[48] to adopt customized "laundry list" reports.[49] Such an innovation may meet with resistance internally and complaints externally, unless properly implemented. They can only meet with success if universally adopted, actively endorsed by the practice, and reinforced by appropriate referring physician education. The use of voice recognition dictation (VRD, see Chapter 14) has led to the creation of widely used templates or macros that can result in a more uniform reporting style across specialties.

The most traditional measure of radiologist quality has been peer review. The initial JCAHO foray into QA (as discussed previously in this chapter) failed largely because of the lack of earnestness on the part of radiologists in this area. Such an endeavor will only succeed if formalized. At NYU, a system of peer review has been established in each section, whereby an individual section member is assigned, on a rotating monthly basis, the task of reviewing 20 random reports generated by that section during the month in question. The cases are reviewed independently, a brief report is given, and the two interpretations are then compared and mediated by the section chief. Variations, if verified, are then discussed by the chief with the individual radiologist. The results are known only to the radiologist in error, the reviewer, and the section chief. This is intended, in the spirit of CQI, not as an exercise in finger-pointing but as a learning opportunity.

Opportunity 8: Delivery

Jane Beauman is a 43-year-old mother of four, who presents to FPO for an MRI and MRA of the brain to evaluate a headache, the worst headache she has ever had in her life and which began last week. Her MRA shows a long area of intense spasm in the right middle cerebral artery, just above the cavernous sinus. "Now I see why," I remark to myself. "There's a small middle cerebral aneurysm, maybe 2 mm, causing the spasm." I report the exam, glad that I didn't miss a subtle finding.

The next night, Ms. Beauman presents at the NYU Emergency Room in a semistuperous state. While waiting to be examined, she slips into coma. The CT scan performed at that time demonstrates a large subarachnoid hemorrhage centered above the right cavernous sinus. Within three hours, she is dead.

In her deposition two years later, Ms. Beauman's doctor claims that she had never received the MRI report before her death.

Our product, in its simplest terms, is the answer to the referring physician's clinical question ... the received report. A major impediment to the successful completion of the "product" has traditionally been the delays in report sign-offs and transmission. Although use of VRD systems can involve a painful learning curve (see Chapter 14), and can slow efficiency, they have significantly impacted the turnaround time in the delivery of the product. This, together with the use of automatic faxing of reports, has cut average delivery time of reports at the NYU Faculty Practice from 36 to 48 hours to well under 24 hours.[50]

A definition of "important" and "critical" results should be made internally, as a first step. "Important" results are those that may shorten or negatively impact the patient's life, such as the presence of a lung mass, aortic or cerebral aneurysm, or fracture. "Critical" findings are those that could potentially kill the patient if not treated in an emergent fashion. Critical findings have been clearly elucidated at NYU (Table 15-7). A plan of action has been drawn up, which establishes what the critical findings are, how and to whom they should be communicated, and how they should be documented.

When an important finding is made, the patient's accession number can be entered into a specific link, whereupon the physician's office will be notified of the finding and of the report. This call is then documented in the database and an e-mail is sent to the radiologist to confirm the physician receipt of the finding. Certainly, a direct call to the physician's office is also to be encouraged. If that is done, the time and person spoken to must be documented in the final report or addendum. The automated system established at NYU solves several practical issues; the potential on-hold wait time, the inability to contact the physician, the problem of documentation, and, most importantly, the all-too-common issue of distraction, whereby the radiologist forgets to make the call.

Critical reports are handled in a slightly more elaborate manner. In this instance, the radiologist must make and document the call, and document that the clinician understands the import of the call and finding. The frequency of critical findings is tracked in a "critical occurrence cloud," which can be viewed over various intervals of time. The more frequent the event, the larger its typeface in the cloud.

Opportunity 9: Clinician/Patient Response

Early the next morning, Dr. Luong's office calls. "Now I have to go back and get a CAT scan today," Maria muses. "It's probably easier to go to the place nearby in Brooklyn. It's got to be easier than yesterday!"

We'll never see Maria again.

The ultimate definer of quality is the consumer—the patient, the referring clinician, the insurer, and the employer. The cost of attracting a new patient may be 10 times as much as the cost of retaining an existent albeit unhappy client.

Patient response should be routinely monitored with the use of patient satisfaction forms, given to each patient who enters the diagnostic center. Such satisfaction surveys only succeed if a high percentage of patients respond to them and if the survey questions are precise and concise, include patient demographics, and allow multiple responses. "Key quality characteristics" are those qualities of services that the customer finds most important. Unsolicited complaints and telephone hotlines are limited in their ability to proactively meet patient needs. Focus groups, benchmarking, personal interviews, and structured surveys are more appropriate scientific tools, in keeping with TQM, in measuring and guaranteeing patient satisfaction.

Table 15-7 Critical Findings

Active bleeding	Ischemic bowel
Acute stroke	Major vascular injury
Aortic dissection	Major retroperitoneal hemorrhage
Appendicitis	Mediastinal emphysema
Brain tumor (mass effect)	Ovarian torsion
Carotid artery dissection	Placenta previa (near term)
Cerebral hemorrhage/ hematoma	Placental abruption
	Portal venous air
Cervical spine fracture	Pulmonary embolism
Complete bowel obstruction	Ruptured aneurysm
Critical carotid stenosis	(or impending rupture)
DVT or vascular occlusion	Significant line or tube misplacement
Depressed skull fracture	Spinal cord compression
Ectopic pregnancy	Tension pneumothorax
Epiglottitis	Testicular torsion
Fetal demise	Traumatic visceral injury
Free air in abdomen (if no recent surgery)	Vascular occlusion
	Volvulus

Monthly reviews of the results should be performed. Unsatisfactory issues should be addressed by the team with the use of multivoting and ranking, to determine which issues to tackle first. With a TQM program, however, it is not just the individual issues that should be addressed, but the whole constellation of concerns of associated contributors.

The strides made in correcting these deficiencies should be communicated to patients, referring clinicians, and insurers. A radiology booklet, available both in the waiting room and on the Internet, while serving as an underlying informational/advertising function can also keep patients abreast of the importance of their input. The satisfaction issues of the referring clinicians should be addressed with periodic, routine visits to the offices made by the center's marketing personnel. The satisfaction issues with respect to the payers can be documented in report cards, such as the benchmark measurements of the NCQA.

Outcomes measurements are a vital feature of any CQI program. To date, the only bona fide program to measure outcomes is that of the MQSA.

Step 4 (ACT)—Team Acts to Improve Maria's Experience

All members of the team are now acting to improve the specific areas of Maria's experience. From the ordering of the study, through greeting at ultrasound, to the report dictated by the radiologist, to the monitoring of Maria's response to the whole experience, each team member is equally important in making sure that the process is seamless.

CONCLUSION

Maria received a quality of care that would have passed accreditation by the ACR, review by JCAHO, and oversight by our over-read tracking program. Nonetheless, she is not coming back.

As discussed in this chapter, total quality improvement addresses the entire process, is patient-centric, and is not interested in blaming individuals. There are a multitude of systems issues in every step of the patient's journey through our practices that needs to be addressed, not just the end product itself.

An initiative taken by NYU Radiology over the last several years has been the incorporation of other freestanding practices into the overall NYU practice. An example is a multispecialty medical complex in New York, with a full panoply of imaging modalities, which did not have in-house radiology. The imaging studies performed at the center are PACSed (PACS—picture archiving and communication systems) to NYU and read at the main site. Ideally, a report is issued within 24 hours of image transfer. The major challenge in this endeavor, as expected, is the balancing of two seemingly contradictory missions: that of the rigorous professional quality demands of an academic practice and the equally rigorous service demands of a customer-centric business. As we've discussed in this chapter, these are the two opposite sides of the coin of "continuous quality improvement." Neither is the correct or more noble way. The reality is that all practices must have professional and consumer quality concerns. If we are to be that savvy provider who rushes to the head of the curve, we must embrace, perfect, and even enjoy wholeheartedly the quality challenge of this dichotomy.

Dos and Don'ts of Quality Improvement Programs	
Dos	**Don'ts**
1. Create process maps and flowcharts to understand your work flow and the individual components that make up the greater whole.	1. Make conclusions, changes based on gut instincts, or gestalts if data is available.
2. Collect and analyze data to assess how to improve work flow.	2. Create scapegoats.
3. Assess and reassess to make improvements constant.	3. Ignore patient safety or patient surveys.
4. Assign responsibility to individuals for action plans and improvement programs—make it personal yet still a group effort.	4. Seek to *meet* expectations, seek to *exceed* them.
5. Endorse training and education for employees, such as Six Sigma, the Toyota Way, Deming, Baldrich, and so on.	5. Think of short-term profits or gains—your company's reputation is long-lasting and so needs a long-term vision.
6. Prevent errors, don't just address them.	6. Fall into hackneyed platitudes—make TQM goals concrete and meaningful and specific to your situation.
7. Establish industry norms and strive to exceed them.	7. Focus on only one of your customers. Remember that in radiology the patients, referring physicians, payers, grant-funding agencies, and administrators are all our customers.
8. Widely publicize and communicate the mission-driven goals.	8. Underestimate the importance of a well-dictated report that addresses the patient care and clinician's issues.
9. Stress teamwork.	9. Underfund resources for error analysis and systems redesign.
10. Celebrate successes.	10. Create an environment in which errors or mistakes are swept under the rug—use them as an opportunity to improve.

REFERENCES

1. Radford GS: The Control of Quality in Manufacturing. New York, Ronald Press, 1922.
2. Shewhart WA: Economic Control of Quality Manufactured Products. New York, D van Nostrand, 1931.
3. Erturk SM, Ondategui-Parra S, Ros PR: Quality management in radiology: Historical aspects and basic definitions. J Am Coll Radiol 2:985–991, 2005.
4. Juran JM: Juran's Quality Control Handbook. New York, McGraw-Hill, 1988.
5. Chambers DW: TQM: The essential concepts. J Am Coll Dent 65(2):6–13, 1998.
6. Dowd SB, Tilson ER, Carlton R: Quality Management Exam Review for Radiologist Imaging Services. Albany, NY, Delmar, 2002.
7. JCAHO: Quality of Professional Services Standards. (1975).
8. Berwick DM: Continuous improvement as an ideal in health care. N Engl J Med 320(1):53–56, 1989.
9. Laffel G, Blumenthal D: The case for using industrial quality management science in health care organizations. JAMA 262(20):2869–2873, 1989.
10. Appel F: From quality assurance to quality improvement: The joint commission and the new quality paradigm. Qual Assur 13(5):26–29, 1991.
11. Schwartz HW: Quality improvement: The JCAHO model. Radiol Manage 14(3):45–57, 1992.
12. National Committee for Quality Assurance: The State of Health Care Quality: 2005 National Committee for Quality Assurance Washington, DC, 2005, p 25.
13. Williamson J: Medical Quality Management Systems in Perspective in Lovich J (ed): . Health Care Quality Management for the 21st Century. Tampa, FL, American College of Physician Executives, 1991.
14. Haas J: Quality management systems: Choosing the best system for your workplace. Biomed Instrum Technol 36(5):311–317, 2002.
15. DeFeo J, Barnard W: Juran Institute's Six Sigma: Breakthrough and Beyond. New York, McGraw-Hill, 2004.
16. www.health.state.mn.us/divs/eh/radiation/xray/archives/qa.pdf
17. www.health.state.ny.us/dbspace
18. Hynes DM: Quality management. Can Assoc Radiol J 45(5):353–354, 1994.
19. Crosby PB: Quality Is Free: The Art of Making Quality Certain. New York, New American Library, 1979.
20. Hillman B, Amis E, Neiman H: The future quality and safety of medical imaging: Proceedings of the third annual ACR Forum. J Am Coll Radiol 1:33–39, 2005.
21. Stockburger WT: CQI for imaging services, part I, an introduction. Radiol Manage 14(3):79–83, 1992.
22. Papp J: Quality Management in Imaging Sciences, 2nd ed. St. Louis, Mosby, 2004.
23. Hillman BJ, Amios ES, Neiman HL, et al: The future quality and safety of medical imaging: Proceedings of the third annual ACR forum. J Am Coll Radiol 1:33–39, 2004.
24. Geraedts HP, Montenairie R, van Rijk PP: The benefits of total quality management. Comput Med Imaging Graph 25(2):217–220, 2001.
25. Applegate KE: Continuous quality improvement for radiologists. Acad Radiol 1(20):155–161, 2004.
26. Hanks GE: Quality control and assurance. Am J Clin Oncol 11(3):411–414, 1988.
27. Shortell SM, Bennett CL, Byck GR: Assessing the impact of continuous quality improvement on clinical practice, what it will take to accelerate progress. Milbank Q 76(4):593–624, 1998.
28. Weinreb JC: Building a team for change in an academic radiology department. Radiology 232:327–330, 2004.
29. Jablonski R: Customer focus: The cornerstone of quality management–management issues. Healthc Financ Manage 46(11):17–18, 1992.
30. American College of Radiology Appropriateness Criteria™ for imaging and treatment decisions. Reston, VA, American College of Radiology, 1995.
31. Swensen S, Johnson CD: Radiologic quality and safety: Mapping value into radiology. J Am Coll Radiol 2:992–1000, 2005.
32. www.massgeneralimaging.org/roe/
33. Kohn LT, Corrigan JM, Donaldson MS (eds): To Err Is Human: Building a Safer Health System. Washington, DC, National Academies Press, 1999.
34. Pijl ME, Doornbos J, Sickles EA, vanHouwelingen HC, et al: Quantitative analysis of focal masses at MR imaging: A plea for standardization. Radiology 229:534–540, 2003.
35. Wilcox JR: The written radiology report. Applied Radiology Online 35(7):2006.
36. Berlin L: Pitfalls of the vague radiology report. AJR Am J Roentgenol 174:1511–1518, 2000.
37. Weissberg R, Buker S: Writing Up Research: Experimental Research Report Writing for Students of English. Englewood Cliffs, NJ, Prentice Hall, 1990.
38. American College of Radiology: ACR Standard for Communication: Diagnostic Radiology. In: Standards. Reston, VA, American College of Radiology, 1995.
38a. ACR practice guideline for communication of diagnostic imaging findings. In: Practice Guidelines and Technical Standards. Reston, VA, American College of Radiology, 2006:3–7.
39. Clinger NJ, Hunter TB, Hillman BJ: Radiology reporting: Attitudes of referring clinicians. Radiology 169:825–826, 1988.
40. Langlotz CP, Caldwell SA: The completeness of existing lexicons for representing radiology report information. J Digit Imaging 15(suppl 1):201–205, 2002.
41. Naik SS, Hainbidge A, Wilson SR: Radiology reports: Examining radiologist and clinician preference regarding style and content. Am J Roentgenol 176:591–598, 2001.
42. Lafortune M, Breton G, Baudouin JL: The radiological report: What is useful for the referring physician. Can Assoc Radiol J 39:140–143, 1988.
43. American College of Radiology.: ACR Practice Guidelines for Communications: Diagnostic Radiology. Reston, Va, American College of Radiology, 2001.
44. Sobel JL, Pearson ML, Gross K, et al: Information content and clarity of radiologists' reports for chest radiography. Acad Radiol 3:709–717, 1996.

45. Tuddenham WJ: Glossary of terms for thoracic radiology: Recommendations of the nomenclature committee of the Fleischner Society. Am J Roentgenol 143:509–517, 1984.
46. Available at mirc.rsna.org/radlex/service.
47. American College of Radiology: Illustrated Breast Image Reporting and Data System (BI-RADSTM). Reston, VA, American College of Radiology.
48. Shively, C: Quality in management radiology. Imaging Economics.
49. Langlotz CP: Automatic structuring of radiology reports: Harbinger of a second information revolution in radiology. Radiology 224:5–7, 2002.
50. Seltzer SE, Kelly P, Adams DF, Chiango BF, et al: Expediting the turnaround of radiology reports: Use of total quality management to facilitate radiologists' report signing. AJR Am J Roentgenol 162(4):775–781, 1994.

Performance Measurements and Incentive Systems for Radiology Practices

Felix S. Chew and Annemarie Relyea-Chew

One of the most important duties of the leader of a radiology practice or department is to create the opportunities for his or her people to do their very best. Sometimes it becomes necessary to try to measure precisely how well they are doing and learn whether their perfromance is improving. If their performance is not as good as it should be, it may become necessary to change their behavior or to motivate them. In this chapter we will discuss performance measurements and incentive systems in the context of the academic radiology practice, with specific regard to radiologists. We will also consider general principles that are applicable to other settings.

fulfillment of a task or achievement of a goal. For many tasks, no single performance measurement is sufficient. The more complex the task, the more complex the system of measurement must become. For example, measuring the performance of a salesperson with regard to the seemingly simple task of selling items from inventory becomes complicated when you consider the many ways in which goods can be sold and bills collected, and the role of salespeople in representing the company to the public and in cultivating repeat and future customers. Measuring the performance of a diagnostic radiologist can be equally complex, probably even more so.

PERFORMANCE MEASUREMENTS

A performance measurement is a means to measure the job performance of an individual or group (unit) against some criterion for

EFFECTIVE PERFORMANCE MEASUREMENTS

The principle behind measuring performance is to define performance and then examine what actions yield from that performance. Those

BOX 16-1

Attributes of Effective Performance Measurements

1. The measurements are congruent with the goals of the organization.
2. The measurements focus on value drivers and critical resources.
3. The measurements are simple and understandable.
4. The measurements are likely to be uniformly interpreted.
5. The measurements are broadly applicable across the range of activities.
6. The measurements can be obtained in a reproducible, timely manner.
7. The measurements are cost effective to obtain.
8. The measurements are difficult to manipulate.

Adapted from lecture notes by Gregory W. Fischer and Patricia W. Linville, Fuqua School of Business, Duke University, Durham, NC.

actions can then be monitored and measured. Eight attributes of effective performance measurements are summarized in Box 16-1.

First, the measurements should be congruent with the goals of the organization. Measuring any type of activity—or even giving the appearance of measuring the activity—will tend to improve the level of that activity (the Hawthorne effect, in which behavior changes or performance improves following any new or increased attention). It makes little sense to direct attention to something that is not congruent with the goals of the organization. Measurements should focus on the value drivers and critical resources, rather than on the correlates. For example, if an activity with a definable work product were measured by the hours worked rather than the product produced, you might see an increase in hours of work but not necessarily an increase in production.

Effective performance measurements should be simple and understandable. Once a performance measurement system is in place, measurements will be obtained over time and used to identify trends and outliers. Interpretation of trends depends on the simplicity and understandability of the underlying measurements.

The measurements should be interpreted by all parties who come into contact with them: those who make decisions based on them, as well as those whose work is being assessed because of them. If the managers have an interpretation that is different from that of the workers, the two groups will not be able to communicate and thus synergize successfully.

Effective performance measurements should be broadly applicable across the range of activities that are undertaken by the organization. Broad applicability allows the organization to compare the performance of different activities with each other. The measurements should be obtainable in a reproducible, timely manner. If the measurements cannot be obtained in this way, they will not be useful in evaluating performance or managing resources. If the measurements are not reliable, then trends and differences become impossible to interpret.

The measurements should be cost effective to obtain. If the cost of measurement is greater than the possible benefit, then it makes little sense to expend the resources to obtain them. Finally, the measurements should be difficult to manipulate. Gaming the system by manipulating the measurements is often an attractive alternative to improving performance.

PERFORMANCE MEASUREMENTS FOR RADIOLOGISTS

How do you measure the performance of a radiologist? What is it exactly that radiologists do, and how can that be measured? In a complex organization like an academic radiology department, the division of labor and physician specialization is critical to the goal of accomplishing tasks that no single person can do. What are some of the performance measurements that are being used for radiologists, and how effective are they?

Clinical Performance Measurements

Relative Value Units

The resource-based relative value scale (RBRVS) is a measure of work done by medical professions that is directly related to reimbursement (see Chapter 8). This scale is expressed in relative value units (RVUs). Reimbursement rates from third-party payers are typically expressed in terms of dollars per RVU, so that the greater the number of RVUs, the larger the payment. RVUs are therefore an obvious performance measure related to something important to any organization: money. With each report that a radiologist generates and signs off, RVUs become available for reimbursement. It might appear that RVUs would be an excellent performance measurement for radiologists. However, RVUs are related more to the *total* resources required to produce a radiologic report than to the actual amount of work performed only by the radiologist.

The original RBRVS was based on a combination of the physician's work input, the opportunity cost of specialty training, and the relative practice costs.[1] The physician's work input was further estimated along four dimensions: time, mental effort and judgment, technical skill and physical effort, and psychological stress (Box 16-2).[2] The radiology implementation of the RBRVS included physician work and practice costs but assumed that all radiologists had the same opportunity cost of specialty training. The inclusion of practice costs meant that studies that required a large capital investment in equipment with rapid obsolescence, such as MRI or CT, would have high RVUs, regardless of the effort required on the part of the radiologist. Studies that didn't require large capital investments would have low RVUs, like radiography and sonography.[3] RVUs were created at a time when certain imaging technologies were newer and much more expensive than they are now, therefore magnifying the differences between activities that require high and low capital investments. Even within the context of expensive equipment, RVUs have not kept pace with newer technology, so that the RVUs generated by interpreting a digital mammogram are essentially the same as those generated by interpreting a film-screen mammogram, even though the difference in capital investment is quite large.

The use of RVUs as a performance measurement for radiologists also raises the issue of equity across subspecialty practices, some of which may be heavy with CT or MRI, while others may be heavy with radiography.[4] Arenson et al's study of RVUs in academic practice indicated the need for an adjustment factor of 0.50 for angiography, 0.58 for CT, and 0.58 for MRI, relative to radiography.[5] RVUs can also be adjusted for the proportion of time an individual spends doing clinical work, to derive a figure that represents RVUs per full-time equivalent (FTE) radiologist. This is particularly apropos to part-time workers or physicians whose salary is being covered in part by extramural funding.

A challenge is that as the RVUs are adjusted, their relationship to actual dollars generated and productivity weakens. For example, adjusting RVUs for percent of effort covered by NIH funding can be a challenge in that radiologists' salaries often far exceed the NIH cap. While RVUs do have most of the attributes of an effective performance measurement, when applied to an individual radiologist, they fail to focus on the value drivers and the critical resources. For a radiologist, the key value driver is his or her ability to transform imaging studies and radiologic expertise into radiologic reports, and the critical resource is his or her time. The radiologist's knowledge, judgment, and skill are not critical resources because they are not depleted by use. RVUs would be a more suitable performance measurement for an entire radiology practice, or perhaps for a separate organizational or business unit that encompasses capital investment, operational costs, and labor. RVUs clearly do not reflect other value parameters of teaching, research, citizenship, and administrative duties.

Financial Measurements

Gross charges represent the amount of money a department bills for its services; these are divided into technical and professional

---

BOX 16-2

Dimensions of Physician Effort

1. Time
2. Mental effort and judgment
3. Technical skill and physical effort
4. Psychological stress

Adapted from Hsiao WC, Braun P, Yntema D, Becker ER: Estimating physicians' work for a resource-based relative-value scale. N Engl J Med 319(13):35–41, 1988.

components. Gross charges depend on the fee schedule. Although gross charges are correlated with cash collections, RVUs, and radiologist's work effort, they do not really focus on value drivers or critical resources, and no organization exists simply to generate gross charges. Gross charges are an intermediate work-in-progress that is generated by a radiology practice's activity, but they are not an effective performance measurement. Gross charges are directly related to RVUs, with all of the attendant problems, and gross charges can be easily manipulated simply by raising or lowering prices. Charges and revenue need not be conjoined.

Several other financial measurements that are easily and commonly obtained by radiology administrators include gross collections, net collections, and individual profit-and-loss. Gross collections represent the cash that a department collects from its gross charges. Gross collections do not take into account the cost of actually collecting the money and they rely on individuals (bill collectors) within the administrative group independent of the physicians who are being judged by that parameter. Net collections do take into account the cost of collecting the money, and are related to the payer mix and the cost of the billing, collections, and accounting operations. The cost of collecting from some payers is less than others, and the net amount that is collectible is also different for different payers and for different procedures. Bad debt and uncollectible bills are also related to the payer mix: some payers cannot or will not pay their bills. An individual profit-and-loss figure can be implemented in different ways, but most commonly it is a single number that represents the net collections that are based on a radiologist's RVUs less the total compensation for that radiologist, often with an adjustment for the radiologist's percent of nonclinical effort. In this scenario, at least extramural funding data are collected and compensated administrative support can also be counted.

Because all of these measurements are directly related to RVUs, none of them focuses on the value drivers or critical resources for radiologists, and are therefore not effective performance measurements. Furthermore, in radiology, as in other areas of medicine, financial measurements are largely outside the control of the individual physician, so using them

would violate the controllability principle. The controllability principle holds that a worker should be held responsible only for actions that are under his or her control. Collection rates are controllable by interpreting physicians only to the extent that incomplete reports and delays in signature/verification can adversely affect the coding and billing cycle, which may then reduce collection rates.

Examination Volume

The number of examinations interpreted during a specified period of time can be used as a performance measure. Examination volume may be divided by the proportion of time a radiologist is on clinical assignment to derive examination volume per FTE radiologist. Although this would appear to be simple and understandable, the manner in which the measure is derived can lead to variations in the count. A single radiograph of both hands might be counted as one or two examinations, and an enhanced CT scan of the abdomen and pelvis with 3-D reformations might be counted as one, two, three, or four examinations. In determining the number of exams reported, you can count patients studied, cases completed, reports dictated and signed, CPT codes billed, or accession numbers reported, and each will likely yield a different number.

Agreement on the explicit description of the measurement for examination volume and how it is derived is important. The number of studies read by an individual radiologist is easily counted by any of these methods, but how does this hold up as a performance measure? The number of studies read has many of the attributes of an effective performance measurement. Reading studies is certainly congruent with the goals of any radiology practice. It does focus on the value driver for radiologists—the ability to transform imaging studies and radiologic expertise into radiologic reports—but it does not take directly into account the critical resource: time. Different types of studies take different amounts of time to read or perform, and the same study done on a complicated patient will typically take more time than the same study done on an uncomplicated patient. Even most independent assessments of hospital quality provide a certain "acuity index" that measures the degree of complicated/complex diagnoses seen and treated. Thus, the number of studies read by an individual is not necessarily applicable across the range of radiology subspecialties, nor is it applicable across the range of practice settings or case mixes.

Radiology Reporting

Radiology information systems record when patients are scheduled, when they arrive, when their examinations become ready for interpretation, when their reports are finalized, and all of the intermediate steps. Work flow analysis may be used to identify bottlenecks in the system. Rapid report turnaround time (RTT) is an often-cited metric for quality, usually measuring the time from exam completion to finalized report (report turnaround time) or from preliminary report to finalized report (signature/verification time). Because the billing cycle cannot begin until a report has been finalized, slow RTT may affect cash flow. The total amount of work done (RVUs, number of studies read, or other metric) would be the same regardless of the turnaround time.

Time On Task

Can time be used as a performance measurement? If the time spent covering a clinical service is the measurement, the radiologist might consider the elapsed time from when he or she begins the work to when he or she is free to leave as the time spent, while another observer might look at the time actually spent interpreting images, performing procedures, and conducting consults. While the time of a radiologist is a critical resource, there is not a direct relationship between time on task and the production of radiology reports, nor is there a direct relationship between radiologist time and departmental revenue. The intensity of the work, the case mix, and the efficiency of the radiologist are important. Finally, time on task is easily manipulated: a radiologist can start early, work through lunch, and stay late, without doing any additional work. Also, some radiologists simply work faster than others.

Performance Measurements in Use

A nationwide survey of radiology departments in the United States by Ondategui-Parra et al at Harvard revealed that performance measurements for departments could be divided into five categories: productivity, reporting, access to examinations, customer satisfaction, and finance.[6] Productivity indicators studied included examination volume, examination volume per modality, professional RVUs, professional RVUs per FTE employee, gross charges by modality, collections by FTE employee, technical RVUs, technical RVUs per FTE employee, and examination volume by resource and/or device. Radiology reporting indicators included report turnaround time, transcription time, and signature time. Customer satisfaction indicators included patient complaints, patient satisfaction, patient waiting time, referring physician satisfaction, and employee satisfaction. Financial indicators included expenses, days in accounts receivable, collections by modality, average RVU per examination, cost per RVU, hours worked per RVU, and supply cost per RVU. While most of these metrics are better suited to measuring departmental performance, a few of them are applicable to individual radiologists, and 40% of the departments that responded to the survey indicated that they used one or more of these metrics to monitor the performance of and provide feedback to individual radiologists.[7]

Other Issues

There are other issues with certain clinical performance measures. First of all, they generally focus on only one aspect of a radiologist's clinical activities—quantity—and do not address quality. Second, they can be measured individually, and therefore may hurt cooperation and coordination between radiologists, encouraging competition rather than cooperation. Third, they do not address legitimate clinical activities, such as consultations with referring clinicians or patients, self-directed learning, quality assurance, problem-solving, systems-based practice, or risk management. The mere existence of a system of performance measures that includes RVUs or RVU-derived metrics may tacitly delegitimize difficult-to-measure activities of critical importance to an organization unless they are counterbalanced in some way. Under a pay-for-performance model, you get exactly the performance you pay for.

Academic Performance Measurements

The goals of an academic radiology practice extend beyond clinical service and revenue, and include the creation and dissemination of radiologic knowledge (research and teaching). Both research and teaching are highly complex, multifaceted activities that do not necessarily have a single, clearly defined work product. Radiology practices, and society in general, devote considerable resources to these activities. How can these activities be objectively measured? There are two general approaches: process measurements and outcome measurements. Process measurements look at the way in which an activity is being performed, perhaps measuring infrastructure and training, resources applied, intermediate work steps, or workers' attitudes and behaviors. Process measurements may also look at "markers," or things that can be measured that are associated with good processes or good outcomes, but that are not a product of a process or an actual outcome. Outcome measurements consider only the final work product or goal of an activity.

Faculty members in academic radiology practices tend to be highly subspecialized, so that no two individuals have exactly the same job. In the realm of the dissemination of radiologic knowledge, some faculty members might specialize in clinical teaching of students, residents, and fellows at the workstation. Other faculty members might emphasize the creation of educational materials, such as textbooks or computer-based teaching files, while still others might specialize in lecturing to practicing radiologists at continuing medical education courses and national meetings. All of these activities should be highly valued by the department. But is there a method for measuring the quantity and quality of this activity that is equitable and comparable across the entire range, or should each type of activity have its own set of measurements?

Time On Task

One obvious metric for teaching effort would be to count the number of hours spent teaching. However, even this seemingly simple metric has pitfalls. For example, if teaching were combined with patient care or research, one would need to apportion the hours among the different activities. Does class size matter? If a teaching subsidy were based on hours of instruction received by students, then perhaps time spent teaching large classes should count more than time spent teaching small classes or time spent mentoring individuals. Faculty preparation time should always be counted. Although one could count faculty time spent creating teaching materials such as Web sites, alternatively, one could count student time spent learning from them.

Teaching Evaluations

Teaching evaluations are commonly obtained in academic settings and sometimes used, or misused, as a metric for teaching. Teaching evaluations are necessarily subjective, even if rendered in numerical terms, and often reflect the short-term entertainment value of a session, not the true goal of learning, retaining, and applying new knowledge. Because the outcome from teaching can be difficult to quantify, teaching evaluations often focus on process and can be difficult to interpret.

Publications

Keeping up with the study of publications has always been one goal of academic life, and is integral to the process of scholarship. Publications come in many forms, and not all publications are equal. Publication of original research—the creation of new knowledge—is considered to be the highest form of academic publication, and often requires the greatest degree of time and intellectual effort. Not only does the research have to be conceived, planned, funded, and accomplished, but the paper also has to be written and shepherded through the publication process. Other types of publications include descriptive articles, review articles, and educational articles. Articles can be long or short. Articles can be published in the peer-reviewed literature as well as in non–peer-reviewed periodicals, textbooks, monographs, or online.

Authorship is variable. First authorship is commonly thought of as the best form of authorship to claim,[8] but coauthorship has long been the most common form of authorship. We studied authorship in radiology journals and found that over a 35-year period, the percentage of papers with four or more authors increased from 3% to 61% in *AJR* and *Radiology* while the percentage of papers with only one author fell from 52% to 5%.[9] Coauthorship may be driven by the complexity of current research, requiring the participation of multiple specialists, but it may also be driven by incentives for faculty to publish more. Through the proliferation of coauthorship, more authorships can be created without increasing the amount of research or writing that is being done, but coauthorship is potentially a good thing from an educational and mentoring point of view.

Citations

The number of citations to published papers is one quantitative measure of quality and influence. A citation is the event that occurs when one paper includes another paper in its list of references. For the medical literature, the science citation index (ISI-Thomson, Web of Science) indexes citations, including many publications that are not included on the National Library of Medicine's Medline. The existence of a citation means that the cited paper was useful or influential in some way to the furtherance of knowledge; frequently cited papers would have greater usefulness or influence than infrequently cited or uncited papers. Citations are therefore of potential use as a performance measure for research productivity. Counting the total number of citations measures the impact of a person's work, but may be inflated by a small number of heavily cited papers. Counting total citations would also give greater weight to review articles than to original research, because review articles tend to be more heavily cited. Calculating citations per paper does not distinguish high from low productivity, and ISI's definition of a citable item may not match the common understanding of a paper.

You could also count the number of significant papers, as defined by a particular citation threshold or the impact factor of the journal publishing the article; the citation threshold would have to be set arbitrarily, and perhaps adjusted for seniority. As well, you could create some arbitrary set of papers—say, the top five or ten—and count the citations to those papers. Hirsch's *h*-index is an alternative citation-based measure.[10] The *h*-index is based on the distribution of citations received by a given researcher's publications. Hirsch, a physicist, writes: "A scientist has index h if h of his/her Np papers have at least h citations each, and the other $(Np - h)$ papers have at most h citations each."[10] That is, a scholar with an index of h has published h papers with at least h citations each. The higher the *h*-index, the better.

In diagnostic radiology, most papers are infrequently cited or not cited at all, but when they are cited, there is typically a lag of one or more years between publication of the cited article and publication of the citing article.[11] This hurts the young academician who is just starting his or her publication record. Once a citation has been recorded in the literature, it never goes away; therefore, using citation metrics does not indicate what a faculty member has been doing lately. Citation conventions differ among different fields, so comparing the citations in the radiology literature with the citations in a basic science field would be inappropriate.

Grant Support

Counting grants submitted, grant application scores, grants funded, and dollar value of grants can be one way of quantifying performance in the research area. However, among clinical diagnostic radiologists, grant support is relatively rare, so this metric is simply not applicable to the majority of radiologists. Percentage of effort funded, however, is an important parameter to evaluate since it will determine the adjustment to the RVUs expected of that individual. Grants must also be viewed in the context of a means to an end. The end is not to get a grant but rather to do significant research that is shared with and by the medical community. A grant is a means to performing that great research, not the outcome itself. Without publishing the work from a grant, no general good is derived from the research, and the effort and dollars are wasted.

PERFORMANCE MEASUREMENTS FOR NONRADIOLOGIST PERSONNEL

Performance measurements for nonradiologist personnel should reflect the specific nature of their job. Depending on the size, setting, and organization of the radiology practice or department, jobs for technologists, nurses, support staff, and administrative personnel will differ from one place to another, and therefore performance metrics must also differ. Even within a single institution or practice, these metrics may not be comparable across jobs, even if they are intended to measure the same thing.

In constructing performance measurements for these positions, you should take great care to ensure that the measurements focus on value drivers and critical resources. Let us consider patient transporters. Particularly in large hospital settings, many radiology practices have found it cost effective to maintain their own dedicated staffs of patient transporters, rather than rely on a hospital-wide service. If you consider the pure mechanics of bringing patients from one location in the hospital to the radiology department, you might come up with metrics such as waiting time, response time, transit time, number of trips, or idle time. You might also calculate numbers, such as cost per patient trip or cost per transporter per day. The possible implementation of these metrics brings to mind visions of transporters unsafely racing patients through the hospital to reduce their transit time. To reduce idle time while maintaining the short transit times, the transporters might move at a snail's pace when not actually moving patients (going with an empty wheelchair to fetch a patient, for example) or simply become hard to find (and presumed to be working).

These and other behaviors that would directly address the metrics would be nonproductive for the practice. A better way to design a metric would be to consider how radiology transporters contribute to the practice. Transporters do that by helping to maintain a smooth and continuous flow of patients through the various imaging areas and devices, so that the use of capital equipment is maximized and patient waiting time is minimized. It is therefore not the *actual* transit, idle, or waiting times that are important, but the predictability and reliability of the service. If an MRI technologist knows exactly how long it will be before a patient will arrive at his or her scanner once the transporter service has been notified, then he or she can maintain a continuous flow of patients through the scanner. An average time from request to arrival of 30 minutes, with a 90% range from 25 to 35 minutes, would actually be preferable than an average time of 25 minutes, with a 90% range from 5 to 45 minutes. In the latter case, the scanner is much more likely to sit idle while waiting for a patient to arrive, and a scanner that is idle is not contributing to the practice. In addition, the variability will also result in some patients waiting longer for the scanner, and an unhappy patient is one that is not likely to return.

It is for this reason that reporting mean times without also considering variation can miss significant process failure. One further point about patient transporters is that they do not work in isolation; they work as part of a team (along with schedulers, patient assistants, and technologists) that maintains patient flow. Team metrics might be more appropriate than individual metrics.

INCENTIVE SYSTEMS

An incentive system is a method of controlling behavior. Incentive systems are deployed by managers to manipulate the behavior of their employees. In this context, the behavior that employers seek to control is job performance. A distinction should be drawn between methods for determining employee compensation and systems for controlling behavior. Methods for determining employee compensation will necessarily have incentives, but their purpose is generally to gain the services of employees, and not to control their behavior. For example, a compensation program based on salary plus step increases for longevity provides an incentive for employees to remain with the organization, but it does not provide the manager with a means to control actual behavior. A system of salary plus bonuses, in which the bonuses are always distributed according to a fixed formula (e.g., fully vested partners get a certain share that is always larger than that of partially vested partners), also does not provide a means of control. Even a compensation system based on wages plus tips (a system that we have not yet encountered with respect to radiologists) does not really provide a method for the manager to control the behavior of employees.

An incentive system may provide monetary compensation to employees, but it does not necessarily have to. The theoretical underpinning of incentive systems is "expectancy theory." Expectancy theory holds that behavior is controlled by its expected consequences: an individual will act in a certain way based on (1) the expectation that the act will have a given outcome and (2) the attractiveness of that outcome to the individual. In this circumstance, rewards would be strongly linked to performance.[12] As we discuss later, expectancy theory and incentive systems are not without controversy.

Managers have a legitimate interest in controlling the work performance of employees. Indeed, one of the key tasks of leadership in any organization is to get the best performance possible from individuals and teams. Quality of work, productivity, customer satisfaction, risk management, quality of work environment, and so forth, are directly related to the behavior of employees. Successful organizations have often used explicit direction, supervision, training, and organizational culture as the predominant methods of social control.

Radiologists are individuals who have completed a long period of training. The four-year residency program can also be viewed as a period of acculturation to the professions of radiology and medicine, during which trainees internalize the tacit knowledge that governs professional behavior. Selection for entry into each stage of education and training for a radiologist is highly competitive. Once in practice, radiologists usually work independently of one another as consultants to other physicians. As a group, radiologists are highly compensated relative to other medical specialties, and enjoy high status. In one sense, the existence of an incentive system as an attempt to control the behavior of a group of independent professionals like radiologists can be regarded as a symptom of managerial failure. We will discuss the attributes of good incentive systems, and then consider some of the ways in which they may fail. We will then consider the question of just how good a good incentive system can be, and what is necessary to motivate people.

GOOD INCENTIVE SYSTEMS

All happy families are alike; each unhappy family is unhappy in its own way.

LEO TOLSTOY, *ANNA KARENINA*

Good and bad incentive systems are like the happy and unhappy families that Tolstoy refers to in the opening words of *Anna Karenina*. Good incentive systems are good in the same way, but bad ones can fail in a variety of different ways.

The first attribute of a good incentive system is that the people who are its targets must be able to do the task or achieve the goals for which there is an incentive. Not only must they have the ability, training, skills, resources, and opportunity, they also must accept the task or goals as appropriate. Second, the targets (i.e., employees) must agree that if they do the task, they will actually receive the reward. For example, if the reward is a year-end bonus, the targets must expect that the organization will still be in business, that it will honor its commitment to provide the bonus, and that the targets will still be employed. Third, the targets must consider the reward for completing the task to be attractive, valuable, and equitable, relative to the effort that would be required to receive it. For example, if someone would have to work extra hours in the evening and on the weekends to complete the task, and the expected reward is small in comparison to the usual compensation for that amount of effort, that person is unlikely to even accept the task. Similarly, if the reward is a golf outing at the boss's country club, and the target does not play golf or enjoy spending time with the boss, that person will not accept the task. Fourth, the incentive system must reward the right behavior. For example, if the incentive system is designed to improve customer service, but actually rewards sales, then

Characteristics of Good Incentive Systems

1. The people who are the targets of the incentive system have the ability and resources to complete the task.
2. If the task is completed, the people who are the targets of the incentive system will actually receive the reward.
3. The reward is valued by the people who are the targets of the incentive system.
4. The incentive system rewards the right behavior on the part of the people who are the targets of the system.
5. The incentive system encourages the people who are the targets of the incentive system to work well together.

Adapted from lecture notes by Gregory W. Fischer and Patricia W. Linville, Fuqua School of Business, Duke University, Durham, NC.

sales may improve, but customer service will not. Finally, the incentive system should encourage people to work together. A good incentive system will enhance coordination of effort among targets with different roles or skills. It should improve knowledge transfer, and it should be perceived as equitable by the targets. These five features of good incentive systems are summarized in Box 16-3.

BAD INCENTIVE SYSTEMS

An incentive system may fail if goals are not set appropriately. If goals are set too high, so-called "stretch goals," the targets may rightly decide that they cannot do the task with their current level of training, information, and resources, and may simply choose to ignore the goals. In the process, management can lose credibility. If the goals are easily attainable, the targets may engage in sandbagging, in which they appear to have barely reached the goal. They may, in fact, have withheld additional progress that they have made beyond the goal, waiting for the next incentive period. For example, if a radiology assistant professor has been given the target of three publications per year, he or

she may hold manuscripts back once the target has been reached, just in case he or she comes up short the following year.

An incentive plan that does not actually provide the target with the reward once his or her goals have been reached will fail; in fact, the plan will fail if the targets simply have the perception that they might not receive the reward, whether or not that is the case. For example, if employees are to receive stock options for reaching their goals, but the stock price of the company is dropping, they may decide that the options will be worthless by the time they get them. In another example, employees might receive credits toward a defined benefit retirement plan. If the employees think that they will not stay with the organization long enough to retire, then the incentive will have no value to them.

A reward that has insufficient value for the target will not provide motivation. If the target does not like the reward—that is, if there is insufficient upside relative to the risk and effort required to get the reward—the target will not bother to try to attain it. Financial compensation is often the reward that is attached to an incentive system, but other rewards may be as valuable or perhaps even more valuable than cash. Status and recognition can be valuable rewards, as might a prized parking spot or desk location. However, idiosyncratic rewards that have value to some but perhaps not to others should be avoided. An example might be gift certificates to a store that sells items few people would need or want: for example, a golf outing at the boss's country club or perhaps skydiving lessons.

The incentive system will fail if it does not reward the right behavior. This pitfall can be described as rewarding A while hoping for B. Common examples would include rewarding sales while hoping for profits, rewarding short-term performance while hoping for long-term performance, and rewarding quantity while hoping for quality. The details of the performance measurements used to determine whether the goals have been achieved are critical in rewarding A and actually getting A. It is natural for targets of an incentive system to study that system to get the most out of it with the least amount of effort. Thus, employees may engage in sandbagging, in which they direct their efforts only toward the things that are rewarded, and not particularly toward the common goals of the organization. In this incentive-incompatibility problem, the individual's goals are not congruent with the those of the organization, and the situation may itself be the direct result of the incentive system.

A good incentive program will encourage people to work together more effectively, and a poor one will actively discourage people from working together. The complexity of activity in radiology practices and the subspecialization that this complexity has engendered requires that people at various levels work together effectively. An incentive system that forces co-workers to compete with each other will not foster cooperation and knowledge transfer. If the system is "zero-sum"—that is, one person's gain is always another person's loss—then the situation is even less likely to foster cooperation. A zero-sum system may be perceived by some as inequitable, particularly if the performance measures do not capture the subtle differences in the work effort and work product of various subspecialists. Equity issues are also raised by the question of controllability. If incentive rewards are distributed according to factors that are out of the control of the targets, the system will be perceived as unfair, and will fail.

WHY INCENTIVE PLANS CANNOT WORK

In his classic article in the *Harvard Business Review* and in other writings, author and educator Alfie Kohn presented six reasons why even good incentive plans cannot work.[13,14] First, money or other rewards do not motivate people. People clearly need money, and money can obtain certain behaviors from people, but can it make them want to behave in those ways? Increasing pay can certainly keep people from moving to another employer who pays more, but will their work quality actually increase if they are paid more? Kohn states that "no controlled scientific study has ever found a long-term enhancement of the quality of work as a result of any reward system."[15] Second, rewards are manipulative, and can be therefore punitive in effect. Failing to receive an expected reward

is generally viewed as a punishment. An environment in which specific behaviors are identified and are either being rewarded or punished is one in which people will feel controlled. Third, individual rewards rupture working relationships by fostering competition. When co-workers begin to view one another as obstacles to their own individual success, cooperation is replaced by competition, and teamwork fails. Fourth, rewards don't solve problems; they merely obtain short-term compliance within the existing framework. Relying on incentives to improve suboptimal performance ignores underlying problems that may be the cause of that suboptimal performance. An incentive system cannot be a substitute for giving workers what they need (more training, more resources, etc.) to do a good job. Fifth, rewards discourage risk-taking and kill creativity. No one will think outside of the box when the rewards are inside it. People will focus their attention on completing the task that leads to rewards, not on better ways to do the task. They may find that the task isn't even necessary. Finally, rewards undermine intrinsic motivation. People who do outstanding work do it because they love what they do. To be paid—even well paid—no doubt pleases them, but the excellence of their work is not the result of a paycheck. When extrinsic motivations, such as rewards, become substitutes for internal motivations, job performance will suffer, particularly when it is tied to interesting or complicated tasks. The existence of an explicit incentive may suggest to people that without the incentive, they would not perform the task; therefore, it is not a task worth performing, except to get the reward. Under those circumstances, how well will the task be performed? Kohn's arguments are not without controversy. These points are summarized in Box 16-4.

WHAT MOTIVATES PEOPLE?

If incentive systems only buy short-term compliance with simple tasks, how does one obtain excellence over the long term? If the workers are motivated to do excellent work, that is, they want to do excellent work, the job of management is to provide the workers with the

BOX 16-4

Why Incentive Plans Cannot Work

1. Rewards are not a primary motivator.
2. Rewards are manipulative.
3. Individual rewards rupture working relationships.
4. Rewards don't solve problems.
5. Rewards discourage risk-taking.
6. Rewards undermine intrinsic motivation.

Adapted from Kohn A: Why incentive plans cannot work. Harvard Business Review (September–October 1993).

necessary knowledge, training, resources, and environment, and then to get out of the way. A number of theories and constructs about human motivation may shed light on how to nurture the intrinsic motivation required for excellence.

One model of human motivation is called "Theory X and Theory Y."[16] Theory X assumptions are that people inherently dislike work, must be coerced or controlled to do work to achieve objectives, and prefer to be directed. Theory X is consistent with expectancy theory, in which awards motivate behavior, and generally with incentive systems. Theory Y assumptions are that people view work as being as natural as play and rest, and will exercise self-direction and self-control toward achieving objectives that they are committed to. They will also learn to accept and seek responsibility. Theory Y suggests that incentive systems are not necessary because people are self-motivated.

Equity theory holds that an individual will act to correct inequities between his or her work (and the consequent rewards) and the work (and the rewards) of comparable coworkers.[17] An individual will compare his or her work inputs (time, effort, diligence, etc.) with his or her work outputs (money, status, security, etc.), and then compare those with individuals doing similar jobs. If he or she observes that there is an inequity, he or she will act to correct it by changing the inputs, the outputs, or both. Actions an individual might take to correct a perceived inequity might include lowering productivity, reducing quality, increasing absenteeism, and simply quitting.[17] On one

hand, equity theory suggests that people will bring themselves down to the lowest common denominator and thus is consistent with the failure of incentive systems to motivate. On the other hand, there may be a positive motivation for low-achieving employees who see the example of more productive coworkers.

The "three needs" theory holds that individuals have (1) a need for achievement, (2) a need for power, and (3) a need for affiliation.[18] The strength of these needs is different among different individuals, and one need tends to be dominant for a particular individual. The implication for management is that people with different dominant needs will respond to different types of motivation.[18] This theory suggests that incentive systems may work for some, but not for others.

The "two factor" theory holds that happiness with a job is determined by two types of factors: (1) motivation factors and (2) hygiene factors.[19,20] Motivation factors lead to job satisfaction when favorable, while hygiene factors lead to job dissatisfaction when unfavorable. In this model, job satisfaction is possible only in the presence of favorable motivation factors and in the absence of unfavorable hygiene factors. Motivation factors include achievement, recognition for achievement, the work itself, responsibility, advancement, and growth (Box 16-5). Hygiene factors include organizational policy and administration, supervision, interpersonal relationships, working conditions, salary, status, and security (Box 16-6). Favorable hygiene factors do not bring job satisfaction, only the absence of dissatisfaction. Incentive plans fall under hygiene factors, specifically organizational policy and administration, and

BOX 16-5

Intrinsic Motivators Related to Job Satisfaction

1. Achievement
2. Recognition for achievements
3. Work itself
4. Responsibility
5. Growth or advancement

Adapted from Herzberg F: One more time: How do you motivate employees? Harvard Business Review (January 2003).

supervision. Thus, a poor incentive plan will cause job dissatisfaction, but a good one will not bring job satisfaction or motivation. Hygiene factors can be thought of as organizational infrastructure: if it is good, no one notices, but if it is poor, everyone suffers.

MOTIVATING RADIOLOGISTS

Radiologists are individuals with high levels of intrinsic motivation. No incentive system or reward can possibly explain why they would voluntarily subject themselves to nine or more years of difficult and all-consuming education and training to become radiologists. The profession of medicine, and radiology in particular, has great potential for long-term job satisfaction. Physicians have responsibility for the care of their patients and for the health care of society at large. There are endless opportunities for professional growth and achievement, and the daily work is continually stimulated by the advancement of knowledge and new technologies. In academic settings, research and teaching provide additional opportunities. Thus, because the typical work of a radiologist already encompasses the intrinsic motivators that lead to long-term excellence, and because radiologists have already demonstrated their strong intrinsic motivation to qualify in their profession, an underperforming, dissatisfied radiology practice usually does not need performance measurements and an incentive system, but rather needs attention to hygiene factors. The most important of these—organizational policy

and administration, supervision, interpersonal relationships, and working conditions—do not involve rewards or money.[20]

MOTIVATING NONRADIOLOGIST PERSONNEL

Although compensation for radiologists comprises the largest type of salary cost for a radiology practice, the performance of other personnel can make or break a department. The same principles apply, but because of the content of these jobs, considerably more attention needs to be focused on internal motivational factors.[20,21] Radiologists and other physicians tend to view their employment as a career, with long-term aspirations within the scope of their employment that extend well beyond bringing home a paycheck. However, other personnel in the radiology practice may view their employment as a job, with a short-term focus on bringing home a paycheck, and a long-term focus on finding a better job. Departmental management should strive to make each job meaningful by providing opportunities for achievement, responsibility, and growth.

The importance to efficient overall departmental work flow (and therefore costs and revenue) of jobs, such as patient scheduler and patient transporter, cannot be overemphasized. People in these roles will represent the department to the public because they will generally have more interaction with patients than most members of the professional staff. For example, the job of patient transporter can be transformed by creating teams that are responsible for the round trips of patients from a specific hospital unit to a specific imaging area and back rather than an undifferentiated (anonymous) pool of individuals who are given the next available one-way trip. Teams can be given responsibility for their own quality improvement. Training can also be an important motivator, so that employees feel more comfortable with the idea of managing unexpected situations. Patient transporters should be trained in basic cardiopulmonary resuscitation, not because we would really expect them to run a code when more advanced health care providers are available, but because it would give them confidence in handling patients and it would communicate to them—in a way stronger than words—that we regard them as an important part of the team that provides radiologic care. Transporters are not just people who push wheelchairs from one place to another, they are an integral part of a health care team, taking care of individual patients. A potential upward path from patient transporter to other jobs within the department may help retain employees within the department, and save on the costs of turnover. It would be hard to overstate the value of an employee who started as a transporter, learned how to use the computer and became a patient service representative, went to community college and became a technologist, and then went to night school and became a manager. A department that enables employees to do this is not just providing jobs, it is developing careers.

CONCLUSION

Incentive systems are methods of manipulation and control. Good incentive systems have specific characteristics, such as rewarding the right behavior and encouraging cooperation and teamwork, while bad incentive systems can fail in a myriad of different ways. The performance measurements that are used to operationalize good incentive systems have specific attributes, such as congruency with the goals of the organization and focusing on value drivers and critical resources. Good incentive systems will buy short-term compliance with the behaviors that are rewarded, but because they do not change attitudes and have negative effects on motivation, cooperation, creativity, and problem-solving, they cannot enhance the long-term quality of work. Bad incentive systems may also change behavior, but the predominant effects may be unintended. Radiologists—individuals with high levels of intrinsic motivation—have jobs that are interesting by their very nature. Departmental chairpersons should address subpar performance on the part of their radiologists not by attempting to manipulate them through performance measurements and incentive systems, but rather by attention to hygiene factors and organizational infrastructure.

Dos and Don'ts of Performance Measurements and Incentive Plans	
Dos	**Don'ts**
1. Use measurements that focus on critical resources and value drivers.	1. Use measurements that are *not* congruent with organizational goals and values.
2. Use measurements that are simple and understandable.	2. Use measurements that are *not* applicable across the range of activities.
3. Use measurements that are timely and cost effective.	3. Use measurements that mean different things to different people.
4. Use measurements that are difficult to manipulate.	4. Spend resources measuring things that don't matter.
5. Recognize achievement with growth and advancement.	5. Employ external rewards as a primary motivator.
6. Give workers responsibility at all levels.	6. Reward one behavior while hoping for another.
7. Recognize and nurture internal motivation.	7. Disrupt teamwork with individual incentives.
8. Attend to workplace hygiene factors.	8. Attempt to solve problems with incentives.

Acknowledgment Much of the material in this chapter was drawn from notes taken by one of us (FSC) during a course on "Managerial Effectiveness" at Duke University's Fuqua School of Business. The course instructors were Professors Gregory W. Fischer, PhD, and Patricia W. Linville, PhD. The material was then adapted to the particular circumstances found in radiology practices and supplemented with readings.

REFERENCES

1. Hsiao WC, Braun P, Dunn D, Becker ER, et al: Results and policy implications of the resource-based relative-value study. N Engl J Med 319(13):881–888, 1988.
2. Hsiao WC, Braun P, Yntema D, Becker ER: Estimating physicians' work for a resource-based relative-value scale. N Engl J Med 319(13):835–841, 1988.
3. Moorefield JM, MacEwan DW, Sunshine JH: The radiology relative value scale: Its development and implications. Radiology 187(2):317–326, 1993.
4. Arenson RL, Lu Y, Elliott SC, Jovais C, et al: Measuring the academic radiologist's clinical productivity: Survey results for subspecialty sections. Acad Radiol 8(6):524–532, 2001.
5. Arenson RL, Lu Y, Elliott SC, Jovais C, et al: Measuring the academic radiologist's clinical productivity: Applying RVU adjustment factors. Acad Radiol 8(6):533–540, 2001.
6. Ondategui-Parra S, Bhagwat JG, Zou KH, Gogate A, et al: Practice management performance indicators in academic radiology departments. Radiology 233:716–722, 2004.
7. Ondategui-Parra S, Bhagwat JG, Zou KH, Nathanson E, et al: Use of productivity and financial indicators for monitoring performance in academic radiology departments: U.S. nationwide survey. Radiology 236(1):214–219, 2005.
8. Chew FS: Coauthorship in radiology journals. AJR Am J Roentgenol 50(1):23–26, 1988.
9. Chew FS: The scientific literature in diagnostic radiology for American readers: A survey and analysis of journals, papers, and authors. AJR Am J Roentgenol 147(5):1055–1061, 1986.
10. Hirsch JE: An index to quantify an individual's scientific research output. PNAS 102 (46):16569–16572, 2005.
11. Chew FS, Relyea-Chew A: How research becomes knowledge: An analysis of citations to published papers. AJR Am J Roentgenol 150(1):31–37, 1988.
12. Vroom VH: Work and Motivation. New York, Wiley, 1964.
13. Kohn A: Why incentive plans cannot work. Harvard Business Review (September–October 1993).
14. Kohn A: Punished by Rewards: The Trouble with Gold Stars, Incentive Plans, A's, Praise, and Other Bribes. Boston, Houghton Mifflin, 1999.
15. Kohn A: Challenging behaviorist dogma: Myths about money and motivation. Compensation and Benefits Review 30(2):27–37, 1998.
16. McGregor D: The Human Side of Enterprise. New York, McGraw-Hill, 1960.
17. Adams JS: Inequity in social exchange, in Berkowitz L (ed): Advances in experimental social psychology, vol 2. New York, Academic Press, 1965, pp 267–300.
18. McClelland D: The Achieving Society. Princeton, Van Nostrand, 1961.
19. Herzberg F: Work and the Nature of Man. Cleveland, World, 1966.
20. Herzberg F: One more time: How do you motivate employees? Harvard Business Review (January 2003).
21. Nicholson N: How to motivate your problem people. Harvard Business Review (January 2003).

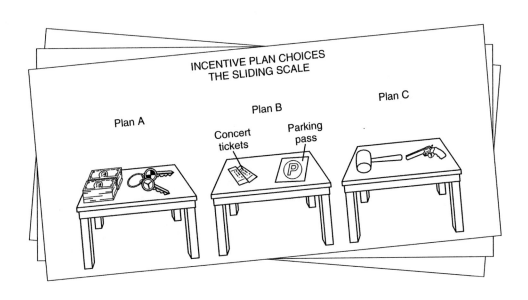

BUILDING AND MANAGING A PRACTICE: GROWING THE PRACTICE

Assessing Growth Opportunities for Your Imaging Practice

William P. Shuman

INTRODUCTION

Why grow a radiology practice? Growth is challenging, hard work, and uncomfortable because it involves analysis, discovery, change, and risk. By contrast, maintaining the status quo is usually easy and comfortable because it involves continuing to do what you already know using familiar techniques. However, if you're standing still in a changing environment, you are actually falling behind. As such, maintaining the status quo may actually increase risk and decrease security, and that should make you uncomfortable. In the immortal words of Alvy Singer (played by Woody Allen) in the movie *Annie Hall*, a radiology practice "is like a shark. . . . It has to constantly move forward or it dies."

Growth in a competitive market comes only when you are doing many things right. Targeting growth focuses your thinking; it makes you concentrate on how to make your practice work better—that is, better than your presumably good competition—to serve the needs of current and future customers. Pursuing growth as a goal motivates you to understand your potential customers, and to incrementally refine your practice's added value and products. You can respond more quickly to new information and change in ways that improve your chances of greater success.[1] The improvement of your practice as a result of the pursuit of growth will most likely decrease risk and increase security. So, actually, growth should make you feel *more* comfortable, not less.

That said, not all growth is good. Doing more of a losing service is a losing proposition ("loss leaders" not withstanding). But doing more of a service that is positive to the strength of the practice is the type of growth we will discuss in this chapter. Such positive growth might produce more profit, more service value, more academic and political impact, a stronger position in your market and improved positioning for future sustainability, a better quality of life for employees and partners, or better recruiting—any or all of these results will strengthen your practice, justifying the effort to produce growth, and making growth a goal worth pursuing for your practice.

Growth: Keeping Your Current Customer Base

Your practice will not grow if you are losing your current customers faster than you are gaining new customers. Losing current customers (or failing to grow the business from your current customers) means you have problems with your service and your product offerings—these problems would probably preclude capturing new customers anyway. (These efforts can all be categorized under the heading of marketing, which includes identifying the requirements and desires of your customers and then ensuring that the products and delivery of services are meeting the needs of the customer—see Chapter 18.)

Getting things right with your current customer base is an important first step. Who is your current customer base? First, of course, are the patients you serve. While some patients are passive and go where referring clinicians instruct them to go for imaging, an increasingly large segment of the patient population is more discriminating and will actively select an imaging service based on what they have heard and what they have experienced. This trend in patients taking greater ownership of their health care creates an opportunity for your practice because these patients will return to you if they have had a sufficiently good experience. And if they are happy enough with their experience, they may even recommend you to your friends or to their doctors.

The second critical part of your customer base is the referring providers. These may include PAs and nurse practitioners as well as family practitioners. And they run the full gamut of subspecialists, some of whom are large consumers of imaging services (neurologists), to others who rarely refer (dermatologists). A wise imaging practice does not fail to consider chiropractors, podiatrists, and rehab therapists as customers as well (Box 17-1). Again, a very satisfied referring provider will not only send a steady stream of business but also will advocate on your behalf (Table 17-1).

Satisfied customers are a valuable asset in three ways. First, they are loyal. If you survey your physician and patient customers using a scale of 1 to 5 (5 is high) for their rating of satisfaction with your service, those who give you a score of 3 may return but could be dissuaded by your competition. Those who give you a score of 4 almost certainly will return. A score of 5 guarantees return and guarantees that no competitor could pull them away (see Table 17-1). They may even help to grow your business by telling their friends about their fantastic experience at your facility, effectively serving as an unpaid marketing division. Thus, the second way a satisfied customer is valuable is that they spread the good word about your business. A customer who gives your imaging center a score of 4 will give a good recommendation if asked. A customer who gives you a score of 5 will beat the drum for you and drag their family and friends into your imaging center. The third way they are a valuable asset is cost. Keeping current customers takes about 25% fewer marketing dollars than capturing new customers.[2]

So how do you drive your customer satisfaction scores from 3 up to 5 (understanding that if you get a score of 1 or 2 in a competitive market, those customers, be they patients or physicians, often will not return to you)? The answer is twofold: (1) clear bidirectional communication with your customers, and (2) rapid effective response to what you learn from them through this bidirectional communication. You need to begin by setting up communication conduits. This means having a physician liaison who can take your "message" out to physician customers and then bring back information from them. That liaison needs to be a great talker and a great listener, and he or she needs to go into offices armed with a bevy

BOX 17-1

Who Are Your Customers?

The "Paying" Customers

Patients
  Passive: Go where they are told
  Active: Go where they perceive good
    service
    Internet users
    Technologically knowledgeable
    Time constrained
    Demand the best
    Come back to good service
    Tell their friends and doctor

Referring Physicians
  Primary care
  Specialists
    Heavy users
      Orthopedics
      Neurology/neurosurgery
      Oncology
      General surgery
      ENT
      Pulmonary
      Nephrology/urology
      GYN/OB
      Rehab medicine
      Internal medicine
      GI
      ER/emergency medicine
      Sports medicine
    Not-so-heavy users
      Psychiatry
      Dermatology
      Cardiology
      Plastic/cosmetic surgery
    Nonphysician providers
      Chiropractors
      Podiatrists
      Nurse practitioners, PAs, nurse
        midwives
      Rehab/occupational therapists
      Employee health programs

The "Nonpaying" Customers

Your employees
Affiliated and nonaffiliated hospitals
Large clinics and multispecialty group
  practices
Payers—insurance and government
Large employers and industries
The general public (future patients)

Table 17-1 Customer Satisfaction Survey: Scoring Schema

Score	Descriptor	Subsequent Behavior
1	Very dissatisfied	Will not return; advises others to avoid
2	Dissatisfied	Will not return
3	Neutral	Indifferent; can be lured away
4	Satisfied; good experience	May return; recommends if asked
5	Very satisfied; impressed	Always returns; recommends you

of communication tools, such as brochures about your specific services, order sheets, Rolodex cards, pens with your scheduling number embossed on them, and educational materials. The physician liaison should visit most referring offices regularly, and should be the type of person who is welcomed by the office staff. Whenever the physician liaison hears from any customer about an aspect of service that is less than great, he or she should rush the news back to you and you should initiate a fix of the problem. A substantial component of a physician liaison's salary (40%) should be tied to practice growth (i.e., both retention of current customers as well as adding new customers). Incentivization tied to growth is a powerful driver of performance for the liaison.

Another communication conduit is the formal, written survey given to physicians and patients to fill out: it should be concise and specific (so that it is convenient and quick to complete). The survey should be clear that its purpose is to improve customer service: it should always end with "Would you recommend our service to your family or friends?" Surveys should be repeated as often as possible without becoming an annoyance, and results should be tracked over time. Fill rate (i.e., percentage of responders filling out surveys) is one metric to ensure you are not overdoing it: specifically, a drop in the percentage of responders who fill out a survey is a sign that the surveys have exceeded "tolerable frequency."

Read these surveys closely for new ideas, especially the "Specific Comments" sections. Survey results and trends should be reported to everyone in your organization; they can become a powerful driver toward great service across your whole organization. Survey results can reinforce a culture of "full-time marketing" by everyone on your team. To improve your satisfaction scores, you must respond effectively to what you learn from the surveys and by being in touch with your customers. Seemingly trivial issues can be critical discriminators. For example, parking must be free (or cheaper than the competition), plentiful, and convenient. Navigation to and within your facility must be simple and direct. Cleanliness and a pleasant "eyewash" appearance of the facility are more important than we would like to admit. Friendly, supportive professionalism on the part of all personnel encountered by any customer is an absolute must. Same-day or next-day access to any imaging modality at the patient's convenience is critical. Easy, hassle-free scheduling, preferably computer-based or with Web-based order entry, is very powerful (Box 17-2). After you have mastered these relatively simple issues, only then do more complex ones such as quality of interpretation, swiftness of reports, image availability, and level of technological sophistication become relevant (Box 17-3).[3] If you hear any complaints about any of these service issues (simple or complex) or get satisfaction scores below 4 when asked about them specifically, you must initiate changes to improve these issues swiftly and effectively. Your goal should be to astonish the customer with your service. After an appropriate interval, go back to the source—the customers—and ask if they have perceived a substantial improvement in service. Inquire, survey, iterate, and inquire again.

Outbound communication from your practice to your existing physician and patient customers usually takes four forms: newsletters, educational material, public relations media, and advertisements. All are important. Newsletters not only keep your physician customers up to date on your offerings and recent

---

BOX 17-2

Critical Service Discriminators We Hate to Acknowledge (Because They Don't Involve How Medically Smart We Are)

Convenient facility location
  Right off the freeway (easy access)
  Near providers' offices or hospitals
  Minimal traffic congestion

Parking
  Needs to be free or nearly free
  Lots of it, preferably indoors
  Near the front door
  No stairs

Facility "eyewash"
  Pleasant, warm, attractive décor
  Spotlessly clean (successful sniff test)
  Comfortable whether sitting or standing
  Upbeat without being too opulent

Facility function
  Easy navigation, good signage, clear directions
  Plenty of changing and waiting areas
  Appropriate temperature
  Modesty and privacy absolute

Interactions with personnel
  Every employee must focus on every patient as unique
  Every interaction is pleasant and supportive
  Change the duties of or fire the rude or brusk employee
  Last question: "Is there anything else I can do for you?"

Scheduling
  Same day or next day for every modality
  Walk-ins and add-ons accommodated
  Every call answered before the third ring by a trained scheduler
  One call to complete the scheduling process
  Strong support for preauthorization
  "What to expect" preps, directions, and instructions faxed or online
  Reminder call the day before
  Computerized order entry whenever possible

Price
  Be neither the cheapest nor the most expensive
  Have a mechanism to handle the underinsured and uninsured

"Day after" call
  Staff calls patient to ask how things went, if patient has any questions or any problems

Critical Service Discriminators We Know and Love (Because They Are Close to Our Hearts)

Value-added quality of interpretation
  Did you answer the clinician's question?
  Recommendations for further investigations
    or action
  Correlation with other imaging and with
    clinical information

Rapid report availability
  Measured in minutes or hours, less than
    24 hours
  Correlated with clinical practice needs
    15 minutes if will support care
    Support same-visit diagnosis and
      therapy

Easy, quick image availability and review
  Hand carry the films back
  Great PACS placed in the high-volume
    referring provider's office
    Functionally intuitive PACS design
      supported by repetitive training
    User-friendly Web access for low-volume
      referrers
  Give film, CDs, and PACS access to any
    provider who might use
  Integrate with their medical record, EMR if
    available

Latest appropriate imaging technology
  Develop the perception and reality of being
    the technological leader
  Support efforts at appropriate use

Education
  Offer education about imaging at the site of
    patient service
  Speak and give talks wherever it will have an
    impact
  Participate in patient and public education

improvements, but they can contain very useful practice "pearls," which make them welcomed and read. An example would be the emerging ability of coronary CTA in determining which patients with chest pain have a coronary artery etiology. Newsletters need to be regularly distributed (even weekly) and can be in both paper and e-mail formats; they should invite responses and suggestions. Other educational materials or courses/lectures that improve appropriateness of use, work processes, or service quality establish your practice as reputable and put you on the high road. Public relations is a whole field unto itself, and should not be ignored or undervalued. A key news article in your local newspaper or a lecture about a new technology given by a radiologist at a community event can elevate awareness about your enterprise.

More traditional modes of advertising can get the word out about your new technology, your level of service, how to access your offerings, and can raise your profile by creating a "buzz." The many forms of advertising include mailed brochures, open houses, radio/TV spots, local magazine or newspaper ads, and news items in all media. All advertising should be viewed as an expenditure, and the return on investment should be closely tracked.[4] To accomplish this, any new business must be tracked to the advertisement that stimulated it. If advertising is modality-specific (e.g., a new PET/CT service), you can use your RIS (radiology information system) to track case volume changes from existing providers in addition to tracking new referring providers, as these temporally relate to the advertising. More generally, each advertisement must have embedded in it a mechanism that reveals to you the specific customers which that advertisement brought in. For example, the reply or scheduling phone number can be unique to that advertisement and thus be tracked. Or a specific call to action can be included in the advertisement ("ask about our free Internet mammogram reminder program"), which reveals the source ad. There might be a free parking coupon (numbered, thus able to track) included in a mailing, or a coupon for free educational materials such as breast self-examination instructions or facts about colon cancer screening. The call to action in the advertisement might invite a visit to a unique website for information or to initiate scheduling (Box 17-4). Advertising is effective communication, which helps retain your current customers, with a positive and documentable return on investment.

BOX 17-4

Ways to Track Results from a Specific Advertising Initiative

Track case volume change temporally related to advertising
Use your RIS
More business from existing referring providers
New referring providers identified

Imbed a cue tied to that advertising
Unique phone number for questions or scheduling placed in ad
Unique website address for information or initiating scheduling in ad
Coupons unique to ad
Free parking
Free educational materials
Discounts or "two for one"
Specific call to action in ad
"Ask about our . . ."

Growth: Adding New Customers

Practice growth results from the powerful combination of keeping your current customers while adding new ones. Once you are effectively retaining your current customers and getting those high survey satisfaction scores from them, your ability to identify and attract new customers goes up sharply. With new physician customers, the first challenge is finding regions or specialties you might want to target, where they are, and who they might be. Once you have identified potential new customers, the second challenge is "flipping" them over to using your imaging organization, away from their entrenched referral patterns. And the third challenge—as with your current customers—is retaining those new customers by iteratively discovering the high level of tailored service that makes them very satisfied (what drives them to a satisfaction score of 5).

How do you find out who and where are the new customers? It is true that every practice group will probably want to serve a portion of poorer patients as a part of good community service. Our imaging skills and technology are

---

BOX 17-5

Strategies for Identifying New Imaging Business Opportunities

Find underserved areas
Map population distribution and density in proposed service area
Map existing imaging facilities by modality and "perimeters of service"—1, 5, 10, 20 miles

Medicare payer data is helpful
Compare population density with available imaging capacity looking for gaps in coverage
Map density of high-volume referring physicians versus locally available imaging capacity
List communities by population versus nearby imaging capacity and compare to national per capita use averages by modality (available from specific equipment manufacturers)

Find well-served areas with weaker competitors
Target survey referring staff of specific hospitals and imaging centers about service quality and satisfaction
Target advertise to specific well-served market areas with response cues embedded in advertising (see Table 17-5)
Physician liaison visits to offices in specific referral areas
Stay tuned to the "buzz on the street"

---

too important to health to be restricted. However, although the less affluent patients can also be profitable, the greatest likelihood of a strong return on investment are the affluent or well-insured customers. They will ultimately generate revenue to maintain your mission of serving the underserved. Thus, it is this segment of the population that should be the new patient target.

So how do you identify such populations of potential new patients and the physicians who might refer them? There are two techniques: first, locate areas underserved by existing imaging enterprises, and second, compete more effectively in well-served areas (Box 17-5). Locating underserved areas for imaging often requires engaging market analysis consultants, but some identification can be done on your own. "Average" per capita use of imaging services by modality can be obtained from Medicare and insurance data and segmented by area incomes, real estate valuations, zip codes, townships, and so forth. Often such data are available from imaging equipment manufacturers. This "need for services" use data can then be compared with available imaging capacity by modality and by locality within various distances—typically 5, 10, and 20 miles. Relatively underserved areas can be thus identified and further compared to referring physician office density (by subspecialty) in the same areas. A great discovery would be a relatively affluent, well-insured population, which is underserved per capita for CT and MR within a 20-mile radius and has a locally high density of the type of physician specialists who typically refer for those imaging exams. In today's world that would be a rare find, but lesser degrees of new business potential are not infrequently uncovered by such techniques. Once an "opportunity" underserved area is identified, you have two options. Either place an imaging center there locally (if potential demand makes a viable business plan possible on the capital investment) or target that area for your advertising, for visits by your physician liaison, and for all your other marketing activities, such as directing the new business to your existing facilities. Alternatively, assessing the market with the installation of a mobile scanner may be an easily reversed option; it can be maintained either as a long-term solution or to gather additional data on market potential.

You should also look for new imaging business from areas which are better served in terms of the match between imaging capacity and imaging use by that population. Not every hospital or imaging center is paying close attention to physician and patient customer satisfaction or to customer needs. (But you will be after reading this chapter!) Searching out markets in which customer loyalty or satisfaction is not high can be very rewarding for your business. Sources of such information might include your own surveys, word of mouth, inquiries made by your physician liaison, or discussions with your existing customer base located in those areas. Even imaging centers or hospitals that provide good service may

have a segment of unhappy or dissatisfied customers—advertising to your competitors' customers can produce new customers for you, especially if you are paying close attention to service satisfiers. Remember also the adage that surveying the people who are *not* coming to your facility may be more valuable than surveying those who are, since the former may provide more frank, worthwhile critiques.

Any time a patient comes to you from a new referring physician who has not previously sent business your way, it is very important that your database quickly identify that new physician so you can follow up to measure satisfaction, and give attention to and offer your marketing tools to him or her right away. Your physician liaison should be in that new referring physician's office the next day, starting a new relationship by making sure everything went well with the patient encounter. Your attention to service needs should delight the new referring physician and you should be very convincing that you're in the imaging business to support the business of the physician's practice and work processes. It helps too if you can convince and make clear to the client that you are using imaging as a tool but your goal is to support the health of his or her patients. Your means is imaging; your end is improved health care.

Fortunately, in both the underserved and well-served markets, growth of outpatient imaging nationally has been substantial and steady over the past five years, running roughly twice that of inflation. Much of that growth has been driven by the high utility of definitive and timely imaging diagnostic information in medical practice. Whether incremental imaging costs result in net savings in health care delivery is actively being investigated. Notably, the Deficit Reduction Act has led to concerns that the growth in imaging will not be sustained. Rather than lessening the use, which remains debated, it is clear that there will be increasing efforts at providing imaging in more efficient and cost-effective ways.

Most new patients choose an imaging facility based first on where their provider sends them, then on location, and then on reputation (Table 17-2).[3] Only after all of that do they

Table 17-2 Why Patients Choose an Imaging Facility (What really matters to them...)

Issue	Percent Who Mention as Important
Referring physician preference	58%
Location	38%
Reputation	38%
Insurance accepted	21%
Technology	18%
Word of mouth	8%

Adapted from Riskind P: Using service metrics in outpatient imaging to optimize your practice. Presented at American Roentgen Ray Society Annual Meeting, Vancouver, BC, 2006.

Table 17-3 Why Referring Providers Recommend an Imaging Facility

Issue	Percent Who Mention as Important
Quality of interpretations	92%
Ease of scheduling	70%
Turnaround time of reports	68%
Insurance accepted	62%
Location	60%
Relationship with radiologists	57%
Hours of service	53%
Reputation	40%
Friendliness of staff	38%

Adapted from Riskind P: Using service metrics in outpatient imaging to optimize your practice. Presented at American Roentgen Ray Society Annual Meeting, Vancouver, BC, 2006.

consider whether their insurance is accepted, level of technology, and ease of scheduling. In the absence of the referring physician having an equity stake in an imaging center, referring physicians choose an imaging facility based overwhelmingly on the quality of interpretation (Table 17-3).[3] Their lesser choice factors, like those for the patients, are ease of scheduling and acceptance of insurance plans, and also relationships with the radiologists, report turnaround time, location, hours of service, and responsiveness of staff. These choice factors employed by patients and by referring physicians are those on which you should prioritize your efforts at service improvement.

In an article about creating competitive advantage for an imaging center, Patricia Riskind talks about the importance of the "What's next?" attitude.[5] Organizations need to avoid complacency and to stay ahead by constantly looking for new directions and anticipating new challenges, asking, "What's next?" This attitude may involve decisions to offer new technology sooner than the competition. It also involves measuring and anticipating any changes in both physician and patient customer expectations. And it means staying very aware of moves by your competition. Repeat customers are especially influenced by a reputation of those practices that stay out in front of change. Be at the "bleeding" or "leading" edge!

So, once you have sought new business for your existing services (modalities) from underserved areas, and have sought new business from being more competitive in well-served areas, what's next for further growth? The answer is: Come up with new services. These new imaging services can be offered to your existing customer base and to new customers, broadening your footprint in your market. An example of a new, more competitive service might include annual breast imaging evaluations in which final results are available the same day. This means giving results (verbally or in writing) the same day for negative mammograms and offering same-day definitive workup (additional views, ultrasound, MR, biopsy) for positive mammograms. Another example of a new service is cardiac CT. You might develop the ability to offer definitive workup of atypical chest pain or of multirisk patients with same-day reports and recommendations to their primary care providers. Targeting these providers—not cardiologists—may prove more fruitful in that "turf wars" are avoided. Also, keeping the control of the patients in the hands of the PCPs is considered an advantage, not to mention collegial. With this approach, you can help these providers sort through clinically difficult and potentially dangerous problems in a definitive, rapid, and appropriate way. They won't lose the patients to follow up to the cardiologists. Both the providers and their patients like that a lot. Yet another new service could be the use of your existing IT infrastructure to get Web PACS images and reports onto the office PC of any referring physician within one to two hours of an imaging exam. This approach dramatically improves the work flow in the referring offices because the patient can come back to them (straight from your imaging center) for a decision about therapy in the same day. In an era in which many practitioners try to see four to six patients per hour, this rapid, convenient desktop access to definitive diagnostic imaging information is powerful support for their productivity. It can be a key element in your efforts to alter entrenched referral patterns.

The other extremely powerful IT initiative for your imaging enterprise is a highly functional, well-developed website. A great website is not only a convenience for current customers (scheduling, patient information, educational information for patients and physicians, etc.), but it can support development of new business by serving as the source where your advertising directs potential customers for more in-depth information about you and your service offerings. This is where your health care philosophy and your business focus can be detailed in depth to educate potential new customers and help convince them to convert to your service. Your website can be loaded with links to educational materials, to your newsletters, to descriptions of your facilities and expertise. Your website must be updated regularly and its impact must be refined by iterative testing. The key words in your website should be chosen based on what search engines are likely to be looking for; an Internet consultant can help with this process of keyword selection.

Your website also can include survey questions for physicians and patients, tabulating and reporting the results to you in real time. This is also where you state your mission, your goals, your focus on excellence of service, and your branded message. And this is one place where you place your call to action: "Give us a try, call our scheduling number, call our physician liaison or our radiologists, call our IT section to try our PACS in your office."

New radiology services can go beyond diagnosis and include therapy. Vein ablations, biopsies, stent placement, fibroid embolization, cryotherapy, high-frequency ultrasound—all are new and may be very cost effective. Joining with other specialties can help offerings of additional new therapies: Radiofrequency ablation of superficial liver lesions, ultrasound-guided cryotherapy of the prostate, even left atrial ablation using 3D CT guidance. It is important to provide information to customers about impending diagnostic imaging technology to immediately capitalize on competitive advantage. If a challenging case arrives prior to complete mastery of the diagnostic procedure, a consultation with colleagues can be obtained so that excellence in care is maintained. However, with new therapeutic procedures, it is important not to advertise new services until radiologists are well versed and comfortable with those new procedures. When they are fully ready to offer the new therapy, then capitalize on your group or hospital branding and on your good relationships with referring physicians to kick off the introduction. If you hire a new radiologist with a new skill set, use that opportunity to announce the new service provided at your facility, be it diagnostic or therapeutic. As with all marketing efforts, most imaging center growth is centered around relationships. To grow referrals, administrators invest in equipment and ensure resources needed for ease of scheduling; radiologists invest in quality and relationships.

Regardless of the types of new diagnostic or therapeutic services that you begin to offer to grow your business, all must be supported by an integrated, vigorous advertising campaign that both gets the word out in your community and also builds a perception of you as the dynamic, impactful, supportive, efficacious, leading-edge imaging enterprise focused on service in your medical community. This is your branding and all your advertising supports your brand awareness. Your branding is a service promise that you must make and keep.[6] In this sense, "marketing is in everything you do," because your ability to keep your service promise is impacted by your hiring, training of personnel, purchase of equipment, the architecture of your facility, IT functionality, the knowledge of your radiologists, business office, coding/billings/collections, and the character of your interpersonal interactions at all levels. Keeping and exceeding your service promise creates your branding. With your branding as a key tool, you can seek new markets with a good chance of success.

Your advertising needs to be regular, repeated, integrated, easily recognized, well designed, quick to understand, ethical, and broad in distribution among targeted audiences. While you and your physician liaison can drive the advertising campaign, help from advertising and graphics consultants is essential. It is easy to be penny-wise and pound-foolish with advertising dollars, that is, it's easy to underinvest. Anywhere from 4% to 10% of your gross income should be committed to advertising.[7] The goals of your advertising should be established first (Box 17-6) and an impact on income estimated if the goals are reached. Only then is a budget chosen which is large enough to have a good chance of meeting your advertising goals and is sized proportional to the potential return. A multiplier of 5 is not uncommon for marketing dollars; thus, for example, if you project that you can increase your profit by $100,000 through meeting a specific advertising goal, consider

spending at least $20,000 on advertising to get there.

It is essential to quantitatively measure the financial impact of your advertising, so you know the specific return on the investment you have made, and thus can iteratively tailor

---

BOX 17-6

Some Examples of Specific Advertising Goals

Increase MR exams from 2500 to 4000 exams per year
  The drive to full capacity

Increase awareness of appropriate new indications for cardiac CT
  Begin a new program that will grow over time
  Early prominence grabs large market share

Create a new image of technological leadership
  Splash advertise every new cutting-edge machine
  Build perception of leadership over time

Target female patients (medical decision makers for the family)
  Broadcast a full range of breast imaging services
  Advertise specific skills in obstetrical ultrasound (especially high risk)
  Highlight a full range of gynecological imaging at the highest technology level

Grow PET/CT exam volume at an annualized rate of 35%
  Build relationships with and service levels to oncologists

Increase local CT market share from 18% to 30%
  Plenty of available slots
  Latest isotropic technology

Advertise your focus on the specific services providers want
  Cite ease of your scheduling and computerized order entry
  Your great PACS
  Preauthorization support
  Subspecialized radiologists

---

an advertising campaign over time toward the greatest support of your incremental service improvement and growth.[8] If you do not measure the impact of your advertising, you stand a good chance of wasting a lot of money. How to measure the specific dollar impact of your advertising is covered in a number of good marketing texts.[8,9] The most effective advertising is targeted and is not broad in spectrum. For imaging enterprises, advertising should be aimed not only at specific subspecialties of referring physicians, but also at patients and their families, contracting entities (hospitals, employers, payers), advocacy groups (heart disease or cancer or women's health, etc.), and even at your own employees. Your advertising needs to state clearly what imaging services you offer and why you are special and different from your competition. You might even list what you offer and what the competition does not (e.g., subspecialized, fellowship-trained radiologists, same-day appointments, reports in under four hours, all insurances accepted, multiple locations of service, evening and weekend hours available). Advertising should position you as the premier purveyor of quality and of appropriately advanced technology; it should state the level of service you offer in some detail and how that service is driven by your mission. Price is usually not a central issue, but stating that you take various types of insurance, are recognized by HMOs or employer plans, or even that you accept credit cards might help. Emphasize your value to the customer; for example, you provide rapid reports, education, knowledgeable consultations, PACS transfer of images, no waits for patients, free parking, on-time exams. Such value is powerfully persuasive and goes a long way toward making your competition less relevant in your market.

CONCLUSION

So now you have done it all. Because you chose to go after growth, you first improved your product line and service, guided by information from your patient and physician surveys. Since your team members were highly motivated to do a better job by growing the business and thus improving survey scores, they too worked together to come up with ideas and suggestions about how to better serve your existing customers. You have built up your imaging capacity in each modality so it is 15% greater than your current demand; as a result, you can always say yes to a request for same-day service and you still have room to grow. Your scheduling is quick, effortless, and pleasant—even computer based. Your parking is ample, close at hand, and free or inexpensive. Navigation to and from your facility is no problem. Patients get easy-to-understand instructions every time on their exam prep, on what to expect during their exams, and on how to find you. When they arrive at your facility, patients see an attractive, immaculately clean, and smoothly operating department staffed by cheerful, skilled employees who treat each patient as unique and special. Referring physicians marvel at the swiftness of your reports and at being able quickly to view imagines on the PC in their own offices. They appreciate your guidance on the appropriateness of exams and your subspecialized interpretive skills for the need for follow-up studies. You have succeeded in the drive to a score of 5 on your satisfaction surveys from both patients and referring physicians. Your customers are amazed by your service.

Now that you have secured your current customer base, you are ready to go out after new markets. Your attractive, informative, repetitive advertising campaign uses several media and targets your current customers plus wisely selected new markets. You use consultants to help you analyze new opportunities, new market localities, new services, and to create new advertising. You are able quickly to detect changes in your market environment and changes by your competitors and to respond effectively to those changes. As your business increases, you have an even more positive impact on the quality of health care in your community. Your political and economic clout increases and you are viewed as leading the move toward quality and cost effectiveness. You will wisely use your new influence to increase your focus on service. You are changing, your imaging organization is getting stronger, your future is a bit more secure, so—inevitably—you will grow.

Dos and Don'ts of Assessing Growth Opportunities	
Dos	**Don'ts**
1. Create concise reports that answer the clinical question, offer recommendations, and show your subspecialty expertise. 2. Provide report turnaround in one to three hours. Call in unexpected positive findings immediately. 3. Provide same-day imaging every time it is requested, or, at the latest, by the next day or at the patient's convenience. 4. Inculcate a culture of friendly, supportive service in every employee. "Is there anything else I can do for you?" Everyone "owns" the customer satisfaction scores. 5. Develop a targeted multimedia marketing campaign guided by your physician liaison. Track results and return on investment. 6. Choose new growth opportunities carefully after in-depth research of your market. Use consultants. 7. Be consistently the first or nearly the first to introduce appropriate new technology. 8. Survey, survey, survey. Know how your patient and physician customers see you. Fix the problems they report. 9. Pay attention to your facility—easy access, spotlessly clean, comfortable, pleasant "eyewash." 10. Make your scheduling quick, pleasant, and supportive—a knowledgeable person always answers before the third ring.	1. Ignore the maxim: "Radiology is about relationships—with providers." 2. Have too few schedulers with too little training, performing time-consuming scheduling on a cumbersome phone system. 3. Accept a goal of 24-hour report availability, irrespective of your providers' practice needs. 4. Have a different generalist radiologist in every seat every day (i.e., no "ownership"). 5. Fail to inculcate courtesy and focus on service into every employee. 6. Accept scheduling backlog due to scanner or staff shortages, or inadequate imaging capacity for local demand. 7. Maintain a facility location far from the concentration of referring providers or hard to access. 8. Fail to develop strong IT support of user-friendly PACS and RIS, located in referring providers' offices. 9. Underfund your advertising budget. 10. Neglect the small details: parking, facility navigation, facility cleanliness, "eyewash," attention to courtesy, privacy.

REFERENCES

1. Stewart TA: Growth as a process: HBR interview with Jeffrey R. Immelt. Harvard Business Review 84:60–70, 2006.
2. Scott M: The art of Woo. Radiology Today 5:4–20, 2004.
3. Riskind P: Using service metrics in outpatient imaging to optimize your practice. Presented at American Roentgen Ray Society Annual Meeting, Vancouver, BC, 2006.
4. Stevens M: Your marketing sucks. New York, Crown Business, 2003, p 49.
5. Riskind P, Foreman MS: Game on: Creating competitive advantages. Radiology Management (July–August): 44–48, 2004.

6. Scott M: Marketing's ever-growing role at hospitals: It's not like it used to be. Radiology Today 6:17, 2004.
7. Meyeroff W: Enhancing your imaging image. Medical Imaging (December 2005), pp 1–10.
8. Stevens M: Your marketing sucks. New York, Crown Business, 2003, p 126.
9. Levinson JC: Guerilla Marketing. Boston, Houghton Mifflin, 1998, pp 8–16.
10. Sexton D: Financial analysis for smart marketing decisions, in Marketing 101. Hoboken, NJ, Wiley.

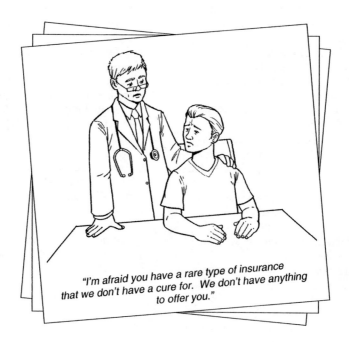

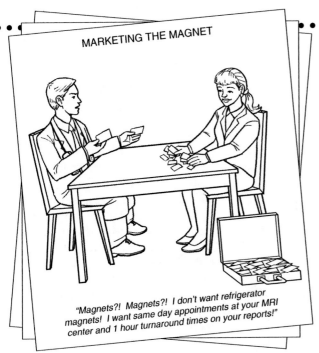

CHAPTER 18

MARKETING THE MAGNET

"Magnets?! Magnets?! I don't want refrigerator magnets! I want same day appointments at your MRI center and 1 hour turnaround times on your reports!"

Marketing

Joseph Robinson and Dennis Condon

INTRODUCTION

The goal of this chapter is to stimulate your thinking, give you some practical tools, and help assure your success as a radiologist in an outpatient imaging center business venture. There are a few things that are critical to the success of any entrepreneurial endeavor, and some that are specific to medical imaging.

To grow a *profitable* business, every business needs to:

- Understand its market
- Be intimate with its customers
- Make smart capital investment decisions
- Control expenses

In addition, outpatient medical imaging needs to:

- Be a master of imaging technology
- Market unique medical expertise, education, and technology
- Focus on customer service

- Effectively use information technology (IT)
- Stay on the cutting edge, but be cautious of the "bleeding edge"

So, if you take away only one thing from this chapter it should be that your active engagement in planning and marketing of the practice and yourself is key to the center's success.

DO YOU NEED ANYTHING BEYOND MEDICAL EXPERTISE AND GREAT TECHNOLOGY?

The short answer is yes, and I can see many of you cringe as you think to yourself, "That's not what they told us in medical school or during my residency." You're right, and your expertise and the reputation you have managed to build up to this point in your career are the reasons why you should consider opening your own center or becoming a partner in an existing site. I don't discount expertise, but I know each of you can name a site somewhere that does not have the best reputation, often for a variety of reasons. You have also heard about the centers that are successful. How are they successful? How do they make that happen? Does it have to do with the right place and the right time? Perhaps, but although blind luck does sometimes happen, it cannot be the basis for a business plan that will raise the monies required to start your center and is certainly not a strategy for success.

Rise early, work hard, strike oil.

J. PAUL GETTY

The early bird catches the worm.

ANONYMOUS

Planning and hard work separate the winners from the losers in business. Planning includes:

- The hard work and preparation that went into your education.
- Researching and understanding the market where you want to open your center.
- Researching and understanding the direction of the technology you plan to put into your center.
- Selecting the right business people to help you get started (e.g., contractors, architects, finance experts, etc.).
- Developing a marketing plan *before* you open your center.

HOW MUCH DOES TECHNOLOGY MATTER?

Technology is important. For example, MRI (magnetic resonance imaging), molecular imaging, computer-aided diagnosis, 4D ultrasound, flat-plate detectors, liquid metal bearings, PACS (picture archiving and communication systems), RIS (radiology information systems), and redundant server technology are all examples of technology we know, and, as imaging professionals, love. Each year, technology advances enable us to redefine the practice of medicine in new and amazing ways. This has never been more the case. MR is making the move to "ultra high field"; CT is seeing tremendous growth based on new detector technology and faster computers. Molecular medicine, led by imaging, promises a new age

of treating and diagnosing disease. We can actually store images and reports together digitally and access them quickly to deliver better patient care. Roentgen may have started all of this in 1892 when he imaged his wife's hand, but we are now entering what I would consider a golden age of technology, that hasn't been seen since the early days of MR and CT.

However, you also have to be cautious not to get too caught up in the race for the latest in technology. The latest and greatest, without a demonstrable or at least a credible claim toward improved patient diagnosis or treatment, will be of no interest to your referring clinicians. How many of us got caught up in the CT slice war when fundamentally the only two jumps of significance may have been to isotropic voxels at 16 slice for optimizing volumetric reconstructions and 64 slice for cardiac imaging. The jump from 4 to 8 slice brought revenue to the local sales rep and more data to an ever-filling archive. If you don't plan on doing cardiac CT or have a significant volume issue to take care of, it doesn't matter to your customer if you have 16, 32, or 40 slice; it's all multislice to them. All those buzz words we love—phased array coils, multislice/multichannel, gradient echo imaging—do not mean the same to your customers (referring clinicians, etc.). What they want is the best diagnosis, fast. Technology does matter, but only to the extent that it can offer new applications that your customers understand and images that mean something to them clinically (Box 18-1).

You might be thinking, "This guy doesn't get it. Having the highest technology in the area *is* my marketing strategy." Having the "highest technology" can be a strategy, but it's an expensive one and short lived, as we have seen in the recent evolution of CT. The message is clear for the outpatient imaging owner: Don't spend your money on unproven or nonreimbursable technology. Invest in reliable, proven technology from a manufacturer that has:

- Good local service
- Robust remote diagnostics
- Open IT architecture (make them prove it; don't simply accept a DICOM conformance statement)
- A reasonable price

BOX 18-1

What Can Be Effective and Good Business?

- Solid, proven technology, like 1.5T MR. There is hardly a customer today that would not prefer MR performed at high field (≥1.0 Tesla), unless it cannot be tolerated.
- Multislice CT technology that is "field" upgradeable as you grow your business and reimbursement catches up.
- Flat-panel mammography with CAD. It is good medicine and your customers understand it as a differentiator.
- DR or CR for X-ray. It's vital for an electronic patient record.
- PET/CT if there is a need in your market.
- Ultrasound that enables 4-D imaging and is ergonomically designed for your operator.
- Outpatient interventional radiology.

neuroradiology, body imaging, musculoskeletal diagnostics) will matter most to the specialists within your market. Technology matters if you are perceived as "low tech" or behind the times by the referring community. However, there is a paradox in terms of what serves as excellence in quality, and service from the majority of your radiology customers' perspectives. As stated earlier, imaging services are typically treated as a commodity with implied adequacy of the product. Most of your customers do not have the time to understand the imaging technology nuances that radiologists get excited about. Again, what matters most is the level of customer service you offer to them and their patients. Customer service matters the most to the average primary care physician. Primary care physicians and specialists need to be targeted differently. This will be covered in more detail later.

The only unacceptable brand of equipment should be one that cannot interface with your IT network, and you should never limit yourself with proprietary vendors. Why does this matter to your marketing effort?

- Unreliable service means excessive, unplanned downtime—a "business killer." Turning away business because your equipment is down has the obvious short-term impact, but the long-term impact can be exponential when you lose referrals to your competition because you are not perceived as dependable by your customers.
- Bleeding-edge technology is a potential drain on your finances. Understand the difference between cutting-edge and bleeding-edge technology. The "cutting edge" brings newly emerging technology reliably into practice; "bleeding edge" technology can bring even more ground-breaking technology to bear but is not reliable in terms of consistent uptime. Also, bleeding-edge procedures often come to fruition prior to the approval of reimbursable codes. This can create an undue burden to boost volumes of reimbursable procedures to make up for the expense, *and* clog your schedule with exams that do not pay.

The opportunity to differentiate yourself technically or with specific expertise (e.g.,

WHAT SEPARATES THE WINNERS FROM THE LOSERS IN THE MARKETPLACE?

Timing, Skill, and Location

If you are the first imaging center in a given market you have a distinct advantage. You can establish referral patterns that will be hard to break. You have the opportunity to establish personal relationships in the community that will sustain your practice no matter who else enters the market.

There is also an advantage to "early adopt" reimbursable technology, such as PET-CT or computer-aided detection for mammography. Being the only game in town, even if initially, can foster the impression that yours is the only group that has the content expertise, even after other groups begin to offer the same service. As importantly, it can lead new groups of physicians to refer to your group. If you're getting your business right, this may be all the opportunity you need to earn their business across the spectrum of routine and cutting-edge services.

However, one note of caution: similar to "bleeding edge," "early adoption" is only an advantage if the marketing efforts of your practice are supported by the "white papers" of medical journal articles of the appropriate specialty. Virtual colonography, for example, has generated enthusiasm in specific markets, but broad adoption has been slow. This can be partially blamed on the spotty reimbursement, but it is also heavily influenced by gastroenterologists getting mixed reviews in the medical journals questioning how best to use the procedure. Should they start ordering it? When and what procedures could it replace? Imaging centers that felt they had to have the capability spent their money too early.

There are examples in various markets in which demand has been created. Demand creation can be done, but not by a radiology practice marketing group working alone. In short, bringing a service early to your market increases the odds of success.

Your Skill Matters

It's not just being the first into a market that will win the day; it's a combination of technology and the skill of your team to execute flawless implementation. The radiologist must be the leader and invest time through the relationships he or she has created in the referring community, academic affiliations, and local payers to make it happen. You need to make a decision and a commitment to establish a team if you are going down that road. If you aren't willing to invest in the right people with the right resources, this strategy will no doubt fail.

Location—How to Choose?

Your own domain market knowledge can be the most valuable starting point when choosing your location. You know based on your experience in the area that community "X" has to send their entire outpatient imaging 30 minutes down the road to community "Z." You feel that patients and referring physicians in community X would prefer to stay local and maybe have access to some services that the imaging center in community Z does not offer. Great place to start, but banks don't like to make loans on thoughts and feelings; they like data. Depending on the market, there can be simple

ways to get the data, but sometimes more complex methods are required. Let's start with the simple ones:

- Local phonebooks will list imaging centers and potential referring physicians in communities X and Z. It's easy and free. There are also databases available for sale such as local state chapters, local physicians' directories for your area, or Verispan.
- Maps or a simple map program, such as Microsoft MapPoint, can be used to lay out where the competition is located, showing patients how far they need to travel to get to community Z, such as listing access roads for your potential center. A good, experienced commercial real estate broker can find you what you need. For example, you can explain to them that you need 10,000 square feet of space, preferably on grade, in a medical office building, in community X. Ideally, the building should be occupied by primary care physicians and high-value specialties such as orthopedics and neurologists.

When you have found a potential location based on your requirements, get out and knock on doors. Talk with the physicians in the community—this will also support your marketing plan that we will discuss later—and ask them:

- Where do they send their imaging today?
- What kind of imaging exams do they order?
- What do they need from a radiologist?
- What volumes do they refer weekly?
- What would be important to them in a local imaging center?
- What do their patients need?
- Would they support you if you opened a new center in the area? (Very important question!)

If they are supportive, ask them for a simple, nonbinding note on their letterhead stating that they are supportive of a new center and there is a need in the area. This can be a great piece for your overall business plan when you go to banks, and it creates a sense of buy-in on the part of the local physicians. Based on the data you've collected, you can make an intelligent, informed decision on your location that will have a high probability of success.

SELLING VERSUS MARKETING— WHAT'S THE DIFFERENCE?

A simple way to think about the difference is this:

Selling is asking for and/or representing your business in a personal manner. Sales executes the plan by converting prospects into clients. Marketing is the tools and direction for your business success; marketing tells a sales department and/or business where to go and what to say.

Many people view selling and marketing as the same thing; it is not. First, there's a myth about selling that should be cleared up. Many physicians view selling as an activity they do not engage in. It is perhaps one of the reasons they became doctors. But the reality is that in most doctors' everyday life, they are selling something, that is, themselves, a special interest, a diagnosis, and so forth. If you can gain an understanding that selling goes on beyond retail stores and car lots, then you have made a giant step toward embracing your role in the sales activity of your outpatient center or practice. Selling can and does take many forms. It is certainly what goes on in consumer businesses around the world every day (Box 18-2).

Representing Your Business

This can be as simple as being an "ambassador" for the practice; project what you want people to think about you and your practice. For example:

- Are you easy to talk with?
- Are you prompt in returning phone calls?
- Do you project a sense of caring for patients and referring physicians and their problems and issues?
- Do you understand their problems and issues?

BOX 18-2

Selling Is . . .

- Representing your business.
- Direct and indirect communication with your customers.
- Asking for commitments.

If you take the time to communicate directly with patients, referring physicians, and your staff, show you care about their problems and are approachable internally and externally, you are being a good "ambassador" of your business. If you stop and think about it for a moment, are these not the characteristics you like in the people you do business with on any level, such as your accountant, local mechanic, or hospital administrator? They may not meet all the standards you set, but you know when they do and you want to continue to do business with them, because you like or respect them and you feel that respect is mutual.

Direct and Indirect Communication with Your Customers

The customers with whom you want to have direct as well as indirect communication include:

- Patients
- Referring physicians
- Payers
- Health care administrators

The first lesson is to communicate directly; there is no substitute for picking up the phone, or having a live interaction. Most people love live contact, and it can be a unique differentiator! Do not rely solely on e-mail, which is impersonal and too often fraught with misunderstanding because inflections cannot be properly understood or defined and response times are often inadequate. It can, however, be difficult to directly communicate as frequently as you would like, so sometimes indirect communication must be used. Included in this category are:

- Patient reports
- E-mail
- Advertising
- Letter correspondence

Answer these questions before communicating. Do your reports reflect an understanding of the patient and the referring physician? What messages do you want to send within your e-mail, or deliver in your advertising mailings, or correspondence?

Each one of these communication points is an opportunity to sell. Opportunities cost time and money; therefore, they need to make an impact. Talk to patients whenever possible, understand and incorporate what the orthopedic surgeon needs to see in his or her report. When you do these simple things, you are selling! And the great part is that most of these efforts will also make you more effective as a physician. Internalize the golden rule of sales that says:

All things being equal, people will do business with, and refer business to, those people they know, like and trust.

BOB BURG

Asking for Commitments

Ok, some readers may be thinking, "I could maybe do the other things listed above, but asking for commitments? That's what used car salesmen do." So how do you ask for a commitment, and from whom should you get it?

I have always found that the best way is simple and direct. For example, "Dr. Neurosurgeon, I understand, based on our conversation, that it takes the local hospital five days to get your reports and they do not always tell you everything you need to know and often the films get lost. . . . If I could get your patients' films and reports delivered to your office electronically within 24 hours of the exam, could I depend on you to send me more of your patients?" Or, a little less direct, but a similar message, "I know you told me the hospital does not get reports out for five days. At Beautiful Day Imaging, I can get you films *and* reports in 24 hours. Will you give us a try?"

As you can see, you can be as direct or as soft as you like, but ultimately you are asking for at least a minimal commitment. No one expects that you or anyone else will put up a nice center, offering high technology and personal service, without needing to have patient volume that will support the commitment; they won't be offended when you ask.

The marketing department should produce collateral—brochures or pamphlets showcasing your practice—and other advertising, but if that is all you have them do, you are not taking advantage of the power they can provide. Marketing should use internal data, such as billing systems information, to analyze what's working and where the holes exist.

Scenario: Your marketing team analyzes your referring physician information and points out to you that most of your MR business is coming from only two neurology groups, even though there are four neurology groups in your area and three orthopedic groups in town. Based on this information, you may determine a need for a collateral piece, such as a one-page summary of *your* expertise, and the technology that supports you, with specific images. The marketing department should also be working with the sales team to understand what you are doing well with the two neurology groups who *are* referring, and carry that message to the other two neurology groups in town who are not.

You, as the physician practice builder, should understand this as well. Make personal contact with those not referring to you and use the information that marketing/sales has learned from customers when you call or visit.

Scenario: Marketing may have learned that there will be an opportunity with PET reimbursement in diagnosing Alzheimer's disease. This makes neuro PET imaging a target for growth. Include the use of PET for Alzheimer's disease and your group's expertise as part of your discussions with the neurologists.

Marketing can and should be measuring and analyzing your market and results. They should also be using any available external data to understand what your market is doing; this could be regulatory information and market share data from independent firms or information about the market in general that can be gleaned from payers. Think long and hard before investing in any activity that cannot be measured and tracked. In the above scenarios for MR and PET, you have used marketing to increase your referrals.

Should You Be Doing Both Marketing and Sales?

Yes, but that does not mean that you need to have more than one person doing both when you are getting started. Ideally, everyone in your practice should be selling:

- To patients, through fast, friendly service and a pleasant environment

- To referring physicians, through office sales calls with a dedicated salesperson
- Through you, the radiologist, with phone calls and live visits
- Through a site manager who should be involved directly in the sales process, as well as with live referring physician calls, and ensuring operational excellence at your site

On the marketing side, someone needs to produce collateral for distribution to referring physician offices and your own office directly to patients. The goal is to generate prospects. The collateral should be focused on the values you want your center to represent:

- Outstanding service
- State-of-the-art technology
- Physician quality
- Research
- Contributing to the health of the community and/or offering unique services not available at hospitals or other imaging centers
- Your specific training and experience
- Fellowships
- Hospital/academic center affiliations
- Research and/or clinical trial engagements
- Recognition that your center (or an individual at your center) has received for clinical excellence or quality focus

Remember, you and the technology can be key differentiators for the practice. Do not downplay what differentiates you. For example, an academic-affiliated center should market subspecialty readings and leveraging research, that is, "tomorrow's advances made available today."

There are several possible messages that should be tailored to your center, and the community needs or community opportunities. The combination of a clear message, communicated with effective collateral through your sales channel or channels, is the foundation for a good sales and marketing program. Both sales and marketing teams should work with you to form an effective business growth team.

KEYS TO SUCCESSFUL OUTPATIENT IMAGING CENTER MARKETING

The only real reason to open an outpatient imaging center is bringing forward a value proposition that exceeds what is currently available. Your value proposition should both satisfy and hopefully exceed the following generally recognized needs of your customers: the referring physicians and their staff, patients, payers, your staff, your partners, and yourself. Understand that the customers are your "pillars" of any good outpatient imaging center; then satisfy their needs.

Satisfying Different Customers

Your goal is to delight the customer—to exceed expectations with a better service or product than they imagined getting. Focus on what the customer desires or requires (1) that he or she is not now getting done in a satisfactory manner or (2) that could be done much better. Realize that sometimes the customer must be shown a better way. Let's look at some of the basic needs of these customer groups.

Referring Physicians

Referring physicians are seeking technology that can advance the care of their patients. They want:

- Instant access to quantifiable, unambiguous interpretations.
- Accurate interpretations with diagnostic certainty—delivered fast.
- A satisfying experience for each patient that makes each feel as if he or she is the only patient in your practice, each and every time.
- Consultative support from a professional who is appreciative of their referral.
- Instant access to a radiologist who understands that there is no such thing as a stupid question.

Physicians want their choice of a referral to your imaging center to reflect well on them with respect to the patients' opinion and care. You are "representing" the clinicians when their patient is sent to you. They picked you. You need to continuously help them understand why your center is a better choice.

Referring Physicians' Office Staff

The office staff of your referring physicians want:

- Instant access with no unnecessary questions or delays. This means referring to you cannot be a hassle (precertifications are seen as your responsibility, despite their offices' possessing the necessary data to validate the need for the study).

- Good service with good explanations of what you need to get the study ordered and the patient out of their office in an expeditious manner.
- Convenience for their patients, so they don't have to explain why they are sending them miles out of their way for an exam.
- "One-stop shopping"—They don't want to have to explain to their patients why they have to have multiple stops for their plain film, mammogram, DEXA scan, MRI, and so on: "No, you need to go to another office to have a general radiograph to clear you for metal artifacts before we send you to the MRI."
- Instant access with no holds to get information they need from you to service their patients, including reports faxed or verbally transmitted as needed.

The key to both of these customers—the physicians and their staff—is that they will refer to people they trust and respect and who serve their interests best.

Patients

Patients sometimes vary in their needs based on their clinical condition, age, cultural beliefs, and educational level. The basic need required by most is compassion; other needs and wants are:

- Dignity and respect while in your care.
- A good explanation for why they are having an examination done, and what the equipment will do to or for them.
- Treatment as though they have choices (they are not just a package that has been delivered to your doorstep).
- Quality medical care, defined by first impressions, such as an interpretation of the scan and results conveyed to their doctor the same day, and an attractive, clean environment that is aesthetically pleasing and includes conveniences and amenities such as plenty of parking.

Patients enjoy being surprised by good service from people who look in their eyes and truly care about them. Delight them with coffee, donuts, today's newspaper, and a masseur or masseuse in the waiting room!

Payers

Payers desire covered lives. The insurance business boils down to a numbers game and is based on limiting risks. In the end, these publicly traded companies must also focus on providing an increase in shareholder value. To do this effectively they need:

- Patients to want their policies.
- To be known for providing access to convenient high-quality care.
- No-hassle service.
- You to play by their rules (e.g., preauthorizations, paperwork for use approvals, appropriate coding).
- You to comply with laws and ethical standards at all times.
- Access to services that are stamped with approved, known quality standards, such as ACR accreditation.
- The highest quality services with improved outcomes.
- All of the above to be provided at the lowest possible cost.

Staff

Your staff, which includes radiology technologists, center management, sales/marketing, radiologists, and clerical workers, desires:

- Recognition for their role in improvements in patient care.
- Appropriate reimbursement for their level of expertise and service.
- Recognition as part of a team that can improve the life of multiple patients.

Your Partners

Financial and medical partners have different needs. Both groups' needs must be met; some require more time than others, but they both need to understand each other's expectations:

- A venture capital firm ultimately wants a high return on investment. You should know how high is high.
- A medical partner wants immediate access to resources and possibly a piece of the pie. Again, know how much and whether you can still swallow that pie, legally, ethically, and morally.

Leading Your Center Team

It's not sufficient to just be the best at imaging. If that were the case, all patients would flee to academic medical centers with the latest and greatest technologies. It's the continual search for a better value proposition. True leaders in the outpatient imaging market are continually preparing for the aha moment from the market, which occurs when true customer satisfaction is achieved. As Tom Peters, known as "the guru of management," would say, you need to create "raving fans." These "fans" talk up their experience at your site and create new customers for you. Because they rave about you, they do the marketing for you.

If you already have raving fans from your other sites of service, what are the major risks associated when establishing a new outpatient imaging center? High start-up costs are some of the biggest challenges when opening a new center. The key is to have sufficient demand quick enough to support the revenue needed to operate a multimodality, full-scale outpatient imaging center. That demand may be created by the raving fans. If sufficient volume isn't generated, the outpatient imaging center can be a substantial drain on resources, despite the best intentions.

Here are some data points you must have in advance. What are the strengths of the existing imaging providers and hospitals? What are the weaknesses of the current providers? Is it better to align with hospital services and others, or create a competitive environment? Either way, you must do a comprehensive analysis of strengths, weaknesses, opportunities, and threats (SWOT, see also later under "Comprehensive Environmental Assessment") to render this new service. These need to be looked at realistically (Table 18-1).

Also, every business needs great leaders and your center is no exception (Box 18-3). Strong leadership is important and it starts with you (see also Chapter 3).

When you wake up and don't plan to make a difference, go back to sleep.
    COACH HERMAN BOONE FROM THE FILM *REMEMBER THE TITANS*

Operations at an outpatient imaging center must be appropriate and exceptional. You must

Table 18-1 SWOT

Strengths	Weaknesses
• Only high-field MR for 30 miles • Report turnaround time	• New to the community • No PET/CT
Opportunities	**Threats**
• Patient convenience	• Local hospital

BOX 18-3

A Leader . . .

• Makes others feel important.
• Promotes the vision.
• Stays involved and is close to the action.
• Delegates responsibility while always working on innovating and seeking means of removing obstacles to success.
• Motivates others to achieve their goals.
• Tends to be a person who is highly competitive.
• Sets the team's goals and is continually seeking means to grow.

---

plan to have the right modality at the right place at the right time with the right resources—consistently. You can see what defines "great service" in Box 18-4.

WHAT TO DO TO INCREASE YOUR CHANCES OF SUCCESS

The first thing you need to do is build upon your knowledge base. To be successful you must have as much market knowledge as possible. To gain market knowledge you must identify and quantify your sources of human intelligence. Physicians, hospital staff, patients, and staff all have different viewpoints on the marketplace; they also have a large circle of acquaintances that may have access to generally unobtainable market information. For instance,

---

BOX 18-4

What Defines Great Service?

- Operational Excellence
  - Scheduling templates
  - Staff expertise
  - Appropriate asset use
- Quality Defined by the End User
  - Report turnaround time
  - Exam protocols
  - Clinically valued reports
- Appropriate Pricing
  - Overall value
  - Appropriate contrast usage
- Focused Technology
  - Noninvasive strength
  - Interventional access when appropriate
  - IT capabilities
  - 3-D, 4-D exposure

---

they may have knowledge about competitors' plans to:

- Expand services
- Create a new line of business by buying a new piece of equipment
- Package their services differently

You must capture that knowledge and solicit data from some generally overlooked sources, such as:

- Certificate of need filings
- State building project lists
- Bond rating agency information
- Web searches or newspaper articles
- Insurance companies
- Large-scale employers

While this task may seem overwhelming the key is to make sure you focus on those sources that give you the best data. Tap into those with the most market knowledge more frequently (e.g., cultivating doctor relationships), while staying in touch with and surveying the other sources less frequently, or even on an ad hoc basis (e.g., patients and staff).

You can do all of this in many different ways; however, the most structured would be through surveys, focus groups, and interviews.

- Surveys take time to develop and administer but are generally the easiest means of getting large samples of data (see Appendix 18-1).

- Focused interviews are generally honed from the data you receive in the survey or through personal contacts. Focus groups normally take about an hour and really drill down on specific details of inquiry (e.g., physician satisfaction, definition of quality radiography, etc.).

Physician referrers are also an important source of competitive information. They will willingly tell you what the competition is doing that you aren't, but they will also tell you what they want to have happen. Some suggestions may be possible to achieve immediately, and others should be stored as future goals and reassessed for accuracy and clarity. These data can be obtained by simply scripting your staff and partners to ask the pertinent questions. For example:

- Which facility or provider offers you the greatest clinical information?
- Which facility offers the best clinical response to your needs, through better clinically relevant reports, turnaround time, and so on?
- Do we have and offer the right equipment for that specific marketplace?
- Are there any improvements under way at area hospitals or diagnostic imaging centers that you believe are important?
- Which facility do you feel makes it easiest for you and your staff to take care of your patients?
- Which of the following aspects makes it easier?
  - Access to radiologists?
  - Access to rapid and easy scheduling?
  - Internet and phone access?
  - Rapid telephone and report responsiveness?
  - Clinically appropriate solutions based on report data?
  - Convenience of locations?
  - How long do your patients have to wait for an appointment?

So now you have all of this competitive and market data. What's next?

Develop a Plan and Use the Plan

In marketing there are generally four "Ps" that must be defined: Product, Price, Place, and Promotion.

- Product—What are you selling? (the service you would like to provide and the report in which you deliver your results)
- Price—What are you charging for this service and to whom does it matter? (patient, payers, businesses, consider copays, direct)
- Place—Where will this service or these services be offered? (hospital, mall, ambulatory surgery center, self-standing diagnostic imaging center)
- Promotion—What is your position in the marketplace and how will you differentiate yourself? What will you do to gain mind share from your referring physicians, payers, and patients? Will you be the most convenient, a technological leader, a subspecialty read provider, and/or lowest cost? What personalized materials (items with your center's name, telephone number, and website address printed on them) will you hand out to promote your services:
  - Pens
  - Magnetic memo holders
  - Mouse pads
  - Shower breast examination cards (during cancer awareness month)

Provide a consistent, regular rotation of promotional materials to your customer base, keeping in mind that referring physicians, their staff, and patients refer to people they like, they trust, and who are competent to serve them and their patients' needs. To build that trust and stay true to those expectations it is advisable to create a marketing plan.

It is not your customer's job to remember you. It is your obligation and responsibility to make sure they don't have the chance to forget you.

PATRICIA FRIPP

Marketing Plan Template

Developing a marketing plan template is essential to remaining focused on your objectives and ensuring everyone else in the organization does as well. The marketing plan's purpose is to provide an overview of your diagnostic imaging center's marketing plan process. This document describes the imaging service as it currently exists. This can include clinical information, customer information, market dynamics, and so forth.

Goals and Objectives

Develop program goals and service objectives for your imaging center that describe the short- and long-range objectives:

- Short-range goals are the specific items you would like to achieve over the next year.
- Long-range goals are those items that are less specific and may be three to five years out. In this section, write out the specific reasoning behind marketing this service and what potential marketing changes may have to take place if the market conditions change.

Target Markets

Create or expand primary and secondary markets for the imaging center, describing who your potential customers are for the specific services you are offering, and in what geographic area they are located. This is the section that differentiates your physicians by specialty and separates the targeted patients by demographics, so that you can focus your marketing efforts and get the best return for the specific investment.

Comprehensive Environmental Assessment

What does the competitive landscape look like? List all other providers of these services in your primary and secondary markets. Include those you consider competitors, and even those that you consider complementary or friendly (hospitals perhaps). You will have to list the strengths, weaknesses, opportunities, and threats (SWOT) from all of these players (see Table 18-1).

- Strengths—Those factors that make it advantageous to use and continue to use their services.
- Weaknesses—Any inadequacies you can find regarding their provision of services.
- Opportunities—Describe what you believe allows your diagnostic imaging center to market at this particular time.
- Threats—List the dangers to the success of a particular competitive service, for example, their alliances, changes in technology (PET to PET-CT or PET-MR), as well as any perceived responses by your competitors.

How successful are your competitors now, and why? What would you have to do to provide

Table 18-2 Quantitative Data		
MRI Referrers	Volume Potential per Week	RVUs
Dr. A	25	50
Dr. B	10	18
Dr. C	3	4

equal or better service, and what would make those individuals who currently refer to them switch? What is the market potential? You must look at this from a qualitative and quantitative approach.

Qualitative data identifies the individuals, neurologists, orthopedists, primary care physicians, chiropractors, and so forth, that could be considered prospects for your services. Quantitative data include the number of potential customers and volume of their services purchased, including an estimate of potential revenue derived from each (Table 18-2).

Recommended Market Strategies

This section lists the expected approach you will use to market your services. What will be your primary message? Subspecialty reading? Faster turnarounds? Clinical care you can trust? Customer service?

Work Plan

These are the tactics you will use: communication vehicles, direct mail, billboards, radio, Internet, conferences, and so on. Decide who will be responsible for each step, how long each step will take, and how you will evaluate success.

Budget

What will your budget be? This is the total dollar amount required to implement the plan. Part of your plan has to be the creation of a sales force. When it is all said and done, regardless of your product, people buy from people. This means you have to dedicate resources to this endeavor and invest in an appropriate sales or practice liaison position (see Appendix 18-2).

HOW TO BUILD A MARKETING GROUP

Paying the Salespeople

How to pay salespeople can be controversial, but it shouldn't be. I firmly believe there is only one way to pay a salesperson—pay for performance. This means to pay salespeople a bonus or commission based on clearly defined performance metrics. The pure marketing person or group can be paid this way as well, or paid by way of an overall bonus, based on a group of metrics that are defined. For example, you have someone performing a sales function to grow volume in specific modalities; you also have a budget that you have put together as part of your business planning process. The budget may be dollars, but those dollars are derived through procedure volume. The modality volume budget should be the key metric on which that salesperson's compensation is based. This may not be the only metric you choose to pay on, but it should be your key to drive performance. You may also want to pay salespeople on the number of calls they make per day/week/month, as well as educational luncheons and dinner events. It is also a good idea to have some incentive for keeping internal systems updated, such as a contact management tool. A sample compensation plan is found in Appendix 18-3.

In a pay-for-performance model, targets are based on the budget; if they overachieve the volume, they can make more; if the volume is underachieved, they will make less. If you choose to have a marketing bonus plan (I recommend you do), it should be based on overall volume target achievement and some portion of internal requirement that you and your center manager define as important for your business success. This plan should be paid quarterly and annually as well.

You may ask yourself, "Why should I pay any type of bonus or commission more frequently than once a year?" Simple answer: Good sales and marketing people will perform best when the "carrot" is not so far out in front of them that they cannot see it. Commission or 100% annual bonus puts the target so far out that they are not as motivated by it as you want them to be. They may leave the company before the bonus is distributed. Or they may wait to leave until after the bonus is provided. Mass exodus on January 1! Goals for a whole year can look daunting for many employees; if you divide them into quarterly bites, they can see that carrot more clearly and drive themselves every day to meet their goals. They get frequent rewards, seen as an affirmation of their good work. They have a better self-image.

What Should Your Sales Team Be Doing?

One thing you need your salespeople to do is be is the "voice of the customer." To be that effective "voice of the customer," they should be:

- Making 10 to 15 customer visits per day.
- Scheduling at least one luncheon per week.
- Setting up educational events for your area physicians a few times per year.

These activities are designed to deliver the key messages that define you and your practice, educating the customers on what procedures you offer with new technology developments, and, most importantly, asking them to send their patients to your practice! When your sales teams are making their calls they should be asking questions about scheduling, report turnaround, and patient satisfaction. The answers to these questions are the "voice of the customer" back to the practice, to let you know how you are doing and where there may be opportunities for improvement.

After they have made their calls, had luncheons, and so forth the work of the salespeople is not finished. Internally, they should be communicating the issues and opportunities, working with marketing on sharpening the message, changing collateral, planning an event, and so on, and they should be an integral part of the team that helps to fix customer problems when they arise. Also, at the end of each day they should use a CRM (customer relationship management—see later under The Power of Information) tool of some type to record who they visited and what they did that day. Accountability is a philosophy that should pervade the firm.

Should the Team Be Working Strategically?

This may seem like a stupid question, but it's not and here's why. If sales and marketing people set out to accomplish all the tasks described above, there may be some moderate success, but to have real success there also needs to be some specific planning that will help everyone to work "smart" and have better, more predictable success. What you don't want is the "shotgun approach." This is when sales and marketing people have no clear direction and make calls based on where they want to shop during the day, or where their favorite coffee shop is located. Strategic marketing is the heart of how marketing shoud be done. Also, remember the concept of opportunity costs. Yes, the shotgun approach may be "working"; they got you a 7% increase in MRI. However, the "opportunity" (with a better-directed team approach) was a 14% growth rate. You lost that additional 7% opportunity. So don't celebrate so quickly.

WHAT IS "STRATEGIC MARKETING" AND HOW CAN IT WORK FOR YOU?

Targeting for Success

Strategic marketing simply means to have a plan that fits into the strategic plan for your practice. For example, if you are going to make an investment in 64, 128, or 256 slice CT, then CVCT is a strategic direction you want your practice to take. Hopefully, *before* your purchase, you have researched the direction of CT and see that coronaries and runoffs are going to be big for CT. Your study also tells you that currently these patients are getting diagnostic catheterizations performed at the local hospital. You also know that the patients undergoing the catheterizations are likely coming from primary care physicians in your area. To be successful with your 64 slice CT and get patients for these new applications you are going to need to do a few things:

- Develop the clinical message (e.g., why non-invasive imaging matters as far as risk to patient).

- Train a physician in interpretation and clinical scenarios.
- Get some outstanding images that reinforce the message.
- Create a list of specialties/primary care physicians that see the kind of patients that will "feed" the scanner.
- From the specialty list, create a specific target list from current referrers and those who do not refer any patients.
- Get the collateral and target lists into the hands of your sales and marketing team and radiologists to start making calls and setting up *key* luncheons that you should attend to tell the story.
- Closely monitor the results of the calls and the quality of the service.

It's not just having a better tool; it is providing better results—remember, you are the product!

You now have a strategic plan that will lead to success if you execute it well, monitor it closely, and follow it up. You should be doing this with every service you offer, that is, identifying key referrers that will feed the modality, developing and then executing a plan, and closely monitoring the results (Box 18-5).

You will not see the results you want everywhere, so you need to be prepared to listen to the voice of the customer, and then follow up and make changes accordingly.

Last, the interventional catheter doc does not have to be your enemy. By performing coronary CTA, you will identify patients that are more appropriate for diagnostic catheterization and intervention, as well as patients that may have been less willing to undergo an invasive procedure without a high pretest probability. As such, you become the coveted referral source to the cardiologist. Pay for performance, tackle business strategically, and track results.

BOX 18-5

Metrics Worth Tracking

- Weekly—Call volume, overall center volume, special procedure volume
- Monthly—Procedure volume by modality, volume by referring physician, sales expenses
- Quarterly—All pay for performance metrics

THE POWER OF INFORMATION

What Is CRM?

Customer relationship management (CRM) is how you formulate and track your customer service strategies. Customer service strategies are often difficult to define in health care, due to the many different constituents that you have to appease. They all have different priorities with different time concerns and constraints. Improving customer service is achieved by gathering intelligence regarding all of these individual needs and meeting them each and every time. To do that you have to gather the information and educate everyone within the practice as to what needs to be achieved. Institute an assessment system to ensure that what you say you are offering is indeed being offered. (Behavior that motivates profitable growth should be compensated well financially.)

CRM, and now electronic CRM, improves efficiency and effectiveness by streamlining data collection and automating responses. The goal is to find problem areas before they occur and fix them. At a minimum, with a good CRM system, if you don't catch a problem before it happens at least you can resolve it with an effective means of communicating. Thus you can implement an effective resolution right away, or apply that solution to another related problem synchronously or in the future.

The goal of CRM is to build customer loyalty by building a learning organization that can effectively deal with each customer as if each were the only individual in your practice. You can only imagine how difficult it is to satisfy everyone in health care. First, the patients, who may not be themselves when they are sick. Then the referring physicians, who have multiple patients and concerns to think about—in this era of managed care a physician has to see so many patients an hour to be fairly compensated, making things more difficult for both doctors and patients. The payers need to have justification for all studies and need them to be provided in a cost-effective manner, however ill defined. And finally, patient family members, who want these services available for their loved ones in a convenient and expeditious manner.

CRM allows you to define customers' needs and then create products and services based on those needs, which are effective and efficient, faster than your competitors can. With CRM, you can develop services that not only satisfy but also delight your referring physicians. When done right, it is an effective system to deal with issues as they arise and consistently provides actionable working solutions.

How to get started? First, you have to identify all of your customers, and all of their needs and expectations; this is key. Most people—both in health care and patients—assume all health care providers are the same. Patients are accustomed to long waits in waiting rooms and long delays in getting results from their doctors. Doctors are used to not having information in a timely manner and when they need it. It's time to change. First walk in their shoes, *all* of their shoes. What does each person expect and how can you make the experience with your practice go beyond what he or she has experienced anywhere else? Do it by consistently educating, communicating, and holding yourselves and your staff accountable.

CRM systems deal with the basics of communication, that is, how to speak to your customers, both on the phone and in person. For example, CRM teaches you how to effectively deal with angry or disappointed patients, to diffuse the situation and "make things right" by emphasizing *active* listening. This means listening without the intent to respond—listening with the intent to understand, or "reflective" listening.

The most effective CRM goes beyond the obvious and creates new protocols and procedures, establishing customer service guidelines, skills, and expectations. All of these must be part of your organization's culture and incorporated into your job descriptions and accountability rankings or reviews. It is not effective to have everyone except one staff member or one radiologist follow the rules and meet expectations, because all it takes is one bad encounter to ruin the team's effort, and hence reroute a referring physician's referral choice.

What Are RIS and PACS?

Every radiology practice requires two items: a RIS (radiology information system) and a PACS (picture archival and communication system).

These systems are essential for transferring knowledge to your referring physicians. The RIS generally sends transcribed results. The PACS generally transfers images to your referring doctors and hospitals. This topic has been covered in greater detail in Chapter 13.

A key to an effective practice is the ability to meet growing IT needs. Make IT an integral part of every facet of your practice.

In the spirit of CRM, we must be able to deliver the desired data to the consumer by the means in which they would like to receive it. It could be a report or an image, and, sometimes, it's a conversation. Everyone at the practice needs to know what the customers' preferences are so that they are consistently delivered, each and every time.

CREATING YOUR GROWTH PLAN

Specific Action Plans by Modality and Specialty

The growth plan is the culmination of the strategic plan by modality and is the master playbook to grow the practice. Also known as a business plan, we refer to it as a growth plan because it focuses on exponential growth and not just on the budget, for example. If you don't *plan* for growth—and expect it—it won't happen; you'll just be meeting the budget.

When creating a growth plan you should always involve key stakeholders such as yourself, the practice manager, the operation director, the IT staff, the finance department, sales and marketing, and, depending on the size of your practice, lead techs by modality. The growth plan should be developed by the executive leadership—sales and marketing. You are paying them to do this job, so they need to make it happen. As well, growth plans need to be based on as much hard data as you can get your hands on, for example:

- Lists of referring physicians, broken down by specialty
- Referral volume history by physician, preferably by month
- CPT codes and reimbursement dollars for key practice procedures
- All available market trend data

After you have gathered your information, answer, to the best of your ability based on that data, the following:

- Which modalities will be your focus, both over the long and short term?
- What specific procedures, by modality, will make you successful (identified by Current Procedural Terminology [CPT] code)?
- Which opportunities should you quantify?
- Which specific referring physicians will you target to grow the identified volumes?

Next, determine your goals for volumes and growth. Complete a SWOT analysis by modality (see Table 18-1) and a simple action plan as your activity guide (see attached example). Review your growth plan at least once per quarter, and track your progress against your plan (your billing system can be the best source to accomplish tracking through basic reports).

INVEST IN THE RIGHT PEOPLE

One of the most important issues you will face in developing and marketing your center is determining the need for and hiring the right physician practice liaison. Much can be said regarding the perceived need and differences in expectations for the role.

As previously stated, there is a huge difference between marketing and sales. One of the most important decisions you'll make is this one: "Which person do I need the most, a salesperson or a marketing liaison?" Most practices are convinced that the physician (radiologist) is the best "seller" of services, and therefore they just need someone from marketing or sales to "maintain the relationships." Radiologists will say, "I'm too busy doing the work to speak with doctors regarding what we have to offer." Keep in mind that the ultimate goal is to have a growing business—if you're depending solely on your radiologists to market the business, when they get busy, how and when will they find the time to communicate effectively with referring doctors? When it gets busy, who will fill that void?

Whatever your preference, it serves you well to write down what you would like either person to do; weigh it out—you need that person

to be able to do both the selling *and* maintaining of relationships.

So now, after deciding on a dedicated sales or marketing person, rather than on the radiologists to grow your practice, you've decided that you need help. You have determined what the tasks are that you want this individual to do for your practice and your referring physicians. You can now write a job description (see Appendix 18-2).

Performance-Based Incentive Plan

As mentioned previously, this is a critical part of attracting the right individual and aligning his or her behavior with the goals of your practice. If you want a sales/marketing person or team to be focused on growing your volumes, you must have incentives that will make that happen. How best to pay employees in any area can always be debated. Don't compromise on this one (Table 18-3).

We all have names of our favorite supervisors or technologists that we know have great interpersonal skills and/or excellent leadership skills, but back away from your comfort zone. Don't recruit these people who are effective in their native environments. What you require from marketing is a different skill set for the job. Marketing is a specific skill set, and not everyone can do it successfully. This is a job that functions as a replacement or a surrogate for you with regard to your customers. This is a critical position to the long-term growth of your imaging center: the person you hire must know the practice better than you do. Is this person capable of well representing the interests of the practice? Can he or she argue for the customer and will he or she be heard? Does this individual have the skills to define potentially dangerous or divisive issues? Can he or she keep a cool head under stress and not give away the store? These are some of the questions that you will need to ask yourself regarding the person you decide to hire.

The Interview Process

First, who will be interviewing the prospective inside or external candidate? Potential employees should be interviewed by the key stakeholders in the practice: the radiologists, the directors of marketing, operations, and finance,

Table 18-3 American Radiology Services, Inc., 2006 Action Plans

| Objective: | Grow MRI Volume (sample) | | | | |
| Initiative: | 3-D Marketing Program (sample) | Page 1 of 1 | | | |

Initiative Captain	Initiative Team	Statement of Objective	End Result Statement	Key Action Items	Responsible Individuals	Dates	Resource Requirements
Dr. Jones	Chief MR Tech Sales Marketing	Start and grow 3-D marketing effort to grow orthopedic volume	3-D images personally delivered to target ortho physicians	Establish process flow for data to be routed and reconstructed within 6 hrs	Chief MR tech	1/7/2007	Meetings with key stakeholders
			Recognition by referring community of a unique service	Train key tech to perform 3-D recons	Chief MR tech Radiologist	1/7/2007	Budget for offsite training program
			Create the platform to take 3-D to other procedures through a centralized service	Create target list of ortho physicians	Sales/ marketing	1/30/2007	Billing support
			Orthopedic imaging volume growth of 50%				

and a host of supervisors. Also, ideally, try to have the candidates screened and interviewed by a mentor or other practice liaison/marketing representative.

This process should be unlike many of your other interviews for practice staff, which are focused on hiring people to work for you, doing simply what you tell or ask them to do. This position warrants an outside perspective: the person you choose will be telling *you* what the customers want, need, or prefer. You'll then have to assess whether or not you can meet those demands. Obviously, the bearer of this news must have the capacity to decipher wants versus needs versus potential market opportunities. The individual you hire has to discover and disclose what your customers want from you. He or she must bring knowledge of the marketplace to you and then help to make growth happen.

The patient liaison (or marketing or salesperson) that comes aboard must have the knowledge to clarify issues as defined by doctors, doctors' office staff, and payers and be able to articulate clearly what these needs are. He or she must be capable of analytical thought to provide suggestions and summarize situations. In addition, the individual practice liaison must determine who in the outpatient imaging center can make the desired outcome happen. This person must have a good to great working knowledge of radiology terminology and practice. They must have instant access to resources that can make needed services happen.

CONCLUSION

Everybody must be on the same team. Everybody must know what the elements of your marketing strategy are. The who, what, why, where, when, and how:

- Who works on the marketing message and promotion?
- What is the key message?
- Why did you choose them?
- Where and to whom do you promote this item?
- When do you launch a campaign and with whom?
- How are you going to market and then measure your success or failure?

The key is focus—by you and your team. The bottom line is that marketing is probably the single most effective tool you have for succeeding in a highly competitive marketplace. Marketing encompasses the entire scope of your practice—how you price, produce, position, and promote your product—and impacts every decision you make in your organization. Finally, everyone in your organization is *in* marketing and you are always marketing, every day. Get good at it, and be committed.

The difference between involvement and commitment is like ham and eggs. The chicken is involved; the pig is committed.

MARTINA NAVRATILOVA

Dos and Don'ts of Marketing	
Dos	**Don'ts**
1. Be engaged in your center marketing; you can make it happen!	1. Overpromise and underperform.
2. Be the best in your market at customer service.	2. Ignore your relationships with your payers and referrers.
3. Have a plan and work the plan.	3. Follow your instincts to do what you would like— it's not about you.
4. Pick the right people and pay them for performance.	4. Try to fix everything at once—go through change systemically.
5. Measure everything.	5. Try to be all things to all people—find your niche.

APPENDIX 18-1. SAMPLE SURVEY QUESTIONNAIRE

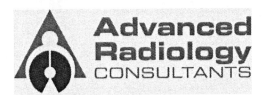

Referring Physician Questionnaire:

Name_____Phone_____

1) On a scale of 1-5 (with 5 being most important factors and 1 being least important) please rank the following:

____ *Practice reputation for quality care*   ____ *Physician's competence*
____ *Patient feedback after consultation*   ____ *Timely appointments*
____ *Board certification*   ____ *Prompt, informative reports*
____ *Office location*   ____ *Relationship with physicians*
            ____ *Other (Please specify below)*

_____

2) Do you regularly refer some of your patients to other radiology practices?
                      _____ Yes   _____No

3) If yes, what is the single most important reason?

_____

4) Please rate our service to you and your patients in the following areas:
    (On a scale of 1-5; with 1 being not important and 5 being very important)

        a) Overall quality care   *b) Friendly, courteous staff*
          1   2   3   4   5   1   2   3   4   5

        c) Consult information   *d) Timely appointment scheduling*
          1   2   3   4   5   1   2   3   4   5

        e) Timely, written communication   *f) Office location and hours*
          1   2   3   4   5   1   2   3   4   5

5) What would it take to increase your referrals to Advanced Radiology Consultants?
_____

6) Do you have any suggestions that would help us improve our service to you?_____
_____
_____

Your staff?_____
_____

Your patients?_____
_____

(Appendix continued on following page)

APPENDIX 18-1—*continued*

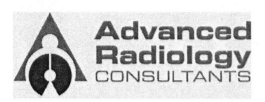

Referring Office Questionnaire:

Name_____Phone_____

1) What criteria do your staff use for making a referral for radiology services?
(Please rank from 1-5, with 1 being very important)

_____ *Physician's request*　　　　_____ *Patient's request*
_____ *Timely appointments*　　　　_____ *Office location and hours*
_____ *Exclusive contract with managed care*　　_____ *Other (please list below)*

_____

2) What can we do to make your job easier?_____

_____

_____

3) Which managed care plan has the highest volume of patients in your practice?

_____

4) Please rate our overall service to you and your patients.
　　(On a scale of 1-5; with 5 being very important and 1 being not important)

　　　　a) Overall quality of care　　　　*d) Friendly, courteous staff*
　　　　　1　2　3　4　5　　　　　　　1　2　3　4　5

　　　　b) Consult information　　　　*e) Timely appointment scheduling*
　　　　　1　2　3　4　5　　　　　　　1　2　3　4　5

　　　　c) Timely, written communication　　*f) Office location and hours*
　　　　　1　2　3　4　5　　　　　　　1　2　3　4　5

5) Advanced Radiology has multiple means of report delivery: fax, mail, and now Internet. What are your preferences?
Please check all that apply:

Fax #_____　　　　E-mail:_____

Fax only_____ Mail only_____ Internet only_____ ALL_____

Are there any problems with our report delivery? _____

_____

6) Advanced Radiology is one of the few radiology groups that has a dedicated Practice Liaison. Please comment on this
service to your group—do you have any recommendations or suggestions?

APPENDIX 18-2. POSITION: PRACTICE LIAISON/SALES

Outline for a Job Description

Summary of Duties

Summarize the duties that will make your practice successful, such as:

- Visit new and existing customers.
- Provide customer satisfaction administration.
- Develop and distribute key practice information and collateral.
- Be the "voice of the customer."
  - Assist management with short- and long-term goals that will help meet growth objectives.

Supervision Received

Report to Marketing and Business Development Director. Work closely with the president of the imaging center.

Supervision Exercised

None at this time.

Typical Working Conditions

Outline the typical working conditions that he or she will experience within your practice and covering his or her territory.

Duties and Responsibilities

Here you want to be specific enough to drive the behavior you need to achieve your goals, such as:

- Recommend and implement the marketing plan.
- Provide customer input to management with recommended solutions.
- Perform "X" number of sales calls per day.
- Develop and coordinate customer educational events and luncheons.
- Oversee and participate in local trade shows as required.

Knowledge, Skills, and Abilities

You need to invest in someone that has imaging knowledge and demonstrated sales success.

Education, Training, and Experience

This is really up to you. I would recommend that a four-year college degree and/or equivalent experience be a requirement. Sales experience, preferably in imaging, should also be required.

APPENDIX 18-3. MARKETER'S BONUS PROJECTION (SAMPLE), 2007 TO YEAR END

Category	Factor	Weight	Paid
A	Site Volumes	0.70	Quarterly
B	MBOs	0.15	Year-End
C	Maintenance	0.15	Quarterly

POTENTIAL BONUS EARNINGS $40,000

Category:	A	B	C
Weight:	70%	15%	15%
Annually	$28,000	$6,000	$6,000

Performance Level:	Bonus Rate	Quarterly		
85%	25%	$1,750	$375	$375
	27%	1,890	405	405
	29%	2,030	435	435
	31%	2,170	465	465
	33%	2,310	495	495
90%	50%	$3,500	$750	$750
	53%	3,710	795	795
	56%	3,920	840	840
	59%	4,130	885	885
	62%	4,340	930	930
95%	75%	$5,250	$1,125	$1,125
	79%	5,530	1,185	1,185
	83%	5,810	1,245	1,245
	87%	6,090	1,305	1,305
	91%	6,370	1,365	1,365
100%	100%	$7,000	$1,500	$1,500

BONUS RESULTS

Annual Bonus Earned   -
Year-End Bonus Earned

Amount Above Target ($1K per point)

Total Projected 2007 Bonus Sample* [   ]   Base Salary [$40,000] Yr End Projected [   ]
Cumulative Year-End Earned

- -

PERFORMANCE CARD (sample)

Site Volumes	MRI	CT	PET	Total
2007 Volumes Budget—TC & HC	20,333	17,801	1,352	39,486
2007 Projected Volumes—TC & HC	16,484	17,804	926	35,214
Raw Performance Level	81%	100%	68%	89%
Weighted Performance Level	4%	5%	62%	71%

MBO				
2007 Target	25	25	25	75
2007 Actual Performance	25	25	25	75
Performance Level	100%	100%	100%	100%

Maintenance				
2007 Target	25	25	25	75
2007 Actual Performance	25	25	25	75
Performance Level	100%	100%	100%	100%

Percent Above/Below Targeted Volume	-23%	0%		-12%

Site: **My First Office**
Marketer: Annie Smith

CHAPTER 19

Teleradiology in Practice

Gautam Agrawal

INTRODUCTION

The practice of teleradiology is one of the most rapidly evolving, dynamic, and changing areas of medicine. Teleradiology is a fraction of a larger telemedicine field that has evolved because of the widespread availability of computers, high-bandwidth access to the Internet, and communications standards in medicine. Without each of these components, the practice of telemedicine and teleradiology would not exist. It is critically important that radiologists grasp this single point when discussing teleradiology: the rules have changed.

Radiologists are no longer bound by space, time, or specialty expertise. Indeed, the strengths of teleradiology rely on time-shifting work to more tenable hours. Radiologists can now work in San Francisco and practice radiology in rural Michigan or vice versa. Pools of experts can be gathered, to bring more accurate diagnoses to patients and providers. We are limited by our own imaginations.

I would guess at this point you're thinking, "I've heard this song and dance before." In late 2000 or early 2001, the high flyers of the Internet boom stocks like Amazon or E-Bay had valuations greater than Sears and K-mart combined. At the same time, these Internet stocks had yearly revenues less than that produced by Wal-Mart in a single day. Pundits espoused the "new economy," forsaking all that was old and traditional. The reality for radiology is that "bricks and mortar" practices will not come crashing down. There will be no "rapid revolution" in how things are done. We will always need radiologists on the ground. Changes will occur, but they will be more gradual than the doom and gloom scenarios of "outsourcing" that have been played out in the popular radiology "press."

The goal of the chapter is to provide an overview of the practice of teleradiology. After a brief introduction, a more detailed discussion of technical services, quality of service (QoS), medicolegal issues, and economic considerations is provided.

DEFINITIONS, PERSPECTIVES, AND MODELS

When people ask me what I do for a living, I say I practice radiology. A common response is something like, "Oh, you're the one who takes my picture if I break my leg." Sometimes it is easier to simply nod your head and avoid further comment. I know you have all had this experience, and it is even worse when family members are involved. After explaining that you are actually a *real* doctor, the next question is: "Where do you work?" When I reply "from my living room," the step that I took forward is reversed by the two I've just taken backward. I explain I practice "teleradiology" and that when little Jimmy breaks his arm 2500 miles away from me in North Carolina, his doctor "e-mails" me his electronic films in real time, and I call the doctor and tell him that Jimmy's radius is fractured. Herein lies a practical definition of teleradiology. Teleradiology is the consultative process by which images and patient information are transmitted to a remote location where interpretations are rendered and then returned to the requesting care provider.

Interestingly, if one considers the larger field of "telemedicine" as the delivery of medical information from one remote location to another, then the roots of the field may have originated in the Middle Ages or earlier. In Europe, bonfires were used to convey information that towns were affected by bubonic plague. This is a simple example of a public health communications system. With the development of national postal systems in the 18th and 19th centuries, remote consultative medicine could be practiced on a time scale of days or weeks. With the advent of the telegraph in the mid-19th century, medical information could be transmitted on the order of minutes to hours. During wars, medical casualty information or supply information was rapidly conveyed over great distances. The invention of the telephone ushered in a new era of communications and remains the mainstay of all telemedicine practiced today. In the last decade of the 20th century and to the present day, a growing fraction of remote medicine is practiced by entirely electronic means through sophisticated communication networks that can transmit data, voice, and video information with nearly instantaneous access to results. Widespread availability of the Internet has spurred use. How long before radiologists can predict the future?

Perspectives

On a more serious level, telemedicine and teleradiology at their core foster collaboration. Radiologists, no longer bound by physical barriers, are able to aggregate diverse subspecialty expertise into a consolidated platform to provide rapid optimal patient diagnosis even to the most remote locations. Support can be given to local radiologists for techniques, protocols, diagnostic strategies, and radiographic interpretations.

Herein is the "rub," and it is central to the hesitancy of many groups to consider outsourcing consultative readings to teleradiology practices. Outsourcing poses important perceived threats to local groups, particularly if the groups are not heavily subspecialized.

The first and foremost threat is that of expertise that may not be present locally. When local subspecialty clinicians begin to receive subspecialty-level consultative readings they tend to quickly begin relying on these to the exclusion of the "generalist" local group. The local group in many ways may become effectively supplanted. This may not be an active, predatory process, but rather a natural extension of the services provided. Teleradiology, for its ability to facilitate physician cooperation, must be recognized as a double-edged sword that can amplify local deficiencies. Our experience has shown us that the way to mitigate this problem is to provide the services through the local group. To provide an example, a local radiologist decides that his or her experience at interpretation of magnetic resonance imaging (MRI) of the finger is limited. The study is sent in the form of a "consultation" to the contracted group. A complete or detailed report is provided, which the local radiologist can use as a template for his or her report. We've seen this model work successfully, and it keeps the local radiologists "in the loop."

A second threat is that of superior work flow. Before the "golden" days of picture archiving and communication systems (PACS), radiologists could hide behind their poor departmental work-flow designs. "Tech forgot to send the case," "printer is malfunctioning," or "some technical issue with the study" were excuses that could be given to clinicians. Now, with distributed PACS, clinicians can access studies within seconds of acquisition. This forces radiologists to perform better and faster. Add to this an outside teleradiology group generating reports on a near real-time basis and you have a milieu for frustration with local radiology groups. On a practical level, we have seen that local groups have often had to analyze and remediate their own work-flow processes after bringing in teleradiology providers. Outside groups often have the ability to produce printed results within minutes of study acquisition. If the local group cannot produce a product like this with similar "turnaround," they may be forced into an awkward situation with their referring clinician base. Indeed, it is not uncommon to hear that the local clinicians have "saved" cases for the teleradiology consultants instead of the local radiologists.

Mitigating these effects requires careful contract negotiation and construction. Having the contracts directly with the remote radiology group rather than allowing the hospital direct contracting may allow the local group more control over their interactions. In addition to risk mitigation, this fosters a greater collaborative effort and a partnership relationship between the local and remote groups. When partnered together in a long-term arrangement, a subspecialty-driven teleradiology practice can bolster and enhance services provided by the local group. Finally, the local group should consider an analysis of their own work flow before starting teleradiology services. It is always better to approach improvement of QoS proactively rather than reactively to outside pressures.

Models of Teleradiology Practice

Teleradiology practices are varied and diverse, and the future will probably bring more unique practices and models. There are at least six general models of teleradiology practices: solo practitioner, standalone practice, overnight services, overread services, global services, or a hybrid combination of these (Table 19-1).

With "bricks and mortar" groups consolidating, similar things are likely to happen with teleradiology services as groups merge to grow volume and coverage areas. These will probably become the dominant players in the market as the technologies and platforms become ubiquitous and the "culture" of physician acceptance of remote reading matures.

It is important here to address a developing practice model that I believe will have significant implications in the future of teleradiology. Because of the massive disparities in salaries between the private-practice domain and academic medical centers, there has been a mass exodus of academic clinicians from the ranks of radiology departments nationwide. This has left departments struggling to maintain staffing with ever-growing workloads superimposed on ever-growing academic pressures to publish. Teleradiology may shift some of the balance back to the academic medical centers by allowing hybridized academic practices. Innovative practices can be arranged in which the radiologist practices part time in a nonteaching clinical role and part time in a teaching role. The academician can provide subspecialty overreads during daytime hours. Large academic centers can serve to further aggregate expertise for difficult or unusual cases. The immediate benefit to the hospital systems is that patient referral may increase. The secondary benefit is that it brings large case sets for retrospective studies and facilitates the academic mission of the institution.

The remainder of this introductory section is designed as a mini-outline for the larger subsections of the chapter. We will discuss the "keystones" of teleradiology, namely technical service, QoS, medicolegal considerations, and economic aspects of the practice. Toward

Table 19-1 Basic Features of Teleradiology Practices by Type

Type of Teleradiology Practice	Basic Features
Solo practitioner	Single radiologist or small radiology group Practitioner(s) don't maintain "bricks and mortar" imaging facilities Examples: independent contractors, remote locum tenens
Standalone practice	Single radiologist or radiology group Practices have and maintain their own physical imaging facilities but perform readings remotely
Overnight services	Provide "emergent" overnight preliminary or final reads, often aggregating studies from many facilities May or may not have ownership stake in imaging facilities from which they are reading Used to facilitate quality-of-life issues for contracting physicians
Overread services	Provide subspecialty overread consultations for difficult or unusual cases Can be used as a third party for accreditation purposes. Outside groups may contract with provider to screen radiology interpretations for quality.
Regional or global radiology network services	Large radiology practices with large-scale regional networks Examples include hospital systems like Kaiser Permanente or military Emerging model related to regional archival of breast imaging
Hybrids	Probably will become the most common "model" of teleradiology practice A practice may own some of the imaging facilities and equipment, provide night coverage for numerous hospitals, and provide some level of overread services for other practices. In addition, routine daytime studies may be interpreted.
Future models	Possible scenario would be educational teleradiology practices in which there is direct tutelage of practicing radiologists A true online active CME or "mini-fellowship" program in which radiologists can improve their skills from their own homes

the end of the chapter, a discussion on some practical aspects of our experience will be presented.

Technical Services

In teleradiology, you live or die by your technology. Optimally, it must work 24/7 × 365, be able to have full redundancy, and survive a nuclear holocaust. Granted, these are slight exaggerations—but not too far from the truth. When considering the technology platform, I approach it from the work flow, evaluating the following five components: capture, transmission, archival of images, retrieval of images, and reporting of the study.

One needs a mechanism of capturing image data in an electronic form. In years past, this may have come from scanned films, which were then transmitted in a standard image file format. Today, the vast majority of modalities are conformant to the DICOM standards (see below). As such, the image data and header are in a reasonably well-defined format, which can be used and manipulated in a nonproprietary way.

Once the data are captured, they must be transmitted to a central repository from which they can then be accessed. Typically, this is done over leased lines (T1, T3, OC-3, etc.) or via internal networks. Determination of which type of leased line is needed requires knowledge of study volume, study sizes (i.e., number of slices, size in megabytes), and degree of compression. The American College of Radiology (ACR) standards for teleradiology state that teleradiology is not appropriate if the available teleradiology system does not provide images of sufficient quality to perform the indicated task. From a storage and retrieval standpoint, this means that compression should not be excessive such that image quality is degraded. This leaves considerable room for interpretation. However, in our practice we use only true lossless compression. It is important to stress that the transmission system must have some level of error checking. This can be accomplished by a variety of means. On a technical level, bit-level error checking can be accomplished by a hardware transmission layer protocol. On a practical level, technologists should have a mechanism to verify that once a study is sent to the remote site, it is received in total, including all sequences, series, and images.

Once the study information is at the data center, it must be archived in a mechanism that is easily understood and easily accessed. The PACS and radiology information system (RIS) or hospital information system (HIS) will be used to specify how and when studies are to be interpreted. Once the study is placed into an active work list, the radiologist will retrieve the examination and render an interpretation. ACR guidelines emphasize that the image display should be of sufficiently diagnostic quality. This latter point is of a "sufficiently" vague nature. For our practice we require all remote readings to be performed from diagnostic workstations with minimum 2- to 3-megapixel diagnostic 10-bit medical-grade monitors. We have found that regular commercial monitors lack the contrast resolution and brightness to provide optimal interpretation.

Once the study is interpreted, the radiologist must render a report. This can be as simple as a manual handwritten facsimile or phone consultation. There is no doubt that the trend is to provide a legible typed preliminary report for urgent cases. Obviously, for a final reading, a fully rendered electronic or typed report is a requirement. To facilitate rapid report turnover, one could consider dedicated high-speed transcription services or natural speech recognition technologies. The latter are becoming popular among administrators, much to the disdain of radiologists. These technologies are maturing, and accuracies are improving. There is no doubt this will become the standard of reporting in the future as technology continues to improve. Once a report is rendered, the RIS/HIS can deliver the reports via facsimile, e-mail, or pager, or make them available for online viewing. The degree of integration will determine the overall efficiency in the system.

Quality of Service

There are at least two components of QoS to maintain: technical and professional. These will be discussed in more detail later in the chapter. Suffice it to say that written procedures and policies should be in place that guide or govern failures or breakdowns in either system.

On a technical level this means that multiple backup systems must exist to guard against data loss, violation of patient privacy statutes, or the interruption of data transmission. On a professional level this means that accuracy is reviewed regularly and periodically. Continuing quality assurance safeguards and policies for remediation of mistakes in interpretation must be in place. Continuing medical education and active follow-up of patient results and outcomes are an important part of this process of proactive quality assurance and quality improvement.

Medicolegal Aspects

Legal considerations are also important in teleradiology as in all medical disciplines. Because this is a new and rapidly evolving field, little if any legal precedent is available to guide actions. This leaves practitioners guessing about the probable legal requirements to practice medicine regarding licensure, liability, confidentiality, security of information, and retention of records. There are few if any practice guidelines but a plethora of opinions on what can and cannot be done. Before starting a teleradiology practice, particularly if it will involve multiple states, consider retaining the services of a lawyer who has specific medical expertise in this area.

Economics

When discussing the economics of teleradiology, one can consider both quantitative and qualitative measures. Additionally, the practice of teleradiology may be considered from the standpoint of "in-house" (within the practice) or outsourced teleradiology.

It is important to recognize that there are a combination of basic factors that, when assessed critically, will define the economic feasibility of teleradiology for a particular practice. These include:

- Capital equipment expenditures
- Software licenses and continuing maintenance
- Numbers of studies being performed and incremental revenue gain or loss
- Radiologist staffing
- Additional technologists or support staffing
- Incremental licensing and credentialing
- Incremental legal costs
- Incremental malpractice costs

The detailed economic analysis exceeds the scope of the chapter; however, guidelines and practice information will be provided in subsequent sections.

TECHNICAL CONSIDERATIONS IN TELERADIOLOGY

For me, the technical aspect of teleradiology is so critically important that it supersedes all other aspects. I liken it to a certain Olympic basketball squad (no names please); by all standards each of the players is among the best in the world. But, as a team, they often lack the cohesiveness of smaller, less well-known squads. If the technology platform is not optimized and working well, your radiologists will be riding the bench.

In the next series of sections we will discuss the technical aspects of a teleradiology practice. To provide a basic framework we will start with study acquisition and close with the final finished product, the radiology report.

Modality Equipment and DICOM Compliance

In 1983 the ACR and the National Electrical Manufacturers Association (NEMA) formed a joint committee to specify standards for Digital Imaging and Communications in Medicine. The incarnation of this effort is the DICOM standard, which undergoes periodic review, revision, and updating.

This DICOM standard serves three overriding purposes: (1) to promote communication of digital image information, regardless of device manufacturer (interoperability), (2) to facilitate the development and expansion of PACS that can also interface with other systems of hospital information (usability), (3) to allow the creation of diagnostic information data bases that can be interrogated by a wide variety of distributed devices (availability).

Importantly, in all purchases of new modalities, conformance to the DICOM standard should be insisted on. However, there is no validation or testing done for equipment by the DICOM Standards Committee or other independent third parties. Because of this, the term "DICOM compliance" should be taken loosely, with the understanding that configuration issues both related to the acquisition and display of images will probably be present and may require attention.

Modality Equipment—Noncompliant Devices

When equipment is not DICOM compliant (particularly older equipment), there are several options to allow the performance of "teleradiology." DICOM converters are devices that convert the output of a modality, usually with both hardware and software add-ons, into a

DICOM-compliant format. The device will "sit" between the modality and the PACS, converting the proprietary study into one that is in conformance. This is a gross oversimplification but is adequate for our purpose here. The devices are proprietary and costly, but still only represent a small fraction of the cost of replacing a modality. Another possible solution for nonconforming devices is to scan printed or developed film. By digitizing the films and "wrapping" the data with DICOM header information, the study can then be transmitted rapidly. More pedestrian (literally) ways of performing "teleradiology" include mailing printed film or compact disks. Immediate consultation is obviously more difficult in this last scenario. On a practical level, our experience with such noncompliant devices is that they just don't perform well. Scanned films, particularly plain radiographs, lack the truest representation of the image, and subtle findings can often be missed.

Workstations

The ACR makes recommendations only on teleradiology when used for rendering the official final interpretation. However, from a conservative standpoint, it is the author's opinion that these should apply to "preliminary" reports as well, because medical decisions are made on the basis of these preliminary reports. Although there is no defined body of case law on this topic, the author believes that one could not be faulted for having equipment at the remote site that matches the capabilities of the on-site facility.

The ACR also breaks imaging into "large matrix" and "small matrix" sets. The small matrix refers to imaging from computed tomography (CT), magnetic resonance imaging, nuclear medicine, digital fluoroscopy, and angiography, in which matrix size is typically at 512×512 pixels and 8 bits of gray-scale depth. Large matrix refers to digital radiography, mammography, and digitized film. The spatial resolution should allow 2.5 line pairs/mm display at 10 bits of gray-scale depth.

On a practical level, one will usually have a mix of both large- and small-matrix studies unless the practice is very highly focused.

So, display solutions should meet or exceed display characteristics for large-matrix imaging.

Monitors and Display

Practitioners considering teleradiology practice have asked on several occasions what type of equipment they should buy. The simple answer is, "Buy the best!" On a practical level, don't skimp on monitors or workstations. These are your patients and your practice, and it should reflect the quality of the group. We have seen multiple examples of early stroke, subtle fractures, and bowel mucosal ischemia that were not apparent on commercial monitors when compared alongside diagnostic workstations. Remember, it requires only a few of these "missed cases" to undo a fragile trust that clinicians have placed in this "newfangled teleradiology technology."

According to the ACR, when display workstations are used for official interpretation with both small- and large-matrix data sets, the following characteristics should be provided:

- Luminance of the gray-scale monitors of at least 50 foot-lamberts (approximately 170 candelas per square meter [cd/m^2])
- Capability for selecting image sequence, window and level adjustments, panning, zooming, rotating, or flipping images
- Capability of accurately associating the patient and study demographic characterizations with the study images
- Capability of providing correct labeling of patient orientation is preserved.
- Capability of calculating and displaying accurate linear measurements and pixel value determinations in appropriate values for the modality (e.g., Hounsfield units for CT images)
- Capability of displaying prior image compression ratio, processing, or cropping
- The display should contain the following information:
  - Matrix size
  - Bit depth
  - Total number of images acquired in the study
  - Clinically relevant technical parameters

- Lighting in the reading room that can be controlled to eliminate reflections in the monitor and to lower the ambient lighting level as much as is feasible

On a practical level, data have shown that the conspicuity of lesions on radiographs is improved more by luminance than by resolution. From our experience, performance is improved with dedicated 2- to 3-megapixel gray-scale 10-bit monitors with average continuous luminance greater than 175 foot-lamberts (approximately 600 cd/m^2). Typically, a third color monitor is available for images that are optimally viewed in color (i.e., duplex ultrasound, perfusion or functional CT/MRI data, or nuclear medicine studies).

Processors and Computing Power

With the explosive growth of multidetector CT and thin-section acquisition with isometric voxels, study sizes have continued to increase. Moreover, 3-D real-time rendering can be used, often with great ease to answer or better delineate results in more anatomic or physiologic scan planes. Volume rendering, shaded surface display, and other 3-D techniques can be extraordinarily taxing on workstations. From a practical standpoint at basic minimum we have found the following design to be acceptable:

- Dual core or dual processor (particularly important for multithreaded radiology environment)
- Minimum of 2 gigabytes (GB) of system memory but preferably 4 GB
- 64-bit operating system is preferable but not mandatory as software is not yet optimized.
- Hard-drive subsystem using Wide Ultra2 SCSI (small computer system interface)
- Video card that can render and texture map screen sizes of 1 megapixel minimum with 24–30 frames per second at >60 Hz refresh. Typically a dual core or dual link (SLI, Crossfire) will improve performance. The video card bus should be PCI express.

From the author's experience, large proprietary systems based on UNIX are too costly to justify. Preferable are off-the-shelf workstations, which can be an order of magnitude cheaper. Importantly, the choice of a 3-D platform would ideally be optimized for a Windows-based workstation.

3-D Applications

Computing demands have caused workstations to become behemoths; however, the majority of the cost of 3-D imaging will be in the software platform and licensing. For this reason it is important to choose and negotiate the contract carefully. In a distributed teleradiology environment, where radiologists may be reading from different locations, it may not be cost effective to buy 3-D software licenses for each workstation. There are two potential solutions to this issue:

- License structure could be negotiated according to the number of concurrent users, with an unlimited total number of users. In this way, the 3-D platform can be installed freely on all workstations.
- Images can be rendered at a remote single site in real time by the practicing radiologist, and manipulations can be delivered in real time via the Web or internal network to any number of workstations.

CT Angiography Overnight

This section is a side note but is particularly appropriate to teleradiology. If there is a battleground on which radiologists may have the upper hand, this may be it.

Radiologists have been losing "turf" to cardiologists in coronary and cardiac imaging for decades. The process is starting anew with CT coronary angiography and probably will continue to progress. One area where radiologists may be able to maintain, gain, or create ground is in the overnight evaluation of the acute chest syndrome.

The "triple scan" can be used to evaluate for dissection, coronary artery disease, and pulmonary embolism simultaneously. On a practical level, it would consume considerable time to awaken a cardiologist in the middle of the night to perform this scan. However, because the radiologist (and in particular the remote night radiologist) is practicing overnight, this provides a unique opportunity to aggregate studies from many institutions and create overnight/emergent 3-D laboratories dedicated to the acute chest syndrome. No large-scale implementation of such aggregate studies has been seen yet, but these are probably on the horizon. The main limiting factors are the study sizes, which can exceed 500 MB.

Data Use and Archiving

All right, now that you have the data, how are you going to store them? With the continuing trend toward imaging larger data sets, greater storage needs are developing. The rapidly declining storage costs have been offset by the greater imaging sizes, limiting any cost savings. Archival of images can be done through the practice locally or remotely. Because of the continuing cost pressures and capitalization of these devices, innovative companies have developed models to help reduce these costs. A third-party vendor may host the PACS/RIS in addition to archiving data for a set cost per study. The latter concept has been referred to as an application service provider. For smaller and medium sized groups these application service providers may prove to be an effective solution with costs as low as $5.00 to $8.00 per study without capital outlay. Hybrid models using a mix of local and remote storage can provide lower operating costs with higher capital costs. It is important to analyze the local practice, use, and operating and capital budgets in determining which model to use.

From a practical standpoint, archival of data for preliminary or final interpretations is similar. Clients are often surprised that we archive data indefinitely for overnight teleradiology services. Medical decision making is often based on "preliminary readings." As such, we must hold ourselves accountable to the full medicolegal extent of interpretation. I believe it is recklessly irresponsible not to archive teleradiology data, and practicing overnight services are no exception. Archival of data also allows us to make comparisons with old examinations, which can greatly improve specificity. Because our archive has become so large, on a

practical level this author might compare approximately 5% to 10% of cases in a given night to an old examination contained in our archive.

Because it is difficult to separate pediatric and nonpediatric data, we archive all data indefinitely. As a side benefit, on several occasions our referring radiologists and their PACS administrators are pleased to hear this. We can and have restored locally corrupted data. This further strengthens our collaborative efforts with local groups.

PACS

The writer uses many four-letter words when dealing with PACS, because it has been both a blessing and a curse. It can improve speed, productivity, accuracy, and collaboration. However, PACS will also expose work-flow deficiencies within radiology departments that otherwise may have been hidden. Such deficiencies occur daily in which clinicians have seen, and often acted on, information based on their access to the images before the final report has been generated. This means that radiologists will continue to see erosion in their roles in patient care unless they can provide a value-added report in a time frame that is concordant with or before care is delivered or decided. This is the future pressure of radiology, and this will be the future standard to which radiologists will be held. Patients prefer same-day consultations going from imaging to clinic. Radiologists then have the pressure of either delivering the report in a very rapid fashion, or having the clinician act on what they see as the result, without the radiologist. Both scenarios are suboptimal, but to maintain our value to the clinician we must provide both speed and added value in the report. Voice recognition systems help preempt the clinician self-interpretation.

It is absolutely critical to take the PACS system out for a "test drive" before purchasing it. This is especially relevant in teleradiology, in that PACS systems are traditionally not designed for teleradiology. See how other groups have implemented PACS and use it for teleradiology by doing a site visit. Don't go to a "show site." Call up your radiology friend and visit that site. Some platforms, particularly from the larger vendors, are not designed for the distributed teleradiology practice environment but are optimized for a more traditional practice.

Usually the big players are just that—big players. They have staying power and stability of presence if nothing else. Their products are not necessarily more stable, more user friendly, or more highly functioning than some of the smaller PACS vendors. Indeed, we have found smaller vendors to be much more aggressive and willing to customize to the particular environment. PACS is becoming a commodity, so there are a zillion vendors out there; the marketplace is consolidating, however. RSNA is a good time to see some of these in action; it is *not* a good time to make deals unless all of the legwork is already done.

When you are ready to purchase your PACS, consider that there are two common ways to structure contracts: buy the product outright or use the pay-as-you-go model. Purchasing outright often involves high capital outlay with lower continuing costs. These are more prevalent in traditional practices. A pay-as-you-go plan can offer little or no capital outlay but much higher continuing costs. The latter may be more financially prudent in small teleradiology practices. In either case, prudent financial analysis is imperative.

When purchasing user licenses, the traditional model was to purchase a set number of licenses to be placed on dedicated workstations. Often these licenses are costly and are machine specific. Because PACS has allowed us to practice in a distributed environment and teleradiology more often is in a highly distributed environment, license purchase should be very carefully considered. On a practical level, this means that a referring generalist clinician, a subspecialty clinician, or a radiologist may require (simultaneous) access to the images from a wide variety of locations. This may be within the same city or even different countries. Because of this new distributed demand, more innovative licensing arrangements have become available. Licensing arrangements can be made that are based on the number of concurrent users. An unlimited total number of users have access. The most flexible licensing is a pay-per-study model in

which a case is archived with a single cost. For the life of that study there is unlimited access by clinicians and radiologists. In any of these models it is imperative that an analysis of utilization (who, what, and when) is considered before purchase. It is the author's opinion that the "pay-per-click" licensing platform will continue to gain popularity for small and medium-sized teleradiology practices as a result of the low capital costs and flexible utilization.

HIS/RIS/PACS/Decision Support Integration

Tightly integrated HISs, RISs, PACS, and decision support software are among the most important topics for high-quality care. This integration was formerly confined to traditional hospital practices, but it is coming to the forefront in teleradiology practices, because clients prefer to have "final interpretations." If one is to truly render an optimal "final" interpretation, access to the most complete medical record will improve specificity and accuracy. Herein is a massive logistical challenge for large teleradiology practices. It is costly to integrate HISs from diverse hospital systems into a single platform that can be used by the radiologists. In the final analysis, it is unlikely that this can be done reasonably without greater standardization of medical information storage, akin to DICOM standards for imaging.

That being said, even in a distributed teleradiology environment, the teleradiology group may be a central player in a hospital or imaging center infrastructure because of significant utilization. Even if the practice is not hospital based, we need to view the platform as extending across a distributed environment. This environment can be far reaching, including doctor's offices, hospitals, billing offices, transcription, imaging centers, etc. The platform may serve people in multiple countries, let alone multiple states, or cities.

Decisions about radiology-specific platforms, software, PACS, and RIS should no longer be considered "radiology department" decisions. Close coordination must be concerted with local and enterprise information technology staff in each platform decision.

Your local referring clinician may use your platform for access to his or her patient's images. Changes you make to your system may affect the ability to view those cases. So, these decisions must be carefully made and an implementation plan developed.

Decision support in radiology is a concept to be given serious consideration. As radiologists, our interpretations serve as our main "product." The question we must consider involves how best to extend the functionality of that product from the words on the paper to added value to clinicians. Because the lines between teleradiology and traditional radiology are being blurred, this applies to *all* radiology practices.

Because fully electronic reporting and retrieval of reports is becoming more widespread, we must enhance the quality of the final product. As a more concrete example, a patient has a CT scan of the abdomen with a mass in the kidney. The report's impression will include renal mass. Hyperlinks will automatically provide a differential diagnosis. The radiologist will comment on the most likely cause, in this example, perhaps a renal cell carcinoma. A link to the most current medical concepts and treatments with references on renal cell carcinoma will be threaded into the report. It can also link directly to patient education materials that the doctor can give to the patient. As medical treatment and diagnosis become more and more complex and specialized, this decision support will facilitate and optimize the primary care provider's role in current management and treatment concepts. Is it strange that the *radiologist* may provide the most current medical practice and treatment options in their report? As I stated in the first paragraph, the rules have changed and this is value we must add (teleradiology or otherwise).

Voice-to-Text Technology

Now that we have the images via the PACS, we must generate a report via the RIS. It is inevitable that one day we will exclusively use speech recognition software for this purpose. Today is a different story, and as long as these technologies keep confusing "Indication: fell off of patio, neck pain" for "Indication: fellatio, neck pain" we're in for some growing pains. (In case you were wondering, this actually occurred in one of my dictations, and I fortunately caught it before finalization.)

The economics, feasibility, accuracy, and viability of speech recognition dictation are dealt with extensively in Chapter 14. However, there are a few important concepts to be aware of when implementing these systems:

- The savings you get in transcription costs will probably be offset by productivity losses. Those savings may be applied by hiring full-time equivalents (FTEs) or support staff to recapture productivity losses. Our experience is that these systems do not save money. They cost shift only.
- Workstations must be robust. Do not use the minimum requirements or even the "recommended" setups. We have found significant accuracy performance benefits by greatly exceeding the "recommended" system configuration. Buying fast multicore or multiple-central processing unit systems with greater memory will improve performance. Often dedicated soundcards with high signal-to-noise ratio inputs can provide further benefits.
- Don't skimp on sound dampening equipment for the room in which voice dictation is used. Echoes can be a significant source of errors with typical voice recognition systems.
- Consider using noise cancellation "over-the-head" headsets rather than handheld speech microphones. These over-the-head sets stabilize the microphone-to-mouth distance and will reduce variance in recorded volumes due to repositioning of the handset. Consider budgeting for large numbers of alcohol wipes with the shared microphones. Of course, you may choose to purchase an individual headset system for each radiologist.
- The voice recognition platform should be integrated into the RIS. Ideally the RIS will be tied directly to the PACS, and the selection of a study will automatically open a dictation session.

In deciding which platform to use, it is important to recognize that there are very few actual speech recognition engines. There are several companies that will sell speech recognition software with their own "jazzed-up" front end, but the underlying speech engine may be the same. It is important to know what the underlying speech engine is, who makes it, and who supports it. Always "test drive" the product thoroughly before purchasing it. Most vendors will encourage you to try the product in house for a few weeks/months. Take them up on this offer. Use the software in the exact environment that you plan to read from to see how it performs.

This has been a very contentious area for radiologists. Some adapt very well to the natural speech conversion environments; others fail miserably. Reasons are varied, but to militate against a mass exodus or uprising of your radiologists, provide an alternate mechanism for report generation through the speech technology platform. As an example, most platforms will allow you to send a digital voice file of the report to a transcription service. Incentive plans may need to be instituted for those who use speech recognition software. We have seen some academic institutions provide incremental cost savings of speech recognition reports directly to the radiologists. In some instances it can amount to $2.00 to $4.00 per report. This will be then tied to a radiologist bonus. Typical radiologist volumes can be 10,000 to 30,000 cases per year and can quickly add up.

QUALITY OF SERVICE

It should be stressed that an important concept in teleradiology (more so than routine radiology) is QoS. Greater emphasis and care ultimately must be placed on teleradiology service, because it is a fledgling discipline. People still cling to their mistrusts and will use every example that they can find to point out how the system "doesn't work." Our experience has been that surgeons tend to have greater mistrust of this as a group, but this is a gross generalization. For this reason, providing higher quality of service than is provided locally remains the mantra of teleradiology. QoS can be divided practically into two broad areas: technical and professional.

Technical Quality of Service—Hardware and Software

Continuing routine technical maintenance and conformance testing are required in the

transmission, archival, and retrieval of data. The display systems should also be tested regularly for conformance and uniformity using standard test patterns. Practices may consider using a medical imaging physicist to regularly test devices. Routine testing of modalities and acquisition of data are proscribed by ACR criteria.

With emergent or overnight teleradiology, patient care depends on timely availability of images and rapid interpretation. The ACR recommends that written policies and procedures should be in place to ensure continuity of teleradiology services. This should include internal and external redundancy systems, backup telecommunication links, and a disaster plan. On a practical level, one could consider maintaining two physically separate central data centers. Generally, these would be separated by significant distances (more than 50 miles) and be serviced by redundant leased lines arising from separate points of presence. In the event of failure or outage, data are redirected automatically to the backup site in a seamless fashion. In the event of simultaneous failure, a disaster plan involving local radiologists or other physicians will have to be evoked.

Professional Quality of Service

It is important to recognize that on a professional level, the patient examinations originate at the point of acquisition by the technologist. It is for this reason that the ACR recommends that examination at the transmitting site must be performed by qualified personnel trained in the examination to be performed. In all cases this means a licensed and/or registered radiologic technologist, radiation therapist, nuclear medicine technologist, or sonographer. This technologist must be under the supervision of a qualified licensed physician. On a practical level, it is critical that the remote and local radiologists work together to improve protocols, technologist education, and study quality. We have found that informal mechanisms (i.e., radiologist to radiologist) foster the collaborative nature of the relationship. A formal mechanism for addressing study questions and answers should be in place optimally.

At minimum, basic physician competency should be demonstrated by board eligibility. Optimally, board certification and subspecialty accreditation (when applicable) would be a basic prerequisite. According to ACR guidelines, the physician should have basic understanding of the basic technology of teleradiology, its strengths, limitations, and use of the teleradiology equipment.

When images are interpreted preliminarily, as is the case in many overnight teleradiology situations, there must be a mechanism and polices of peer review in place. These policies will guide physician notification schemes, "missed diagnoses," or "opinion differences." The content and character of this review is not accusatory and is meant to improve patient care outcomes in the future. The review should include the following components:

- Identification of the appropriate study, patient demographics, and report
- Identification of the radiologists rendering the preliminary and final reports
- Identification of the physician managing the patient at the time of the preliminary report and the physician or care provider responsible for the subsequent care of the patient. If the patient is not under the direct care of a provider, identification of the patient contact information.
- Review of the discrepancies in the report and review of the images by an expert third party
- Assessment of validity of the discrepancy (i.e., was the final report correct?)
- Identification of the changes in clinical management and potential actions resulting from those changes
- Remediation and education of the radiologist(s)
- Communication of the results of the review to the care providers involved

When images are interpreted on a final basis, periodic random review should be undertaken. One mechanism by which this can be done is with patients who have had repeat examinations separated by time. Concordance or discordance in results can be recorded and collected for examination. Another mechanism to consider is third-party review of random caseload.

MEDICOLEGAL CONSIDERATIONS

It is important to recognize that because of the rapidly evolving and fledgling nature of teleradiology, there is a relative paucity of legal precedent. A few of the more basic considerations are detailed in this section.

Multistate Practices

When the practice of teleradiology crosses state boundaries, the radiologists must meet the appropriate medical licensure requirements. From a conservative viewpoint, practitioners should be licensed not only in the state in which they reside but also in the state(s) in which they are practicing. The practitioner should be credentialed at the facilities if it is routine practice to do so in the setting in which care is delivered. In particular, this usually applies when care is delivered to hospital-based settings.

Liability may be a more difficult issue, but again from a conservative standpoint, the practitioners should meet the most stringent minimum liability standards of the state in which they are practicing or residing. Liability policies should be sought that have the flexibility to introduce new states and new radiologists without undue burden. There are a limited number of national providers of malpractice insurance. Costs can be higher in these situations, and prudent cost analysis should be performed before entering into teleradiology agreements.

International Practices

Considerable media attention has been devoted to international teleradiology practices undercutting U.S.-based practices. However, there are important considerations that one should be aware of when outsourcing to an international teleradiology-based practice. The first and foremost is that of minimum basic credentialing and requirements for licensure. From a conservative standpoint, the practicing radiologist should be licensed in the state in which care is delivered. Additionally, appropriate board certification should be insisted upon for all radiologists practicing internationally but delivering care within this country. It is uncertain whether licensing is required in the nation where the radiologist resides and practices.

At minimum, liability coverage should be acquired for the state in which the care is delivered. It is important to recognize that an even more limited insurance carrier base may be available to cover radiologists practicing overseas but delivering their care in the United States. Additionally, one important liability consideration is that of extradition in the event of a medical malpractice lawsuit. It is unlikely that most nations will extradite a physician to stand trial in a noncriminal lawsuit. In particular, India, China, and Israel do not extradite for civil lawsuits such as malpractice. In the event that there is a medical malpractice suit, the group that has hired the international teleradiology practice may be subject to risk irrespective of malpractice committed by the local group. Moreover, it is likely the hospital will bear the brunt of the risk. Careful consideration of this point should guide practices in choosing a teleradiology partner.

Periodically multiple bills are introduced in Congress that try to restrict international teleradiology practice. Close attention must be paid to current and developing legal trends that may affect the transmission of data overseas. These are often centered around security and compliance with the Health Insurance Portability and Accountability Act of 1996 (HIPAA).

Because much media attention has been directed to the "outsourcing" of U.S.-based teleradiology, little information has been presented on U.S.-based teleradiology practices practicing on an international level. It is the author's experience that throughout the world, U.S.-trained and board-certified radiologists carry significant credentials that are sought after. In this model, high-quality patient care can be delivered to remote or rural areas as well as urban and high-growth areas. Patients will often pay a premium to have a study interpreted by U.S.-trained and board-certified radiologists. Because of this, globally based teleradiology practices in the United States are growing significantly. Licensing, credentialing, and malpractice requirements should meet the basic standards of the country in which care is delivered.

Time to Reporting

One important parameter that is often misunderstood in teleradiology is time to reporting. Many teleradiology practices will proclaim very low times to reporting. Most teleradiology practices will use the time from which they received the study. This can present difficulties, because the receipt of the study could be significantly later than the study acquisition time. These delays can be related to technologist errors, reconstruction time, or transmission time. Additionally, a report transmitted may not be received at the local site, particularly if it is faxed—for a multitude of reasons, including fax transmission errors, local phone exchange errors, and the fax results being lost. It is for this reason that times to reporting are not as accurate or as short as many practices claim. The main importance of this is in the overnight emergent teleradiology field, where typical practices will have reports generated in less than 30 minutes.

From a practical viewpoint, reporting should be accurate and timely, and if there are subsequent questions or interactions between the care provider and the radiologist direct access to the radiologist should be rapid. Some practices, including overnight practices, will report every result directly to the referring physician by telephone. Such reporting methods are uncommon among overnight providers and are highly sought after by clinicians. They improve patient care because of the direct interaction between physicians. Additionally, when results are directly communicated, the time to reporting and reliability of reporting are improved. It is crucial to document any communication in the official reports, including time, date, and persons involved.

Final versus Preliminary Reports

From a medicolegal standpoint, it is important to recognize that reports can be "final" or "preliminary." The former has no overread or second radiologist and will generally be a complete report as per ACR reporting standards. The latter is an abbreviated report designed to answer the immediate clinical question. These are typically reserved for the overnight teleradiology practices or "curbside" consultations.

Although these have slightly different medicolegal implications, the most important report in an emergent setting is arguably the one on which the initial medical decision making was based. For nonemergent findings, the final report has clear precedence because of its completeness.

Insurance is more costly when rendering final reports as compared with preliminary reports. From a medicolegal standpoint it is important to recognize that a remote group practicing teleradiology without the patient history, former studies, and relevant clinical information rendering final reports is probably not providing optimal patient care. This has important implications if a practice is outsourcing to a remote group. Often practices will prefer that when the overnight cases are rendered as final, they will not have to review and read the cases the following morning. Unless there is integration of the RIS/HIS/PACS between the local and remote practices (as discussed previously), reports are often created without incorporating old examinations and history. Clinicians will then ask the local group to again present the results routinely with these data. It behooves clinicians to be cautious when entering into agreements with remote teleradiology practices in which "final readings" are performed without the appropriate relevant clinical history and prior studies.

Accreditation

There are two major bodies that will accredit teleradiology practices: the Joint Commission on Accreditation of Healthcare Organizations (JCAHO) and the Healthcare Facilities Accreditation Program (HFAP). JCAHO is clearly the larger of the two accreditation bodies.

From a teleradiology perspective, accreditation by one of these bodies can rapidly facilitate credentialing for the hospital setting. Many hospitals that participate in either of the accreditation programs will accept the certification of those programs for credentialing. For smaller or geographically well-localized teleradiology practices, this accreditation may not prove to be cost effective. For larger, multistate practices with many radiologists, the added value of

JCAHO or HFAP certification may save costs and time in credentialing. This writer is not aware of any defined medicolegal requirement to obtain either certification.

Health Insurance Portability and Accountability Act

HIPAA regulations give us the basic minimum set of confidentiality guidelines by which to practice. However, the teleradiology platform (inclusive of acquisition, transmission, archiving, and reporting) must operate with security protocols to protect the confidentiality of patients' private health information. Measures must be installed to safeguard the data and to ensure against intentional or unintentional corruption/loss of data or theft. At the acquisition level, the local HIPAA conformance is in place. The moment the study has begun to be transmitted we must insure that the data can be encrypted. There are two basic methods of transmitting data over a wide area network: network address translation with encryption and virtual private networks (VPNs).

In a nutshell, a VPN is a way to transmit data securely using inexpensive public lines (such as the Internet). VPNs have two components: tunneling and encryption. The "tunnel" is a mechanism by which two computers may communicate with each other directly over a public network (like the Internet). The other component of the VPN is the encryption, which protects data traveling on this public network so that even if data are intercepted, they are rendered useless. VPNs may be more difficult to implement initially but have strong security features. On a practical level, we favor the use of VPNs because of their enhanced security as compared with less robust network address translation with encryption.

Archived data are also encrypted, reducing the possibility of loss or theft at the data center. We use proprietary encryption protocols for archival that are not widely available, so that any data lost or stolen from the data center are effectively rendered unreadable. Access to images and reports is also via secured protocols. Results are transmitted via facsimile to secure facsimile locations (namely emergency departments and local radiology departments). Results are accessed electronically via the Web using standard Web-based security protocols including user name and password and appropriate logging of data access.

E-mail Security Issues

It is important to note that routine e-mail is not secure. The transmission of patients' private health information via unsecured e-mail is a direct violation of the terms of HIPAA. However, e-mail transmissions can be used if a link to the report is provided in the e-mail and the recipient must securely log into the Internet location containing the reports. The access to private health information must be logged electronically. Use of secured and encrypted e-mail is acceptable.

ECONOMICS

Cost Effectiveness

The economics of teleradiology can be classified into at least two large subdivisions: in-house and outsourced. Each has its unique and common defining economic pressures. Clearly the economics are viable enough that the industry has become a multi-billion dollar operation worldwide. However, the medical literature lacks accurate published information on the cost-benefit or cost effectiveness of teleradiology. According to the literature, the main proven patient benefits come in rural or underserved areas in which the availability of an expert radiology reading may avoid an unnecessary patient transfer or may improve timeliness of study results.

Full-Time Equivalents and Costs

The cost effectiveness from the standpoint external to the local group (i.e., the community) is different from the economics and benefits to the local group. The benefits from the radiologist standpoint can be both financial and qualitative. For example, if the local radiologist must be awakened repeatedly overnight, it becomes difficult for that person to practice effectively the following day. As such, many practices will allow the radiologist to take the day off after being "on call" (or to have limited duties). From a financial standpoint, this means that covering 365 days per year will effectively remove at minimum 1 FTE from the work force. After calculating benefits, vacation, and the like, this result may be closer to 1.25 FTEs (for 365 days). For a small to medium-sized hospital, 5 to 10 studies will be acquired overnight. If this is done on average for a year, at industry standard costs of U.S. $50 to $55 per study equivalent, costs will be approximately U.S. $100,000 to $200,000 per year in coverage. This is clearly well below the salary and benefits of the typical FTE radiologist yearly and on a cost basis, one can justify the expenditure. With the FTE now available to work during more productive daytime hours, it allows the group to leverage its size to take on larger and more lucrative contracts.

Hiring and Recruiting

Qualitative benefits to the local radiology group exist as well. Certainly, radiologists often have chosen their field in part because of lifestyle considerations. Overnight call duties for radiologists are often discordant with their expectations of lifestyle afforded by the profession. Groups that cannot meet those expectations may suffer in a competitive hiring environment for a limited radiologist pool. Radiology practices may find it difficult to hire new employees without having overnight services in place. This gives further incentive to consider outsourcing portions of the practice.

In internal teleradiology, there are significant costs related to the setup and infrastructure of maintaining a teleradiology platform. These are often treated as capital outlays and on a net-present-value basis can exceed the cost of operating expenses for outsourcing. The largest costs are usually related to the software and licensing as well as continuing communications, networking, and hardware that must be purchased. A prudent cost analysis and comparison must be made against the outsourced model.

Competition

The practice of teleradiology is becoming more competitive. The competition comes from the multitudes of teleradiology practices based in the United States as well as practices based abroad. Moreover, the competitive edges that were unique to some groups are no longer present. Wide variability in both the pricing models and quality of groups still exists, and it is important to have firsthand knowledge of a remote group, its radiologists, and the quality of their reports before outsourcing radiology. The remote group represents and reflects the local group, and reference checking is thus imperative. The features you should consider when hiring a remote teleradiology practice are outlined in Box 19-1.

There is rapid expansion of the field and fragmentation of the teleradiology market into many players of varying sizes. As the field

matures, teleradiology practices will probably consolidate to maintain scales of economy and to be able to remain competitive. This reflects the same trend in "bricks and mortar" radiology practices that has been occurring over the past 10 to 15 years.

Marketing and Contracts

Marketing first and foremost begins with market research. It is important to identify needs both locally and regionally before beginning a teleradiology practice. Third-party firms can be hired to do this, but simply knowing your local/regional market serves as a good stepping stone. Talk with local radiologists at your local ACR chapters; get out there and make contacts.

That being said, we have seen marketing from a variety of different media outlets. Some of the bigger teleradiology providers send numerous marketing materials to prospective clients. Advertisements can be placed in journals or other radiology media outlets.

At the end of the day, marketing for our practice comes down to past performance and reputation. Greater than 90% of our new business is unsolicited and by word of mouth. Before signing with an overnight provider, clients should check and recheck references. When outsourcing, remember that this remote group reflects on your practice. It is the equivalent of a bad hiring decision. As with PACS systems, "don't go to the show site." Find the list of the clients that have dropped or changed services. This will be your best source of information about the reality of the practice. There are several practices that have changed names repeatedly over the years. Be wary of these, because they often have tarnished their reputation so badly that they were forced to hide their true genealogy.

Contracts should be constructed by a lawyer who has specialty expertise in teleradiology or at least telemedicine. Lawyers with such expertise are rare indeed, but with some searching you can find them locally. In most metropolitan areas at least a few lawyers will have dedicated practices in telemedicine. You will hemorrhage money with their fees, but in the end their experience will be worth every penny.

BOX 19-1

Important Points to Consider When Outsourcing Teleradiology Overnight

- Cost structure for exams
  - Are services provided on a per-case basis or per hour of coverage?
- Credentials of remote group, including subspecialty training
  - Look for experience, board certification, subspecialty training, and certification.
- How are results communicated to the referring clinician?
- Are the results given directly from physician to physician? This latter point may help practices with emergency departments and hospitals that are reluctant to "buy in" to the concept of teleradiology.
  Overnight practice hours
  - Do these coincide with the hours that are needed?
  - Are these changeable and flexible (i.e., one day, might need more coverage, one day need less)?
- Daytime, daytime holiday, or weekend daytime practice hours
  - Check for availability.
- Are subspecialty "overreads" or consultation readings performed?

Administrative Infrastructure

How much support staff do you need? Good question! That depends on what you're doing. Reading 10 cases a night via teleradiology is not going to require a staff of dozens of people, but reading 10,000 may. There are no specific guidelines to the degree of overhead, but as size of the practice grows, the fractional percentage of overhead seems to grow, not shrink. This is not dissimilar to our federal government.

We have heard of groups spending 30% of their gross revenues on administrative support staff. This can include receptionists, technical support staff, operators, credentialing specialists, billing specialists, and a whole bevy of other people whose job titles are more impressive than what they may actually do for the company.

The basic recommendation is to keep your beginning practice clean and free from these administrative staff people unless they are absolutely needed. These positions can be added as needed. Incentive-based pay can improve productivity and minimize overall costs.

Licensing, Credentialing, and Billing

The area of licensing, credentialing, and billing is one gigantic quagmire. If you can avoid dealing with this and give it to one of the more junior guys in the group, you should. All kidding aside, this is critically important and deserves the highest attention.

Licensing is often a rate-limiting factor for teleradiology practices. Licenses are expensive both to obtain and maintain. Some states require personal interviews or additional testing before obtaining a license. As a general rule of thumb, plan for 3–6 months to obtain licenses. Also, with each additional license, subsequent licensing becomes more tedious (as the new state now requires all of the verification of each of the previous state licenses). There is a geometric progression of complexity that is difficult to overcome. As practices start to read thousands of studies per night, licensing requirements begin to abate, because radiologists can read significant volume from one or two states.

Credentialing is just as cumbersome as licensing, if not more so. With state medical licensing there are a limited number of states (50). With at least 5000 hospitals in the United States, there is a nearly unlimited variety of credentialing applications, forms, and other quirky information required. Each of these has its own ways and means of credentialing physicians. Our longest credentialing process took 13 months to complete. The hospital checked in excess of 500 references for our group and radiologists before approving credentialing. I would have guessed that around the 200-plus mark, they may have said, "you know what, these guys are probably OK" and pushed it through. On average, however, the credentialing process will require 2–3 months per site.

Credentialing can be facilitated by JHACO or HFAP accreditation as discussed earlier. Certain hospitals will accept third-party or independent primary source verification of physicians from facilities with this accreditation. These sites can often complete credentialing in a matter of weeks. Realize that credentialing is a self-made problem. Each hospital creates its own policies on the degree and type of credentialing necessary. Hospitals may not adapt or yield to alternative practices, or make exceptions. As an example, we have had hospitals insist that our physicians obtain basic life support training before being credentialed. It's going to be hard to perform remote cardiopulmonary resuscitation on a patient 2500 miles away from my living room, but "rules are rules." You've got to sympathize with the people who have the job of making sure that check boxes are completed.

Depending on the type of teleradiology practice, you may need to bill third-party payers, insurance companies, or Medicare/Medicaid. A discussion of this is out of the scope of this chapter and is discussed in other chapters. For "overnight" teleradiology services, billing is often much simpler. Contracts are entered into by a hospital or local radiology practice. Billing is performed directly with the local group on a fee schedule that has been previously negotiated. At the end of a billing cycle, caseload is typically submitted and a bill is rendered. The payer will remit funds, generally speaking, within 30 days in full. Wouldn't it be nice if Medicare or insurance providers worked like this?

Life of a Teleradiologist

First and foremost, there is no such thing as typical lifestyle, work hours, pay, or caseload for teleradiologists. Teleradiology practices are diverse, some with daytime hours only and 24- to 48-hour report turnaround, and others with 24/7 coverage with 30-minute report turnaround. The hours, practice environment, and lifestyle are what you make of them. Some groups will call every result to the referring clinician at the time of interpretation. Others will generate reports only and send them to the referring clinician. We've seen small practices in which radiologists will read 40 or fewer cases a day to much busier practices in which radiologists can read in excess of 150 cases per day. Equally variable are the work hours and length of the work day. Some practices will have short work schedules in which radiologists may read for 4–6 hours, or longer days in which radiologists are reading for 10–12 hours. Vacation time is equally variable, with some groups offering 34 weeks of vacation for 17 weeks of work. Other groups offer as few as 8 weeks of vacation for the year. Some teleradiology practices require that you read from a central reading facility, whereas others allow you to read from home. At the end of the day, the only thing that can be said about the life of the teleradiologist is that it's what you make of it. There are no hard and fast rules, and everything is open to negotiation. All that is required is a little searching for a practice that fits your goals.

FUTURE DIRECTIONS AND CONCLUSIONS

The end is really the beginning in this case. Teleradiology will continue to remodel the shape of how medicine is practiced throughout the world. With greater pressures for high-quality care served even to the most remote locations, teleradiology has the power to effect medical change. Innovative new hybrid practices may emerge such as academic teleradiology practices. Technologies will continue to improve, and faster and cheaper access to higher bandwidth will facilitate more widespread collaboration. The mainstay of radiology, our static reports, will have dynamic content that can be updated to provide the most value to our referring clinicians and patients. In the end, as in the beginning, our future progress and success in this field depends on our ability to maintain quality both on a professional and technical level.

The Dos and Don'ts of Teleradiology Practice	
Dos	**Don'ts**
1. Understand that the rules have changed.	1. Don't be cheap. Spend adequately on technology, but don't waste money. Costs are high, but lawsuit costs are higher. Capital is king, so guard it carefully.
2. Carry moral ascendancy. Your actions should always be preceded by the question, "Is what I'm doing right"? All of your dealings should be forthright and honest, not just truthful.	2. Plan way ahead. Credentialing and licensing can take as long as a year. Decisions about growth are limited in great measure by licensing and credentialing.
3. Have passion for what you're doing. At the end of the day, radiology and medicine are concerned with improving the health and lives of our patients. Approach each case with the notion that this is someone's mother, or child, or loved one.	3. Build in redundancy. Make sure the platform is redundant three times over. Reliability is a paramount concern when you're remote.
4. Be willing to accept risk. Ventures like this are risky, but you should be willing to see your ideas through to the end. Playing it safe and avoiding risk is a good way to remain mediocre.	4. Don't go it alone. There are lot of people with experience in both practice management and teleradiology practice management. Seek them out and ask their advice.

Dos	Don'ts
5. Emphasize quality of service. The difference between the truly successful practices and the average practice is that successful practices live, breathe, and preach quality, whereas the less successful practices only pay lip service to it.	5. An ounce of prevention is worth a pound of cure. Reacting to problems is not optimal. Proactive management and addressing potential sources of problems before their manifestation are preferable.
6. Learn to walk before trying to fly. Appropriate business planning, financial analysis, and marketing and implementation plans should be examined carefully before spending a single cent.	6. Procrastination is an enemy of success. Something that must be done now probably should have been done weeks ago. Get on it.
7. Understand that radiology is a distributed environment. The lines between "traditional" and "teleradiology" practices have blurred. Traditional groups practice teleradiology daily, even though they don't think of themselves in this way.	7. One bad apple spoils the bunch. Be meticulous in hiring practices, even at the cost of growth. Remember, the people you work with are a reflection on you.
8. Innovate. Remember, we have a blank canvas now. We can choose what we want to paint. We can define or redefine the practice of radiology.	8. Failing to recognize the changing landscape of medicine can be your downfall. It is important to keep current on national and state health care policies. This will change your practice and could potentially have disastrous results.
9. Obtain a good lawyer. Have a legal team who is adept in the practice of multistate teleradiology.	9. If you build it, they may not come. Have contracts either in hand or nearly so before starting teleradiology services. When you start you need to have some cash flow.
10. Incentivize employees. If you give people a reason to do better, they will.	10. Losing sight of the patient is a real danger. At the end of all this, we are physicians and our interests are with the patient. Make sure that your actions are guided by this principle.

SUGGESTED READINGS

Aas IH: Organizational cooperation in teleradiology. J Telemed Telecare 11(1):45–50, 2005.

American College of Radiology: ACR Technical standards for teleradiology (October 2005).

Collmann J, Alaoui A, Nguyen D, Lindisch D: Safe teleradiology: information assurance as project planning methodology. J Am Med Inform Assoc 12(1):84–89, 2005.

Craig J, Patterson V: Introduction to the practice of telemedicine. J Telemed Telecare 11(1):3–9, 2005.

Hailey D, Roine R, Ohinmaa A: Systematic review of evidence for the benefits of telemedicine. J Telemed Telecare 8(Suppl 1):1–30, 2002.

Herron JM, Bender TM, Campbell WL, Sumkin JH, Rockette HE, Gur D: Effects of luminance and resolution on observer performance with chest radiographs. Radiology 215(1):169–174, 2000.

Hoffman T: Teleradiology: an underdeveloped legal frontier. ACR Bull (September 2005).

Jarvis L, Stanberry B: Teleradiology: threat or opportunity? Clin Radiol 60(8):840–845, 2005.

Larson DB, Cypel YS, Forman HP, Sunshine JH: A comprehensive portrait of teleradiology in radiology practices: results from the American College of Radiology's 1999 Survey. AJR Am J Roentgenol 185(1):24–35, 2005.

Mun SK, Tohme WG, Platenberg RC, Choi I: Teleradiology and emerging business models. J Telemed Telecare 11(6):271–275, 2005.

Soegner P, Rettenbacher T, Smekal A, Zur Nedden D: Guidelines for teleradiology practice: results of the Tyrolean teleradiology pilot project. J Telemed Telecare 9(Suppl 1):S48–S50, 2003.

Thrall JH: Reinventing radiology in the digital age. Part I. The all-digital department. Radiology 236(2):382–385, 2005.

Thrall JH: Reinventing radiology in the digital age. Part II. New directions and new stakeholder value. Radiology 237(1):15–18, 2005.

Thrall JH: Reinventing radiology in the digital age. Part III. Facilities, work processes, and job responsibilities. Radiology 237(3):790–793, 2005.

Tie M, Koczwara B: Quality improvement through teleradiology: opportunities and challenges. Australas Radiol 48(4):476–479, 2004.

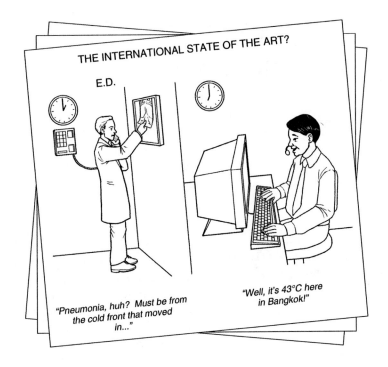

Medical Entrepreneurship in Diagnostic Imaging

Frank James Lexa

Whatever can be done, will be done.
If not by incumbents, it will be done by emerging players. If not in a regulated industry, it will be done in a new industry born without regulation. Technological change and its effects are inevitable. Stopping them is not an option.

ANDY GROVE

INTRODUCTION

This chapter has four parts. First we will explore the current opportunity for medical entrepreneurs in the United States with an emphasis on our field of radiology. Topics for discussion include both the nature of entrepreneurial activity in imaging as well as the economic and financial issues that influence its success or failure. This part also surveys the current investment climate for innovative health care ventures.

In the second portion of this chapter we will examine the structure of the process, beginning with the generation of new ideas, and then map the development paths and sources of investment for embryonic companies through entry into the marketplace. There are many routes to medical entrepreneurship, and there are diverse paths to success. Our focus will be on how and when ideas receive outside funding both public and private—with emphasis on how those decisions affect the entrepreneurial process, in particular the trade-offs inherent in accepting funding.

The third portion of the chapter will first enumerate and then address many of the common challenges that face American medical entrepreneurs. We will concentrate on the issues that must be faced initially for radiologists in establishing a business—in other words, actions that you must take before investing your time or your (or someone else's) money in a high-risk, high-reward venture. The seeds of both success and failure are often sown early, and most nascent ventures can ill afford to waste their resources. Much of the ultimate success (or lack thereof) of many businesses can be traced back to this early developmental period. Just as in biologic development, insults and problems at the earliest stages can be far more destructive than problems and bad decisions later on. The birth and neonatal phases are particularly risky for highly innovative companies. One of the reasons for dividing the process of business development into stages is that relatively predictable challenges arise at each step. A smart entrepreneur is one who anticipates and meets these issues directly instead of waiting until they are overwhelming.[1]

In the fourth and final section we will systematically address 10 difficult questions that you will have to answer if you really think that you are ready to take on the challenges of entrepreneurship in the diagnostic imaging field. This chapter is based on articles that originally appeared in the *Journal of the American College of Radiology* during 2004 and 2005.[2,3]

THE ENTREPRENEURIAL OPPORTUNITY

Entrepreneurism in America: The Environment

The United States is a highly entrepreneurial society that produces legions of innovators in a wide spectrum of fields and disciplines. Furthermore, a combination of freedom and relative openness also make the country a magnet for attracting some of the most capable individuals from around the world to come and try to make their fortunes here.

Entrepreneurial activity consists of successfully creating change and innovation in the world. It is far more important than most people realize; it is far more pervasive than most people think, and finally, in interesting ways, it is both easier and more difficult than is commonly perceived. As Andy Grove pointedly states, there is an inevitable thrust to the waves of change that sweep through society. This phenomenon is particularly characteristic of our technology-driven field of radiology. One of the exciting aspects of American society is the way that the nation welcomes and even expects regular innovation in many aspects of its economy.

In this regard, diagnostic imaging is a particularly striking industry subsector. The cliché, "better, faster, cheaper" is practically embedded into the culture of diagnostic imaging. It is what we have learned to expect every year at the RSNA (Radiological Society of North America) meeting or other similar technology trade shows. Many of us entered radiology because of the combination of excitement and novelty that comes from working with leading-edge technologies. We expect our products and devices to improve on a regular cycle and they usually do, even if better and faster don't always translate into cheaper (or vice versa).

However, in discussing health care and business in the same chapter, it must also be stated at the outset that medicine is a unique facet of American business. There are special standards and scrutiny applied to health care goods and services that don't occur in other realms of the economy, such as entertainment or information technology. In fact, the results of entrepreneurism in medicine have an admittedly checkered history. At times in the United States this has taken a nefarious turn to "snake oil"—both metaphorically and, at times, literally. This perceived conflict is quite powerful in the corporate setting, particularly in the delivery of services where good medicine and good business are perceived to be at odds by many. This pits ethics against self-interest and economic considerations, with some types of entrepreneurship being blamed for rising costs.[4,5] Indeed, it is important to note that not all innovations are warmly welcomed by the stakeholders in the health care enterprise and in fact are often strongly opposed.[6,7]

With that said, new technologies and other innovations are often welcomed and as noted above even regularly expected by those of us in high-technology medical fields. Overall, in fact, there is an enormous engine for innovation in the United States. At the height of the last economic surge, over $100 billion a year was spent on venture capital alone to help entrepreneurial ventures make it to the market (Table 20-1). As in other exciting, cutting-edge fields there is often marked variability and cyclicality to the magnitude of this investment.[8] Life science is a critical component of venture investing. In 2004, for instance, 28% of the venture activity occurred in the life sciences.[9]

However, even in a much quieter period, venture activity can still be quite substantial. For example, even in a much tougher time—calendar year 2003—over $19 billion in venture capital (VC) was still put to work by American firms domestically in the hope that these investments in new entrepreneurial enterprises would be successful enough to bring the high double-digit and even triple-digit rates of financial return that VC investment firms target.[10] The VC market had its best first quarter since 2001 in the beginning of 2006, with $6.02 billion invested.[11]

Table 20-1 U.S. Venture Capital Investments by Fiscal Year

Year	No. of Deals	Avg. per Deal Sum (Million US$)	Investment (Million US$)
1996	2,469	4.36	10,762.30
1997	3,080	4.74	14,591.99
1998	3,550	5.84	20,718.89
1999	5,396	9.91	53,487.98
2000	7,812	13.36	104,379.88
2001	4,451	9.11	40,537.78
2002	3,053	7.11	21,692.68
2003	2,876	6.82	19,613.81
2004	2,991	7.28	21,768.86
2005	3,027	7.35	22,261.59

Adapted from PricewaterhouseCoopers/National Venture Capital Association MoneyTree Report, Data: Thomson Financial — Updated 31 Dec. 2005. Available from: http://www.nvca.org (accessed 7 September 2006).

The health care and medical sectors are a significant component of the annual venture dollars invested in the United States, composing more than a quarter of the money invested in the high-risk, high-reward component during the past year by VC funds.[12] This reflects the roles of both entrepreneurs and their investors working together to drive the engine of medical innovation.

The U.S.-based health care industry is a particularly dynamic sector of the domestic economy.[13] It has a sector rate of change that is one of the highest within the U.S. economy. It absorbs and in some ways relies on and even expects a regular diet of new products and services. Few industries in America are as welcoming of new products and services as the health care field. Although this openness to change clearly seems to vary among the diverse consumers of health care technology, patients and physicians in particular expect that there will be a constant stream of steady improvements as well as occasional breakthroughs.

To get a sense of the magnitude of the innovation that occurs in this market, some statistics prove particularly illuminating. The number of patents issued in the United States has been growing substantially in the past decade.[14] In a recent year, the U.S. patent office issued almost 200,000 patents, a large number of which have direct or indirect biomedical applications.[15] Although the Food and Drug Administration is sometimes criticized for slowing the process, the agency approves a large number of new biomedical compounds and devices annually. Large U.S.-based corporations spend substantial amounts on research and development each year. Medical firms, particularly pharmaceutical and biotechnology companies, are among the most aggressive and consistently innovative in the American corporate landscape.

At face value, diagnostic imaging seems to be an obvious lucrative area of investment. Imagine the pitch to an overseas investor: the American health care market exceeded $2 trillion in 2005,[16] with an aggressive growth rate that is expected to continue to at least 2020 or 2025. Moreover, diagnostic imaging is a particularly compelling sector of that market, with a recent year-over-year growth rate of more than 20% (personal communication, Cherrill Farnsworth, Health Help, Inc.). To top it off, this is a highly dynamic sector with multiple stakeholders and a hunger for all types of new technologic innovations. Although we are all chastened by recent downturns in reimbursement (at this writing there are serious cuts planned from the Deficit Reduction Act) and from threatening competitors to traditional imaging, the above pitch is still one of the most compelling in venture investing. This author has used more detailed versions of these investment proposals in recruiting overseas backers with considerable success. We will now turn to the process of entrepreneurship and examine how this is driven at the level of an individual radiologist or team with a great idea.

AN OVERVIEW OF THE ENTREPRENEURIAL PROCESS— HOW THE FUTURE IS CREATED

Imagination is the beginning of creation. You imagine what you desire, you will what you imagine, and at last you create what you will.

GEORGE BERNARD SHAW

The Beginning: Idea and Vision

The entrepreneurial process takes many paths, and there is a plethora of choices from beginning to end. Although there is tremendous diversity and certainly no single road to success, this discussion will cover some of the most common challenges that entrepreneurs face in the process of successful innovation in America and how they address them. All entrepreneurship begins with an idea or, as it is more commonly said today, a "vision."

An important additional point to clarify here is that entrepreneurship in medicine occurs along a spectrum of innovation. At one end is the incremental "better mousetrap"—an improved service that can attract business through better performance, improved safety, lower price, higher doctor or patient acceptance, or a combination of such positive features. At the other extreme is the truly revolutionary technology that is so novel and so dramatic that it disrupts and ultimately will destroy an entire existing industrial sector—the proverbial "buggy whip manufacturer" sent to the dustbin of history by the rise of the age of automobiles.

More recently, and more germane to those of us in radiology, is the end of pneumoencephalography with the introduction of the computed tomography (CT) scanner. This is a dramatic example of relatively rapid replacement. Most novel technologies in our field do not come with this degree of speed and finality. The legendary economist and student of capitalist economic systems, Joseph Schumpeter, termed this latter phenomenon "creative destruction," and it is an integral component of many of the most successful and significant efforts of entrepreneurs.[17] Sometimes predicted destruction does not occur if both technologies are robust and neither has peaked in maturity. For example, in our field in the late 1980s and early 1990s many predicted that magnetic resonance imaging (MRI) would replace CT scanning for almost all applications in neuroradiology, particularly brain imaging. A combination of the relative strengths of the modalities and an impressive effort in continued innovation on the CT side has instead kept them both on the playing field as of this writing. In fact the exponential nature of the improvement in CT capability with persistent doublings every couple of years has already shown that CT may replace many of the indications for not only MRI but also diagnostic angiography.

This issue of integrating new products or services into the existing market and society is not a trivial one and in fact can substantially slow or block beneficial new technologies and services. Incremental or intermediate forms of innovation (e.g., this year's faster software upgrade for your scanner, or a better vascular catheter, or a safer formulation of a pharmaceutical) are all relatively easy for existing users to accept. Many types of entrepreneurial activity, however, require greater adjustment and face resistance—occasionally severe—from the existing markets. For example, a novel form of software or a revolutionary machine with the power to displace an entire subspecialty of physicians would obviously face market resistance from those who would be replaced, no matter the overall performance or economic advantages. The phenomenon is most acute when the early adopters are also those who will have to adapt and change the most. It is particularly problematic when they are also those most at risk from being "creatively destroyed." A relatively recent example of this in medical services is the rise in use of refractive surgery and its effect on traditional producers and retailers of eyeglasses and contact lenses. In this case, the people most threatened are also those in a position to act as gatekeepers for many of the customers.

For example, carefully consider some potential examples: a robust pharmaceutical treatment for atherosclerosis that makes coronary angioplasty/stenting as well as carotid endarterectomy and stenting unnecessary, a software algorithm that can replace the need for most MRI and CT technologists by allowing automatic on-site or remote control of a scanner, or a computer-aided diagnostic system that can read radiology images faster and more accurately than humans can. These are real (albeit heavily disguised) versions of representative technologies that early-stage entrepreneurs have disclosed to the author's investing teams in recent years as part of the initiation of the entrepreneurial process. They would all represent significant threats to a substantial fraction of the market that they target—particularly the current users.

At the least, these challenges would force existing users to adapt themselves and their work to the changing technology, not only to co-opt the displacing technology from others, but also, and more importantly, to avoid becoming obsolete as the technology is implemented. This class of more dramatic entrepreneurship requires not only the idea and vision, but also a great deal of effort to help the market to accept a new disruptive, displacing product.

A fascinating related phenomenon is how imaging entrepreneurs deliberately or inadvertently change the medical landscape by restructuring a radiology service or subindustry. This is not necessarily the result of changing a technology or the invention or introduction

of a new device. Instead, this shift is a result of an aggressive rethinking of how an industry is ordered and how the relationships between customers and providers can and should work. Restructuring a service or industry may result in substantial change in work or even wholesale "disintermediation" of a group or groups as the sea change occurs.

An example of the former is the use of picture archiving and communications systems and teleradiology systems to disaggregate the performance of imaging from professional interpretation. This creates the opportunity to separate these functions in time and space. As we have seen, it also opens the doors to threats of outside encroachment on these traditional radiology roles. In the United States this has facilitated a much wider diffusion of imaging technology away from traditional sites where radiology existed. It is now common for nonradiologists and even nonphysicians to own imaging equipment and separate these functions. These systems, in combination with smaller, simpler scanners, have facilitated the ability to make the acquisition of images essentially ubiquitous. This is a genuine disruption of the type described by Christensen in his ground-breaking work on the way that low- or even poor-performance technologies by new entrants can displace the use of superior systems by market leaders like us.[18]

Whereas a little more than a generation or two ago most sophisticated imaging was relatively concentrated in comprehensive, full-service medical centers, we are now moving into a world in which it is possible to have fairly advanced imaging performed in many free-standing or shopping mall sites. In the not too distant future, these technologies will probably diffuse into drugstore chains and perhaps into a significant fraction of physicians' offices.

There is also a potential silver lining or two in this technologic change for those of us in radiology. One is that access to imaging has improved for people who might not have otherwise had such access, and more importantly, it may facilitate the ability for us to read scans from outside the United States.

In radiology, a significant form of "disintermediation" fostered by our members has been the way that mammographers have taken on a much greater clinical role in the management of breast disease. By becoming "breast imaging physicians" with closer attention to patient care and the implications of our imaging activities, they have significantly expanded the nature of a radiologist's range of skills. They successfully transformed their role in patient care and avoided being commoditized. Mammography is one of the few radiology activities that is relatively insulated from both domestic encroachment and the risk of overseas outsourcing. Mammographers have also succeeded in raising the public profile of radiology and radiologists. This is a badly needed effort in our profession.

In our field, another significant example of the "disintermediation" phenomenon is the evolution of a direct-referral or self-pay pattern among our patients. Most radiologists who trained more than a decade ago probably did not foresee that they would have patients calling them directly to schedule a study and arriving with a credit card to pay for their imaging session. The reduction or elimination in some cases of the referring physician's role and/or the payer in the process of a patient receiving an imaging study from a radiologist is a fascinating business case study of this process of "disintermediation." The overall transaction is simplified, barriers to the provision of service are reduced or eliminated, and the overall cost of service provision can be reduced. This example includes most of the components of the strengths, weaknesses, opportunities, and threats embedded in a genuine revolution in how patients and doctors interact. It is also a compelling reminder that most revolutions are not single events or points in time. Instead, they are longer sagas that are works in progress as we experience them. Now we turn to how ideas morph into revolutions.

The Entrepreneurial Process—Team

Ideas, big or small, evolutionary or revolutionary, high or low tech, all begin with an entrepreneur. Having an idea is not enough; there must be a person (or usually persons) willing to invest their time and energy to make the idea

a reality. Successful entrepreneurs are a breed apart. Those of us in the venture community who work with them search for certain characteristics that correlate well with recurrent business successes.[19]

However, the point must be made that it is exceedingly rare to find a single person with all of these traits. Often there is a split along the lines of those described in the founders of Apple Computer, with Steve Wozniak providing the technologic expertise and capability, whereas another person, Steve Jobs, supplied the corporate managerial and marketing skills.[20] More commonly in the 21st century, larger entrepreneurial teams start companies, and the team members (hopefully) among them embody the required characteristics and skill sets to successfully innovate while also being able to work well together. This combination of team creation and design is one of the most critical issues in successful entrepreneurship.[21] Teams that fail to fill all their key roles will flounder no matter how well they work together, whereas those teams whose members can't work together will also fail no matter how individually talented or gifted they may be.

The Entrepreneurial Process—First Funding

The next early step in the entrepreneurial process is the search for financial support. This can take many forms at the beginning, but rarely are conventional banks the right answer for beginning entrepreneurs.[22] If the team and the idea have come out of an institution such as a university, government laboratory, or hospital, then there may be funds already in use or funds (with strings usually) available. This is often enough to at least carry out some very preliminary work. In most situations these institutional funds are somewhat limited. For those who are on their own, usually the founders pay for the earliest costs out of their own pockets. This is often difficult but can be the best way to develop an opportunity while maintaining complete ownership and control. The issues related to different types of funding are summarized in Table 20-2.

Usually around this stage, entrepreneurs look to banks for funding. At face value it makes perfect sense; they have lots of money, and they do loan it out. The apocryphal quote from a different kind of entrepreneur probably says it best. Willy Sutton, when asked why he robbed banks, gave name to Sutton's Law: "because that's where the money is."[23] So why aren't banks usually the right answer? The problem for imaging entrepreneurs is that banks tend to be very conservative in their loan processes. The risk of failure in early-stage ventures is extraordinarily high and usually exceeds the tolerance of your friendly neighborhood commercial lender. They might be more generous if you are willing to put up your house for collateral—not always the wisest choice at this stage for you or the venture. Additional problems with bank funding include the comparatively small sums available relative to the needs of an early-stage company and the fixed repayment schedule that might not match well with the speed of your success.

This leads to a third funding source for ventures at this stage. Many entrepreneurs look to "friends and family" financing rounds that raise money from those who know, respect, and are comfortable with members of the team. In these rounds, some ownership of the eventual company is usually sold; however, these can also be arranged as loans (debt financing) to the entrepreneurs instead of as equity transactions. Each of those financial structures has its advantages and disadvantages from the entrepreneur's perspective. Loans must be repaid, win or lose, unless you, the entrepreneur, have very generous friends and family who will just forgive the loans, or unless you declare bankruptcy and default on the debt—in which case you probably won't be invited over for Thanksgiving. However, there are serious advantages. If you issue debt, you don't dilute (diminish) the founder's ownership of the resulting corporation. If you succeed in repaying the loans you still own the entire company.

The alternative is to issue equity or perhaps mixtures of debt and equity. Selling shares in a company at any stage shares the risk; both the entrepreneur and the investors win, or else both sides lose. The downside is that this can be an expensive way to raise money. As a result of the high risk to your investors, you may have to give up a substantial chunk of the company at this stage to acquire a reasonable amount of capital.

Table 20-2   Non–Venture Capital (VC) Funding Sources for Early Ventures

Funding Source	Advantages	Disadvantages
Founders	Control, ownership	Risk, limited sources
Banks	Retain ownership	Limited sources, collateralization, strict repayment schedule
Friends and family	Friendlier terms	Limits on sources, personal costs, relationship strains
Angels	VC-type terms	Can be expensive
	Industry knowledge— smart money	Often small sums
Greenhouses and technical development funds	Aid with nonfinancial issues	Often highly specialized
	Networking	May have political issues

For example, imagine that you have a great idea and you need $100,000 to build a prototype of a new imaging device so as to get your company going and arrive at the stage where the firm would be able to attract a serious, next-stage investor. Your brother-in-law is willing to back you, but after his last investing fiasco, he wants at least 25% of the company in return for supporting you. If you succeed and eventually go public (see below for details about the process) in 5 years at a stock market valuation of $100 million, that equity will then be worth $25 million. That block of equity shares that your brother-in-law owns is going to be a generous windfall to him. More important, it will probably be sorely missed by you and your team at exactly the time that you will want to use equity to further develop your company.

A fourth source available in some locales and now showing up in many regions and on the Internet are angel investors or "angels." These are individuals with the wealth and usually the industry expertise to help small companies.[22] They are often organized into networks and clubs where they work together to fund and advise young entrepreneurs. They are often specialized by industry sector and/or geography and in the right circumstances can be a fortuitous first step for the novice entrepreneur, in that the financing may include valuable advice and help with opening doors, additional hiring, and other serious challenges for young, growing companies.

A fifth source at this point can be government-sponsored funds and organizations that specialize in helping new businesses get started. These are often called greenhouses, incubators, small business development corporations, and the like. They often combine elements of financial support with advising and other needed services, as well as in some cases physical space for new business enterprises. Here in the Philadelphia metropolitan area we have several such organizations, including a state-supported incubator, a "greenhouse" fund that supports early opportunities, a local innovation start-up fund, as well as an organization financed by the state dedicated to helping entrepreneurs find and grow high-technology jobs within the state,

through a combination of advising, funding, and support networks.

These services can be excellent resources at this stage, because most entrepreneurs need more than just funding. This basket of services gives them needed advice and guidance, as well as helping them to spend wisely what funds they do acquire. VC funding is also available at this stage; however, recent trends suggest that traditional American-based venture funds have been "upstaging" their activity and commitments with an evolution toward more mature companies and away from the earliest stage ventures. Venture funding mechanisms will be discussed in greater detail below.

The Entrepreneurial Process— Intellectual Property Protection

Usually before the above processes become too advanced and certainly before much else occurs, the entrepreneurs must determine how to protect their ideas. Again, those working for institutions may have to work with attorneys in-house or with a technology transfer office to work out issues of patent application and maintenance. Everyone, regardless of the setting, must look carefully at how to protect his or her ideas. Patent applications are commonly used to protect technology ideas but are not necessarily the right route for every idea and every entrepreneur. In the right circumstances a strong patent portfolio can be very valuable.[24] All entrepreneurs should probably at least explore legal protection before setting out into the public domain. This can help with deciding if the costs of a patent (which can easily exceed US $10,000 in early costs) are worthwhile and clearing up any issues of ownership if the idea was generated while the entrepreneur was in the employ of a hospital or university or other entity that may try to claim partial or complete ownership of the intellectual property (IP). It is far better to sort this out at the beginning and obtain clear title. More than one medical entrepreneur has ignored this at his or her peril. Large institutions have deep pockets and long lives. You can take all the risk yourself and put in long hours to create your dream and then years later find yourself in a nasty fight with a rapacious entity that is demanding a big piece of the prize.

The value of your IP and your ownership bears on another critical decision. Not all ideas require building a new company to best capture their economic value. Sometimes there is much greater return in licensing the technology to existing companies or selling it outright at the time of discovery. The amount of potentially valuable IP that can be protected and the costs and other issues related to developing it yourself are critical components of this important decision point. Many people assume that every idea merits a company. The first IP disclosures the author made were in the MRI contrast sector. Our tech transfer office wanted to start a company, but every VC investor we met with believed (correctly, as it turned out!) that this was a compelling licensing play but a lousy company creation opportunity. The key issues here revolve around the time value of money and the risks of development and the competition. A full explanation of the analysis is beyond the scope of this chapter, but the main points are summarized in Table 20-3.

Patents or no patents, entrepreneurs still need to be cautious about disclosing sensitive information about their ideas, particularly so-called "enabling material." This term refers to data that a competitor could use to your disadvantage either directly through copying or indirectly to better compete against you. The entrepreneur and the other team members need to be careful in business meetings, scientific publications, and particularly on the Web with such information. Nondisclosure agreements are a common tool for keeping information protected while using it in business formats, but they may also hinder the rapid and/or effective dissemination of company information and slow your business development progress. In fact, many financing sources including some VC firms may see a nondisclosure agreement as a hindrance to becoming involved with the team.

The Entrepreneurial Process—Early- to Middle-Stage Funding

Emerging companies—particularly those making good progress—eventually outgrow the founding and seed stages. Their funding and other needs at this point usually exceed what the government programs, angels, friends and family, and the founders can supply (unless you have remarkably wealthy relatives and acquaintances).

This is where more traditional VC takes the lead. Deal amounts vary substantially by sector, geography, and stage, but here we are usually talking more about millions of dollars rather than the thousands for the earliest funding rounds. In the United States there are over 800 venture firms.[25] Although the United States has one of the oldest and best organized venture financing industries, there is also a strong and expanding global venture industry, some of which also has a strong interest in investing here in the United States.[26] Venture investing works in a somewhat analogous fashion to the earlier brother-in-law or angel examples, albeit at a much larger scale and scope with more formalized processes and procedures.

Table 20-3 Company Creation versus Licensing Opportunities

	New Company	Licensing
Advantages	Ownership Higher value Control	No risk to you Lower time/effort requirements Keep day job
Disadvantages	Funding requirements Higher risk	Lower return Entrepreneur often sidelined

Initially the entrepreneur will directly contact a venture capitalist or work through networks of contacts, through trade fairs or venture conferences and the like. Those who have promising ideas are invited to present their ideas and answer questions about the company to the entire venture firm or at least to the key partners. When the team goes to several VC funding sources to try to raise funding this is called a "road show." If the idea seems promising, then the firm will begin a formal process of due diligence. The partners will take a closer look at the venture, the markets, the competition, the technology, and so forth, so as to decide whether or not to fund. The lead venture capitalist and his or her staff will work closely with the potential entrepreneur to look at the idea, the team, and the market to evaluate the overall opportunity.

This is a highly pyramidal process, and anyone embarking on this route must understand the odds. Of the 1000 or so ideas that an individual venture capitalist looks at each year, only a handful are actually funded. When the VC firm finishes its due diligence, a decision is made to offer funding to the entrepreneur. This offer is called a term sheet. Although it includes many important features, the paramount ones from the entrepreneur's perspective in an equity deal are the amount of money offered and the percentage of the company that the venture capitalist will now own in return for investing. Returning to the brother-in-law example, if he had given you $100,000 on a company valuation of $400,000, that would have given him 25% ownership. This is called the valuation, and it is obviously of great import in negotiations. However, it is interesting to note that the money alone is often not the key factor that entrepreneurs use in evaluating investing offers.

In fact, a recent study showed that actually a fair amount of money at this point is left on the table by entrepreneurs. These individuals make their choices more on the basis of allying with firms that have other strengths related to expertise, personnel, market knowledge, experience, and the like, that bear on the ultimate success of the venture, rather than just

the up-front dollar amount.[27] This raises the issue that much of what the venture capitalist should be providing to the entrepreneur goes beyond simply money. This so-called smart money means that the capitalist is also helping with hiring, market targeting, regulatory issues, networks, key contacts, and so on.

Many VC firms will structure the outlay of the payments of their commitments. That is to say that whereas they may make a commitment of $1 million to you in return for their ownership shares, you don't just get a check for the full amount and everyone shakes hands and leaves the boardroom. Instead, the commitment may be divided into several payments that are tied to concrete milestones your company must meet, including developing a prototype and performance measures. This is one of many types of controls that will be included in the governance of the investment by those who have put in a large stake. Significant investors will often ask for a seat on the board of your company, as well as substantial access to operational personnel, financial data, and inclusion in major corporate decisions. Taking on VC funding is more akin to a partnership with the venture firm rather than a "silent partner" type of "dumb money" investing. This is another major reason why you need to carefully consider from whom you take money at this stage. For better or worse, you are going to be intimate partners for a while.

Private VC is often the logical source of potential funding for companies at this stage. However, there are many other sources as well, including small business innovation research programs run by the government, corporate development funds, and corporate partnering. The government may also play other roles at this stage. Here in Pennsylvania, the government has also invested in venture health care funds from some of the money from the Tobacco Settlement to help companies at this stage of development.[28] Another source at these stages can be to partner or ally with a larger corporation that can provide funds, access to technology and markets, or other important success ingredients. These can take the form of using corporate VC moneys, an in-sourcing agreement, or a direct purchase or acquisition of all or part of the entrepreneurial company by the larger entity. Sometimes that model can be combined in a hybrid with a traditional VC model in the form of a corporate-sponsored venture fund that combines both financial and strategic goals in a single entity.[29]

The Entrepreneurial Process—Middle to Late Stages

VC also continues to play a role as companies grow and need additional financing. These often take the form of several rounds, usually lettered in order beginning with a Series A round. As the rounds get further along, they also generally increase in size, sometimes requiring the combined activity of several venture funds in a "syndication deal" to handle the large cash amounts and enhanced operational oversight of the growing investment. These later stage rounds were traditionally considered less attractive than getting in on the deal at the beginning. However, recent data suggest that this has at least temporarily reversed as VC firms shift their focus to later stage investing.[30] One of the most difficult decisions required of an involved VC investor is whether to continue investing versus stopping and terminating an investment. Academic studies of this process suggest that doing this well is actually one of the most important determinants of success and failure overall in venture investing—in fact surpassing the ability to manage a successful investment.[31] This decision of terminating a bad investment—of admitting a mistake—is apparently quite difficult, but again is a hallmark of investors who are consistently successful at the venture game as opposed to those who have a run of luck.

The Entrepreneurial Process—Harvest Strategies and Exit

The final step in the process is to decide how to end the venture. Hopefully, the venture has done well and a profitable conclusion can be achieved for everyone involved. The most coveted end is to go through an initial public offering (IPO) of the stock as a publicly traded company. This usually creates the greatest selling event but is also one of the rarer courses, particularly in slower economic times. This is often described as an IPO "window," and in fact the public market's appetite for technology IPOs seems to be increasing.[32] The majority of start-ups in the United States do not make it all the way to an IPO but instead follow other paths. Other options include a private sale to another entity in the field as discussed earlier or keeping the company in the private domain so long as there are capital reserves and there is enough income to keep the company going. Many companies also reach a point at which the entrepreneurs may decide to move on and perhaps sell part of the company off to a larger entity and continue to work on a subset of their ideas in a small, more entrepreneurial environment.

CAN YOU HANDLE THE TRUTH? ARE YOU AN ENTREPRENEUR?

Optimism is a strategy for making a better future. Because unless you believe that the future can be better, it's unlikely you will step up and take responsibility for making it so. If you assume that there's no hope, you guarantee that there will be no hope. If you assume that there is an instinct for freedom, there are opportunities to change things, there's a chance you may contribute to making a better world. The choice is yours.

NOAM CHOMSKY[33]

If you are serious about being an entrepreneur, there are many important questions that you must ask yourself at the outset of your planned venture. In this section we will discuss what it means to be an innovator and how you can avoid many of the most common mistakes that entrepreneurs make. One of the first issues we need to address is that not all medical change is initiated by classic "entrepreneurs."

It should be said at the outset that this writer abhors most business clichés. Like many other people with a medical and scientific background, my eyes rolled when I heard about "the vision thing." I think that speakers who use "bandwidth" in any context other than electrical engineering are probably lacking in "bandwidth" themselves. Although no paradigms will shift in this chapter, one buzzword that must be mentioned at this point is "intrapreneur." That term appears here because it makes a useful point about what we as practicing physicians can do without leaving our day jobs. Intrapreneurship reminds us that a great deal of innovation can and does occur within existing organizations. Remember, not everyone needs to drop their current practice and go off to join a high-tech start-up or be able to invent the next imaging platform. It is also possible to innovate incrementally (or sometimes even fairly dramatically) within the context of your current practice.

This society lionizes entrepreneurs who are able to start billion-dollar companies, and this has led to a Hollywood stereotype of the lone genius who quits his dead-end job and, after starving for a few years, becomes an overnight software billionaire. That does happen, but that image tends to overshadow the enormous amount of significant change in the U.S. economy that is led by those who invent, improve, and change things within existing institutions—that is, intrapreneurs. This role of intrapreneur is in fact a very powerful driver of American business change and improvement—one that is often both unsung and undervalued by the general public.

Also, keep in mind that in some ways it is both harder and riskier to be an intrapreneur than an entrepreneur. Let's say that you have a "brilliant" idea, and you convince your department chair to invest in a new imaging system or center. If that center does terribly and ultimately fails, that could be a "career-limiting" or even "career-ending" decision for you. Arguably, this is not dissimilar to being unable to reimburse your father-in-law for the start-up funds he lent you (i.e., career limiting). However, as stated above, entrepreneurial funding also provides one the opportunity to distance oneself further from personal risk. It is worth repeating here that there are risks all along the spectrum of innovation. However, keep in mind that as a physician in active practice, you have extraordinary opportunities to observe the landscape and

search for great opportunities. This section will address the early challenges facing innovators of all types. Here we will suggest ways that by asking the right questions as you face these challenges you can improve your chances of becoming a successful entrepreneur or intrapreneur.

"In the Beginning…" What to Ask Yourself before You Even Get Started

At its core, the process of entrepreneurship is about having a powerful idea for how to improve the world around you and then making that change occur. In the case of a device it is everything from having the idea through building prototypes, testing, to regulatory approval, manufacturing, and sales. Most ideas are incremental—the better mousetrap, the cheaper, faster, and/or better way of doing things. It is not enough to have an idea; you also need to figure out how to make it occur and have the drive to make it happen. There is a sort of mantra that is of value to use with entrepreneurs at this stage: Remember that the vast majority of new ideas don't work, most visions turn out to be illusory, and most new businesses in the United States do not succeed. You have to ask yourself repeatedly: "Why are you (or why am I or these ideas) different? Why will I beat the odds?"

This is not to discourage entrepreneurship or encourage nihilism—far from it. As I discussed in an academic article, the opportunity for us in medicine is enormous.[2] As I stated both there and earlier herein, I think that there are tremendous opportunities and that radiologists should be leading the way. As you will see from some of the examples that follow, there have been enormous successes by physician innovators.

Rather, I bring it up for the opposite reason. Great entrepreneurs can't afford to waste their time on bad ideas. Bad choices need to be discovered before you invest much of your time, money, and credibility. Developing the skills to discriminate between good and bad opportunities frees you to focus on the high-probability ideas that might be big winners.

The mantra has a second purpose. It screens out those who may be generating reasonable ideas but who don't have the drive to see things through to fruition. As one of my VC partners once said to me, "Ideas are cheap. We invest in people and opportunities, not ideas" (personal communication, Charles Burton, 1999). To be an entrepreneur means to be the driving force behind making the idea materialize.

The writer's investment team met several years ago with a physician who had this limitation. He had an innovative idea for a better design for endoscopy equipment. The problem was that the idea needed a great deal of work on both the technology and the business sides. Most important, it needed a leader and champion to see it through to success. This inventor wanted us to set up the company for him and then send him royalty checks every quarter while he stayed on the sidelines. When we explained how much work it would take to turn his idea into a company, he decided to move on. He wasn't interested in putting in the effort and didn't seem suited for the actual work of entrepreneurship despite having a clever idea. We (and the rest of venture and medical device communities) haven't heard from him since. He relegated his own ideas to the dustbin of history. To paraphrase Thomas Edison, "the perspiration makes a much bigger contribution than the inspiration."

People who give up just because you give them the reality check in the mantra aren't going to become great entrepreneurs. They may have very good ideas, but they won't be able to bring them to the light of day in our highly competitive society. You may be able to build a great team with and around them, but someone else will have to lead the venture.

Another example of this occurred when our team worked with a prominent engineering professor who had an interesting idea for a medical imaging device. He was a full professor at a famous university, with an impressive background and a busy lecturing and meeting schedule. We went through the process of company creation with him. He was taken aback by the commitment he would need to make and even more so by the risk of failure. He hadn't failed at anything in his life thus far. He was concerned about tarnishing his record with a black mark. He was frozen with fear that his friends, family, and colleagues would laugh if he failed. He decided to play it safe and not pursue his own dream. The university later sold his patents for pennies on the dollar to someone who was willing to run with them. Entrepreneurship is not for people who want a sure thing. Those who can't handle failure (often repeated) and can't get back on their feet after a defeat should stick to their day jobs. Glory in this arena goes to those with both brains and guts.

There is also a third purpose to the mantra, and this is where you can glimpse a real entrepreneur. When you ask them the hard questions (see next section below) about their enterprise, they come back with answers and modifications that improve on the original idea. It gets better and better as they work on it. They push, adapt, and improve to do whatever it takes to make it work. These are the women and men who can build the future.

SO YOU ARE READY TO START— TEN CRITICAL CHALLENGES

Ten Key Questions to Ask Yourself as You Embark on a New Venture

So you think that you have a great idea and you have passed the initial screening that we outlined above. Now you are ready to push ahead and ask the hard questions that will bring your idea and plan into focus. This process is important regardless of where you are on the innovation spectrum. Whether you think you are the next Bill Gates or a new Thomas Edison or just have an incremental idea that you think you might be able to patent or could sell to other radiology practices, this is the point at which you have to do some hard testing before you start spending your money or your time. If you think that this is easy, check the list of major pitfalls at the end of the chapter.

Here are some of the key questions to ask yourself at this stage and some types of good and bad answers that you should consider. These questions and your answers will help immeasurably both in refining your plans and in avoiding the most common pitfalls that trip up entrepreneurs in our society. It is also important to emphasize that you need to find trusted mentors and advisors at this point. You need to get the opinions of those who have been involved in your field (ideally people who also have experience with ventures at this stage) as a reality check on your thinking.

1. How valuable is this idea? In particular, think hard not just about how valuable it is to someone else but how much of that potential value will actually accrue to you. That you have a better mousetrap doesn't mean that you will either be able to sell it, or if you do, that you will be able to capture much of that value. How big is your market, how much of it can you get, and how will you do it and keep it? These are truly big questions, but if you are going to invest your capital and your time, make sure you do it for a worthy goal. Too often entrepreneurs come up with an interesting idea or innovation, but don't consider: (1) how innovative it is, (2) how many other people will find it both interesting and valuable, and (3) how much of that perceived value can be translated into a desire to pay for it. This is a particular problem in the medical field, where the person who receives the value and the entity that pays for it are usually not the same. Several years ago this writer met with someone who wanted to revolutionize the treatment of varicose veins. The problem was that most of the value was received by the patients, but the entrepreneur wanted to sell solely to large institutions. These major hospitals were reluctant to purchase a novel and expensive device that would have a long road to receiving reimbursement from the government. We helped redesign the device and the service offering so that there was a better opportunity to sell this to physician's offices where the benefits would be more appreciated.

2. What do I need to do to be able to take this forward? Is this something that I can (or should) do myself in my home office or garage, or do I need to enlist a team of people to do this with me from the very beginning? The first approach worked well when Bill Cook founded Cook Incorporated in 1963. He used his spare bedroom as the first factory for his innovative wire guides, catheters, and needles. This grew into the radiology giant Cook Group Inc. and made him a multibillionaire.[34] A similar use of available domestic resources was made by Andreas Gruentzig. He worked in his kitchen to develop the balloon angioplasty catheter in the early 1970s.[35] The answer for you needs to encompass many variables. Take into account your time and attention, additional personnel, funds, lab space, specialty services (e.g., IP). A related question is: Do I want to do this or does it make more sense to try to patent this idea or license it to someone else—either a person or a company that has the resources to pursue it? It is beyond the scope of this chapter to go into all the issues that determine what can and should be patented, but this is an issue that almost all medical entrepreneurs must address. Also, remember that not all valuable ideas can or need to be patented (Box 20-1). Those types of innovations need different types of development and protection. Finally, keep in mind that a great entrepreneur is not just an inventor. He or she usually combines several characteristics: a restless desire for change, a hunger for ideas and talented people, remarkable determination, an ability to tolerate uncertainty and failure, and an attitude exemplified by the words of Winston Churchill, "we shall never surrender."[36] If you aren't that person, then you need to consider some other choices. Either surround yourself with someone or some people

BOX 20-1

Outline of the Patent Process—A Very Simplified Recipe

Step 1: You have a million-dollar idea.

Step 2: Do some basic research yourself: who has done this before, why is my idea different, how will I do it, and so on. If it has possibilities, proceed.

Step 3: Meet with an attorney. If there is genuine value you need expert help at this point.

Step 4: The attorney (usually with a lot of help from you) will do background research, checking for "prior art" (i.e., other inventors in the past who have disclosed the same or similar inventions). If there is merit, you proceed.

Step 5: File a patent application.

Step 6: Wait to hear from the government to respond.

Step 7: Either good news (patent granted) or bad (rejection, which is much more common). In the former case you are up and running; in the latter you return to step 4 and appeal.

Step 8: Patents need to be both maintained and defended, so your legal work isn't over.

who meet that description or consider some of the other alternatives discussed above, like selling/licensing your ideas rather than developing them yourself. This is also the time to ask yourself if you are ready (or want) to quit your day job if that becomes necessary for your venture. Do you want to take the risk of devoting all your time and energy to the venture? It is also the time to ask yourself if your family is ready for you to do this. If you are still working off educational debt, just took out a big mortgage to buy a house to accommodate several new additions to the family, have uncertain prospects for making partner in your group, and have a nonworking spouse, you may want to take a deep breath and rethink how you approach this. This writer once worked with a radiologist with a great idea for providing novel types of services. He had

already borrowed $4.5 million against his estate to develop this project and was in a state where he could lose his house if this didn't work out. On top of that he had several of the other issues described above. We built a partnership that spread the risk for him so that he wouldn't be destitute if the venture wasn't a smash success. A final related question is: How much development do I need to do to be able to sell it to someone else at an intermediate point if I don't do it all myself? This helps break you out of the all-or-nothing mentality that many entrepreneurs have at this stage.

3. Has someone else already tried this or something like it (and what happened and why will I do it better)? One of the big mistakes that entrepreneurs make is assuming that they will succeed where others have failed—without having a compellingly different story from that of the losers. You should ask yourself these questions several times: Why will I be different, how has the world changed, what did they do wrong, has the competitive landscape changed? An old cliché is that it is better to learn from other people's mistakes than from your own. Turning this around, one of the worst forms of failure is that which could have been avoided by doing your homework. Many of the entrepreneurs the author encounters come from companies that have rejected their ideas. For example, we met with a former pharmaceutical executive who had an interesting, but very "far out" idea for diagnostic imaging in the veterinary field. His own company and several others had rejected the idea for a variety of technical, financial, and market reasons. The entrepreneur needs to ask himself or herself why he or she is right and nearly everyone else is wrong. In this case, we were able to help re-craft the idea and focus it on a market segment that was highly receptive to the idea. Learn what has caused other people to fail, and figure out what you can do better to succeed where they failed. Sitting back from the perspective of an investor, it is amazing to this writer

how many mistakes are preventable and how often failure is copied.

4. What known or foreseeable obstacles are there and how will I overcome them? The specific pitfalls that face entrepreneurs are many, and the most common ones are covered here in these 10 questions. Finding them and anticipating solutions is one of the cornerstones of effective planning. The author briefly worked as a business advisor for an overseas company that wanted to enter the U.S. marketplace with a novel medical product in the obstetrics/gynecology area. They were entirely focused on refining the engineering and were doing an admirable job of improving the product. The problem was that they were focusing on that to the extreme detriment of the other dozen issues at hand. In particular, they weren't paying any attention to how they would distribute and market it in an alien nation. Good entrepreneurship involves a juggling act. You usually can't focus on just one challenge at a time. In fact, you often have to focus on them all simultaneously. Moreover, anticipating problems and either preventing or ameliorating them is one of the most important characteristics of successful entrepreneurs. Although this team would certainly get a grade of "A+" in technical development, they would get poor to failing marks elsewhere. In particular, they did a poor job of introducing the product and didn't think carefully about how to get their product into large chain stores and how to promote it. Success is usually not so much a matter of doing one thing superlatively; rather, it is a matter of simultaneously avoiding doing badly or even failing on a plethora of issues that can trap you.

5. What is my competition? Ask how you will be able to distinguish yourself from your most important competitors and if there is room for you, the new entrant (barriers to entry)? An additional important question that you will ask repeatedly over the lifetime of the enterprise is how will the competition react to what I do?

Unless your competition is asleep at the wheel (and even if they are, they almost certainly will wake up eventually) and/or remarkably stupid, they will eventually go after you once you succeed. You have to be willing and able (as in chess or in any other competition) to think several steps ahead of your competition and stay ahead throughout the game. This writer and his students worked with a company that wanted to introduce a personal health care product that would compete against one of the giants in the field. Normally this would be considered suicidal—the health care equivalent of trying to go head to head with Microsoft in home computer software. However, by carefully considering how to get a foothold and how to compete in a novel way, we were able to find ways to compete successfully with the giant. This is more impressive when you consider that our investment would have been less than a rounding error in the annual budget of the current leader.

6. Who are my customers, and how will I reach them? The medical enterprise is a complicated one, with multiple customers and multiple ways to approach the system. This is both an advantage and disadvantage. On one hand, there are many potential customer groups. Your product or service may be attractive to physicians or patients or perhaps another stakeholder group. However, the more subtle point is that the value of your entrepreneurial effort has to be seen by the ultimate payers or you won't make the sale. We looked at a very interesting software package for improving medical services. It had substantial value for the patients and some practitioners, but was targeted at large institutions that saw little bottom-line value for them. We encouraged the inventors to develop products that better matched perceived value to those who would write checks: an institutional product for the large entities and more innovative products focused on health care providers and health care consumers.

Patients may love your idea, but their managed care organization may not care and if the companies are the buyers, you are at an impasse. In that case, you need to figure out how to use stakeholders such as physicians or patients to make it worthwhile for the target organizations to buy the service or product. This is a very common problem for physician entrepreneurs. They invent something of potential value, but don't look hard at this issue of the value proposition. They target the wrong group and then wonder why the world doesn't beat a path to their door.

7. This leads into a closely related question: What will the "selling proposition" to my customers be? Even if there is alignment between those who value your product and those who will pay for your innovation, you still need to work on how you will reach them and how you will craft the message. This is not trivial and is one of the most common reasons that scientific and medical start-ups get into trouble. It is also a particular problem for overseas entrepreneurs. These are marketing issues, and although they will loom even larger in later stages, you still need to consider this carefully and even test-market your ideas at the earliest possible stage. It is worth reminding yourself that you live in the most marketing-driven society on the planet and that without marketing expertise it is very unlikely that you will achieve your potential. Dr. Albert C. Barnes was an early 20th-century pharmaceutical inventor who developed many drugs, including Argyrol (a mild protein silver compound used as an anti-infective; Argyrol Pharmaceuticals). He was more than a researcher. His success also depended on his innovative approaches to directly marketing his products to physicians and hospitals.[37] This led to spectacular success, and one of his legacies is the Barnes Foundation in suburban Philadelphia, which is one of the finest Impressionist and Post-Impressionist art collections of its kind in the world.

8. Do I own this idea or at least part of it? This sounds like a trivial, almost stupid question, but it is neither stupid nor trivial. Many medical ventures involve IP (or should). This question encompasses several investigations that the entrepreneur needs to make at the outset and builds on several of the earlier points. First—and it always seems amazing that this is an issue—is determining whether you even own your own ideas outright. Two places to look are either your employment contract or the university policies and procedures manual. Sample language in a contract that may entirely preclude your ownership is "Any remuneration earned by employee while in the employ of employer shall be forwarded to employer."[38] Many physician-inventors come to me with ideas, and then we find out that their university or a previous employer actually owns some or in a few cases all of the potential IP underlying the inventor's idea. Make sure that you know your employment contract, and consider those issues as you develop and disclose your inventions. Second, once you think that you have an idea that depends on IP, you need to obtain help with patenting. This is necessary both to make sure that you have something different from previous inventors and if so then to take action to adequately protect your work. Sometimes in these cases the university can be a great partner in helping you obtain good legal help and paying or at least defraying the costs. A good patent application requires a great deal of time and a substantial amount of money. Moreover, there are continuing issues after the initial application that require additional time, attention, and expense to maintain a patent. If you decide to go it alone, make sure that you have complete ownership or at the least know exactly where you stand. An entrepreneur who consulted the author recently had tried to convince his university to patent his idea. The technology transfer office spent months evaluating it and concluded that it wasn't worth their time to pursue it. He

thought that their refusal gave him clear rights and then spent more than US $10,000 of his own money to acquire the patent and begin his venture. After several years and some financial success, he received a letter from the university claiming that they owned a substantial chunk of his enterprise. This is still continuing, but suffice it to say that the only real winners in these situations are the lawyers and their ilk. Universities and other large institutions usually have longer life spans than inventors do. Making sure that these issues are resolved in black and white is the only way that you can prevent a nasty surprise either now or in the future. Another way to quickly lose ownership of your patentable ideas is to present them in public before you file. As physicians and scientists, we routinely speak in public about our ideas and publish our work. The rise of the Web and other venues for public disclosure has made this much more treacherous. Be very careful about public disclosure. While working for an IP firm in the 1990s, one of this writer's assignments was with a brilliant scientist from the Pacific Northwest who had a bundle of very compelling patent ideas. However, when our team of attorneys started to interview him, it turned out that he had presented some of these at conferences and that precluded their patentability. He lost well over half the aggregate value of these ideas by not obtaining good advice and obtaining IP protection before going public.

9. What is my ultimate goal? It may seem early to be discussing this, but smart entrepreneurs do this from the very beginning. Often physician-entrepreneurs ignore this question, assuming that they can do this later. Although we will revisit this question at every stage of the venture, it is a good one to raise at the very beginning. One of the greatest challenges that physicians and scientists face in a new venture is to take on the nontechnical challenges of the venture. There is a natural tendency to continue doing what you are good at doing. We recently completed a project with a company that was composed of very smart imaging research scientists. They really didn't have a goal for the company. They just wanted to do research and development work on their system. When a management team was brought in, they had very different goals for when, where, and how to run the company. My group helped mediate between these two groups and develop clear, timely goals for the company, including a way to sell part of the company within 2 years. In fact, for many new entrepreneurs, setting ultimate (not just short-term) goals may be the most critical focusing element to help them think profoundly about the business and its goals. As Stephen Covey writes in his *Seven Habits of Highly Effective People*: "begin with the end in mind."[39]

10. A final question, perhaps the most important because it encompasses the previous nine elements, is: Is this the right time for the venture? For entrepreneurship, as in many areas of life, particularly surfing and personal relationships, timing is everything. The right idea, the right market, the right competition (or lack thereof), and the like make all the difference. In addition, the right answer here may be that you are too late or perhaps that you need to wait until you improve the idea or until the market changes, or perhaps change the environment yourself. Sometimes the timing is perfect, but sometimes it is terribly wrong. However, sometimes to succeed, you can improve things and develop the market both for your innovation and for the funding. When John Abele and Peter Nicholas founded Medi-Tech in the late 1970s, they had to both develop novel links to physicians as well as convince the financial markets that medical devices were worthy investments.[40] Their efforts led to the extraordinary success of the Boston Scientific Company.

CONCLUSIONS

Entrepreneurism is a particularly exciting facet of American business in the early 21st century. In our field of radiology, it drives the development of new devices, new applications, novel types of service delivery, advances in information technology, and new ways of working. This brief overview has outlined the landscape for entrepreneurial development and the types of funding that are currently available to medical entrepreneurs in the United States, the commonalities in how entrepreneurial activity takes place, and how entrepreneurial ventures end when they are successful.

In closing, remember the wisdom inherent in the two earlier statements: "Ideas are cheap" and "Most new businesses fail to succeed." The odds are long, and the way is not always easy. However, a great idea whose time has come is invaluable and if executed well can result in enormous dividends.

As stated at the outset, there is no single simple formula that will guarantee success. However, there are many predictable challenges and hazards in early- and seed-stage ventures that you can expect to encounter and must be ready to confront. The questions posed here are difficult ones, but they may well save you time, money, and heartache. If you handle these well and can address these issues, your enterprise will have a much greater chance of succeeding. Never forget, there is a world to win!

The Dos and Don'ts of Entrepreneurship

Dos	Don'ts
1. Know your customers. Be relentless in asking how you are providing value to them. This is one of the most important ingredients in success in modern business.	1. Lack commitment. Ideas are cheap: the drive to change the world is rare.
2. Regularly reassess your plan. Nothing is written in stone. The world changes and your opportunities will change. Your plan and your tactics need to change too.	2. Ignore the competition. You always have competition, and you always have to pay close attention.
3. Find and develop the best team members you can. People really will be your biggest assets. Even the brightest stars need a group to help them. The smartest ones know this and seek out support.	3. Have inadequate resources. Entrepreneurship is an intensive process. You can't do it all by yourself in the garage. Bring in the financing, partners, and institutions you need in time for them to help you.
4. Test your ideas and refine them constantly. In addition to being open to new ideas, you must actively seek them out. Smart people and organizations are good learners. As the cliché goes, "survival is not mandatory." Those who can adapt are the ones who win.	4. Lack a plan. Stumbling along is a sure-fire recipe for entrepreneurial disaster.
5. Learn to handle failure. Successful people in the entrepreneurial world often fail. The point is they try, they learn from their mistakes, and they get up again. The successes are what matter.	5. Think small. Little incremental projects may be fun, but big, aggressive world-changing ventures are much more satisfying.

LIST OF ABBREVIATIONS AND GLOSSARY

Debt—A loan of money now to be repaid under terms in the future. May often be combined with equity (see below) or converted to equity in early-stage financing.

Entrepreneurship—Broadly defined, the process of innovation, particularly the creation of a new business involving risk. From a French root, meaning to undertake.

Equity—Owning shares in a company. For entrepreneurs, selling equity—a portion of the company—is a common method of acquiring capital for expansion.

Firm (venture)—Group of individuals organized to invest in entrepreneurial ventures. Usually involves a substantial level of involvement in directing and operating the company in addition to providing funds.

Fund (venture)—Investment fund set up by a venture firm to aggregate capital from investors and then invest with promising entrepreneurs. Generally a fairly illiquid investment with a time horizon of 10 years, occasionally more. A venture firm may run several funds at the same time, and each fund may be invested with multiple entrepreneurial opportunities.

Initial Public Offering (IPO)—The first offering of stock in a young company to the public. This is the "listing" that occurs with a stock exchange and is one of the most desirable ways to recoup an investment with a start-up company.

Venture capital (VC)—Form of high-risk, high-reward investment generally targeted at innovative companies with a high potential for the creation of a public offering.

REFERENCES

1. Mark Henricks, Entrepreneur.com, quoting John Osher. Available at: http://www.entrepreneur.com/ext/home.
2. Lexa FJ: Medical entrepreneurism: the current opportunity in America. J Am Coll Radiol 1(10):762–768, 2004.
3. Lexa FJ, Lexa FJ: Physician-entrepreneurship: a user's manual, part 1: critical questions for early-stage medical ventures. J Am Coll Radiol 2(7):607–612, 2005.
4. Hanlon CR: The ethics of entrepreneurial medicine. J Am Coll Surg 190(4):459–465, 2000.
5. Fletcher T: The impact of physician entrepreneurship on escalating health care costs. J Am Coll Radiol 2(5):411–414, 2005.
6. Markels A: A prescription for controversy. U.S. News and World Report (October 6, 2003), p 50.
7. Rice B: Your latest legal threat: consumer fraud. Med Econ 81(2):30–32, 2004.
8. Lutz S. Venture capital financing sets record pace in '95. Mod Healthcare 26(6):36, 1996.
9. MoneyTree Survey by PricewaterhouseCoopers, Thomson Venture Economics and the National Venture Capital Association. Available at: http://www.nvca.org/presscenter.html, 2005–2006 Year in Review (2006), accessed June 25, 2007.
10. National Venture Capital Association. Available at http//www.nvca.org (June 25, 2007).
11. Data from VentureOne and Ernst and Young. US venture market recovers to 2001 levels. Available at http://www.altassets.com/news/arc/2006/nz8493.php (27 April 2006).
12. National Venture Capital Association. Available at http//www.nvca.org/presscenter.html, 2005–2006 Year in Review (2006), accessed June 25, 2007.
13. National Center for Health Statistics. Health, United States, 2003 National Health Expenditures, Table 112, p 306. Posted by the Centers for Disease Control. Available at:http://www.cdc.gov/nchs/products/pubs/pubd/hus/trendtables.htm (26 April 2004).
14. Snapshot, USA Today (May 14, 2004), p 1.
15. United States PTO. Available at http://www.uspto.gov/patft/index.html (13 February 2004).
16. http://www.cms.hhs.gov/nationalhealthexpenddata/02_nationalhealthaccountshistorical.asp.
17. Schumpeter J: Capitalism, socialism and democracy, 1942.
18. Christensen C: The innovator's dilemma, when new technologies cause great firms to fail. Harvard Business School Press, 1997.
19. Hines JL: Characteristics of an entrepreneur. Surg Neurol 61(4):407–408, 2004.
20. Weyhrich S: The Apple-1 vol. 2.0, 20 October 2001, in Apple II history (copyright S. Weyhrich 1991–2003). Available at http://apple2history.org/history/ah02.html (4 May 2004).
21. Katzenbach JR, Smith DK: The wisdom of teams: Creating the high-performance organization. New York, McGraw-Hill, 1993.
22. Evanson DR: Where to go when the bank says no. Princeton, NJ, Bloomberg Press, 1998.
23. Willie Sutton. Available at http://en.wikipedia.org/wiki/Willy_Sutton. Accessed (1 June 2006).
24. Praiss DM: Creating a winning patent portfolio. Nat Biotechnol 19(Suppl): BE5–7, 2001.
25. National Venture Capital Association website: Available at http://www.nvca.org/faqs.html (30 April 2004).
26. Business.com. International venture capital firms and funds. Available at http://www.business.com/directory/financial_services/venture_capital/firms_and_funds/international_regions/ (3 May 2004).
27. Hsu David. What do entrepreneurs pay for venture capital affiliation? J Finance 59(4):1805–1844, 2004.
28. http://www.pennsylvaniabio.org/index.php?option=com_content&task=view&id=58&itemid.
29. Fletcher L: Eli Lilly enters venture capital arena. Nat Biotechnol 19(11):997–998, 2001.
30. Grimes A: Late-stage start-ups get more money. Wall Street Journal (Tuesday, 27 April 2004), pp C1–C4.
31. Guler I: A study of decision making capabilities and performance in the venture capital industry [thesis]. University of Pennsylvania (HB 0042003. G971), 2003.
32. Tam P-W: Tech IPO's kick into high gear. Wall Street Journal (Tuesday, 27 April 2004), pp C1–C4.

33. Chomsky N: "Wired" Magazine (January 1998), p 167.
34. Cook Group. History and innovators. Available at http://www.cookgroup.com/history/index.html. (21 November 2004).
35. Coronary stenting history and new developments, p 1. Available at http://www.ptca.org/archive/bios/gruentzig.html (26 November 2004).
36. Winston Churchill speech on Dunkirk, House of Commons, 4 June 1940.
37. The Barnes Foundation. The life and work of Albert Barnes. Available at:http://www.barnesfoundation.org/h_bio.html
38. Armon BD: Bringing your medical device to the marketplace. Physician's News Digest. Available at: http://physiciansnews.com/business/1102armon.html (November 2004), accessed 20 November 2004.
39. Covey S: Seven habits of highly effective people. New York, Simon and Schuster, 1989 p. 95.
40. Swain E: Boston Scientific: making the most of its first 25 years. Available at http://www.devicelink.com/mddi/archive/04/08/019.html (27 November 2004).

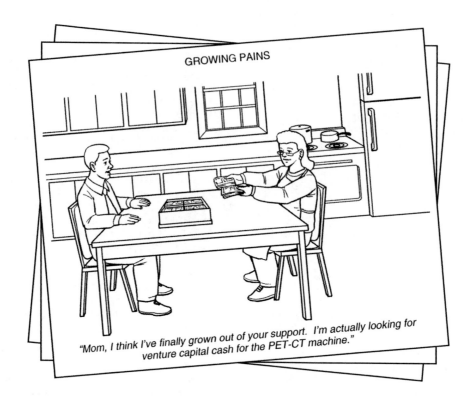

GROWING PAINS

"Mom, I think I've finally grown out of your support. I'm actually looking for venture capital cash for the PET-CT machine."

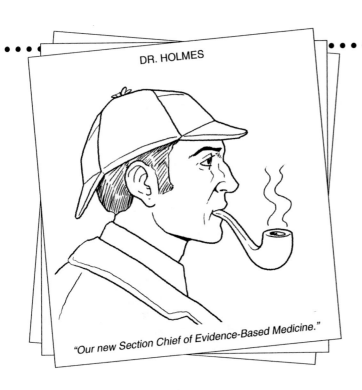

CHAPTER 21

DR. HOLMES

"Our new Section Chief of Evidence-Based Medicine."

Evidence-Based Imaging

C. Craig Blackmore

There was, for starters, the tendency of everyone who actually played the game to generalize wildly from his own experience. People always thought their own experience was typical when it wasn't. There was also a tendency to be overly influenced by a guy's most recent performance: what he did last was not necessarily what he would do next. Thirdly—but not lastly—there was a bias toward what people saw with their own eyes, or thought they had seen.

MICHAEL LEWIS, MONEYBALL

INTRODUCTION

Health care costs continue to spiral upward in the United States. As of 2005 the United States spent 15.3% of its gross domestic product on health care.[1] This is nearly double the developed-country average of 8.3% and 50% higher than the number two nation, Switzerland. Nonetheless, the World Health Organization 2003 report stated that the United States has only the 37th best health care in the world,

and ranks 47th in life expectancy and 42nd in infant mortality.[1] What then is the value that is obtained from the enormous U.S. expenditures on health care? Clearly, medical practice in the United States is neither as efficient nor as effective as other parts of the developed world.

The standard doctrine for medical care in the United States, as well as other western nations has been that of the individual practitioner and individual experts. Physicians are taught how to practice through rote memorization and patterning of behavior from acknowledged "experts" in the field. The expert is assumed through his or her personal experience to have accumulated sufficient expertise and knowledge to be able to determine the appropriate care for a given patient under a given clinical circumstance. Knowledge from these experts is passed on to medical students and other medical practitioners through lectures, texts, and direct observation. Strangely, critical thinking and critical evaluation have only a limited role in this traditional medical model. This "eminence-based medicine" philosophy has been challenged in the past decade through the promulgation of evidence-based medicine and its corollary, evidence-based imaging.[2-5] Evidence-based imaging is defined as medical decision making based on the best medical imaging evidence integrated with physician judgment and patient preferences.[3] Evidence-based imaging is based on the premise that no single individual can accumulate sufficient unbiased experience to be able to make and form choices with respect to the appropriate care for patients. Individual experience is generally biased by that which was seen recently and by fear of rare events rather than knowledge of common events. Furthermore, human health and illness are so complex that logic and personal experience are never sufficient to untangle their intricacies. Instead, medical practice should be based on careful review and analysis of information that is published in the medical literature. This literature database is potentially less biased and based more on objective findings from multiple individuals, and thus is a more appropriate choice upon which to base medical care.

Evidence-based medicine, and its radiology correlate, evidence-based imaging, is an iterative process. The medical practitioner: (1) formulates a question that is relevant to clinical practice, (2) searches the medical literature for relevant data, (3) critically analyzes the reported research, (4) incorporates the data from the medical literature into medical practice. Each of these steps has unique challenges. Fortunately, however, there is a growing body of literature on methods both of performing evidence-based imaging and of developing the resources to allow evidence-based imaging.

FORMULATING THE CLINICAL QUESTION

Formulation of an appropriate clinical question for application of the evidence-based imaging process is deceptively difficult. We tend to think in terms of broad generalizations and often expect that medical practice will be similarly general. For example, one can ask the question:

Which is better, computed tomography (CT) or ultrasound, for imaging in abdominal pain? Of course, in such a general form, the question cannot be answered. First, the patient population must be defined. Are we considering subjects who are men, women, children, young, elderly, thin, obese? Each of these characteristics may affect the choice of CT or ultrasound. In addition, we must understand the precise clinical scenario. Is the abdominal pain chronic, acute, right upper quadrant, left lower quadrant, flank, deep, superficial, mild, severe? In addition, is there fever, white blood cell count changes, positive pregnancy examination, previous surgical history, vomiting, peritoneal signs, sepsis, immunocompromise? We must understand what actions are being contemplated based on the test result. Is imaging being contemplated to determine if the patient requires surgery for appendicitis, enemas for constipation, proton blockers for gastroenteritis, exploratory laparotomy for bowel injury? Finally, what do we mean by CT or ultrasound? Does the study include the administration of intravenous contrast? What are the technical parameters for the imaging evaluations? Only with all this information in place can a specific clinical question be derived that is amenable to analysis using the evidence-based imaging approach. From this example, a clinically relevant question might be: "Which imaging test is more sensitive, multidetector CT with intravenous contrast or transabdominal ultrasound, in adult male and female patients of standard body habitus with signs and symptoms suggestive of but not definitive for acute appendicitis?"

IDENTIFYING THE MEDICAL LITERATURE

There are two general approaches to evidence-based imaging: "bottom-up" and "top-down."[6] Each approach has corresponding resources in the medical literature. The bottom-up approach relies on the actual research data in the form of carefully constructed and comprehensively reported research articles. Practitioners can individually locate, appraise, and apply evidence to imaging practice. In the bottom-up approach the individual practitioner is taking responsibility for the entire evidence-based imaging process and as a consequence has both more responsibility and more control over the relevance and adequacy of the analysis.

A challenge in the bottom-up approach is the difficulty in searching and assimilating the vast quantity of data in the medical literature. There are currently more than 15 million articles published in the medical literature. Some of these studies are carefully designed research with defensible conclusions. Other studies represent conjecture, anecdote, and opinion. Evidence-based imaging requires capturing what is valuable from the medical literature and incorporating it into clinical practice.

For the bottom-up approach, the underlying resources are the National Library of Medicine Medline (www.ncbi.nlm.nih.gov/entrez/query.fcgi?DB=pubmed) and the Excerpta-Medica Embase databases (www.embase.com). These are extensive catalogs of abstracts published in the peer-reviewed literature. Neither resource is completely comprehensive, but these can be supplemented by additional searches of the reference sections of identified articles, of meeting symposia, and of government publications. Medline, Embase, and other search engines are generally easy to use, although performance of a comprehensive, yet parsimonious search will be facilitated by relying on medical librarians and other expert resources.

The top-down approach to evidence-based imaging relies on evidence-based imaging summaries produced by centers that specialize in this function (Table 21-1). Under this approach the evidence is gathered, analyzed, and synthesized or summarized into a form that the individual practitioner can directly apply to his or her practice. Under the top-down approach the individual practitioner is relying on experts to synthesize the evidence. However, if the synthesis is done in a transparent manner, using appropriate tools and methods, the practitioner may maintain a high level of confidence in the results without having to go through the often time-consuming process individually.

For the top-down approach, the single best repository of evidence to drive radiology practice is the textbook *Evidence-Based Imaging: Optimizing Imaging in Patient Care*,[5] which includes a systematic discussion of the evidence (or lack thereof) that drives imaging practice for a host of common clinical scenarios across radiology practice. This book includes 30 chapters authored by experts in the field who

Table 21-1 Sources of "Top-Down" Evidence Summaries

Evidence-Based Medicine Center	Web Address
Center for Evidence-Based Radiology	www.evidencebasedradiology.net
Cochrane Collaboration	www.cochrane.org
Blue Cross Blue Shield Technology Evaluation Center	www.bcbs.com/tec
Oxford-Centre for Evidence-Based Medicine	www.cebm.net
University of York Centre for Reviews and Dissemination	www.york.ac.uk/inst/crd
Agency for Healthcare Research and Quality, Evidence-Based Practice Centers	www.ahrq.gov/clinic/epcix.htm
UK National Health Service, National Institute for Clinical Excellence	www.nice.org.uk
National Public Health Services for Wales, ATTRACT Center	www.attract.wales.nhs.uk
UK National Health Services, National Library for Health	www.clinicalanswers.nhs.uk
University of Western Ontario, Canada (neurology)	www.uwo.ca/cns/ebn/

have both clinical experience and training in the evidence-based imaging paradigm. The author of this chapter serves as an editor for the *Evidence-Based Imaging* text.[5,7]

Fortunately there is an expanding variety of top-down resources in radiology that complement the *Evidence-Based Imaging* text.[8] These include series on evidence-based practice in major radiology journals (including *Radiology* and the *Canadian Association of Radiology Journal*), as well as websites from institutions and medical societies (Table 21-1). Probably the most useful of these is the center for evidence-based radiology in Ireland (http://www.evidencebasedradiology.net). There also are well-established resources for evidence-based medical practice outside of radiology that may have relevance to imaging questions. These include the Cochrane Collaborations (http://www.cochrane.org) and the Oxford Center for Evidence Based Medicine (http://www.cebm.net). In the United States further work in the evidence-based medicine arena has been funded by the Agency for Health Care Research and Quality (AHRQ) (http://www.ahrq.gov/clinic/epcix.htm) and the Blue Cross Blue Shield Technology Evaluation Center (http://www.bcbs.com/tec). These organizations can also provide valuable information. To identify the appropriate literature to guide top-down evidence-based imaging practice, the practitioner would search one or more of the sources to find data that are relevant to the specific clinical question detailed above.

From a practical standpoint, the top-down approach is more easily accessible to practicing radiologists. For example, using the bottom-up approach for the appendicitis example detailed above, search of the primary literature in Medline would reveal literally thousands of citations on imaging for appendicitis. Narrowing the search to prospective clinical trials would still yield a wealth of information beyond the needs of the practitioner. Sifting through all of this information is a daunting task. However, for the top-down approach there are now two meta-analyses on the topic, as well as a chapter in the *Evidence-Based Imaging* text,[5] which includes the meta-analysis results updated with other relevant information. These sources could form the basis for evidence-based practice.

CRITICALLY ASSESSING THE LITERATURE

Critical assessment of the imaging literature is perhaps the most vital component of evidence-based imaging. Unfortunately, most of what is found in the medical literature is biased and incompletely reported, and would therefore form a poor basis for medical practice. There are currently more than 50 journals focused on imaging. However, there is insufficient high-quality research to provide content for such a large number of periodicals. In a critical survey of the cost-effectiveness literature in the late 1990s we found that only 7% to 14% of radiology cost-effectiveness analyses in the medical literature adhere to 10 minimum methodologic standards (Table 21-2).[9,10] Furthermore, in a review in the 1990s the methodologic qualities of studies of outcomes in radiology were also found lacking.[11] The biases that are common in the imaging literature unfortunately have also been shown to have an important effect on study results.[12] Accordingly, few of the studies that are published are of sufficient quality to form the basis for evidence-based practice. Recent promulgation of the CONSORT[13] (Box 21-1) and STARD[14] (Box 21-2) criteria will hopefully have an impact in improving the thoroughness with which medical studies are reported. They may also have an impact on how research is performed.

One of the more important opportunities for bias to creep into radiology investigations is in selection of subjects for a study. In general, because the results of research investigation will be applied to a specific clinical group, the selection of the subjects for the study should also reflect a specific clinical scenario. Readers of the literature must always ask, "Which subjects were selected and based on what criteria?" In general, consecutive enrollment is better than sporadic enrollment. Prospective enrollment will also potentially produce less bias results than retrospective enrollment. However, these are generalizations. A well-performed retrospective study may yield less biased information then a poorly performed prospective investigation. Readers must assess whether the groups that are being compared

Table 21-2 Compliance with Methodological Standards for Radiology Cost-Effectiveness Analyses Published in Radiology and Nonradiology Journals

Criteria	Radiology Journals ($n = 44$)		Nonradiology Journals ($n = 56$)	
	Number	%	Number	%
Comparative options The two or more options being compared are defined in the article.	43	98	50	89
Perspective of analysis May be payer, provider, patient, or society.	6	14	14	25
Cost data Some estimation of costs is provided.	43	98	55	98
Source of cost data given May be reimbursements, micro-costing, accounting costs, etc.	31	70	46	82
Long-term costs included Costs beyond the single episode of care. These may extend out for years depending on the clinical question.	9	20	20	36
Discounting applied where appropriate Accounting for the time value of money.	5	11	18	32
Outcome data provided Information on actual patient outcome. This may be mortality or quality-of-life data.	35	80	29	52
Summary measure or dominant measure identified Summary of costs and outcomes is given in single metric (e.g., quality-adjusted life years)	18	41	27	48
Incremental computational method for summary measure Costs and outcomes are measured as the difference between competing strategies.	9	20	22	39
Sensitivity analysis performed Accounts for uncertainty in the analysis.	8	18	24	43
Average number of criteria with compliance	4.8	48	5.4	54

Adapted from Blackmore CC, Magid DJ: Methodologic evaluation of the radiology cost-effectiveness literature. Radiology 203:87–91, 1997; Blackmore CC, Smith WJ. Economic analysis of radiological procedures. A methodological evaluation of the medical literature. Eur J Radiol 27:123–130, 1998.

BOX 21-1

CONsolidated **S**tandards **O**f **R**eporting of **T**rials (CONSORT) Checklist

Title/abstract
- Detail how subjects were allocated to interventions (e.g., randomized).
- Introduction
- Outline scientific background and rationale.

Methods
- Describe eligibility criteria, setting, and location.
- Detail interventions performed and timing.
- List objectives and hypotheses.
- Describe primary and secondary end points and how measured.
- Describe determination of sample size.
- Mention method of randomization (e.g., random number generator).
- Mention method of concealment of allocation (e.g., opaque envelopes).
- Who generated allocation sequence? Who enrolled participants? Who assigned participants to groups?
- Was there blinding, and if so, how was success of blinding evaluated?
- List statistical methods used.

Results
- Include a flow diagram of study participants through protocol.
- Give dates of recruitment and follow-up.
- Outline baseline demographic and clinical characteristics.
- Include number of participants and whether intention-to-treat analysis was used.
- Summarize primary and secondary results with effect size and precision.
- Include subgroup and ancillary analyses, prespecified and exploratory.
- Describe any adverse events.

Discussion
- Give interpretation of results.
- Assess generalizability (external validity) of results.
- Integrate results with other current evidence.

Adapted from Moher D, Schulz K, Altman D: The CONSORT statement: revised recommendations for improving the quality of reports of parallel-group randomized trials. Journal of the American Medical Association 285:1987–1991, 2001.

are otherwise equivalent with the exception of the imaging test or if there is some systematic difference between them. For example, one could compare ultrasound and CT for identification of hepatoma in subjects with cirrhosis. To make a valid comparison, however, the patients in the two arms should either be selected at random for CT and for ultrasound, or all eligible subjects should undergo both tests. There should be comparability between the subjects in terms of age, gender, body habitus, co-morbidities, duration, and severities of liver failure, and so on. Any systematic difference in these factors might bias the results in favor of one imaging test to another. Less obvious, but equally important is the concept that selection of subjects should not be based on performance of imaging but rather on clinical criteria. For example, when evaluating the accuracy of CT for determining the presence of diaphragmatic rupture in trauma, a study that focused on patients who underwent CT but ignored patients who went to the operating room based on chest radiograph findings without CT might give a lower estimation of the accuracy of CT. Because obvious cases will be apparent on chest radiographs, CT in this situation is generally performed only in those cases where the findings are more subtle. Thus, looking only at the cases that are imaged with CT is a reflection of the accuracy of CT in these subtle cases but is not a reflection of the accuracy of CT overall for the evaluation of diaphragmatic rupture. This problem worsens when two imaging modalities are being compared. From the cirrhosis and hepatoma example described above, one could compare the accuracy of CT and ultrasound by looking only at those cases that underwent both imaging modalities, excluding all subjects who had only a single imaging evaluation. This would mean that the accuracy information for CT and ultrasound was being collected from the same patients. However, there is tremendous potential for bias here, because patients in most practices do not routinely undergo both imaging studies. The only patients to undergo a second imaging study would be those with whom the results of the first imaging study were equivocal or unclear. If the standard protocol is for evaluation with CT in this scenario,

BOX 21-2

STAndards for Reporting of Diagnostic Accuracy (STARD)

Title/abstract
Identify in title that study is of diagnostic accuracy.

Introduction
- State research question or study aims (e.g., estimating accuracy).

Methods
- Describe the study population (inclusion and exclusion criteria, setting and location).
- Describe basis of recruitment of subjects (clinical symptoms, imaging tests, performance of reference standard, etc.).
- Describe participant sampling (consecutive, random, etc.).
- Describe data collection (retrospective, prospective).
- Describe reference standard.
- Describe technical specifications for imaging tests and reference standard.
- Describe categorization of test results (criteria for positive, negative, etc.).
- Describe number, training, and expertise of test interpreters.
- Describe blinding.
- Describe statistical methods for determining results.
- Describe statistical methods for test reproducibility, if any.

Results
- Report when study was done.
- Report clinical and demographic characteristics of subjects.
- Report number of subjects who met inclusion criteria who did not undergo test or reference standard, and why.
- Report time from test to reference standard and any treatment received.
- Report distribution of severity of disease.
- Report cross-tabulation for test results, including indeterminate results.
- Report any adverse events.
- Report estimates of diagnostic accuracy with measures of uncertainty (confidence intervals).
- Report how indeterminate results were handled.
- Report estimates of variability in subgroups, if any.
- Report estimates of test reproducibility, if done.

Discussion
- Discuss the clinical applicability of the study results.

Adapted from Bossuyt PM, Reitsma J, Bruns D, et al: Towards complete and accurate reporting of studies of diagnostic accuracy: the STARD initiative. American Journal of Radiology 181:51–56, 2003.

then it can be expected that the subjects who undergo ultrasound will only be those in whom the CT is equivocal. Thus, the comparison of CT and ultrasound will be made in the group in whom CT is not informative, yielding an unfavorably biased estimation of CT accuracy with respect to ultrasound. Unfortunately, this is a common research design in radiology.

Another important potential area for bias is in blinding. It is well known that the interpretation of an imaging study for research should

be performed without knowledge of the final outcome. Knowledge of final outcome can bias interpretation, particularly in subjective areas such as imaging interpretation. Such blinding is easy to achieve in prospective studies but can also be achieved in retrospective evaluations. Less obvious but also important is that evaluation of the reference standard should be made by individuals who are blinded to the test result. For example, the accuracy of CTA for identification of traumatic thoracic aortic injury can be made by comparing the results of CTA to catheter angiography. However, catheter angiography is an imperfect reference standard, and the result may sometimes be difficult to interpret. If the results of the CT scan are known to the interpreters of the catheter angiogram, then the catheter angiogram interpretation may be biased to agree with the CT results. This will falsely elevate the sensitivity and specificity of CTA.

Another area where bias can creep into the results, particularly of an investigation of diagnostic accuracy, is when equivocal studies are excluded. The reality is that sometimes the result of a diagnostic imaging study is unclear. The standard 2×2 table used to calculate sensitivity and specificity has no place for equivocal results. Sensitivity and specificity are dependent on all results being recorded as either positive or negative. Therefore, researchers must decide a priori how such indeterminate results are to be treated, make this explicit to the reader, and include them in the results. It is unfortunately relatively common to find that researchers when faced with ambiguous results of a test will simply exclude that patient from the analysis. Excluding equivocal cases will make both sensitivity and specificity higher than they truly are and will present the reader with data that are not applicable to the real world where equivocal cases, though hopefully uncommon, do occur.

No research study is ever perfect. One rough guide to the thoroughness with which an investigation was performed and reported is whether the authors accurately and completely report the limitations of their study. A frank discussion of any methodologic flaws within a research study as well as an estimation of the direction and potential magnitude of the effects of these flaws and biases is very valuable to the reader. Discussion of the limitations of a study should be considered an indication of the integrity of the authors and therefore the believability of their results.

For additional information on this topic, the reader is referred to recent series in the journals *Radiology*[15] and the *American Journal of Radiology*,[16] and to specific articles[17-19] and texts on this topic.[20] In general, a grading scheme is applied to summarize the strength and quality of the evidence supporting a given conclusion. "Levels" of evidence are designated to confer the overall confidence that one should have in the results of an evidence-based imaging summary (Box 21-3).[21] Randomized clinical trials and carefully controlled multi-institutional observational studies are valued more highly than case series and uncontrolled data. Unfortunately, such high-quality studies are rare. In addition, the skills required to perform critical literature review are not necessarily emphasized in radiology training and not necessarily well developed in practicing radiologists.

BOX 21-3

Strength of Evidence

Level 1: Strong Evidence
Studies that can be broadly generalized to most patients. Included are prospective, blinded, unbiased comparisons of diagnostic tests with well-defined reference standards when assessing diagnostic accuracy or blinded randomized control trials when assessing therapeutic impact or patient outcomes. This also includes well-designed meta-analyses of studies at evidence levels 1 and 2.

Level 2: Moderate Evidence
Studies with narrower generalizability. Included are prospective or retrospective studies with methodologic deficiencies that are minor and well described to allow assessment of their impact. For diagnostic accuracy, these studies are blinded and performed on an unbiased sample. This level includes well-designed cohort or case-control studies, and randomized trials for therapeutic effects or patient outcomes.

Level 3: Limited Evidence
Diagnostic accuracy studies with multiple or severe flaws in research methods, small sample sizes, or incomplete reporting, OR nonrandomized comparisons for therapeutic impact or patient outcomes.

Level 4: Insufficient Evidence
Studies with multiple, possibly large-impact, flaws in research methods. Included are case series, descriptive studies, or expert opinions without substantiating data.

Adapted from Kent DL, Larson EB: Diagnostic technology assessments: problems and prospects. Annals of Internal Medicine 108:759–761, 1988.

Under the bottom-up approach to evidence-based imaging, the user of research data takes responsibility for the critical literature review. A comprehensive understanding of research design, meta-analysis, and bias is obligatory for bottom-up evidence-based imaging. With top-down evidence-based imaging, the user again relies on the preparers of evidence-based summaries to critically assess the literature. Ideally, an evidence summary includes not only the conclusions but also the limitations and biases in the included literature.

Again using the diagnosis of appendicitis as a top-down evidence-based imaging example, the recently published meta-analysis of the comparison of CT and ultrasound demonstrated superiority of CT.[22] However, the meta-analysis also included critical reviews of the literature on the topic and found consistent flaws in all of the published studies. For the appendicitis imaging literature, a particular problem was verification bias, where the performance and interpretation of the reference standard was affected by the imaging test results. This means that whether patients had surgery or clinical follow-up as a reference standard was determined by the results of the CT scan. Some cases of appendicitis may be self-limited or might resolve with nonsurgical treatment. These cases would be identified as true positives if the CT was interpreted as positive and the patient went to surgery, but they would be interpreted as true negatives if the CT was read as negative and the patient outcome was clinical follow-up. Thus, the estimates of sensitivity and specificity that are published for both CT and ultrasound overestimate the true accuracy of these modalities.[22] The published meta-analysis article serves as both a resource on the accuracy of CT for appendicitis and as a critical assessment of the methodologic rigor of the literature on the topic.

APPLYING THE EVIDENCE

True outcomes data in radiology are rare. The effect on patient health of specific screening studies, particularly mammography, is known. However, this is a relatively infrequent situation in radiology. Other examples of actual outcomes studies in radiology include imaging for low back pain, angioplasty and other interventional procedures, and some emergency radiology imaging studies. Where such outcome information is available, it can be used to directly guide imaging practice. More commonly, however, only information on sensitivity and specificity of imaging is available. The practitioner must translate imaging accuracy into information that is useful to the patient. The imaging efficacy hierarchy first proposed by Fryback is a useful paradigm for understanding this approach (Box 21-4).[23] Under Fryback's model, imaging efficacy can be thought of as occurring through a sequence of steps. At the most basic level, to be useful, imaging must be technology efficacious, meaning that an image can be generated, is free from artifacts, and details anatomy. If this condition is met, then accuracy information can be derived where sensitivity and specificity for an imaging study in detecting disease are detailed. Once accuracy has been demonstrated, this information can be used to define changes in diagnostic certainty in a given patient. In other words, following a test result, how is the likelihood of a given diagnosis changed? If diagnostic certainty has been changed, then treatment may be modified. Once treatment is modified, then there is potential to change patient outcome. Once patient outcome has been altered, societal benefit can be assessed through cost-effectiveness analysis.

From this hierarchy we can see that diagnostic accuracy is an important condition for improved patient outcome but is not sufficient. Where outcomes data are lacking, the imager must be able to infer the effect of imaging on outcome by translating accuracy into diagnostic certainty, and alter medical decision making. Accuracy can be translated into diagnostic certainty through the use of Bayes' theorem. Bayes' theorem states that the probability of disease following a test (post-test probability) is related to the probability of disease before the test (pretest probability) as well as the sensitivity and specificity of the imaging test. Sensitivity, specificity, pretest and post-test probability, and Bayes' theorem are detailed in Box 21-5. If the probability of disease after a test is changed to the point where treatment changes, then there is potential for patient outcome improvement.[24]

From the appendicitis example, if the pretest probability based on the clinical examination is

BOX 21-4

Imaging Effectiveness Hierarchy

Technical efficacy: Production of an image that contains information
- Measures: signal-to-noise ratio, resolution, absence of artifacts

Accuracy efficacy: Ability of test (and reader) to differentiate disease from non-disease
- Measures: sensitivity, specificity, ROC curves

Diagnostic-thinking efficacy: Effect of test on diagnosis probability in a given patient
- Measures: pretest and post-test probability, diagnostic certainty

Treatment efficacy: Potential of test to change management for a patient
- Measures: treatment plan, operative or medical treatment frequency

Outcome efficacy: Effect of use of test on patient mortality and quality of life
- Measures: survival, quality-adjusted life years, health status

Societal efficacy: Appropriateness of test from perspective of society
- Measures: cost-effectiveness analysis, cost-utility analysis

Adapted from Fryback DG, Thornbury JR: The efficacy of diagnostic imaging. Medical Decision Making 11:88–94, 1991.

about 50%, then through application of Bayes' theorem it can be seen that the probability of disease after a positive CT scan is 97% (Box 21-5). Surgeons will operate on patients with presumed appendicitis at less than 100% certainty of disease, because they wish to avoid misdiagnosis with progression or perforation. The threshold for surgery for appendicitis is a level of certainty that is 80% to 85%, because this reflects the rate of positive laparotomies performed historically.[25,26] Accordingly, because the probability of appendicitis increases from 50% to 97% after a positive CT scan, it can be seen that the result of the CT scan converts a patient who will not undergo surgery to one in whom operation is indicated.

Using such an approach allows the definition of scenarios that indicate the appropriateness of imaging. For appendicitis, using Bayes' theorem it can be argued that CT will not change

management when appendicitis is clinically certain, because even a negative CT scan will result in a post-test probability of appendicitis higher than the threshold for surgery. Accordingly, CT is not useful in subjects with high clinical certainty.

This is an example of a rigorous mathematical approach to incorporation of evidence into clinical care. In clinical practice this may be done ad hoc. Clinicians request imaging studies, and radiologists help provide guidance as to the most accurate study for a given clinical scenario. However, the actual effect of the imaging on clinical decision making may be overlooked, resulting in unnecessary imaging. The goal of medicine, and therefore of imaging, is to improve patient health. Accordingly, to incorporate medical imaging data into practice the imager must understand the relationship between those data and eventual patient outcome. The use of evidence-based imaging requires that the practitioner understand how accuracy, the most commonly available data in imaging, translates into outcome.

Evidence-based imaging also allows the radiologist to look beyond individual patient outcome. The highest level of outcome is that of society, as measured by cost-effectiveness analysis. Cost-effectiveness analysis is a method of estimating the value in terms of human health obtained for each dollar spent on health care. In cost-effectiveness analysis, all of the costs and all of the possible outcomes resulting from different imaging approaches can be integrated to produce a summary measure of cost effectiveness, generally using a concept such as quality-adjusted life years. The central tenet of cost-effectiveness analysis is that of opportunity cost, implying that if resources are used for a single intervention in medicine, then fewer resources will be available for all other potential interventions. Cost-effectiveness analysis permits comparison of different potential interventions (including diagnostic imaging) across medicine, and thus may be a useful policy tool. As an example, Mahadevia and colleagues evaluated the cost effectiveness of lung cancer screening with helical CT.[27] Although the accuracy of helical CT and effect on patient treatment and outcome is still uncertain, Mahadevia et al evaluated whether such screening would be cost effective for a range of potential values for

BOX 21-5

Sensitivity, Specificity, and Bayes' Theorem

1. **Sensitivity** (*sens*) is the ability of a test to correctly diagnose in subjects with the disease.
   True positive (*TP*) means that the test is positive and the subject has the disease.
   False negative (*FN*) means that the test is negative and the subject has the disease.

$$sens = \frac{TP}{TP + FN}$$

2. **Specificity** (*spec*) is the ability of the test to correctly diagnose in subjects without the disease.
   True negative (*TN*) means that the test is negative and the subject does not have the disease.
   False positive (*FP*) means that the test is positive and the subject does not have the disease.

$$spec = \frac{TN}{TN + FP}$$

3. **Bayes' Theorem** Permits calculation of the probability of a patient having the disease after a positive test result is known ($P_{post\text{-}test}$) from the sensitivity, specificity, and the probability of disease before the test result is known ($P_{pretest}$).

$$P_{post\text{-}test} = \frac{(P_{pretest} \times sens)}{(P_{pretest} \times sens) + [(1 - P_{pretest}) \times (1 - spec)]}$$

4. Example of application of **Bayes' Theorem** to CT imaging for appendicitis:
   CT for appendicitis: sensitivity = 0.94; specificity = 0.95.
   Pretest probability of appendicitis with clinically equivocal exam = 0.50

$$P_{post\text{-}test} = \frac{(0.50 \times 0.94)}{(0.50 \times 0.94) + [(1 - 0.50) \times (1 - 0.95)]} = 0.97$$

the effectiveness. They found that the most important factors influencing the cost effectiveness of CT screening were adherence to screening, extent of identification of slow-growing tumors that would not affect the patients' longevity, the cost of the helical CT, and the underlying quality of life in smokers. The authors concluded that CT screening would only be cost effective if the continuing studies of CT effectiveness had very favorable results. Given the potentially high cost of screening very large numbers of smokers with CT, it may not be in the best interest of society to fund this intervention.[27] Of course these conclusions are dependent on the final results of the continuing National Lung Screening Trial.

CHALLENGES

The evidence-based imaging paradigm is not without challenges. The greatest of these is the relatively low quality of the published radiology literature despite a vast quantity of articles available. It is to be hoped that publication of the STARD and CONSORT guidelines as well as several research methodologic series in the major radiology journals will, over time, improve the quality of publications. A second limitation in the evidence-based imaging approach is the break with traditional thinking that is required for this paradigm shift to occur. Evidence-based imaging is sometimes perceived as cookbook medicine and resisted for that reason. In fact, in some ways evidence-based imaging is liberating to the practitioner in that the individual radiologist is given license to doubt the gospel of the experts by whom he or she was indoctrinated in medical training.

Evidence-based imaging also cannot exist in isolation. One accepted definition of evidence-based imaging is that it includes the combination of the best current evidence with clinical expertise and patient values.[28] Thus, neither the practitioner nor the patient's contribution is neglected under the evidence-based imaging paradigm, despite the implications of the "cookbook" label.

One indication of the success of the evidence-based medicine paradigm is the rush for developers of clinical practice guidelines to add "evidence-based" to the title or description of the guidelines. Unfortunately, such guidelines may not follow the rigorous process that forms the foundation of evidence-based practice.[29,30] Thus, to accept a resource for top-down evidence-based imaging, the practitioner must be sufficiently savvy to be able to critique whether that resource is in fact a recommendation based on a thorough and systematic review of the literature or on the advice of experts from the more traditional "eminence-based" approach.[2]

CONCLUSIONS

The cost and quality challenges in the medical care system are not going to end. Evidence-based imaging is not a panacea but does represent an important approach to the rationalization of imaging care. Understanding and applying evidence-based imaging is requisite for imaging practice today.

Dos and Don'ts of Evidence-Based Imaging	
Dos	**Don'ts**
1. Use evidence-based imaging resources.	1. Rely on expert panels.
2. Read the literature critically.	2. Believe everything you read.
3. Evaluate for selection bias.	3. Assume all patients are the same.
4. Understand study limitations.	4. Discount retrospective studies.
5. Think in terms of medical decision making.	5. Focus just on accuracy.

REFERENCES

1. World Health Organization. The World Health Report 2006. New York, World Health Organization, 2006, p. 185.
2. Wood BP: What's the evidence? Radiology 213:635–637, 1999.
3. Sackett DL, Rosenberg WMC, Gray JAM, Richardson WS: Evidence based medicine: what it is and what it isn't. BMJ 312:71–72, 1996.
4. Evidence Based Radiology Working Group. Evidence-based radiology: a new approach to the practice of radiology. Radiology 220:566–575, 2001.
5. Medina LS, Blackmore CC: Evidence-based imaging: optimizing imaging for patient care. New York, Springer, 2006.
6. MacPherson DW: Evidence-based medicine. Can Med Assoc J 152:201–204, 1995.
7. Medina L, Aguirre E, Zurakowski D: Introduction to evidence-based imaging. Neuroimag Clin North Am 13:157–165, 2003.
8. Medina LS, Blackmore CC Evidence-based imaging: review and dissemination. Radiology. In press (2007).
9. Blackmore CC, Magid DJ: Methodologic evaluation of the radiology cost-effectiveness literature. Radiology 203:87–91, 1997.
10. Blackmore CC, Smith WJ: Economic analyses of radiological procedures: a methodological evaluation of the medical literature. Eur J Radiol 27:123–130, 1998.
11. Blackmore CC, Black WB, Jarvik JG, Langlotz CP: A critical synopsis of the diagnostic and screening radiology outcomes literature. Acad Radiol 6(S1):S8–S18, 1999.
12. Lijmer JG, Mol BW, Heisterkamp S, et al: Empirical evidence of design-related bias in studies of diagnostic tests. JAMA 282:1061–1066, 1999.
13. Moher D, Schulz K, Altman D: The CONSORT statement: revised recommendations for improving the quality of reports of parallel-group randomized trials. JAMA 285:1987–1991, 2001.
14. Bossuyt PM, Reitsma J, Bruns, D, et al: Towards complete and accurate reporting of studies of diagnostic accuracy: the STARD initiative. Am J Radiol 181:51–56, 2003.

15. Applegate KE, Crewson PE: An introduction to biostatistics. Radiology 225:318–322, 2002.

16. Beam C, Blackmore C, Karlik S, Reinhold C: Fundamentals of clinical research for radiologists. Am J Radiol 176:323–325, 2001.

17. Blackmore CC: Critically assessing the radiology literature. Acad Radiol 11:134–140, 2004.

18. Black WC, Welch HG: Screening for disease. Am J Radiol 168:3–11, 1997.

19. Kent DL, Larson EB: Diagnostic technology assessments: problems and prospects. Ann Intern Med 108:759–761, 1988.

20. Blackmore CC, Medina LS: Critically assessing the literature: understanding error and bias. In: Medina LS, Blackmore CC (eds): Evidence-based imaging: optimizing imaging for patient care. New York, Springer, 2006 pp 19–27.

21. Medina LS, Blackmore CC: Principles of evidence-based imaging. In: Medina LS, Blackmore CC (eds): Evidence-based imaging: optimizing imaging for patient care. New York, Springer, 2006.

22. Terasawa T, Blackmore CC, Bent S, Kohlwes RJ: Systematic review: computed tomography and ultrasonography to detect acute appendicitis in adults and adolescents. Ann Intern Med 141:537–546, 2004.

23. Fryback DG, Thornbury JR: The efficacy of diagnostic imaging. Med Decision Making 11:88–94, 1991.

24. Sox HC, Blatt MA, Higgins MC, Marton KI: Medical decision making. Boston, Butterworth, 1988.

25. Addiss DG, Shaffer N, Fowler BS, Tauxe RV: The epidemiology of appendicitis and appendectomy in the United States. Am J Epidemiol 132:910–925, 1990.

26. Andersson RE, Hugander A, Thulin AJ. Diagnostic accuracy and perforation rate in appendicitis: association with age and sex of the patient and with appendectomy rate. Eur J Surg 158:37–41, 1992.

27. Mahadevia PJ, Fleisher LA, Frick KD, Eng J, Goodman SN, Powe NR: Lung cancer screening with helical computed tomography in older adults: a decision and cost-effectiveness analysis. JAMA 289:313–322, 2003.

28. Sackett DL, Richardson WS, Rosenberg W, Haynes RB: Evidence-based medicine. New York, Churchill Livingstone, 1997.

29. Steinberg EP, Luce BR: Evidence based? Caveat emptor! Health Affairs 24:80–92, 2005.

30. Blackmore CC, Medina LS: Evidence-based radiology and the ACR appropriateness criteria. J Amer Coll Radiol 3:505–509, 2006.

PART **4**

LEGAL AND LEGISLATIVE CONCERNS

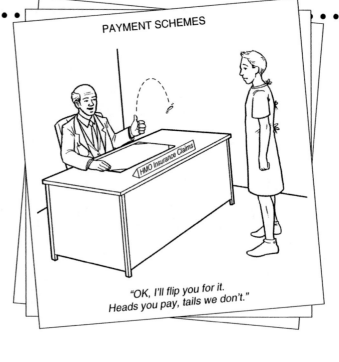

CHAPTER 22

PAYMENT SCHEMES

HMO Insurance Claims

"OK, I'll flip you for it.
Heads you pay, tails we don't."

Contracting with Managed Care Organizations

Andrew Litt

Contracting with a managed care organization (MCO) is now a fact of life for most radiology groups in the United States. MCOs control a portion of the patients in almost every market, from the most urban to the most rural. Although the nature of managed care has changed somewhat over the last 10 years, moving away from lock-in "HMO"-type plans to more flexible point-of-service (POS) or preferred-provider organization (PPO) plans, the overall percentage of patients enrolled in these products has continued to increase. At the same time traditional indemnity plans have declined to the point of near irrelevancy. Although significant regional variations exist, radiology practices tend to see about 30% of their patients from managed care, 30% to 40% from Medicare and other government plans, and the balance from other sources including self-pay. Realistically, most radiology practices cannot survive without patients and revenue from MCOs (see Table 22-1).

What makes this reality even harsher is that most patients have no loyalty to their radiologist. Although some patients may be willing to pay out-of-network co-insurance and deductibles to see a certain surgeon or other specialist, few will consider paying any premium to have their imaging study performed at one facility instead of another. The most a radiologist can hope for is that the referring physician insists on patients having their studies performed and interpreted by their preferred radiologists. Radiology is perceived as a commodity, one place being as good as the next, and individuals don't pay extra for commodities.

Thus, radiology practices must contract with MCOs for their own growth and survival. Whether or not we like the concept of managed care, whether or not we think that managed care executives make too much money, whether or not we object to their rules and regulations, most radiologists have to accept the need to deal with those organizations. The good news is that in many, if not most, cases the MCOs

Table 22-1 Managed Care Plan Types

Type	Description	Out-of-Network Benefits
HMO	Network of providers who have agreed to discount fees	No
POS	Network of providers who have agreed to discount fees plus "wrap-around" major medical benefit	Yes, but with increased costs (co-insurance) to patient
PPO	Network of providers who have agreed to discount fees for increased volume	Yes, but with significantly increased costs (co-insurance) to patient

need us as well. They want as broad a network as possible to make access for their members easy and convenient. They want an extensive book of participating physicians (or its online equivalent) to impress their clients, the employers who purchase health care. They want access to different types of equipment and procedures, and are concerned about being overly dependent on a limited number of radiologists.

Recognizing this mutual, if unstated, need should provide the basis for a productive, positive negotiation. Importantly, this is a negotiation and not a confrontation. Like the foreign diplomats who meet and always report that "productive discussions were held" even when there was agreement on not one item, you must approach this undertaking always keeping the overarching goals in mind. The practice desires a contract with the MCO that provides the best rates and other terms achievable. The MCO wants to secure the participation of that radiology group with the least possible overall cost and the fewest changes to its general program. Whatever each side thinks of the other is irrelevant; one side cannot view the other (at least publicly) as the enemy. The goal is not defeat of the other side (elimination of the MCO would reduce the revenues

to the practice), but agreement and even a sense of partnership on the best possible terms. Roger Fisher, one of the most famous authors on negotiations, titled his book *Getting to Yes*, because that is the objective of the exercise. If an agreement is not reached then the negotiation is a failure. If the agreement takes too much advantage of one side or the other, then it is equally unsuccessful.

Of course, the most important concept here is that you must negotiate to achieve anything. Many physicians, radiologists included, tend to sign every contract put before them, assuming that there is little that can be done to improve on the standard terms. Although negotiating the contract or its renewal is no guarantee of a better outcome, surely there is no downside risk in attempting to rationally and positively work with the MCO toward a better arrangement. That means overcoming the natural tendency most physicians, indeed most individuals, have to avoid a confrontation or a bargaining situation. Other than at the car dealership, most Americans have little opportunity to develop or hone negotiating skills, and professionals tend to view such enterprises with deep disdain. So the key is to overcome the natural reticence and jump into the pool.

PROCESS AND PREPARATION

A well-conducted negotiation generally lasts more than a single moment in time; it is a process that has defined stages. These can be thought of as preparation, discussion, coming to agreement, final contract, and follow-up. An important negotiation like this should not be only one session where the MCO representative presents a contract with rates and other terms, the radiologist demands some changes, a compromise is reached, a contract is signed, and both sides leave, never to see each other again. This will definitely work against the radiologist if for no other reason than most MCO contracting representatives have very little authority to make any changes on the spot. Moreover, the radiologist in this scenario is responding rather than leading and, more importantly, may not even know what he or she really wants as the best outcome (Box 22-1).

The essential first step in any negotiation is preparation, which consists of answering the following questions:

- What are our strengths and weaknesses in this negotiation?
- What are the MCO's strengths and weaknesses?
- What is our best realistic outcome of this negotiation? (Note that "realistic" comes from the same root as "reality"; a payment rate of five times Medicare is desirable but not realistic.)
- What is our BATNA (best alternative to a negotiated agreement)?

The adage that "information is power" is right on target when it comes to negotiation. The more data the radiology negotiator has about his or her own organization and about the other side, the stronger is his or her position at the table. To negotiate effectively demands developing as many "leverage points" as possible, and this requires accurate, detailed information.

Current Conditions

The first priority is to understand your radiology group's current situation with respect to finances, competition, and relationships. What is the existing payer mix? If the contract under discussion is an existing one, then how much revenue (both in actual dollars and percentage of total) and how many examinations come from that contract per year? While you're at it, examine all your existing sources of revenue to see what each individual payer (private and governmental) is contributing. This provides a gauge of the relative importance of the contract under discussion. Is this contract vital to the group's existence or just a potential source of new patients? If the agreement is a new one, you will need to make some estimates about how much the contract will be worth, and this will depend on getting data about this payer as will be discussed later.

After this analysis, examine each payer and evaluate how their current reimbursements compare to a standard schedule. Don't use your fee schedule, because most practices have fees that bear no relationship to costs or to realistic payments. Use the Medicare fee schedule for your area. Compare each payer to that schedule on a current procedural terminology (CPT) code basis, or at least group the CPT codes by modality (roentgenography, fluoroscopy, magnetic resonance imaging or MRI, computed tomography or CT, etc.) and type of study (without contrast, without and with contrast, etc.) and compare the average rates and volumes for those groupings. This should document how the plans compare with respect to both individual rates and utilization, which together equal total dollars, for each modality. Remember to do a separate analysis for professional fees and global fees depending on the relevant site(s) of practice. If you already have contracts that are tied to the Medicare schedule, then some of this work will be done for you, but don't forget to examine the volume data as well. You need to identify those CPT codes or areas that may require special reimbursement treatment (interventional codes are often an example) because either the Medicare rates are too low or the volumes are high.

The next stage in the self-examination process is to review capacity for growth by modality. Which practice areas (CT, MRI, etc.) have room for growth? Are there excessive waiting times for some modalities (e.g., breast imaging)? The goal is to determine if the plan can bring in volume to fill underused resources. This will contribute revenue that predominantly goes straight to the bottom line. Therefore, even if the plan's rates are relatively low, adding new business to an underused facility or modality might make sense. However, if capacity at that site or that modality is limited, it would not be wise to replace existing higher paying patients with the new ones, or to cause further delays and reduced referring-physician and patient satisfaction.

Now that you've looked internally, it's time to look externally. What is your competitive position in your "market" or your geographic region? Are you the preferred choice among all the referring physicians, the "800-pound gorilla," or are you the "also ran," picking up the crumbs the big guy(s) leaves behind? Who are your competitors? Can you estimate how many referrals are going to them instead of to you? Why don't you have 100% of the referrals?

There may not be definitive answers to these questions. The purpose of this exercise is to get some sense of how the MCO may view you. If you have hard data that you can use to educate yourself or the MCO (e.g., patient and/or physician satisfaction surveys), then start with that. In any case, you need to appreciate the viewpoints of local referring physicians with respect to the practice. Do some market research; that is, talk to the leading physicians and find out how they judge your practice. Are you essential to their taking care of patients? Do they tolerate your group but prefer to send patients elsewhere when possible? Do you have special services or capabilities that they really rely on? The perspective of your colleagues is probably similar to that of the MCO. Are you essential to the plan's participating physician list, just a nice addition, or not even desirable? This is the time for brutal honesty. Don't delude yourself! It's not that you won't try to portray your strengths in the best light when you actually negotiate, but you have to consider the probable perspective of the other side. If your site has old equipment, radiologists who are not board certified, and a dirty waiting room, don't expect them to treat you like the major academic center or cutting-edge, customer-focused outpatient imaging center down the street. Conversely, if you are that major player, don't sell yourself short.

Geographic access analysis plays a large part in MCO contracting as well. The plan needs to have a reasonable geographic coverage of physicians in a specialty to meet its members' needs. Radiologists are particularly valuable, because many patients will need to use that service (as opposed to, for example, epilepsy surgeons who can be more geographically disparate). Obviously if yours is the only practice in a rural area you have significant advantage, but even practices in urban or suburban regions may benefit from examining this issue. Although it may be reasonable to expect a patient to drive 5 miles for a radiology study in a medium-sized suburb, that distance may be too great in Manhattan.

Therefore, take out a map and mark out the competition. Where are they located? What is their proximity and yours to the hospital or to the large medical offices, or even to the main residential and business areas? Attempt to demonstrate that you can more efficiently and effectively serve the plan's members because of your location.

Access is not just geographic, however. Your group may provide more evening and weekend hours than the competition. Perhaps there is free parking next to your outpatient center. Are there long waits to be seen at the hospital radiology department, but you can easily accommodate patients in a few minutes? Access can also be electronic, with the ability to request imaging studies online. Additional advantage can be obtained by making reports and images available in the referrer's medical record. Look for any factors that differentiate your practice. Is yours the only facility in the area that offers a 64-slice CT scanner capable of cardiac CT angiography? Do you have the only interventional radiologist performing uterine fibroid embolization?

The last piece of the puzzle is existing relationships. Are you providing essential professional services at the hospital so that its administration will help you secure a better MCO contract? Are you part of the independent practice organization of physicians who may be able to include your contract in their overall agreement? Can you convince key physicians in the community (especially primary care and obstetrics/gynecology doctors) to request (demand?) that your facility be added to the network? For example, insuring adequate access to mammography can help primary care groups meet pay-for-performance requirements and strengthen their motivation to advocate for

---

BOX 22-2

Self-Examination Analysis

1. Payer mix
2. Revenue and examination analysis by payer
3. Relative fee schedules
4. Capacity for growth
5. Competitive position
6. Geographic access
7. Relationships

---

and refer to your group. This is not the time to be the "Lone Ranger"; better to remember that strength is in numbers. Although you often cannot legally negotiate contracts as a group, you can exert influence on each other's behalf (see Box 22-2).

Company Specifics

Now that you have completed a thorough self-assessment so that you have built a thorough understanding of the strengths and weaknesses your group brings to the table, you can focus on the other side in the negotiation. Knowledge about the MCO will provide you additional leverage points. Understanding their needs will afford you negotiating room for trade-offs and compromises.

First, try to obtain some data on the position of this company in your local or regional marketplace. Talk to the individual responsible for managed care negotiations at the local hospital. Check with the state department of insurance. Browse the Web. Determine the number of "covered lives" or members this plan has and the number for the other plans in the area. Is this a dominant company with a significant market share or an up-and-comer trying to break in? Obviously this will affect how much they want you in their network, or for an existing contract, how much they are willing to lose your participation.

Similarly, try to ascertain the kinds of products this MCO is offering. Are they a strict HMO product only, or do they offer a variety of more open-access type plans (POS, PPO, etc.)? If they have these programs that allow

patients to see out-of-network physicians while subject to co-insurance, this may give you flexibility in accommodating those referrals without formal participation. At least you can use this possibility as a leverage point with the MCO. You should also determine if the plan offers Medicare and/or Medicaid products. If they have just added one of these government programs they may be interested in trading something for your participation.

Finally, look on the company's website for any special clinical activity they are trying to promote. For example, many plans are trying to (and are required to) increase their percentage of eligible women who receive annual screening mammography. If you have excess capacity that could help them meet this need, you become more valuable. In general, try to understand how the plan is marketing itself. What is it telling its customers (the employers who pay for health insurance)? How can you fit into the company's marketing message? Does this MCO view itself as the select, high-quality option or the broadest-network-possible option? If the plan uses the word "quality" extensively and you are a largely subspecialty-certified group with the latest equipment, then you have something to offer them. In general, the idea is to look for any key words or concepts that you can use in the conversations with the plan representatives to let them know you are simpatico.

Similar information can be found by talking, if possible, to the key employers in the area that are contracting with that MCO. Try to find out what is important to the plan's customers, and see if you can offer something special. Building bridges here may also be helpful later in the negotiating process. If a major employer group complains to the MCO that your practice is not in the network, or is thinking of leaving the network, that is incredible leverage on that plan.

Once you have some basic information, it's time to do some more market research. Check with your key referring physicians as well as with those large or potentially significant practices that don't send patients. Is this an important MCO to them? Are you not seeing those patients because you don't participate with that plan? Sometimes one has to take these answers with a large degree of skepticism. The key is to try to determine what percentage of their practice(s) comes from that MCO. Often a referring physician will urge radiology groups to take every plan offered, even when that referrer wouldn't accept the plan themselves. They just want to make it easier for their patients and, as importantly, for their administrative staff. The referring physician may be able to even stay out of the network for some plans and either collect the co-insurance and deductibles or waive them. (Note that it is usually not legal to routinely waive all co-insurance payments.) Nonetheless, that referring physician may not want to hear complaints from their patients that you charged them out-of-network fees. It's an unfair double standard that arises from the minimal value and loyalty accorded to radiologists by patients.

It may be worth accepting a plan with a few members and mediocre rates if you believe that it will secure all the referrals from a key physician group. On the other hand, remember that the MCOs know a lot about each other. If you accept plan X with only 20,000 members paying 75% of Medicare, don't be surprised when plan Y with 200,000 members comes looking for a reduction from its current 120% of Medicare rates. One has to make these participation decisions in a broad context. Although it is often possible to decline participation in one key plan and/or several minor players and still receive the rest of the referrals, most radiology groups cannot afford to remain significantly out of network. Therefore, one has to choose carefully. However, in most cases, one should not feel required to accept every plan no matter how unsatisfactory the terms.

The other MCO reputation data you need is the plan's history with payments and customer service. If this is an existing contract, check with your billing staff or vendor. Determine the percentage of claims incorrectly rejected. Having a good reimbursement rate is of little value if a significant number of claims are improperly rejected. Likewise, measure the days in accounts receivable (A/R) for this plan and for your other contracts as well. This statistic, defined as the current accounts receivable (at charges, not expected payments) divided by the average daily charges for that plan, is a good measure of payment performance. Assuming an efficient billing process that is submitting accurate and complete ("clean") claims, the days in A/R should not generally be over 60 and should ideally be 35 to 45 days. If this plan's A/R is significantly longer than that figure, then this will become a significant negotiating point. Although in some cases you may not actually be able to convince them to guarantee better service, you may obtain other concessions such as a commitment to advance the practice some money against future claims. Again, having data to present will enhance your leverage at the table.

Obviously these data are harder to obtain if you do not currently have a contract with the MCO. You can speak to other physicians in the area who are enrolled and get a sense of their experience. However, consulting with other radiology groups about these issues could be considered collusion and should be avoided. This is another area where an independent practice association (IPA) can be quite helpful. An IPA consists of physicians and other health care providers who contract with HMOs to meet the needs of their enrollees but will also see patients from other HMOs or patients from outside an HMO. It can act as a clearing-house for this type of information and can work to resolve outstanding issues and complaints.

Finally, if at all possible check the reputation of the individual plan representatives with whom you will be meeting. Are they the quiet, rational types or the obnoxious, "take-it-or-leave-it" types? You may not be able to change these people, but hearing war stories from others will prepare you for the discussions and should influence your strategy (Box 22-3).

BOX 22-3

MCO Analysis

- Covered lives—market share
- Products offered
- Marketing strategy
- Reputation
- Employer clients
- Referring doctors' participation
- Accounts receivable issues

CONTRACT REVIEW

The next step in the negotiation preparation process is to answer the question, "What is our best realistic outcome of this negotiation?" To do that you need to understand and review all the possible areas of discussion and potential agreement. Although rates are clearly the most significant item on the agenda, they are not the only potential focus. Contracts have pages of terms, most of which will initially be written to favor the MCO. It is important to review these documents in detail before sitting down at the table.

Ask the MCO representative for a copy of the proposed contract and a copy of the provider manual. The latter is relevant, because many of the contract terms will refer to and incorporate the rules in the provider manual (e.g., with respect to precertification of radiology tests) without actually stating those rules in the contract itself. Try to obtain an electronic version if possible.

Participation

First ascertain which specific plans are covered by this contract. It is typical to include the HMO, POS, PPO, and similar products that the MCO has, but be careful about "all-products" clauses that commit you to signing up with any product the company may offer now or may develop in the future. The companies are always adding new plans and "deeming" that existing participating physicians are automatically part of the new product. Although often the practice may wish to participate in the new offering, that plan's specific rules or other provisions may make it unwise to do so. The contract should give the physician group notice of any new products and the opportunity to accept or reject that offering. If the group participates with the plan, it should not be on less favorable terms than the current participation unless there is mutual agreement. In addition, be careful about agreeing to participate in traditional indemnity insurance plans, because the MCO is receiving a much higher premium for those plans and there

is no ability of the plan to steer patients or otherwise affect patient or referring-physician behavior in the indemnity structure. In this type of plan there is no in-network or out-of-network concept, and the co-insurance is the same for all providers. Thus, you should expect to receive your full charge for each service rendered.

This power of steerage gives the MCO its greatest leverage. Therefore, if you agree to participate with the plan, the MCO should agree to not steer or direct any patients away from your practice (e.g., to a lower cost provider). There is little value in having finalized a contract and having your practice listed in the participating provider book, yet still not be seeing any patients.

The next contract issue to consider is that of credentialing. Frequently the MCO will agree to include a physician or group in the network and then take as long as 6 months to credential them for billing purposes. Usually this is not a conscious decision on the company's part but rather part of the overall inefficiency that seems to mar the business practices of these organizations. One should try to understand their credentialing process and perhaps see if another organization (e.g., the local IPA) has been delegated to perform this review on the plan's behalf. Regardless, the contract should stipulate that a physician who provides services under the plan will be paid retroactively for services provided from the date the credentialing data are submitted to the MCO, no matter when the plan finalizes that credential. This protects the physician or group and places the economic risk where it belongs, with the plan. It does not, however, address the headache of delayed payment.

Now that the physicians are covered, you need to make sure that all sites are included. Ideally the MCO should agree that patients seen in any of the practice's current or future sites will be considered as in the network. More likely, they will insist on at least a site assessment before inclusion. This usually is a review of the facility, its equipment, technical staff credentials, cleanliness, and the like. So long as the practice is afforded the opportunity to make corrections to any deficiencies noted, then this is a reasonable condition of participation.

BOX 22-4

Participation Analysis

- Which products?
- Steerage
- Credentialing
- Sites

Increasingly as MCOs try to limit their networks, they may choose to accept some sites and not others depending on their real or perceived geographic needs. You should note any contract language limiting site inclusion and try to negotiate the broadest acceptance possible. Moreover, the term "site" should be carefully defined. If a practice wishes to expand an existing location by adding a modality or additional space within a relatively limited geographic radius (less than a mile usually), that should not be considered a new site but instead expansion of the existing one (Box 22-4).

Clinical Policies

Now that you've reviewed the rules for joining the network, look at the regulations regarding provision of clinical services. Much of this information will be in the provider manual and not in the contract directly. The contract may have a clause that requires the physician to "abide by" any utilization review or other care management processes. This would be more fairly written as expecting the physician to "cooperate with" such processes, because there will be times when it is not possible to strictly follow such systems.

Moreover, it is important to understand and be sure you can follow the utilization rules and/or processes defined. Most plans will usually not waive requirements for prospective precertification of some examination types (usually MRI, CT, and positron emission tomography or PET) or for retrospective utilization review; however, they may be willing to slightly modify their processes to meet your needs depending on the size of your practice and the interests of the referring physicians. The other increasingly prevalent utilization process is that of claims bundling; for example, CT of the abdomen and pelvis is not paid as two studies but at a combined reduced or bundled rate. One must understand the implications of these rules on both the administrative processes of the practice and the potential financial gain for participation. If a significant share of practice revenue comes from multiple-study CT (chest, abdomen, and pelvis), it may be wise to accept an overall lower reimbursement rate without bundling than a higher rate with that restriction. In any case, the contract should state that changes to the provider manual must be made in writing with advance notice. The group should be permitted to reject such changes or at least trigger a renegotiation process.

Another provision you should check in the contract or more commonly in the provider manual is the service standards established by the company. As part of an effort to improve patient access they may require that nonemergency examinations be performed within a set time frame (e.g., 2 days for a CT scan, 4 days for an MRI scan, and 1 week for a diagnostic mammogram). Confirm that your practice can meet these standards and identify any problem areas (usually mammography is one). Similarly, the plans are starting to establish maximum turnaround times for nonemergency reports. Again, check your ability to comply.

Claims Payment

After providing the service, the biggest challenges with managed care participation come in claims payment. MCOs are usually not known for paying promptly and correctly. They will often try to use incomplete or inaccurate claims filings as an excuse, but their information and claims processing systems are often at fault. Some states have introduced "prompt-payment" laws or regulations that require a plan to pay a "clean claim" within a specific number of days (usually 45–60). If they do not pay in this time then interest and penalities may be applied. Although it is unlikely that many plans will accept penalties for slow payment (other than those already imposed by those state prompt-pay statutes), it is sometimes possible to get them to include a "good-faith effort" clause that puts them on record as striving for claims payment within a certain time frame.

This is usually 60 to 90 days unless state law says otherwise.

Even if the plan declines to guarantee payment timing, you must still review the contract and/or provider manual to see what rules the plan is imposing and what constitutes a clean claim. Most plans have a "timely filing" deadline, typically between 60 and 120 days from the date the service was performed. If the claim is received after this date, it will automatically be denied. If the deadline is within reasonable parameters and your billing organization can get the claims out in that time (which they should anyway), don't fight to try to lengthen the process. Even if the MCO representative will agree, it is unlikely that their information technology group can implement this variation for your specific practice correctly, and thus your claims will be denied incorrectly.

The definition of a clean claim and the method of claims submission are also important. Determine if there are any special data items that this plan requires on its claims submissions (for example, some require the Unique Physician Identification Number of the referring physician), and again check that your billing operation can provide them. Similarly, if the plan requires a specific method of claims submission, usually electronic, verify your ability to use their system. Although the MCO is not likely to change either its clean claim requirements or submission method, if their demands are excessive and would require considerable operational changes on your part, you can use this requirement as a leverage point. Moreover, by understanding these issues, you can prepare your billing staff before commencing the relationship and minimize the number of unpaid claims during the start-up phase of the contract. One issue you can negotiate is the right to resubmit a claim not considered clean within a defined period of time (usually 60 days).

The last claims issue of consequence is that of "recoupment" whereby the MCO will deduct money from future claims for claims it previously paid but now believes were processed incorrectly. Insist on a nonrecoupment clause in the contract. If the plan judges that previously paid claims should be revised or if there is any dispute regarding such claims,

then these should be handled independently of any new claims. They should send out a notice describing the problem and requesting a payment from you for the money allegedly owed. It is unreasonable for them to automatically deduct such monies from future payments without giving you the opportunity to object, explain the situation, or even prove that the MCO is incorrect in its assessment. Moreover, this will make analysis of future claims problems extremely complicated.

Dispute Resolution

Ideally the contract should outline a process of resolution of disputes, usually involving an appeals process within the MCO itself followed by arbitration. Time periods should be given for each part of this procedure. The MCO will probably propose binding arbitration, thereby foreclosing any possibility of using the court system to address disputes. There are positive and negative factors to be considered; however, restricting an option is usually not preferable and should not be ceded easily. On the other hand, no dispute is likely to be of such magnitude that the courts become an economical path to pursue.

Even within arbitration there are some important concerns to be addressed. The agreement should specify a panel of arbitrators rather than a single individual. A neutral three-person panel is likely to be fairer. Often contracts will specify how the panel is chosen (one member by each side and one by the other two) and that the panel members must be members of the American Arbitration Association or a similar body.

In this era of large national MCOs, the relevant state law is also important. The contract should specify that the applicable state law governing the agreement is the one in which the practice is located and that any arbitration will take place in that state. A similar legal issue is that of a "hold harmless" or indemnification clause. Each party agrees to hold harmless from liability under the contract the other party for certain acts or omissions. Although these clauses are relatively standard, it may be advisable to have an attorney review this and the contract as a whole before ratification.

Term and Termination

There are many issues to consider regarding the length of the agreement. A short term (usually 1 or 2 years) offers the advantage of allowing the group to remain competitive with marketplace pricing changes. If fees and payments (especially from Medicare) are rising, then a renegotiation will be useful. It also will allow for changes in how or where services are provided. A longer term avoids the need to have renegotiation sessions, which are time consuming, costly if legal help has to be purchased, and not necessarily productive; it also guarantees that the group will retain its current position in the network and its rate structure. Also, if rates are declining, then fixing them for a longer period of time is clearly advantageous.

Many contracts are short-term agreements with automatic renewal (so-called evergreen) clauses. These usually call for a renewal once per year unless one party gives notice to the other within a specified time frame (typically 60–90 days). This can be useful for the group especially if the evergreen provision links rates to some external standard (such as Medicare) or even better a cost-of-living adjuster, thereby allowing for rate changes that match market trends without the need to renegotiate each year. The MCO should never be allowed to make rate changes without affording the practice the opportunity to discuss them and if necessary terminate the contract. If an evergreen provision is included, there must also be a method to address new procedures and/or technologies. Often this is done by establishing an average payment as a function of Medicare and linking the rate for new CPT codes proportionally to that average. However, in this period of significant Medicare instability, one must be careful about linking codes too tightly to Medicare. It is also important to know to which year the Medicare rates are being tied. Some MCOs base their rates on previous Medicare values, instead of current ones, so as to follow their expense stream over time in a uniform way.

The agreement should also include provisions for early termination of the contract. Usually there is a clause calling for termination by either party without cause with a specified notice period, for example, 90 days. There will also be clauses referring to termination with cause (breech of contract), usually on a shorter time basis, but with an opportunity for either side to correct the breech within a specified period of time. The radiology practice should also have the ability to quickly extricate itself from a contract if the payer stops paying the group or goes into bankruptcy, or some other extreme financial situation develops.

NEGOTIATIONS

After all this preparation the radiology group should be very well informed about the group, its competition, and the MCO to be on the other side of the table. Now is the time to construct a list of all the issues to be discussed. Obviously rates are on the list, but don't put them first. Start with the contract terms or provider manual issues you've identified as needing to be changed or adjusted. Include any restrictions in the current contract that would limit your ability to practice or would reduce the number of sites or locations where you could practice.

Once you have created this contract term list, prioritize it in terms of importance and potential effect on your practice. This is not the order for discussing these issues with the MCO representative, but it should provide a mental framework for determining what trade-offs or compromises you are willing to make.

Rates

Now it is finally time to review the rates that the MCO has proposed. Based on the knowledge of your practice pattern by modality and source of patients (which referring physicians belong to this plan), you should examine the specific codes or groups of codes by modality to again look for potential trade-offs or compromises should you need to make them. Any payment rules such as bundling will also enter into this. Remember, the goal is not to discuss these issues at the negotiating table but instead to create a mental framework that you always have in mind during the negotiation. For example, if plain radiography is a relatively small part of your practice, you may be willing to accept a lower rate for those procedures if you can increase the CT or MRI rates. The capacity analysis you performed earlier should enter into this process as well. Can you agree to open your mammography practice for more hours to accommodate more of the MCO's members in exchange for higher MRI rates? Perhaps you can accept a lower MRI rate for an enhanced CT payment, if your MRI system is beyond capacity with no room to grow, but your CT system is underused and this new contract could potentially bring in many new CT referrals but few new MRI scans.

The mix of inpatient (professional only) versus outpatient (global) cases should also affect your framework. If the bulk of your revenue comes from a free-standing imaging center where you bill globally, make sure that this gets the priority over the hospital work. Sometimes it is acceptable to have a "loss leader," that is, a service or location that doesn't really make money and maybe even loses a little but gives you access to a great number of other sources of revenue. For most free-standing imaging practices, plain radiography and mammography are often loss leaders, but this is not always so and may be changing with the recent changes in Medicare payment regulations. Most important is to understand what that loss leader represents and to assure that not all services will fall into that category. It is rare to truly be able to "make it up on volume" if every service does not at least cover its underlying costs.

BATNA

Now that you have prioritized the contract issues and the rate issues, the last thing to do is to consider your BATNA (best alternative to a negotiated agreement). This is an important concept developed by Robert Fisher in *Getting to Yes*. What will you do if you can't come to an agreement with the MCO? Can you afford to walk away from the table and reject the contract? Sometimes the answer will clearly be yes, but often the answer may be no. If this is an existing contract that represents a meaningful percentage of your revenue, your position is weaker than if it is a new contract that might add a small number of new referrals per year. Sometimes it is not a simple binary choice.

Perhaps you can reject the contract and still gain access to many of the same patients through an independent PPO that is "reselling" the physician network. Your group will not be listed in the provider manual and may have to collect co-insurance, but you still can market your new availability to your referring physicians.

One can think of BATNA as the balance of power in a negotiation. For example, if you need a new TV there are many options available (buying from local electronics stores, Internet stores, etc.), so you have many alternatives for your BATNA and your power is greater. If you need Internet access for your home there may be a small number of options (dial-up companies, cable systems, DSL providers), so you retain some choice but it is limited. Finally, if you seek to purchase a rare book, there may only be one store currently selling that item, and your ability to negotiate the terms of the sale will be restricted.

Developing a BATNA means looking for alternatives to give you power at the negotiating table. It is rare to have no other alternative but to meekly accept the terms of the contract as initially presented by the MCO. Sometimes a BATNA will involve difficult changes or adjustments in your practice; perhaps you would have to close an existing site or reduce your staffing. This may still be preferable to accepting a contract with rates that are below your costs. Use this process to seriously think about these alternatives and look for other possibilities that allow you to change your BATNA. For example, if the site where most of this MCO's members would be cared for has old equipment and declining patient referrals, closing that location and opening up another one somewhere else to gain new patients from a better paying plan might be worth consideration. Having real alternatives to the agreement, even if they are not ideal ones, will empower you and give you a confident attitude that will positively change the discussion dynamics in your favor.

The research you have done about the MCO should also inform your suppositions about their BATNA. What will they do if you don't sign or renew the contract? Do they have easy alternatives or more difficult ones? How much of their reputation is based on their physician participation? Can they readily send patients to another practice nearby?

The concept of BATNA is a mutually dynamic one. As the negotiation proceeds, both sides will be adjusting their estimation of their BATNAs on a continuing basis, even if not explicitly. As information is presented in the discussions, the alternatives available to both sides change. Therefore, it is essential not to reveal your "walk-away" alternatives to the other side. Your attitude at the table should reflect your desire to come to a mutually beneficial agreement. Understanding that knowledge is power means controlling how you use that knowledge, not necessarily trying to impress others with that knowledge.

Time, People, and Places

You should also consider the time frame of the discussions. Most radiology negotiators (whether physicians or administrators) have other more primary roles and responsibilities and are uncomfortable with the negotiating process. Hence they seek to have a meeting, get the issues on the table, and get an agreement so they can go back to their regular work. In most cases, this works against the radiology group. First, unlike the radiology representatives, the MCO staff considers this their principal duty and they are generally more experienced and confident with the modus operandi.

Second, relationships are an important part of successful negotiations, and these take time to mature. If you have developed some rapport with your MCO counterpart, it is likely that you will achieve a better result (if only slightly) than if you are strangers. Moreover, because these contracts are usually long-term commitments and other issues and challenges are likely to come up in the future, having a good relationship with a representative of the company is going to provide future potential benefits as well.

Finally, working through your issues in a careful and deliberate manner over a period of time allows you to constantly be judging the strength of the other side and its desire for agreement. It also permits you to develop potential trade-off or compromise scenarios involving multiple factors. The discussions become characterized by an attitude that is less "Take it or leave it" and more "What about this or that?"

You must then consider who the "other side" should be at what point in the process and in fact, who should be present from the radiology group. Typically, the MCO will send a "contract representative" to meet with the group's leader(s) as the first step. These individuals are fairly low in the hierarchy of the company and have little power or authority to make decisions or changes to the contract. Nonetheless, it is useful to begin the process with this envoy and to begin to articulate some of your issues. This should provide some initial feedback on how the company will respond to your needs and requests, which items it is going to be easy to have changed, which will require some further negotiation, and which will be very challenging. This is an important time to try to get an insight into the needs of the MCO. Try to mention some of the things you know about the company and what you perceive its needs are as a test of your understanding. The goal is to probe the MCO's position for leverage points for your side, either based on existing strengths you have or needs they have. Remember not to try to address all the issues in one setting. Let the MCO representative meet you a few times and build that relationship in a positive direction, if possible.

Once you have identified the issues that the local contract person cannot or will not address or adjust, you have to work your way up the chain of command. There is usually a contracting director or supervisor to whom you can refer these issues, and often someone higher in the chain of command as well. Sometimes you will end by meeting with the president of the company or at least the regional director. Take each of these steps deliberately, trying to resolve some issues at each level.

Working horizontally within the company is also important. Some of the issues you want addressed may fall into the realm of "medical policy," or you may be able to push them into that category. These concerns should be addressed at a meeting with the local medical director, a physician who may often be slightly more sympathetic or at least understanding of your position and your needs. This is also the individual to address about what you can offer the company that is clinically unique or at least significant. Most medical directors weren't radiologists before they "went corporate," so try to frame the issues in a way that a general internist or surgeon can understand. Also, attempt to convince referring physicians to write or call the medical director on your behalf; anything that will increase your reputation and/or value with the MCO is worth trying.

Similarly, if you were able to make contact with some of the key employer clients of the MCO, you may wish to engage one or more of its sales representatives in your discussions. Let that individual know why your practice is important for his/her employer client's (geography, existing patient referral patterns, etc.). The sales team can exert significant influence over the contracting group but rarely are engaged to do so.

As you connect with each of these individuals, remember that the goal is an agreement, not a victory. Both sides are entitled to make a profit from the arrangement and to maintain and grow their business. Presumably you have spent all this time preparing and negotiating because you want to participate in their network at a reasonable reimbursement rate under an acceptable set of policy guidelines. Unless otherwise provoked, your tone should always be respectful, measured, and cooperative. This is neither a debating society where you are trying to win points nor a wrestling match where you wish to overpower, or worse humiliate, your opponent. Ultimately some level of partnership and mutual understanding will result in a better outcome for both sides.

All of this careful attention to detail and staging requires the full concentration of the participants. Negotiations should be held in a quiet place, removed from the clinical activities, the telephone, and other distractions. The reading room is the worst place to try to think, pick up the other side's unspoken cues, and reach agreement. That said, it may be useful to have the MCO representatives see your facilities and reading areas, especially if you have recently renovated or have new equipment to show off. A visit to the reading room when multiple consultations with referring physicians are taking place can also impress someone regarding the value of radiology (and your

practice) in the delivery of health care in a specific community. Again, don't assume that the MCO staff knows anything about your practice or radiology in general. The more you educate them regarding your value, the more leverage you will command.

Finally, consider which representatives from the radiology practice are the most appropriate to participate in the negotiation. Generally, one should not negotiate alone. While one individual may take the lead in the discussions, it is useful to have someone else there to observe the other side, to look for their subtle responses and cues, and to make sure the key points are being addressed. Having two people also allows for better "after action" analysis of the meeting and planning for future deliberations. A good combination may be the practice business manager and a physician leader. It is not always advisable to have the president or other chief executive of the practice at the early meetings. This allows the negotiating individual to defer some decisions for further consultation with that leader or executive committee. Also, when and if the discussions include a higher level of authority within the MCO, that physician group leader can participate as a comparably new voice. The planning of who negotiates at what point should dovetail with the planning of which issues to address in what order as described earlier.

Because the negotiations progress over a period of time, it is important to continually update this planning, taking into account what has been already agreed to and what new information has come to light. Keep notes and summarize agreements after each session; do not rely on recall. It is amazing how two people can have such different perceptions or recollections of the same reality. The goal is not to take a year to negotiate each contract (although in some cases that may happen) but instead to use the time to find the best way to convince the other side of the correctness and value of your positions. In addition, you will have to make compromises and trade-offs; doing so over time allows you to achieve more value for each one. Simultaneously you are updating your BATNA and refining your options should an agreement not be reached. It is vital to have alternatives, but at the same time, you should not usually go back and renegotiate points previously agreed to or attempt to add key issues at the eleventh hour. The other side at the table needs to trust in your reasonableness and integrity. Failing to come to an overall agreement should always be as a result of not being able to find common ground, not because of tactics used by either side. The goal is a pact that both sides may not find completely satisfactory, but neither side feels is completely unsavory.

FOLLOWING UP

The negotiation of a mutually satisfactory contract and its ratification or signature should not be viewed as the end of this process. Unlike buying a home or other typical negotiations, the purpose of these discussions has really been to articulate the terms by which the two parties (MCO and radiology group) will work together for a period of time. The goal in some way is the development of a partnership or at least a mutually beneficial relationship. This requires frequent attention. Because the contract will probably have to be renegotiated again, in full or part, at some time in the future, using the intervening time to develop better relationships with that company can be productive over the long term.

Look for opportunities to meet with the contract representative and/or medical director on a regular basis (at least once every 6 months). Discuss how the contract is going, issues that have arisen, claims problems, and the like. Focus attention on how well you are doing for that company and its members. Educate the representatives about new technology or services you may be offering in the near future. Continue to demonstrate the value that you bring to them and look for ways that they can bring additional value to your practice.

There are other ways to build useful relationships as well. Make it clear to the medical director that you are happy to arrange expedited or special care for the company VIPs, relatives, and so on. See if you can serve on their physician advisory board (or similar committee) as the radiology representative. Look for opportunities to support the company's program initiatives (special mammography screening days, etc.). In general, act like you are pleased to be their partner.

At the same time, your billing organization should be closely monitoring the performance of the MCO with respect to the contract rates and terms. If you have negotiated special terms or enhanced rates, the company may have difficulties implementing those out of the ordinary items into their computer systems. The actual payments must be carefully checked against the rates promised on the basis of each individual CPT code. Also, any provider policy changes that you have negotiated must be constantly verified. In most cases the MCO will not purposefully ignore or fail to implement the terms of your contract, but instead will place it in a work queue of changes that their information technology group has to handle and will neglect to follow up to assure completion. Frequent reminders and occasional threats may be necessary to have the claims payments and provider policy issues addressed. Once again, the relationships you have built will provide some support in seeing that these changes are made.

CONCLUSIONS

Negotiating managed care contracts has now become a vital obligation of radiology leaders. Particularly in an era of potential declining Medicare reimbursement, groups confront the need to secure better rates and conditions from other payers. Successful negotiations begin with changing the attitude of the radiology negotiators from either just meek acceptance or aggressive confrontation to rational deliberation. The goal is that of a continuing relationship, preferably a partnership, that is mutually beneficial to both the group and the MCO.

Developing this framework will require thoughtful preparation and planning by the radiology negotiators. The ability to use knowledge as leverage in negotiating means having that understanding of one's own circumstances as well as those of the other side. Developing a BATNA is essential to the projection of confidence and authority at the table and to knowing when the negotiation is not worth completing.

If managed correctly not only will this specific negotiation yield a beneficial contract, but it will provide the basis for future development with that MCO and perhaps with others. The signed document is not the end result but rather just the beginning of the potential gains that will accrue to the radiology practice—financial and otherwise. Frequent searching for hidden opportunities will enhance the ability of the practice to survive in this challenging reimbursement environment, thereby making worthwhile all the time and effort devoted to this process.

Dos and Don'ts When in Negotiations with MCOs	
Dos	**Don'ts**
1. Prepare carefully.	1. Fail to negotiate—just sign the agreement.
2. Honestly assess your practice for both its strengths and weaknesses.	2. Negotiate from a weak position or one without information.
3. Learn everything you can about the MCO.	3. Forget how you can help the MCO.
4. List your issues in advance and prioritize them.	4. Become agitated or angry.
5. Remember this is a negotiation, not a duel.	5. Lose control of the process.
6. Understand that both sides need to win.	6. Lose sight of the goal.
7. Use references to increase pressure and provide feedback to the MCO.	7. Accept less than your BATNA.
8. Have a fall-back position (BATNA).	8. Make up the loss on volume.
9. Keep accurate, detailed notes.	9. Lose the personal connection with the other side.
10. Follow up.	10. Forget to maintain relationships after the contract is signed.

SUGGESTED READINGS

Alexander JM: Managed care contracting for specialists—1999 HFM resource guide. Healthcare Financial Management (1 December 1998), pp 6–10.

American College of Radiology Managed Care Committee. Evaluating a managed care contract. ACR contract evaluation checklist. Available at http://www.acr.org/s_acr/sec.asp?CID=2622&DID=17673 (accessed 17 September 2006).

Deitch CH, Sunshine JH: The relationship of managed care to business, professional and organizational aspects of radiology practices. Am J Roentgenol 182:29–38, 2004.

Fisher R, Ury WL, Patton, B: Getting to Yes: Negotiating Agreement Without Giving In, 2nd ed. New York, Houghton Mifflin, 1991.

Greenleaf T: Tips for negotiating a favorable managed care contract. Imaging Econ 31:31, 2006.

Marcus DD: The negotiation state of mind: specifics in negotiating managed care contracts. J Med Practice Management (2006), pp 184–187.

Mertz GJ: Can you negotiate better reimbursement? Family Practice Management. Available at http://www.aafp.org/fpm/20041000/31cany.html. American Academy of Family Physicians (2004).

Miller TR: The fundamentals of contract negotiations—managed care plans. Healthcare Financial Management (June 1996). Available at http://www.findarticles.com/p/articles/mi_m3257/is_n6_v50/ai_18515374 (accessed 17 September 2006).

Porter S: Negotiation skills tame managed care contracts. News now. American Academy of Family Physicians, Available at http://www.aafp.org/x42654.xml (accessed 17 September 2006).

Russell PJ: Trends in A/R management. ImagingEconomics.com Special Projects. Available at http://www.imagingeconomics.com/supplements/rad_as_bus/1999_jul_rec_mgmt.html (accessed 17 September 2006).

Susnick H: Selecting managed care plans: getting the most for your practice through the use of evaluation tools. J Med Practice Management (2004), pp 179–181.

Tinsley R: Managed Care Contracting: Successful Negotiation Strategies. Chicago, American Medical Association, 1999.

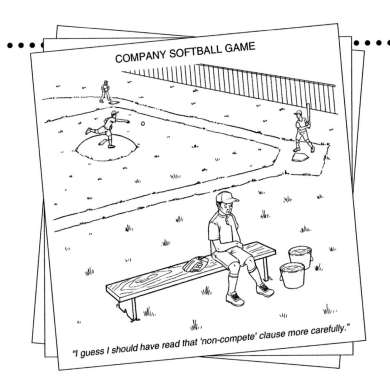

CHAPTER 23

COMPANY SOFTBALL GAME

"I guess I should have read that 'non-compete' clause more carefully."

Employment Contracts

Julie A. Muroff, JD

Almost immediately after this writer began to represent radiologist clients, it became clear that contracting between radiology groups and their members is not a popular topic. Here, unpopular refers not only to the virtual silence on the topic in medical journals and continuing medical education courses but also to the reluctance of so many clients to attend to contracts that had been neglected for decades. Indeed, one client tried to convince the author that, before the engagement of a contentious new hospital administrator, there had been no need for his radiology group to review their employment contracts, "because not much has changed in the past 20 years."

Many years of exploring possible reasons for this aversion have led this author to one

The views expressed herein are the author's alone and do not necessarily represent the views of the United States government or any agency thereof. The discussion in this chapter does not constitute legal advice.

compelling theory: contracts involve lawyers. Having become convinced that the legal profession was to blame for the seemingly universal apathy among radiologists with respect to their employment contracts, the writer has dedicated the past several years to publishing and lecturing on the topic of contracts in radiology practices. The premise is that much of the acrimony that radiologists associate with attorneys can be mitigated by proactively working with them to ensure that group agreements remain sound, from a legal perspective and from a group's cultural perspective. By taking just a few hours on an annual basis to re-evaluate the terms of a group's contracts with each member, and with the group's hospital(s) if applicable, a group may save countless hours and dollars in litigation, not to mention its morale and viability.

This dramatic effect is possible to achieve uniquely through contracts, because they set the tone and establish the foundation for the professional relationships in a radiology practice.

Without a clear directive regarding the expectations and obligations of its members, a radiology group is unable to function effectively. This volatility unnecessarily compromises not only a group's ability to resolve internal conflicts, such as unproductive or otherwise problematic members, but also hinders a group's ability to capitalize on external opportunities, such as joint ventures. Moreover, and perhaps most importantly for the purposes of modern practice, radiology groups cannot protect themselves from turf challenges from without when they are preoccupied with turf battles from within.

For these reasons, among others that will be discussed in this chapter, radiologists can no longer afford to ignore their employment contracts. With a relatively minor investment of time and attention, a radiology group can maximize the potential of employment contracts to bind members to each other and to the group's patients and hospital(s). By involving the group's attorney in the contract drafting and updating processes and by maintaining open communication about the evolving needs and interests of the group, radiologists can minimize conflicts that otherwise may lead to costly legal disputes. Thus, radiologists can be proactive in anticipating conflicts before they arise, instead of being reactive to conflicts that already have escalated beyond the group's ability to contain them.

To that end, this chapter will offer an analysis of employment contracts in radiology practices. Specifically, the chapter will explore the legal definition of a contract in the context of the employment relationship between a radiologist and his or her group, basic types of contracts and some key legal distinctions between them, important provisions to consider including or clarifying in a group's employment agreements, and contractual breaches and remedies. Although the nuances of each applicable state and federal law and each group's culture cannot be anticipated, these basic principles should empower radiologists to use employment contracts to manage their professional relationships more effectively.

WHAT A CONTRACT REALLY IS

The Meaning of a Contract to Your Lawyer

Definition of a Contract

In legal terms, a contract generally is defined as a promise for the breach of which the law provides a remedy, or for the performance of which the law recognizes a duty.[1] Though somewhat stilted, this definition is useful to illuminate two core principles of contract construction: (1) transforming promises into binding obligations and (2) enforcing those obligations under the law. Together, these factors justify reliance on a contract and provide contracting parties with a remedy in the case of nonperformance or breach of a contractual obligation.[2]

A valid contract must express the contracting parties' intent in unambiguous terms. The principal terms of a contract include an offer, consideration, and acceptance. For example, a radiologist's employment contract typically will integrate an offer of employment with the group, conditions for the exchange of medical services for financial compensation, and a signature line to confirm acceptance by the authorized parties. As will be elaborated later in this chapter, it is important to note that acceptance is limited to the specific terms of the offer and consideration expressed in the present agreement and generally does not extend to any prior or contemporaneous arrangements between the contracting parties.

Basic Types of Contracts: Oral or Written

Oral Agreements The indifference of radiologists about their employment contracts is shown perhaps most clearly by the tendency of some groups to avoid formalizing their agreements in writing, relying instead on verbal commitments of employment with their members. Many of this writer's clients considered written agreements to be an unwelcome imposition on the collegial nature of intragroup relationships or to detract from their group's appeal to candidates during the recruiting process. Alternatively, perhaps some groups hoped to achieve greater leverage or flexibility relative to their individual members by declining to commit to specific terms of employment in writing. Although only 7% of the radiology groups polled at a national symposium for radiologists in 2005 acknowledged an exclusive reliance on oral contracts, case law is replete with examples of that proclivity (personal communication from the Educational Symposia, Inc. Economics Data Collection Project, Economics of Diagnostic Imaging: National Symposium 2005). The frequency with which oral contracts, relative to written contracts, have resulted in lawsuits betrays the vulnerabilities inherent in these types of agreements.

There are two main obstacles to relying solely upon oral employment agreements in a radiology practice. The first challenge is a lack of clarity or certainty about the terms of an oral agreement. This ambiguity jeopardizes the legal enforceability of an oral contract and undermines the contracting parties' ability to rely upon it. By its nature, a dispute concerning an oral contract demonstrates that parties may have different intentions, interpretations, or memories about the terms of the same agreement. Unfortunately, these differences are unlikely to manifest until a conflict arises, at which point a third party, such as a judge or a mediator or arbitrator, may need to intervene. Regardless of if or how a dispute ultimately is resolved by one of those third parties, it is likely that the radiologists will remain dissatisfied with the outcome, because they may perceive the decision as arbitrary or undesirable and resent the associated costs and inconvenience.

A second risk of limiting group employment agreements to oral contracts is that the law may require a contract to be written to provide a remedy in certain circumstances, such as for agreements that cannot be performed within a year. This legal requirement is referred to as the Statute of Frauds, which reflects its derivation from statutory precedent in England that was intended to discourage lawsuits based on false or fraudulent obligations. Now enforced primarily through state statutes, the Statute of Frauds remains an important bar to recovery when long-term obligations have not been captured in a written agreement. For example, a court in Illinois found that the Statute of

Frauds barred an oral promise that a new group member would become a partner after 2 years, because it was not possible to perform that agreement within the course of 1 year.[3] As a somewhat morbid, albeit practical drafting note, a court may find that the Statute of Frauds would not apply if an oral promise guaranteed partnership within a physician's lifetime, because it is possible that the physician's lifetime would not exceed 1 year.

Notwithstanding the obstacles to enforcing oral contracts, a legal principle known as promissory estoppel can validate certain oral promises that a promisor should reasonably expect to induce action or forbearance and that actually did, resulting in damage to the other party.[4] For example, a court in Ohio concluded that promissory estoppel should apply when a radiologist (plaintiff) relied upon the oral promise of his colleague (defendant) to negotiate an exclusive contract with one of the group's hospitals.[5] According to the court, the defendant should have anticipated the reasonable reliance of the plaintiff upon the efforts of the defendant, because the group had appointed the defendant to serve as the group's negotiator for the contract. The plaintiff suffered as a result of his reliance on the defendant, because instead of pursuing the contract on behalf of the group, the defendant intended to form a new group that did not include the plaintiff to compete for the exclusive contract. Thus, promissory estoppel appeals to a standard of fairness, because it may prevent the inequity that would result if accepting the definite terms of an oral promise that ultimately was not fulfilled was reasonable under the circumstances of the original promise.

Written Agreements Written contracts are less susceptible to the enforcement challenges of oral agreements, because they are more conducive to establishing the certainty of contractual terms. Thus, written contracts may facilitate a proper assessment of the parties' intent. This benefit is reflected in the parol evidence rule, a legal principle that, if contracting parties integrate their respective obligations into an unambiguous final, written agreement, a court generally will exclude any evidence of prior or contemporaneous understandings with respect to the subject of the written agreement that were not incorporated into that agreement.[6]

The parol evidence rule is acknowledged in most contracts by an integration clause. For example, a standard integration clause in an employment contract between a radiology group and its member may state: "All prior or contemporaneous written or oral statements, negotiations, representations, arrangements, and/or agreements regarding Radiologist's employment with Group are merged into and superseded by the Agreement. Both parties acknowledge that there are no oral or other written understandings, arrangements and/or agreements between the parties regarding Radiologist's employment with Group."[6] Accordingly, by signing a written contract with an integration clause, a radiologist is confirming that the terms of the written agreement alone will dictate the radiologist's obligations and expectations relative to his or her employment with the group.

Although this concept seems straightforward in theory, it becomes quite complicated in a radiology practice, particularly with respect to promises of shareholder status. Case law provides numerous examples of radiologists who allegedly received oral promises of equity ownership in their groups, but whose written employment contracts were silent on the topic. For example, a court in South Dakota held that it was unreasonable for a radiologist to rely on an alleged promise of becoming a "full partner" in his group within 1 year when his written employment contract did not reflect that expectation.[7] The parol evidence rule barred the court from validating the group's oral promise of partnership, because it was made before or contemporaneous with a comprehensive written agreement that did not reference a 1-year partnership track. The court noted that promissory estoppel did not apply, because the alleged statement that partnership would be *considered* after 1 year was not a guarantee that partnership would be *granted* to this particular radiologist. Therefore, in the court's opinion, the group's oral promise did not induce reasonable reliance.

This lesson has been rehashed in courts throughout the United States. For instance, a court in Arkansas rejected a radiologist's claim of partnership despite his receipt of an equal share of his group's profits, his participation in the group's management, and the group's references to him as a partner in meeting minutes and other formal correspondence.[8] The radiologist's designation as an employee prevented him from sharing in the profits of the group upon the termination of his employment. The court explained that the group employment agreement not only did not explicitly refer to the radiologist as a partner but also contained a provision stating that employment by the group does not confer an ownership interest in, or a personal claim upon, fees charged by the group for members' medical services. Additionally, the court noted that the radiologist reported his income as an employee on his tax returns. A court in New Jersey grappling with a similar set of facts and reaching a similar conclusion emphasized that what the parties actually agreed to do in writing takes precedence over how the parties subsequently characterize their relationship if they have not used appropriate measures, such as a written agreement signed by the group and the radiologist at issue, to effectuate a change in the radiologist's status.[9]

Oral and Written Agreements? Many radiologist clients purported to have some vague combination of written *and* oral employment agreements with their groups. This status was shared by 19% of radiologists polled at a national conference in 2005 (personal communication from the Educational Symposia, Inc. Economics Data Collection Project, Economics of Diagnostic Imaging: National Symposium 2005). A common scenario involved the execution of a "generic" group agreement, followed by a number of more "personal" oral promises that were made over the years after the radiologist became more established as a member of the group.

Whereas some radiology practices may recognize a combination of written and oral agreements ("hybrid agreements"), these types of agreements may not be recognized under the applicable state law, or at least not the way that the parties intended. Indeed, there are many circumstances under which contracting parties could come to a different understanding than a court with respect to the validity of hybrid agreements in a radiology group. For example, as was discussed above, the parol evidence rule prohibits the legal validation of prior or contemporaneous oral promises that were not incorporated into a final written agreement. Therefore, contracting parties may think that they have both oral and written agreements, but a court only may recognize the latter if the parol evidence rule applies. Alternatively, a written agreement may specify a process that must be used to make legally valid modifications to the contract terms. For instance, a contract may state that any modifications must be made in a writing that is signed by both parties. If the parties decide to disregard the modification provision and make informal oral promises outside of their written agreement, the validity of those promises may be compromised by the parties' violation of the express terms of their contract. Finally, agreements that are part written and part oral may be categorized as oral contracts under the applicable state law, which may compromise the enforceability of the written terms.[10]

The Meaning of a Contract to Your Radiology Group

The Contract as a Management Tool

Although it is useful to consider the meaning of contracts to lawyers when drafting or reviewing a radiology group's agreements, the focus of this chapter is on the meaning of contracts to radiologists. Accordingly, the rest of this chapter will tackle contract issues from the perspective of a radiology group and its members. It is important to distinguish a group's perspective from that of its individual members, because the needs of a group are not always consistent with the interests of its members. This point raises the first of four basic themes of contract dynamics in a radiology practice (Box 23-1).

The first theme is that the contracting parties are not in positions of parity. Group contracts in general, and the provisions discussed below (see The Muroff Five and Extra Protection) in particular, are intended to protect the best interests of a radiology group as

---

> **BOX 23-1**
>
> **Four Themes of Contract Dynamics in a Radiology Practice**
>
> 1. Contracting parties are not in positions of parity
> 2. Anticipate problems
> 3. Uniformity and consistency
> 4. Meaningful consequences for infractions

---

a whole. The individual interests of group members may be compromised, or even sacrificed, to that end.

Anticipating problems before they arise is a second theme. A radiology group must be proactive in addressing challenges to its legal and business interests so as to avoid setting an inadvertent precedent. In addition to the contractual protections discussed in this chapter, a group should implement concise policies and procedures for dealing with problematic members, disciplinary matters, and partial retirement, among other complicated practice issues. These policies, which will be discussed in Chapter 24, should be consistent with applicable federal and state laws as well as the policies and procedures of the group's hospital(s).

A third theme is to make the group's contractual protections and policies uniformly applicable to all group members. This enforcement approach helps to maximize group cohesion. As will be elaborated below, this strategy also mitigates group conflict and potential liability.

Finally, the imposition of clear and meaningful consequences for violations of a group's contractual provisions and policies is a fourth theme. Certain infractions require measured or graded reactions, whereas others warrant a zero-tolerance position. For example, extended call or abbreviated vacation may apply to unprofessional behavior, such as late or missed call, whereas termination may apply to unlawful behavior, such as sexual harassment. A group's culture, state and federal laws, and hospital protocol should dictate the range of appropriate penalties.

The Muroff Five

Five basic contract provisions can reinforce the employment relationship between a radiology group and its members (Box 23-2; see examples[11-13]). Each of these provisions permits a group to exert a measure of control over its members through the terms of their employment and provides the group with protections against any perceived defiance of this control. Although these provisions represent concepts that are fundamental to most radiology groups across the nation, they are not sufficient, nor are they necessary or appropriate in every case to accomplish a group's objectives. These five provisions must be reconciled with a group's policies as well as those of its hospital(s) and applicable state and federal laws.

Exclusive Employment with the Group

Through the effective use of contracts, a radiology group can dictate the means, manner, and terms of a member's employment. For example, written agreements used by a radiology group can require each member to be engaged in the practice of medicine exclusively as an employee of the group. To that end, a group's employment contract may state: "Employee shall not engage in the practice of medicine except as the Employee of Employer, unless authorized by Employer." This type of clause solidifies the mutual investment between a radiology group and its members.

Likewise, a written contract can memorialize the nature and scope of members' obligations to the group. Many radiology groups use broad, generic descriptions of members' responsibilities, whether for practical or strategic reasons. For example, "Employer shall have the authority to determine the specific duties which shall be performed by Employee as well as the authority to determine the means and manner by which the duties shall be performed." Although such language may seem to maximize a group's discretion, it may be vulnerable from an enforcement perspective in light of the ambiguity of the terms. This ambiguity also may influence a group's ability to enforce a non-compete provision against a former member, as will be explained in the next subsection. Therefore, this author has advised radiology group clients to strike a balance when articulating members' responsibilities by maintaining contract terms of sufficient certainty, yet reserving the authority to designate additional tasks in a subsequent writing signed by both parties.

Exclusive employment provisions also protect the profits and patients of a radiology group. In a written employment agreement, a group can clarify that all patients of a group member will be deemed patients of the group, and the group will retain all rights to bill for services rendered by each member. Additionally, a group can establish ownership of any records and other materials relating to its patients, to the extent appropriate and legally permissible. Furthermore, the group may claim all employment-related income earned by each group member, from lectures, medical-legal work, royalties, and the like, with exceptions that may be designated at the group's discretion.

Aside from these tactical issues with respect to exclusive employment, a radiology group and its members must appreciate technical concerns, including the legal implications of members' employment status. For example, federal antidiscrimination laws generally apply to employees, as opposed to independent contractors. Employment status also invokes tax and insurance considerations. A group should work proactively with its attorney and business manager to anticipate these issues with appropriate contractual language.

Covenant Not to Compete

A radiology group's employment contract typically requires radiologists to agree formally in writing (i.e., "covenant") that they will refrain from engaging in certain activities that would put them in competition with their former colleagues at the conclusion of their employment. These covenants reinforce the understanding, pursuant to the exclusive employment provision discussed in the previous section, that a group member's patients and colleagues belong to the group. Thus, non-compete covenants prohibit radiologists from engaging in the same or similar activities as their former group for a specific period of time and with respect to a specific geographic area that is coextensive with the group's practice. For example, a non-compete covenant may require that, upon termination of group employment, a radiologist must not compete with the group for a limited number of years within a designated radius of the group's site(s) of practice (e.g., the group's city or county, or more commonly, its affiliated hospital or hospitals). The appropriate scope of these restrictions will vary in accordance with a group's state laws, in addition to other factors, such as whether the group practices in an urban or a rural environment.

Because of the high stakes implicated by the group's and members' livelihoods, non-compete covenants tend to be the most common source of litigation between radiology groups and their former members. If a conflict results in a lawsuit, state law will determine the enforceability of the non-compete provision. Although there are specific laws and policies in each state, ranging from whether non-compete covenants are permissible to whether separate consideration is required to validate them, most courts in states that allow these covenants will use a general standard of reasonableness ("reasonableness standard") to evaluate them (see example[14]).

Under the reasonableness standard, a court will consider whether a non-compete covenant imposes a restraint on a former group member that exceeds what is needed to protect the group's interests. Typically, this analysis involves an accounting of the scope of the former group member's duties, the duration of the prohibition, the geographic area affected, and the public interest in continuing to benefit from the radiologist's services. Case law indicates that a group's interest in retaining business usually is sufficient to support a covenant not to compete to protect against a significant risk of diversion by a former group member.[15]

Generally, a radiology group will have the burden of demonstrating the reasonableness of its non-compete covenant under the applicable state law. The former group member's ability to secure employment elsewhere will be a compelling factor in the court's decision. For example, an osteopathic radiologist in Ohio argued under the reasonableness standard that the covenant not to compete for 2 years within the city or county of his former group's practice was unreasonable, because it imposed an undue hardship on him and on the general public that was greater than necessary for the group's protection.[16] The crux of the radiologist's argument was that his subspecialty of interventional radiology was uncommon in the community; the group's hospital was one of the few osteopathic institutions in the area with that expertise. In a similar case in Texas, a radiologist argued that his special skills in angiography and magnetic resonance imaging should be "carved out" of the non-compete covenant with his former group, because none of the other group members or other local physicians shared his experience.[17] However, the Supreme Court of Texas ultimately rejected the radiologist's argument in a decision that reversed the lower court's decision, which demonstrates the inclination of courts to prioritize the collective interests of a group over the individual interests of its members.[18]

Because non-compete covenants typically are enforced to protect the interests of radiology groups, members may take the initiative to protect their individual interests by attempting to negotiate the terms of the covenant at the outset of their employment. For example, in Ohio, one radiologist's attorney successfully circumscribed the geographic restriction of a group's non-compete covenant and added new safeguards for the radiologist, including a clause that prevented the group from soliciting business beyond the boundaries of the non-compete covenant.[19] Although that case demonstrates that some groups are willing to negotiate the terms of their non-compete covenants, a radiologist who demands a negotiation may encounter resistance, if not rejection, by the group if the group's attorney and leadership require all members to agree to the same contractual protections to minimize intragroup conflict and the potential of litigation on the basis or perception of differential treatment of group members. Therefore, radiologists may be concerned that if they challenge their non-compete covenants, or any other terms of their employment, they may jeopardize their status in the group or generate litigation.

In the latter case, state law will dictate a court's options if it deems a non-compete covenant unreasonable. For example, courts in certain states, such as Indiana, may strike the overbroad language in a non-compete covenant to enforce the covenant under the reasonableness standard (see example[20]). These states may be referred to as "blue pencil" states, in acknowledgment of the revisions that their courts may impose on non-compete covenants. Courts in more liberal blue pencil states, such as Illinois, may go a step further by modifying the language in a non-compete covenant to make the terms more reasonable (see example[21]). Conversely, in other states, such as Georgia, a court may decline to modify or enforce a non-compete covenant in its entirety if any portion of the covenant does not comport with the reasonableness standard (see example[22]). These distinctions among state laws are significant, because the risk that a court will modify or invalidate a non-compete covenant may incentivize a radiology group to negotiate the terms of the covenant directly with its members.

Termination with and without Cause

Another contentious yet critical issue for radiology groups to consider is whether employment agreements with group members will recite specific grounds for termination, or if employment will be "at-will," with discretion for the group to terminate members without cause. This decision, and the language that is used to articulate it within an employment agreement, should be made cautiously, with the guidance of the group's attorney in light of applicable federal and state laws. As with non-compete covenants, termination provisions tend to be more palatable to group members when the group's enforcement position is clear and consistent.

Termination-with-cause provisions put group members on notice about the expectations for their performance and behavior during their employment with the group. Although a group has flexibility regarding which causes for termination to designate within its agreements, its discretion ultimately will be limited by federal and state laws. For example, antidiscrimination laws generally prohibit an employer from terminating an employee on the basis of the employee's race, alienage, gender, or other protected status.

A radiology group also may wish to identify certain conditions that will lead to the automatic termination of group members. Conditions of automatic termination may overlap with conditions of termination for cause in the cases of unprofessional or unethical conduct, or the suspension, revocation, or cancellation of a member's license or hospital staff privileges. However, automatic termination can be distinguished from termination for cause, because the former can include circumstances beyond a group member's control. For example, conditions of automatic termination may include the death of a member, or the imposition of prohibitive governmental or legal restrictions on a practice. These circumstances make an ongoing employment relationship untenable, as opposed to merely undesirable.

Whereas a termination-for-cause provision may be appropriate for some groups, most radiologist clients have been employed at-will and can be terminated from their groups without cause. Termination-without-cause provisions can be beneficial to a group as a means of dealing with difficult or unproductive members. However, the absence of an express cause for termination may cause group members to perceive termination decisions as arbitrary at best and discriminatory at worst. Thus, termination-without-cause provisions clearly reinforce the power differential between the contracting parties, because group members may feel vulnerable to the perceived whims of the group's leadership.

With those considerations in mind, this writer has advised radiology group clients to consider a few basic guidelines when implementing termination-without-cause provisions in employment contracts with their members. First, these provisions should apply to all group members to avoid the perception of differential treatment. Second, a general consensus of the group should be required to validate any termination decision. The group's bylaws or policies should designate the requisite percentage, excluding the radiologist whose employment is at issue. Although the latter point may seem obvious, failing to articulate it in writing may lead to enforcement challenges that could be devastating, particularly to a small group. Finally, a group must establish a process to execute a termination-without-cause provision as quickly as possible to protect the integrity of both the group and the terminated radiologist.

Based on the writer's experience with radiology groups, this is a point worth emphasizing: once a member has been terminated, he or she should not be allowed to fester in the group beyond the reasonable yet brief time frame designated in the contract between notice and effective date of termination. It is surprising to learn how many exceptions and excuses have been made for terminated radiologists who, for example, were scheduled for an undesirable call period. Short-term call relief, albeit compelling, is not a sufficient justification for the long-term damage to a group that can be caused by a disgruntled, terminated member. There may never be a "good time" to let a "bad radiologist" go, but the longer a group waits, the further it may be subjecting itself to conflict and potential liability.

Co-termination of Rights

For most radiology groups, the implications of terminating a member extend beyond the immediate practice. For instance, a group may wish to include within its employment agreements a process for terminating a member's hospital privileges at the conclusion of group employment. To that end, a contract between a radiology group and its member may require an executed power of attorney permitting the group's president or designee to execute a resignation from the hospital staff(s) on behalf of a terminated radiologist.

Although the co-termination of a former member's group and hospital rights may be appealing to a group, there can be important legal implications of implementing such a provision. For example, co-termination may influence a departing member's right to a fair hearing with respect to the revocation of his or her hospital privileges. Therefore, a group should consult its attorney, as well as its hospital(s)'s policies and procedures, to ensure that this option is feasible under the group's specific circumstances and applicable state and federal laws.

Protection against Sale or Repossession of Group Assets

Finally, it is important for a radiology group to protect against the sale or repossession of its assets or stock by group members. Options for protection may include structuring the group as a formal business entity, such as a professional association, and/or articulating strategic stock restrictions. The objective is to protect a group from the bankruptcy of its members, or from the vulnerability of a member's property rights due to other life events, including divorce. This protection is important to the group throughout the employment of its members. However, the need for protection becomes even more significant at the point of members' termination, because the group loses its ability to manage or supervise members' activities. In light of the complexities of these considerations, options for protection are best navigated by a group's attorney and business manager or accountant.

Extra Protection

In addition to the Muroff Five, another category of protection that is complicated by divergent state laws, yet is critical for radiology groups to consider, is the anticipation of liability. With the guidance of a group's leadership and attorney, there are a number of precautions that a group can take to reduce its liability exposure. For example, an employment contract may require the group or the new member to purchase liability insurance. This purchase may include extensions or "tail coverage" to protect the group from claims against the group that derive from actions or omissions of a radiologist who is no longer employed by the group. An indemnification or "hold harmless" clause is another protection for a group to consider, because such a clause can shift the economic loss from the party who is responsible for damages by contract to the party who is responsible for damages by action or omission. Confidentiality provisions also are important to preserve the integrity of a group's records and communications. This protection not only may

405

be prudent from a business perspective but also may be legally mandated by the Health Insurance Portability and Accountability Act or other applicable state or federal restrictions on disclosure. Finally, a group's employment contracts can incorporate an alternative dispute resolution provision, as detailed in a later section of this chapter, to mitigate the losses of time and resources associated with litigation.

The group's attorney and leadership can draft appropriate language that accommodates all of the business and legal concerns associated with these protections. Additionally, this team can structure the radiology group as a formal business entity, which will affect the liability of the group and its members. For example, members of a corporation generally are shielded from personal liability for the business entity, whereas members of a partnership may not be.

WHEN A CONTRACT IS BROKEN

Breach

Legal Definition of Breach

Breach of a contract occurs when one party to an agreement fails to satisfy his or her obligation(s) to another party. To prove breach, a radiologist (plaintiff) must demonstrate the existence of a contract, performance by the plaintiff, and breach by another party to the agreement (defendant) that caused damage or loss to the plaintiff.[5] These factors seem relatively basic as a matter of legal theory. However, the interpretation of breach in the context of radiology employment agreements has varied significantly among state courts, and this has generated ambiguity surrounding the translation of these principles into practice.

Practical Examples of Breach

Of value to share with radiologist clients have been several examples of the ambiguity surrounding courts' interpretations of contractual breaches in radiology practices. Because of the complicated and often unexpected outcomes, these cases serve as cautionary tales for radiologists to consider when drafting or updating their employment contracts, or when exploring legal causes of action to pursue against

Table 23-1 Common Examples of Breach	
Category of Breach	**Sample Claims**
Unfair Competition	1. Non-Compete Covenant Conflicts 2. Interference with Business 3. Monopolization
Bad Faith	1. Fraud 2. Discrimination 3. Retaliation

their group or their former colleague(s) (Table 23-1). Thus, the cases reinforce the value of maintaining clear, consistent, and unambiguous terms in employment contracts between radiology groups and their members.

Unfair Competition   Perhaps not surprisingly, claims involving unfair competition tend to generate the most lawsuits between radiology groups and their former members.

Non-Compete Covenants   Conflicts pertaining to non-compete covenants are pervasive among radiologists. Although these types of disputes may have become routine, their outcomes in court can be unpredictable. For example, a judge in Wisconsin found that a radiologist did not violate his non-compete covenant by resigning from his group to submit a competing proposal to a hospital that his group had targeted for an exclusive contract.[23] The facts of this case made the court's conclusion surprising, because the radiologist served as the group's chief liaison in its communication with the hospital, and the competition for the exclusive contract was limited to the radiologist and his former group. Nonetheless, the court reasoned that the employment agreement between the radiologist and his former group defined the radiologist's responsibilities as providing radiologic services, not submitting business proposals.

Interference with Business   The Wisconsin case presented another common cause of legal action between a radiology group and its former members: interference with contractual relations or with a prospective business advantage. Through this claim, a radiology group can try to prevent a former member from undermining its business relationships or prospects.

Although interference is a popular claim in lawsuits involving radiology groups and their former members, it does not have a particularly strong record of success in this context. For example, in the Wisconsin case the court rejected this claim because it determined that the group's proposal for the hospital's business was independently flawed, and because the radiologist offered to hire his former colleagues into a new practice that would benefit from the exclusive contract. Thus, the court seemed convinced that the radiologist did not cause sufficient harm to the business group's to justify any remedy.

Additional misconduct by the defendant, independent of his or her alleged interference with the plaintiff's business, may influence the viability of an interference claim. For example, a court in Massachusetts permitted a radiologist who formed a corporation with a partner and secured a contract with a hospital to withdraw from the partnership and fire his former partner for unsatisfactory performance.[24] The court rejected the former partner's claim of interference, because his termination was not motivated by greed, bad faith, malice, or any other improper motive or additional misconduct with respect to the plaintiff.

Monopolization A third type of unfair competition claim is antitrust or monopolization. To prevail on an antitrust claim, a plaintiff generally must convince a court that a reasonable jury could find that the defendant's conduct was a material cause or a substantially contributing factor of injury to the plaintiff's business interests. Conversely, a plaintiff typically cannot recover damages if the defendant can demonstrate that the decline of the plaintiff's business was attributable to causes other than the defendant's behavior. For example, a court in South Dakota refused to recognize a radiologist's antitrust claim because the court attributed the failure of the radiologist's practice to his unwillingness, as opposed to inability,

to provide the breadth and flexibility of services that his former group offered.[25]

Another court in Arizona permitted a radiologist to advise doctors and patients at his former hospital that he would be opening his own competitive practice, because the radiologist was the only full-time radiation oncologist at the hospital.[26] In deference to the best interests of the affected patients, the court reasoned that the radiologist had a right, if not a duty, to advise referring physicians and patients of the change in the capabilities of the radiology department at the hospital after his departure. The court concluded that this notice permitted the other doctors and patients to make an informed decision about their health care choices.

Bad Faith Allegations of bad faith motivate another common set of claims in lawsuits involving radiology groups and their former members.

Fraud Although most people understand the concept of fraud from a colloquial perspective, the legal definition of fraud is quite technical. Generally, a claim of fraud, or fraudulent misrepresentation, requires a plaintiff to demonstrate that the defendant made a false statement of a material fact, which the defendant knew or believed to be false at the time of the statement. Moreover, the defendant must have intended to induce the plaintiff to act or rely upon the false statement, which the plaintiff did, to his or her detriment.[10] A defendant's concealment of facts also may constitute fraud if the defendant had an intention to deceive as well as an opportunity and a duty to provide full disclosure.[10] Thus, a statement that technically is truthful in part may be deemed fraudulent if the defendant's deliberate omission of other relevant facts is considered misleading.

It should be noted that a claim of fraud typically cannot be predicated on a representation, expectation, or opinion concerning a *future* event. The rationale for this bar may be that, because the future is unpredictable, it is more difficult for a court to distinguish an intent to deceive from an inability to predict. Nonetheless, a court may grant a limited exception if a promise of future action was made with a present intention not to perform it. The misrepresentation of an existing fact, the speaker's state of mind, is the basis for this exception, which may be referred to as fraud in the inducement.[6] Presumably, this type of claim could allow a radiologist to sue his or her group if the radiologist can demonstrate that the group did not intend to keep its promise of making the radiologist a partner, as of the time that the promise was made.

Discrimination Federal and state antidiscrimination laws have prompted a significant number of lawsuits involving radiology groups and their former members. The details of, and distinctions among, these laws are beyond the scope of this chapter. However, a brief analysis of a failure to hire or promote claim based on gender discrimination can illustrate considerations that are common in these types of lawsuits.

In many cases, a radiologist plaintiff is unable to offer direct evidence of gender discrimination with respect to a group's failure to hire or promote the radiologist. Instead, a court may use an indirect, burden-shifting framework that requires the radiologist to demonstrate that he or she applied and was qualified for a job for which the group was soliciting applicants, that the radiologist was rejected despite his or her sufficient qualifications, and that the position remained open and the group continued to seek applications from similarly qualified individuals.[27] The burden then shifts to the group to articulate a legitimate, nondiscriminatory reason for its employment decision.

Next, a plaintiff must present evidence that the group's reason for failing to hire or promote the plaintiff are a pretext, or otherwise must introduce evidence of the employer's discriminatory motive. For instance, a part-time radiologist in Kansas brought a claim of gender discrimination against her group when she did not receive an offer of full-time employment, despite her sufficient qualifications and despite the continued availability of full-time position(s) after the group eliminated her as a candidate.[28] The defendants argued that they did not offer plaintiff the position because they were unaware of her interest in working full

time, and they were concerned about her alleged mistreatment of hospital personnel. In turn, the plaintiff demonstrated that such reasons may be pretextual because she previously told the group's leadership of her interest in a full-time position, and the group continued to send her to the hospitals that allegedly complained of her misconduct instead of seeking a substitute for her at those locations. The subjective, case-by-case analysis that courts use for these types of claims reinforces the theme of ambiguity with respect to the enforcement of contractual provisions in lawsuits involving radiology groups and their (former) members.

Retaliation Retaliation, or retaliatory discharge, is another popular theme of lawsuits involving radiologists and their former groups. Courts may permit this type of claim to offer protection and encouragement to employees who report statutory infractions of rules, regulations, or laws pertaining to public health, safety, and the general welfare by their (former) employers. These reports may generate lawsuits that are referred to as "whistleblower" or "qui tam" actions to reflect the employee's choice to bring his or her employer to justice in light of the compelling public interests that are implicated by the employer's misconduct. Thus, qui tam actions are predicated not only on the employer's harm or damage to the employee plaintiff but also on the harm or damage to the public welfare. If the plaintiff believes that he or she was terminated because of the decision to bring this type of formal or informal complaint against the employer, a retaliation claim may be an appropriate recourse.

To prevail on a retaliation claim, a radiologist typically has the burden of proving that a reasonably prudent person would have concluded that the group was violating rules, regulations, or laws pertaining to public health, safety, and the general welfare, that the group had knowledge that the radiologist reported such violation(s) before terminating the radiologist, and that the group discharged the radiologist in retaliation for making the report.[28] A court may consider the plaintiff's ulterior motives in making the report, as protected whistleblowing must result from a good-faith concern about the defendant's wrongful activity, as opposed to malice or greed on behalf of the plaintiff. Federal protection from retaliatory discharge generally does not extend to independent contractors; however, a group's attorney can determine if state laws offer any protections or introduce any other relevant considerations.

A claim of retaliatory discharge often arises when a radiologist alleges that he or she was terminated for expressing concern about the group's compliance with Medicare. For instance, the plaintiff in the Kansas case claimed that she ultimately was terminated from the group because she refused to sign the group's Medicare compliance plan. Before her termination, the plaintiff explained to the defendants that her refusal to sign the compliance plan was based on her belief that the group was billing her services improperly as a locum tenens physician. The court concluded that the plaintiff's status as an independent contractor would prevent her from enjoying whistleblower protection unless she was able to convince the court, through a separate, subsequent filing, that her retaliation claim should not be dismissed. Accordingly, the court did not speak to the merits of the group's arguments that the plaintiff never filed a formal report or complaint about that billing practice, and that the billing practice reflected a clerical error as opposed to deliberate deception.

REMEDIES

Remedies can protect a non-breaching party's investment in a contract that was not performed in accordance with its terms. The general purpose of remedies is to put a non-breaching party in the same position that he or she would have been if the contract had been performed.[29] This

---

BOX 23-3

Remedies

1. Remedies at law
2. Remedies at equity

---

objective may be accomplished through remedies at law, which include financial compensation, or through remedies at equity, which include alternative forms of relief (Box 23-3).

At Law

Typically, a radiologist plaintiff will seek financial compensation to remedy a breach of contract by a radiology group. For example, a radiologist may demand payment of his or her salary, bonus, and other benefits that were designated in the radiologist's employment contract with the group, yet withheld upon termination.[30] A court may refer to such remedies as actual or compensatory damages to reflect the proportionality of the monetary award to the damage or harm that the plaintiff suffered. Sometimes a defendant's misconduct may warrant additional compensation to the plaintiff in the form of punitive or exemplary damages. Although the standard for punitive damages varies according to applicable state laws, the defendant's behavior generally must be shown to be outrageous or egregious, such that the court chooses to "punish" (punitive damages) or make an example out of (exemplary damages) the defendant by awarding the plaintiff an amount of money that exceeds the scope of the actual harm or damage that was caused by the defendant.

A court's determination of appropriate damages is contingent upon several variables. For instance, a court may consider whether a plaintiff is claiming damages for partial breach or for total breach of the employment contract.[29] In the case of partial breach, the parties ultimately may perform their respective obligations, but under different terms than expressed under their original contract. Generally, damages for partial breach compensate a plaintiff for the loss of time or money that resulted from the defendant's nonperformance, modification, or delay. However, in the case of total or material breach, affecting the heart of a contract, a plaintiff may choose to terminate the contract and refuse to resume any further obligation(s) to the defendant.[29] Although state laws influence these considerations, a group's failure to provide a member with sufficient office space may constitute a partial breach of an employment agreement, whereas a member's decision to change specialties may constitute a material breach. Not surprisingly, a more substantial damage award would be expected in the latter case, relative to the former.

At Equity

Equitable relief may be an option for a plaintiff whose damages cannot be redressed through financial compensation. One type of equitable relief is specific performance, which requires the breaching party to fulfill his or her original obligations under the contract.[31] Although forcing the performance of an agreement may seem desirable, it may not be feasible because employment contracts between radiology groups and their members are classified as personal services agreements.

Courts have argued against the specific performance of personal-services agreements that require such specialized skill, knowledge, judgment, or discretion for many reasons.[32] First, it would be impractical, if not impossible, for a court to provide the continuous supervision that would be necessary to ensure compliance with this remedy. Second, the notion of forced employment may raise concerns under the 13th amendment to the U.S. Constitution, which prohibits involuntary servitude. Furthermore, personal services contracts require a relationship of cooperation and trust between the parties, which could be undermined by judicial intervention. Consequently, as a matter of public policy, courts generally will avoid awards for specific performance in the context of employment agreements, even if the parties agreed to that remedy.

As is the case with most rules, there are exceptions to the trend against granting specific performance of employment contracts. For example, a court in Delaware found that a hospital breached its contract with a surgical resident when it demoted him to a more junior year in its residency program and lowered his status from categorical to preliminary.[33] The court ordered specific performance of the resident's participation in the categorical level of the residency program. In acknowledgment of the unusual nature of its finding, the court limited its holding by emphasizing the unique dynamics of a contractual relationship between a resident and a teaching hospital. Specifically, the educational nature of the residency program seemed to mitigate policy-based objections to specific performance. Moreover, financial compensation could not remedy the irreparable harm to the resident's livelihood that may have resulted from his demotion. Finally, the hospital had a disciplinary committee that could oversee the administration of specific performance, which precluded the court's concern about improper entanglement in the enforcement of that remedy.

Another exception to the general trend against specific performance of employment contracts applies to covenants not to compete. For instance, a court in Illinois held that a non-compete covenant, but not the underlying employment contract, could be enforced by specific performance.[32] Accordingly, the court denied the terminated radiologist's demand of reinstatement to his group and limited specific performance to the non-compete covenant within his employment agreement. This decision to prohibit the radiologist from returning to, or competing with, his former group reinforces the tendency of courts to prioritize the collective rights of radiology groups over the individual rights of group members.

Rescission, or cancellation of a contract, is another form of equitable relief. Rescission may be an appropriate remedy for a plaintiff who wants to avoid the obligations of an agreement that was not performed in accordance with its original terms. For example, a radiologist in Ohio sought rescission of her employment contract with a radiology corporation on the grounds of fraudulent inducement.[19] However, the parol evidence rule barred the radiologist from presenting evidence of the corporation's oral misrepresentations because they were within the scope of, but not included in, her final, written employment agreement. Therefore, the radiologist was unable to provide evidence that the corporation did not intend to fulfill its promises to her at the time that the statements were made. The court rejected the radiologist's demand for rescission and enforced the non-compete covenant in the agreement against her, after finding that the covenant was consistent with the state's reasonableness standard.

ALTERNATIVE DISPUTE RESOLUTION

Alternative dispute resolution is an increasingly popular option for radiology groups that seek to settle their disputes outside of the courtroom to reduce the time and costs associated with litigation. Depending on the type of alternative dispute resolution that is implemented, and the skills of the practitioner, this process also can provide the contracting parties with more control over the outcome of their dispute than they would have had in court. Mediation and arbitration are the two most common forms of alternative dispute resolution (Box 23-4). In fact, some states require parties to a lawsuit to mediate their cases before they are tried in court, and many employment agreements require contracting parties to resolve their disputes exclusively through arbitration.

This section offers only a basic introduction to mediation and arbitration; a group's attorney will be able to help radiologists understand the nuances of alternative dispute resolution under the specific circumstances of the group and applicable state and federal laws and local practices. For example, the group's attorney should explain the process for selecting a mediator or arbitrator and the extent to which the group's attorney will be permitted, if not expected, to participate in the mediation or arbitration processes. The group's attorney also should clarify the expectations of confidentiality regarding information disclosed during those processes.

BOX 23-4

Alternative Dispute Resolution

1. Mediation
2. Arbitration

Mediation

Mediation is the process by which a trained, third-party neutral facilitates the resolution of a dispute by encouraging the parties to communicate about their interests and concerns. The basis of mediation is that this communication will permit the parties to collaborate on an agreement that is mutually acceptable, if not mutually beneficial. To that end, a skilled mediator imposes a *process* for communication but permits the parties to determine their own *outcome*.

Significantly, a mediator lacks the authority to impose a legally binding resolution. Instead, a mediator assists the parties in drafting a written agreement that captures the terms that they have agreed upon voluntarily during the mediation. A court may then enforce the terms of the agreement if one of the parties fails to uphold his or her obligations. A court also may provide a forum for the parties to resolve their dispute if they are unable to reach an agreement after the mediation has concluded.

Arbitration

In an arbitration, a neutral or a panel of neutrals issues a final, binding resolution to a dispute after weighing both parties' perspectives. By agreeing to arbitration, as opposed to mediation, parties may waive their right to a trial as well as their right to appeal the arbitration outcome. An arbitration provision within an employment contract generally will be upheld unless it is demonstrated that the provision was procured by fraud, duress, or mistake, or otherwise was unconscionable.[34] Arbitration remains a popular option for radiology groups in light of its finality and relative expediency.

CONCLUSIONS

The complexity of the concepts, variations, and exceptions discussed in this chapter reinforces the need to be proactive, rather than reactive, in addressing disputes between radiology groups and their members. Understanding the terms and implications of employment contracts is critical to ensure a smooth entrance into, and a relatively more smooth transition out of, these contractual relationships. By analyzing the basic definition and types of a contract, identifying significant contractual terms and protections, and exploring breaches and remedies, this chapter has intended to demystify employment contracts and to enhance group management and cohesion.

Dos and Don'ts of Employment Contracts	
Dos	**Don'ts**
1. Articulate clear and meaningful obligations and expectations of group members in writing within the group's policies and employment contracts, and enforce them consistently among group members.	1. Rely exclusively upon oral agreements within the group, unless there is a clear consensus on the terms and propriety of those agreements under the specific circumstances of the group and under applicable laws.
2. Review the group's employment contracts at least once a year to ensure that the terms are appropriate for the group's current culture and hospital(s) and are consistent with applicable federal and state laws.	2. Use a form agreement or generic contract that is not vetted by the group's attorney and leadership to ensure that it accommodates the issues specific to the group and its state of practice.
3. Maintain a proactive and productive collaboration between the group's leadership and attorney and business manager.	3. Assume that the group's lawyer will proactively notify the group of any laws that could affect the practice, if the group has not communicated that desire or established a continuing relationship with that lawyer.
4. Prioritize open communication among group members and the group's leadership.	4. Ignore behavior that violates the group's policies or contract provisions.
5. Establish a clear process for dispute resolution that will maximize the group's potential to resolve conflicts outside of the courtroom.	5. Assume that a lack of complaints reflects a lack of concerns among group members, especially if there is no outlet or forum for "safe" communication with the group's leadership.

REFERENCES

1. Restatement (second) of contracts. Philadelphia: American Law Institute, 1979, § 1.
2. Williston SA: A treatise on the law of contracts, 4th ed. Rochester, NY, Lawyers Cooperative Publishing, 1990, § 1:1.
3. Taimoorazy v. Bloomington Anesthesiology Service, Ltd., 122 F. Supp. 2d 967 (C.D. Ill. Nov. 28, 2000).
4. Restatement (second) of contracts. Philadelphia: American Law Institute, 1979, § 90.
5. Nilavar v. Osborn, 127 Ohio App. 3d 1; 711 N.E. 2d 726; 1998 Ohio App. LEXIS 1150 (Ohio Ct. App., Clark County 1998).
6. Wall v. Firelands Radiology, Inc., 106 Ohio App. 3d 313, Huron County App. No. H-94-48, 666 N.E. 2d 235, 1995 Ohio App. LEXIS 3785 (Ohio Ct. App., Huron County 1995).
7. Schwaiger v. Mitchell Radiology Assocs., P.C., 2002 SD 97; 652 N.W. 2d 372; 2002 S.D. LEXIS 116; 18 I.E.R. Cas. (BNA) 1761 (2002).
8. Bice v. Green, 64 Ark. App. 203; 981 S.W. 2d 105; 1998 Ark. App. LEXIS 822 (1998).
9. Bloom v. Clara Maass Medical Ctr., 295 N.J. Super. 594, 685 A.2d 966, 1996 N.J. Super. LEXIS 465 (N.J. Super. Ct. App. Div. 1996).
10. Kurti v. Fox Valley Radiologists, Ltd., 124 Ill. App. 3d 933; 464 N.E. 2d 1219; 1984.
11. Muroff, JA: Legal spotlight: contracts 101. Advance for Imaging and Oncology Administrators 16:22, 2006.
12. Muroff, JA, Muroff, LR: Contracts in radiology practices: breaches and remedies. J Am Coll Radiol 1:553, 2004.
13. Muroff, JA, Muroff, LR: Contracts in radiology practices: contract types and key provisions. J Am Coll Radiol 1:459, 2004.
14. Isuani v. Manske-Sheffield Radiology Group, P.A., 805 S.W. 2d 602 (Tex. App. Beaumont 1991).
15. Horne v. Radiological Health Services, 83 Misc. 2d 446; 371 N.Y.S. 2d 948; 1975 N.Y. Misc. LEXIS 2922 (N.Y. Sup. Ct. 1975), aff'd, Horne v. Radiological Health Services, P.C., 51 A.D. 2d 544, 379 N.Y.S. 2d 374, 1976 N.Y. App. Div. LEXIS 10788.

16. Williams v. Hobbs, 9 Ohio App. 3d 331, 9 Ohio B. 599, 460 N.E. 2d 287, 1983 Ohio App. LEXIS 11079 (Ohio Ct. App., Franklin County 1983).

17. Isuani v. Manske-Sheffield Radiology Group, P.A., 798 S.W. 2d 346 (Tex. App. Beaumont 1990).

18. Isuani v. Manske-Sheffield Radiology Group, P.A., 802 S.W. 2d 235 (Tex. 1991).

19. *FirelandsRadiology, Inc.*, 106 Ohio App. 3d 313.

20. Product Action Intern'l, Inc. v. Mero, 277 F. Supp. 2d 919 (S.D. Ind. Aug. 5, 2003).

21. Joy v. Hay Group, Inc., 2003 WL 22118930 (N.D. Ill. Sept. 11, 2003).

22. Georgia White v. Fletcher/Mayo/Assocs., Inc., 303 S.E. 2d 746 (Ga. 1983).

23. Radiology Consultants v. Huberty, 255 Wis. 2d 833, 646 N.W. 2d 855, 2002 WI App 134, 2002 Wisc. App. LEXIS 483 (2002).

24. Malter v. Eldh, 1994 Mass. Super. LEXIS 128 (Mass. Super. Ct. Dec. 2, 1994).

25. Read v. Medical X-Ray Center, P.C., 110 F.3d 543; 1997 U.S. App. LEXIS 6481; 1997-1 Trade Cas. (CCH) P71763 (8th Cir. S.D. 1997).

26. Evans v. Valley Radiologists, Ltd., 127 Ariz. 177; 619 P. 2d 5; 1980 Ariz. LEXIS 282 (Ariz. 1980).

27. McDonnell Douglas Corp. v. Green, 411 U.S. 792, 802–04, 93 S. Ct. 1817, 36 L.Ed. 2d 668 (1973).

28. Parsells v. Manhattan Radiology Group, L.L.P., 255 F. Supp. 2d 1217, 2003 U.S. Dist. LEXIS 5687 (D. Kan. 2003).

29. Farnsworth EA: Farnsworth on contracts, 2 ed., New York, Aspen, 2001, § 12.9.

30. Zannis v. Lake Shore Radiologists, Ltd, 104 Ill. App. 3d 484; 432 N.E. 2d 1108; 1982 Ill. App. LEXIS 1519; 60 Ill. Dec. 209 (Ill. App. Ct. 1st Dist. 1979).

31. Bali v. Christiana Care Health Servs., Inc., 1999 Del. Ch. LEXIS 128 (Del. Ch. June 16, 1999).

32. *LakeShore Radiologists, Ltd*, 104 Ill. App. 3d 484.

33. *Christiana Care Health Servs., Inc.,* 1999 Del. Ch. LEXIS 128.

34. Orcutt v. Kettering Radiologists, Inc., 199 F. Supp. 2d 746; 2002 U.S. Dist. LEXIS 14388 (S.D. Ohio 2002).

Policies and Procedures

Christopher Laubenthal

INTRODUCTION

Imagine yourself preparing to visit a country that you have never been to before. What is on your preparation list? Maybe you will have questions: What am I going to pack? What languages are prevalent? What is the currency exchange? On your preparation list may not be the question: What are the policies and procedures in this land I am about to visit?

Policies and procedures, you might ask. What are these and why should they be on my preparation list? Think of policies and procedures as the code of conduct used by the management profession to organize and direct the human resources and potential of the organization, considered by many as the most valuable resource in an organization. Policies and procedures are the tools that help align and achieve the organization's vision, mission, and values.

As we explore policies and procedures in this chapter, keep in mind the following four questions and how they apply to your particular situation. We will come back to these four questions, because they define the four key elements in an environmental assessment that will assist you in determining the most effective means of implementing policies and procedures to meet your management objectives.

1. What are the governing rules? These can be unwritten and unspoken rules of behavior on one end of the spectrum, to documented "laws of the land," undisputable and known truths to all in the organization. These "laws of the land" may also include local, institutional, or national regulatory requirements. Because yours is a unit within a larger institution—and this is particularly relevant within a health care organization— you will want to understand these external regulatory requirements and the extent to which you will be required to have specific policies and procedures in place at your departmental level.

2. What is the level of organizational structure that matches your practice's level of efficiency and effectiveness? As an example, at the highly organized end of the spectrum, we might think of a military organization with layers of rules and hierarchies. At the other end of the spectrum might be the locally owned and operated corner convenience store, with minimal rules and few structured hierarchies.

3. What are the pressures of the culture and context for the individuals and the groups in your practice? For example, how is your practice structured? If it is part of a larger organization or university, there may be unique factors in public institutions that are implicit in your culture and affect the groups and individuals within your organization as opposed to the situation with private organizations or institutions.

4. What is the level of individual and group perceptions of "right and wrong" behaviors? For example, individual and group perceptions may be aligned to the expected cultural norms of behavior. On the other hand, individual and group perceptions may be more entrepreneurial and may challenge the expected culture of the organization.

Figure 24-1 illustrates these four factors (governing rules, organizational structure, culture and context, and individual and group perceptions) in creating the "policy and procedure boundary." The boundary that you are searching for is the optimal point of efficiency and effectiveness in the alignment of the mission, goals, and values of your practice or department.

With this visual diagram in mind, you might be asking, "What happens when a policy is not aligned to the mission, goals, or values of my practice?" In such an instance, the particular policy would not fall within this optimal boundary, that balancing point of optimizing these four factors—and a reassessment of the four factors would be warranted. Remember that the primary purpose of a policy and procedure set is to align your practice's mission, goals, and/or values and practices of the members of your organization, across the varying factors.

Certainly we have all experienced the tremendous inertia inherent in an attitude of supporting a policy and procedure for the sake of the policy and procedure itself. In such situations a typical response might be: "No, because that is not our policy." Here is another example of moving outside of this optimal boundary in achieving the

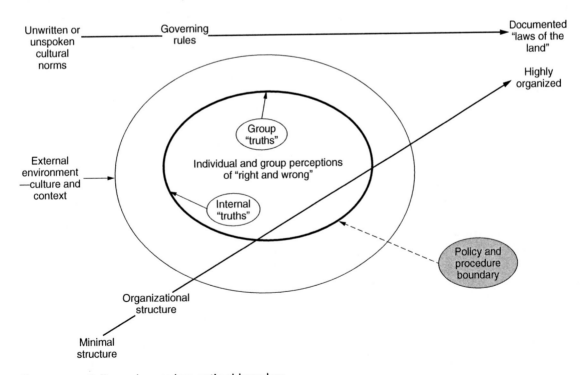

Figure 24-1 Policy and procedure optimal boundary.

required balance in your organization. Refocusing the discussion to finding the optimal balance will naturally return you to the point of commonality—that is, doing what is best for your practice, given your mission, goals, and values.

This chapter focuses on providing a basic understanding of policies and procedures and giving you a tool to use as you assess, create, and implement policies and procedures in your practice. It outlines a journey involving travels into new and possibly familiar territories, in discovery of this optimal "policy and procedure boundary" for your practice. This journey has three parts. First, we will cover the basic definitions of policies and procedures, with some documentation recommendations. Second, you will encounter some tools for conducting an environmental assessment; that is, where do you currently reside along the policy and procedure boundary? This will allow you to begin creating policies and procedures. Third, we will explore the resultant culture and the impact that policies and procedures can create for your practice.

DEFINITIONS

What is a policy? How does that differ from a rule? What is a procedure?

A policy is a plan of action to guide decisions and actions. A policy is a predetermined course of action. The Latin root of the word *politia* is used to denote "civil administration." In the modern business world, a policy sets the boundary conditions for a decision to be made and action to follow. Different from what we might think of as a rule, a generalized course of action or behavior, a policy statement sets the goal to be achieved. It intends to capture achievement and alignment of larger ideals and goals.

As an illustrative example, an organizational policy statement regarding equal employment opportunity might be: "The department is actively committed to providing equal educational and employment opportunity in all of its programs."

In contrast, as stated as a rule: "The department recognizes the requirement to maintain equal opportunities by following Title VI of the Civil Rights Act of 1964 as amended, Title

IX of the 1972 Education Amendments, and Section 504 of the Rehabilitation Act of 1973."

See Table 24-1 for some focus area policies for your practice.

There are nuances in crafting the language of a policy. Beyond these, it is important to highlight that a policy sets a larger scope in providing the framework for decisions and actions. Effective policy statements align organizational philosophy and the human resources within the organization to recognize appropriate actions that meet the policy.

Complementing a policy statement are the procedures. By the strictest definition, a procedure is the manner of proceeding, the way of performing. These are the nuts and bolts, where the details reside. A set of procedures is a series of steps to accomplish an end. It is tactical, action based, and not conceptual. It is the method by which the policy can be accomplished. In the context of "policies and procedures," procedures outline the actions contemplated by management when setting the policy and necessary actions to meet the policy requirement. Depending on the scope of the policy, the procedural steps will be more detailed the narrower the scope of the policy.

As an illustrative example, in the case of a policy with regard to required departmental pre-approval of travel, the accompanying procedural scope would be to outline each of the necessary steps in completing the request for travel form (electronic or paper), the routing of the request, and confirmation return of approved travel, and so on. On the other hand, some policies may warrant a more conceptual framework for the outline of steps representing the procedure content. Such an example might be a policy on principal investigators' disclosure of potential conflict of interest. A properly balanced policy and procedure set parallels the scope of the policy with the level of detail contained in the procedures (Fig. 24-2). By contrast, there is potential risk to create confusion by not balancing the scope of the policy with appropriate procedural instructions.

Several different acronyms can represent an organization's set of procedures. You may hear them referred to as standard operating procedures (SOPs), department operating procedures (DOPs), or quality operating procedures (QOPs). In addition, you may find that there are desktop operating procedures or

Table 24-1 Focus Area Policies for a Radiology Practice

Focus Area	Policy and/or Procedures
HIPAA and IT privacy and security	Training requirements for members in your practice; procedures for handling PHI information; disclosure policies between health care entities; IT system protection and archiving requirements
Communication of critical results	Policy guidelines for communicating critical results to referring physician
Clinical indications for specific studies	Policy for appropriateness of examination selection
Techniques used for imaging exams	In addition to individual examination protocols, policies for selecting the correct technique and projections for imaging examinations
Resident and/or trainee involvement in the practice	Policies and procedures for the training of residents or other on-site trainees
Medication review activities	Policy for review of medications before the administration of contrast agents
Professional and technical (or global) billing activities	Policy and procedures for compliant billing practices
Equipment and radiation safety	Policies and procedures for safe operation of equipment and protection of personnel
Infection control requirements	Policy and procedures for maintaining safe practices for infection control requirements
Human resources and personnel activities	Policy and procedures for human resource and personnel management
Financial and accounting controls and standards	Policy and procedures for handling financial transactions; accounting and reporting; asset and inventory management

worklist operating procedures. These all refer to the set of procedures that describe how one fulfills the policy requirement.

Table 24-1 includes broad areas to consider instead of specific policies and procedures that you will want to have within your organization. There are many good resources available that provide real-life examples of an organization's policy and procedure set, related to these broad areas of concern within an organizational structure. Tailoring a set of policies and procedures to the needs of your organization is key to creating a meaningful and effective policy and procedure set.

With these basic foundation definitions, you might be asking the question, why? That is,

what purpose could a set of policies and procedures serve? Table 24-2 offers some potential benefits of devoting the time and effort in creating and maintaining a set of policies and procedures for your practice or department.

DOCUMENTATION RECOMMENDATIONS

There are several excellent resources on constructing a set of policies and procedures. In fact, there are resources that are tailored to specific industries and to health care organizations. In addition, you will find resources devoted to specific functional

417

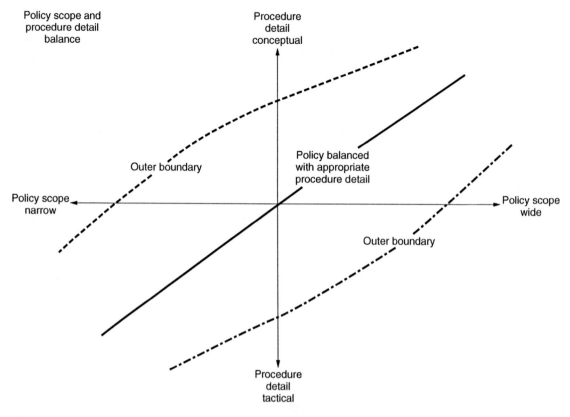

Figure 24-2 Policy scope and procedure detail balance.

aspects within an organization, for example, information technology policies and procedures. It is recommended that you examine several examples and discover the range and possibilities that you want to include in your policies and procedures documents (i.e., template).

In gleaning the resources and adapting these to the experience, this writer always begins a policy and procedure template with the following documentation structure, made up of seven component sections:

1. General policy as it relates to mission/vision/values
2. Background
3. Summary of process
4. Definitions
5. Procedures
6. Guidelines
7. Cross-referenced/other relevant policies and procedures

Depending on the scope of the policy and the complexity of the procedures, it may not be warranted to include all seven sections in the policy

and procedure document. In other cases, where the conceptual framework of the policy is open for varied interpretation and the complexity of the procedures is highly detailed, it may indeed be warranted to include all seven sections in your policy and procedure document. As you review samples from other organizations and develop your own template, you will begin to balance your organizational needs in the structure of the policy and procedure template.

Table 24-3 summarizes each of the seven component sections.

I encourage you to consider various examples of policy and procedure templates within your own organization and from other similar organizations. How do they resonate with your own culture and values? Is the sequence of sections logical? Is there enough information? Here is provided one template that the author has found useful. Practice with this and compare it to others that you glean from other resources. Once you have selected the template, incorporate the same style and consistent format through your entire policy and procedure set. This will add

Table 24-2 Benefits of Instituting Policies and Procedures

Purpose	Benefit
Documenting business processes	Standardization and consistency of administrative support functions
Meet regulatory requirements (local, institutional, national)	Assurance of compliance with local, institutional, or national regulations
Incorporating vision into operations	Reinforcing group mission and vision into daily operational life
Reinforce core values	Opportunity to demonstrate written "proof" of core values of the organization
Sets limits, alternatives, and guidelines	Encourage creativity in developing solutions within specified limits
Sets boundary conditions	Provides explanation, source, and clarity of the limiting conditions; encourages fairness
Quick resolution to misunderstandings	Relieves management of arbitrator role; allows management to focus on facilitator role
Channels actions and decisions along a clear pathway	Provides a systematic approach to decision making
Encourages management by exception	Reserves management involvement to evaluate potential system changes to meet new environmental challenges
Provides consistent and objective decisions	Encourages process fairness within the organization
Limits constant intervention	Allows others to creatively define a solution within a framework; allows management to apply a systematic approach to management
Allows others in organization to make decisions	Encourages all individuals in the organization to make decisions; develops a responsible organizational culture

to the professional appearance of the documents and aid in your audience's reception of the document set.

ENVIRONMENTAL ASSESSMENT

This next section provides a suggested framework for conducting an environmental assessment to determine the best means to optimize your organization's position on the "policy and procedure boundary" presented earlier. The goal of this environmental assessment is to ensure that the policies and procedures that you create and have in place in your organization meet your organizational mission, goals, and values. Remember, this is the reason for having polices and procedures: to align and achieve the organization's vision, mission, and values. To the extent you may find that a particular policy and procedure does not serve such a purpose, you will want to have a process in place for making such a determination and a method for revising or deleting a particular policy and procedure when it no longer serves the primary purpose of your organizational mission, goals, and values.

Table 24-3   Documentation Sections for a Policies and Procedures Template

Section	Description
General policy	This is the statement of the policy (not necessarily a "rule"). Connect to the alignment of larger organizational goals. This section may also include a statement of consequences or sanctions if the policy is not followed.
Background	This section includes an explanation of the larger purpose of the policy, external environmental factors leading to the policy, requirements for institutional compliance (federal or state), and/or organizational intention in creating the policy.
Summary of process	This section summarizes the procedures. It provides an overview of the "process flow" of the procedural steps. It also includes a timeline and sequence reference point for the procedures.
Definitions	This section defines key terminology used in the procedures section. It is useful when there could be varied interpretations of the terminology used in the procedures.
Procedures	This section details the steps required to achieve the policy statement and includes all the details. It is the tactical, action-based section of the document.
Guidelines	This section lists the boundary conditions or other limiting factors that should be considered in carrying out the procedures.
Cross-referenced polices and procedures	This section lists other relevant policies and procedures that reinforce and/or provide additional perspective on the policy and the guidelines.

Your organization's position on this "policy and procedure boundary" is determined by four factors: governing rules, organizational structure, culture and context, and individual and group perceptions. With this in mind, you can optimize the impact of creating policies and procedures that enhance your organization's performance and effective administrative functioning. To this end, below is a step-by-step approach for making an environmental assessment such that you can match your specific organizational needs to the policy and procedure sets in your organization.

Step 1

Make the necessary up-front decision to commit the necessary resources it will take to create the right policies and procedures for your practice.

As is often the case, it is easy to underestimate the necessary resources required to create and maintain a set of policies and procedures. The most important resource is time—the time of your organization's members, your time, and your management team's time. Making a commitment to the necessary creation of new policies and procedures combined with the continuing maintenance of existing policies and procedures is no small undertaking. Usually such activities go to the wayside in the rush of day-to-day issues and challenges. Incorporate your commitment into a routine; develop content experts within your team who review policies and procedures, and amplify this commitment in your communications as a leader of the organization.

Step 2

Investigate the potential benefits of policies and procedures that are critical to the success of your practice and the reception of your policies and procedures among users and providers.

420

Begin this step by asking the question, why have policies and procedures? What benefit will it create for your practice? Will they be aligned with the mission and vision of the practice? This begins to reflect upon your organizational structure and environment and the governing rules inherent in your organization. What is the level of organizational structure that matches your practice's required level of efficiency and effectiveness? What are the unwritten and unspoken rules of behavior? What are the documented undisputable and known truths to all in the organization? As a starting point, you may want to use Table 24-4 to begin the brainstorming.

Step 2 requires some reflection on aspects that may seem obvious. For example, in what phase is your practice currently? Are you in a growth phase or in a stable phase? Into what industry and market niche does your organization fit? Does this apply to your practice? Are there nuances that might be reflected in your mission, vision, and values? Is this uniform across your practice operations? All these and similar questions will help you assess the benefits and appropriateness for creating and implementing a policy and procedure set.

Step 3

Set up cross-functional teams for brainstorming on development of new policies and procedures and for revising existing policies and procedures. (Cross-functional teams might include procedures from different areas within your practice, technical staff, administrative personnel, and other relevant stakeholders.)

In this step you will gather information on the pressures of the culture and the context for individuals and groups in your practice. In addition, in forming the cross-functional

Table 24-4   Evaluation of Reasons for Having Policies and Procedures

Purpose	Appropriate in your practice?	Why or why not?
Need to document business processes		
Meet regulatory requirements (local, institutional, national)		
Incorporate vision into operations		
Reinforce core values		
Set limits, alternatives, and guidelines		
Set boundary conditions		
Need quick resolution to misunderstandings		
Need to channel actions and decisions along a clear pathway		
Encourage management by exception		
Method to provide consistent and objective decisions		
Need to place a limit on constant intervention		
Need to encourage others in organization to make decisions		

teams you will be able to gather information on the level of individual and group perceptions of "right and wrong" behaviors. This will help to define your institutional culture. While focusing the discussions and sessions on policies and procedures, the environmental context for the participants will naturally surface. At the same time you will be able to assess the level of individual and group dynamics with their alignment of organizational goals and objectives. Remember Step 1, and do not be afraid to commit the necessary resources. Use note-taking skills and listening techniques for soliciting process and procedure information from all participants.

Step 4

From the assessments made in Steps 2 and 3, begin drafting a policy and procedure format. Adopt the seven-section documentation format (or other standard template you have created) for assuring standardization and consistency in each policy or procedure document.

Balance what makes sense for the complexity of your operation and your organization. The seven-section documentation format may be too complex for your organization. It may not meet your organizational culture or expectations, as being too formal and limiting. On the other hand, if your organization has had previous experience and familiarity with policies and procedures, the seven-section documentation format may be appropriate for your practice. Bring this discussion forward to your cross-functional teams near the end of their brainstorming process. Always return to the mission of the organization. Are the policies and procedures aligned to the mission and core values of the team? If not, either the policy or the organization will fail.

Step 5

You are ready to begin writing policies and procedures and/or revising existing policies and procedures. As you draft policies and procedures, you may want to keep active a subgroup of your cross-functional teams to help edit and review the initial output, because this will provide a good test of the cultural response to the policy and procedure.

Here are some suggestions to consider as you delve into writing your policies and procedures:

1. Develop a writing style that is easy to read and understand (make your writing gender free and avoid complex jargon). Keep it simple, use action verbs, and be specific. Short and simple statements are best. If you have the resources available, hire a professional writer to set the standard style. The professional can assist by providing helpful tips to the management team responsible for maintaining and revising the policy and procedure set for the practice.

2. Integrate forms management with policies and procedures (nearly all policies and procedures have one or many forms).

3. Coordinate draft policy and procedure reviews using representatives from providers and the management team, from executives, and from other key stakeholders.

4. Institute a consistent policy and procedure numbering system. Format consistently. Establish a numbering system that is easy to reference and modify, if needed.

5. Establish a consistent and clear approval process for finalizing policies.

6. Date it! Develop appropriate chronology tracking for final and subsequent revision dates of the policies and procedures. For example, when procedures are modified, record revision date and archive previous versions. As policies and procedures change, ensure that you have a mechanism in place to document the evolving life of the policies and procedures. There should be a well-defined schedule for review of existing policies on an annual or biannual basis, integrated into the agenda of your policies and procedures committee. Keep it alive, keep it fresh.

7. Use titles and not names in your policy statements and procedures. Revising policies and procedures for the mere sake of updating names will create unnecessary work for your organization.

8. Publish, communicate, train, and mentor your policies and procedures with confidence! Be careful not to underestimate the time and thought required for a communication strategy once you have finalized a policy and procedure or a set of policies and

procedures. The ultimate success and impact of your policy and procedure is directly proportional to the amount of care and nurturing in communication of new policies and/or revisions of existing policies and procedures.

9. Define procedure for implementation, especially for new policies and procedures that may affect current operations. For example, a new policy may drastically affect others in the organization. In such a case, a phased implementation plan may be necessary for the organization to accept and adjust to the new policy and procedure.

With the above pointers in writing your own policies and procedures, plus the outline steps in an environmental assessment of your desired position on the "policy and procedure boundary," do not forget the importance of the commitment and the resources to create the right policies and procedures for your practice. This requires (1) an environmental assessment that functions as a tool to help guide you in determining the right fit for your organization and (2) some highlighted dos and don'ts in crafting your own policies and procedures. In the final section of this chapter we focus on what happens after you have created your own set of policies and procedures for your practice.

THE RESULT

It may be no surprise to you that by replacing the "y" in policy with an "e," you may indeed create something unintended. That is, the successful assessment, creation, and implementation of policies and procedures should not create a police state culture. The basic role of a manager is to develop organizational structures that most effectively channel the human resources to meet the vision and mission of the business organization. The role of the manager is not to police the human resources within the organization but to inspire and lead the enterprise toward optimal performance. The role of the manager is to create value for both customers and employees.

I am reminded of Kaine's curves. On the vertical axis is customer satisfaction, and on the horizontal axis is operational excellence (Fig. 24-3). A compliance-focused organization will underperform on customer satisfaction, though steadily making progress toward operational excellence. A competitive organization will achieve higher customer satisfaction than a compliance-focused organization. An innovative organization will at first achieve the highest customer satisfaction, with low operational excellence, although the innovative organization is best positioned to achieve the highest potential in customer satisfaction and operational excellence. On which of these curves do you envision your own organization and at what point of the curve? Do you want to target a different curve or a different point?

This issue deserves emphasis as the potential downside for an organization layered with policies and procedures and a police mentality for following the rules, a compliance-focused organization. Such a culture may not match your intent of channeling the human resources to meet the vision and mission of the business organization and the optimization of value through customer satisfaction and operational excellence. Do not stifle innovation with restrictive policies and procedures.

On the other hand, if you find that there is a lack of generalized acceptance by the members of the organization of the policies and procedures you have enacted, then some group policing may be necessary (as a collective). This is to be distinguished from individual disobedient behaviors, which should be addressed forthwith. In addition to consistently enforcing your policies and procedures, examine the process of implementing them. Ask yourself the following questions as you consider "process fairness"[1]:

1. How much input did others have in the development process? For example, were opinions requested and given consideration in development of the policies and procedures?

2. How were policy implementation decisions made and procedures implemented? For example: Were they consistent? Based on accurate information? Free of personal biases? Was ample advance notice given?

3. How did managers behave when implementing the policies and procedures? For example, did they explain why? Did they treat others with respect?

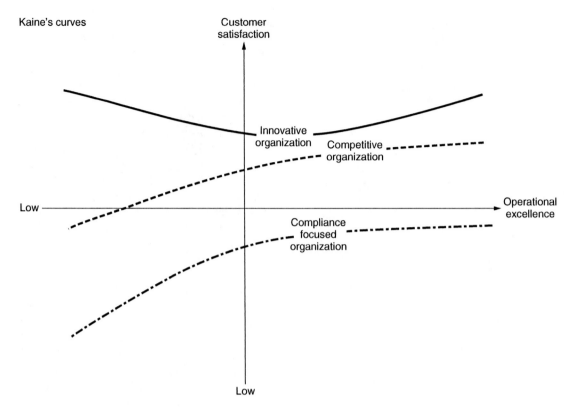

Figure 24-3 Kaine's curves.

Depending on your answers to these questions, you may want to revisit your implementation process. In addition, you may want to incorporate some of these inquiry techniques into your environmental assessment, as appropriate.

With respect to disobedient individual behaviors, once you have established a policy and procedure, it is essential to be consistent with your enforcement and follow-through. If the severity of the infraction warrants disciplinary action, you cannot be afraid of heading into this territory. If not, you risk potential larger compliance infractions and lessen the cultural support of the policies and procedures, as well as the trust in management. The consequences of noncompliance should be added to your policies and procedures manual so that it is explicit and patent to the members of the organization.

You will also want to balance disciplining individual behaviors with the openness to accept that some policies and procedures may be at cross-purposes with your organizational mission, goals, and/or values. To the extent that you have constructed the environmental assessment process in a way that adequately

elicits discussion in your cross-functional teams and that you have taken to heart the tenets of "process fairness," you will create appropriate forums that permit dialogue and thus change to evolve in retaining only those policies and procedures that are truly in support of your mission, goals, and/or values.

In some cases, ultimately, you as the leader of an organization will have to make decisions that may not have adequate consensus. In such cases, to the extent that the members of your organization understand the reasoning associated with your decision, in support of a policy and procedure that may seem to be at cross-purposes with the organizational missions, goals, and/or values, you will engender a culture and context that ultimately support the mission, goals, and/or values of the organization. Remember, in such instances, the focus is not to challenge or change the mission, goal, and/or values of the organization, but to bring them into alignment.

Your policies and procedures should be a living part of your organization. This is not a cookbook that you grab from the shelf during times of need. It should resonate and function within the culture and operations of the practice. You can demonstrate this living nature of your policies and procedures by providing ways that they live up to functional tests, that is, they meet the real needs of your organization's operations and represent your organization's cultural expectations. Incorporate this functional aspect into your management activities; remind people of the relevance of the policies and procedures and their importance in achieving operational excellence and customer satisfaction and furtherance of the organizational mission. As well, do not leave policies and procedures on the shelf, only to be used in times of punitive or corrective actions. Demonstrate how they can be useful in a variety of settings and for a variety of purposes (as outlined in your environmental assessment). The manual can be used as an orientation document for new employees to guide adjustment into the new culture.

To the extent that your policy and procedure set can incorporate self-monitoring activity, the less you will find yourself as a manager becoming a policy enforcer (police officer). An example of a self-monitoring activity is to incorporate into the procedures checks and balances, instead of leaving the authority for the monitoring activity to management. Such a check and balance might be a quarterly or semi-annual report on variations encountered to the procedures or reporting to review panels for policy violations. Incorporating self-monitoring activities into your policies and procedures will also help to reinforce that your policy and procedure set is a living part of your organization and part of the culture of your operations.

Finally, if you consider yourself a start-up company, and many health care ventures and programs can be considered this, take particular caution in considering the possible results of a policy and procedure set in a start-up venture. There are potential downside risks in establishing too many restrictive policies and procedures. At the same time, the risk of failure may be too large without a policy and procedure set for a start-up company, especially in a highly regulated environment. In a start-up there is a delicate balance of devoting enough energy to innovation and high customer satisfaction, while maintaining the minimal required set of

policies and procedures so as to achieve operational excellence. Proceed with an extra commitment to make your environmental assessment a rigorous evaluation of the upside rewards and downside risks of your policy and procedure set within a start-up unit.

In conclusion, this section has demonstrated that the policies and procedures that you implement in your practice compose the institutional roadmap for you to obtain corporate meaning. That is, policies and procedures are a means to an end, in achieving your vision for your practice that will lead and inspire the co-workers in your organization. Your policy set may simply reiterate larger institutional policies, or you may be creating new policies and procedures to enhance your practice operations. In either case, you are creating definition, meaning, and thus the culture of the practice in setting your expectations in how success will evolve. With attention and intention, you can focus the result of your policy and procedure set on that ideal innovative organization, with high customer satisfaction and high operational excellence.

CONCLUSIONS

This chapter serves as a guide on a journey through some familiar and hopefully new territory with respect to a policy and procedure roadmap. We, as members in a global team, form rules that govern the basis of acceptable interactions and processes. From the written laws of the land to the unwritten social norms, human behavior in groups is governed by external forces (governing principles) in combination with individual and group expression of "right and wrong" (moral principles). Groups develop social rules of behavior that impose structure and order, prescribing how individuals act and groups interact. Be it a democracy or a dictatorship, groups of individuals create rules that shape the actions of the people and the outcome or results created by the individuals in a group.

In business organizations, policies and procedures can be that tool set that creates the desired goals in your organization, balancing those external forces and your group's behavior. The basic role of a manager is to develop organizational structures that most effectively channel the human resources to meet the vision, mission, and values of the business organization. It is hoped that policies and procedures will serve as a tool that will enhance your success in your organization. Bon voyage.

Dos and Don'ts of Policies and Procedures	
Dos	**Don'ts**
1. Align policies to mission and goals of your practice.	1. Use policies as a substitute for good management.
2. Use policies and procedures to organize and direct human resources.	2. Forget the culture and context of your practice when formulating policies.
3. Match the stage of your practice to the need for formal structures.	3. Overlay policies and procedures where you expect entrepreneurial behaviors.
4. Use an environmental assessment to build consensus around policies.	4. Silently implement new policies and procedures.
5. Talk about policies.	5. Underestimate the role of implementation and communication.
6. Commit the necessary resources, primarily time.	6. Use names in your policies when referencing positions.
7. Be consistent and clear.	7. Forget what your practice considers fair.
8. Integrate forms management into your procedures.	8. Let your policies and procedures demoralize human resources.
9. Incorporate self-monitoring systems into your procedures.	9. Forget to date your policies.
10. Consider your policies and procedures a living document.	10. Consider your policies and procedures as a cookbook on the shelf.

REFERENCE

1. Brockner J: Why it's so hard to be fair. Harvard Business Review, March:122–129, 2006.

CHAPTER 25

DELINEATION OF PRIVILEGES FORM... NOT!

Delineation of Privileges
Dept of Radiology

	Seen one?	Done one?	Recommended by chair
			✓
Chest X-ray	✓	✓	✓
Mammo	✓	✓	✓
Body CT	✓	✓	✓
Neuro CT	✓	✓	✓
Body Angio	✓	✓	✓
Neuro Angio	✓	✓	✓
Embolization	✓	✓	✓
RF Ablation	✓	✓	✓
Brain Surgery	✓	✓	✓
Brain Transplant	✓	✓	

Name: Dr. Frankenstein
Signature: ___×___

Chair: Mary Shelley
Signature: _mmm~_

Credentialing and Certification

David M. Yousem

Most people view the task of credentialing and certification of physicians as one of the bureaucratic boondoggles that torment the operations of a department. Although these processes are tedious, they are mandated by government and specialty boards uniformly and therefore *must* have some redeeming value, right? Truthfully, the need for credentialing and certification of physicians has, if anything, gained greater importance as society looks to physicians to police themselves in the hopes of improving patient care and guaranteeing patient safety. Intermittently a legislator will raise the specter of a governmental agency providing the review of physician credentials, ethics, and practice standards instead of allowing self-regulation. The more effectively we carry out these processes, the less likely it is that we will lose the privilege of self-regulation.

CREDENTIALING

Credentialing can be defined as "the systematic approach to the collection, review and verification of a practitioner's professional qualifications."[1,2] The goal is to assess and approve for practice the competent and qualified individuals to care for patients at the institution. Credentialing is centered on patient care: is this physician competent and qualified for the patient care duties requested in his or her delineation of privileges? Cassel and Holmboe state that "the practices and standards used in identifying physicians for health plan panels and for hospital privileges ... are the only easily available and widely trusted screens of physicians that are available to patients."[3] Although the central purpose of credentialing and certification addresses these needs of the patients, there are other political roles that the processes may also fulfill that are specific to radiology "turf" issues (see below).

Specific Roles

To safeguard the consumer, the credentialing and privileging committee verifies that:

1. Health care providers are current in licensing, prescribing, and certification.

2. Health care providers have received the necessary education to mitigate risk.
3. Health care providers have not been shown to be incompetent.
4. Health care providers are not impaired by substance abuse.
5. Health care providers meet standards of practice.

Composition

The credentialing committee is made up of physician leaders from various departments, nurse leaders, representatives from the legal office of the institution, and administrative support people. The functions of the credentialing committee include both credentialing of new physicians and re-credentialing of individuals who are already members of the institution's faculty. This committee usually meets on a monthly basis to review the candidates for initial appointments and reappointment purposes. There are often more frequent meetings in the May through August time frame, despite summer breaks, because of the massive influx of physicians every July 1 to residency and fellowship programs. There is also an ever-increasing group of physician extenders, including nurse practitioners, nursing assistants, and physician assistants who undergo the same amount of scrutiny because of their frequent involvement in direct patient care. Representation from these provider groups is useful to the composition of the credentialing committee.

The Process

The credential process is mandated by the Joint Commission on Accreditation of Healthcare Organizations (JCAHO)—newly named "The Joint Commission" as of 8 January 2007—and is, when properly performed, critical to maintaining high-quality care within a medical institution. The credentialing committee sets guidelines for minimum requirements of competency by physicians and permits physicians to perform these professional activities at the governing body's facilities. Reviews for credentialed health care workers must be performed every 2 years.

The process begins with a review of the providers' licenses, past and present. Does the

physician have a valid confirmed license in the state for which he wants to practice, and what is the status of licensure in other states? Collating these state licenses may be an arduous task for teleradiology nighthawk services, because each state's licenses may require renewal at different months of the year and at different intervals. In most practices where patient sedation must be administered a current federal Drug Enforcement Agency number and state-specific drug dispensing license must also be current.

Next comes the biographical history of the candidate from the standpoint of training and education. Any gaps in the chronologic story in the person's career are scrutinized carefully to assure that these gaps were not related to untoward events or situations, such as psychologic or alcoholic treatment, which would raise a warning concerning possible on-going substance abuse or criminal history-related problems. Did the health care provider finish a residency or fellowship in the field in which he or she is wishing to practice? If not, is that appropriate? We recently had to make that decision about an internist who had done 2 years of research in the field of dermatology but never completed a medical residency or a dermatology residency. That physician wanted to practice dermatology and perform dermatologic surgical procedures analogous to those done during the research years. Although it is true that this physician had a medical license and some unique background in dermatologic disease, should the person be credentialed to perform punch biopsies on children's faces? The days of physicians being able to hang a shingle in the country town and practice medicine without formal residency training and supervision are (hopefully) soon to be ancient history. By the same token, board eligibility without board certification remains a "passing" grade at the credentialing committee discussions. In fact, some older physicians may never have passed boards and are still active members of academic medical centers, because board certification, at the time of initial appointment, was never a requirement. Some specialties did not even have boards until very recently. Did Roentgen pass his boards? On the contrary.

The credentialing process also includes a national screening for malpractice suits or

BOX 25-1

NPDB Data Collected

1. Malpractice payments paid on behalf of individuals
   - Not groups or hospitals
2. Restrictions of privileges
   - Not administrative sanctions
   - Not voluntary restrictions of practice
   - Not censures, reprimands, or admonishments
   - Not chemical dependency issues
3. Professional society adverse actions against members
4. Licensure actions taken by state boards

Adapted from West RW, Sipe CY: National practitioner data bank: information on physicians. J Am Coll Radiol 1: 777–779, 2004.

occasions when services were denied to the physician. All questions to which the applicant responds affirmatively regarding any suspension or limitation of licenses or privileges require lengthy descriptions by the candidate about the circumstances surrounding them. The credentialing committee serves as the watchdog for the patient's safety. The Health Care Quality Improvement Act of 1986 established the National Practitioner Data Bank.[4] The NPDB, managed by Unisys, is often referred to during credentialing and certification as a central repository of information relevant to the assessment of the competence of health care providers. The data that are included in the NPDB are listed in Box 25-1.

The NPDB is a confidential source of data not open to the public but available for all credentialing bodies within hospitals. In fact, there is a requirement in the Health Care Quality Improvement Act (HCQIA) that hospitals query every physician on staff at 2-year intervals when renewing privileges. Plaintiff's attorneys who file malpractice suits against health care entities also have access to the database. Managed care organizations, health care entities, and health care societies may have free access to the NPDB files. Individuals may also check out the data pertaining to themselves.

Letters of recommendation with corroboration of training periods are also solicited, usually by the candidate and occasionally by the credentialing board (see sample letter in Appendix 25-1). In most institutions any grade less than good or excellent requires an accompanying explanation.

The physician, in conjunction with the department's own credentialing committee, will submit a delineation of privileges (DOP) form. This is usually a checklist of procedures that the physician feels competent to or would like to perform while appointed to the hospital. There has been a shift in process in review of DOP lists over the past few years, in that criteria for demonstration of competence with the procedures requested is now being required. Previously a physician merely had to check off the box of the procedure he or she wished to perform without providing details such as number of times that procedure was performed in the past, complication rate, and certification of competency by a peer group or subspecialty/specialty board. This request would also have to be approved by the department chairman responsible for the physician and then by the hospital's credentialing committee. Peer review (i.e., assessment of competence) was accomplished predominantly through evaluations and letters of recommendation requested from references.

More recently a minimum number of procedures performed in the recent past (usually 2 years) and/or lifetime is often specified on the DOP form. With regard to radiologists this is very important for individuals who have undergone subspecialty fellowship training. For an individual undergoing a 2-year subspecialty training in neuroradiology or interventional radiology there is a chance that he or she will have performed no barium enemas, upper gastrointestinal series, voiding urograms, or venous ultrasound studies during that 2-year period. This may lead to a hiccup at the credentialing stage when the person is applying for privileges for his or her general radiology private practice community hospital. It is for this reason that some departments recommend also having a lifetime experience criterion on the DOP available, because the experience of prior residency or practice greater than 2 years previously should also count toward competency. If you have read 10,000 chest radiographs in residency but none during the 2-year neuroradiology fellowship, you still would be worthy of being credentialed for that procedure.

Sometimes, however, it becomes the chair's judgment call and that of the credentialing committee whether that individual should be proctored or overseen when performing studies that he or she has not performed over the past 2 years. Should an interventional radiologist who has not performed a myelogram in 6 years be privileged for such upon his third reappointment? In most cases most members of the credentialing committee will accept the chair's judgment; however, the higher the risk of the procedure, the tougher the committee will be with regard to safeguarding the patient.

If a health care organization determines that a privilege request must be denied or current privileges restricted in some way, the physician or credentialed staff member will have to account for such circumstances throughout his or her professional career. This is one of the many standard questions asked by credentialing committees:

"Have you ever had your privileges denied or restricted in your lifetime?"

Often individuals are counseled about the department or hospital's requirements, and they may thus inadvertently request privileges that will not be recommended during the credentialing process. Once again, because of this large impact on the bureaucracy of hospital privileges for the rest of your life, it is advisable to not request a privilege if it is borderline within your competency or experience during the recent past. You may have that procedure denied. Ideally, applicants for privileges should discuss privileging requests with their peer department's leadership to circumvent such problems. By the same token, the credentialing committee recognizes its exposure in potentially denying someone's privileges. Theoretically a physician could file suit if the committee's decision has a lifelong severe effect on his or her career. More importantly though, credentials committees are keenly aware of the effect of their decisions, both on patient care and on health care professionals, and privileging concerns are often easily and amicably resolved. At the same time, a hospital can be held liable if it does not disclose a physician's proven or suspected drug impairment to other institutions. Most institutions do not disclose their "suspicions" of drug impairment unless a formal investigation and due process have occurred.

Many physicians will resign their privileges before undergoing a hospital-based investigation, because the latter may lead to a National Practitioner Data Bank report on the hearing.

There is a role for the credentialing committee removing or curtailing privileges of someone who is currently performing them but is exhibiting concerning behaviors or having untoward complications or quality-of-care issues. This is usually a result of bad outcomes or inappropriate behavior or concern for patients' safety. In one institution's experience, a patient who had a contrast dye allergy received an injection of carbon dioxide by a vascular surgeon to visualize the carotid arteries. The patient developed a stroke in the hemisphere of the injected carotid circulation. When the radiology department was surveyed about their experience with carbon dioxide injections, there was an absence of experience even among the most elderly radiology personnel. The vascular surgeon could not justify the use of the carbon dioxide. The privilege to perform carotid arteriography was withdrawn, and a thorough investigation ensued about the physician's success and complication rate overall. Formal investigations and hearings are governed by institutional bylaws and are usually conducted under the auspices of a legal department or hired counsel. Sanctions may ensue, and the credentials committee is responsible for overseeing the implementation of any monitoring or corrective action plan. Often, practitioners subject to such sanctions choose to leave the given health care institution.

In 2006 JCAHO proposed that the 2007 standards for privileging and credentialing be based on performance data gathered each year. Data-based systems for credentialing are the wave of the future, riding on the heels of maintenance of certification (MOC) requirements. These data systems will need to adjust for the complexity and acuity of cases performed in hospital settings as well as industry standards, the setting of baseline targets, and outcomes assessment. The catchwords for 2007 include "focused professional practice evaluation and ongoing professional practice evaluation." In short, the privileging process will require initial and ongoing evaluations of applicants for their specific privileges. The credentialing process will become more driven by data and by patient safety. Privileges are granted for no more than 2 years at a time, and this means that the credentialing committee will have to find ways to accommodate the additional time required to assess ongoing privilege performance as well as continuing to assess the competence of new practitioners entering the hospital. In some cases this will require two committees: one to evaluate new hires and the other for continuing re-credentialing. JCAHO's 2007 goals also include a requirement to assess a practitioner's interpersonal and communication skills, and professional conduct. Similar to the core competencies of the Accreditation Council for Graduate Medical Education (ACGME), credentialing will therefore require written information and assessments on (1) medical knowledge, (2) technical skills, (3) clinical judgment, (4) interpersonal skills, (5) communication, and (6) professionalism.

Data-driven credentialing documentation for the six core competencies has already circulated through the ACGME and American Board of Medical Specialties (ABMS). Credentialing committees will have to develop quantitative criteria for evaluating these traits as in Table 25-1.

By 2008 JCAHO is asking that hospitals assess their staff physician competency using a Focused Professional Practice Evaluation that includes gathering data from previous and current practice from peers or supervisors.

Table 25-1 Core Competencies and Assessment

Competency	Assessment
Medical knowledge	Maintenance of certification, self-assessment modules, CME credits
Technical and clinical skills	Peer review, outcomes measures
Clinical judgment	Outcomes measures, malpractice history
Interpersonal skills	360-degree evaluation
Communication skills	360-degree evaluation, peer review
Professionalism	Licensure, complaints

Who Needs to Be Credentialed?

All practicing physicians, nurse practitioners, and physician trainees must be credentialed. Residents that rotate to community hospitals must be credentialed to provide care under the supervision of licensed independent practitioners through an affiliation agreement with their sponsoring university program. Affiliation agreements with the community hospitals must define the degree of supervision that the resident will require, the patient care responsibilities at the various levels of training during the residency, as well as insurance information.

The requirements for participating as a licensed independent practitioner for a credentialed training program are listed in the JCAHO document MS.2.30 as stated below.

Elements of Performance for MS.2.30

1. The organized medical staff has a defined process for supervision by a licensed independent practitioner with appropriate clinical privileges of each participant in the program in carrying out patient care responsibilities.
2. Written descriptions of the roles, responsibilities, and patient care activities of the participants of graduate educational programs are provided to the organized medial staff and hospital staff.
3. The descriptions include identification of mechanisms by which the supervisor(s) and graduate education program director make decisions about each participant's progressive involvement and independence in specific patient care activities.
4. Organized medical staff rules and regulations and policies delineate participants in professional education programs who may write patient care orders, the circumstances under which they may do so (without prohibiting licensed independent practitioners from writing orders), and what entities, if any, must be countersigned by a supervising licensed independent practitioner.
5. There is a mechanism and responsibility for effective communication (whether training occurs at the organization that is responsible for the professional graduate education program or in a participating local or community organization or hospital).

6. The professional graduate medical education committee(s) (GMECs) must communicate with the medical staff and governing body about the safety and quality of patient care, treatment, and services provided by, and the related educational and supervisory needs of, the participants in professional graduate education programs.

 If the graduate medical education program uses a community or local participating hospital or organization, the person(s) responsible for overseeing the participants from the program communicates to the organized medical staff and its governing body about the patient and supervisory needs of its participants in the professional graduate education programs.

7. There is a mechanism for an appropriate person from the community or local hospital or organization to communicate information to the GMEC about the quality of care, treatment, and services and educational needs of the participants.

8. Information about the quality of care, treatment, and services and educational needs is included in the communication that the GMEC has with the governing board of the sponsoring organization.

9. Medical staff demonstrates compliance with residency review committee citations.

Note that graduate medical education programs accredited by the ACGME, the American Osteopathic Association (AOA), or the American Dental Association's Commission on Dental Accreditation are expected to be in compliance with the above requirements; the hospital should be able to demonstrate compliance with any residency review committee citations related to this standard.

Credentialing Politics

It is the opinion of these authors that having guidelines in the number of procedures performed is a very useful exercise in the credentialing of physicians. Certainly if someone is requesting privileges for a procedure that they have never performed or for which they have had limited experience it would seem logical from a patient safety perspective that an individual will be counseled to withdraw that privilege or at the very least be monitored

432

during the initial performance of those studies. This should not be viewed as a punitive step but merely as a quality assurance step that serves to enhance patient care.

Many of the turf battle issues between radiology departments and other clinical departments may devolve into a battle at the hospital credentialing/privileging committee.[5] The minimum threshold volume of cases needed to be completed for credentialing that are set up by the radiology department can be equitably applied to nonradiologists who wish to perform radiologic procedures without the accusation of creating a "guild culture." If these thresholds are applied fairly then only qualified individuals will be performing imaging studies including interventional procedures. Thus, the establishment of the procedural numbers should not be arbitrary but instead should be created in a fashion that ensures patients' safety, appropriately restricts inadequately trained individuals who may harm patients, and assures that the specialty of radiology is appropriately maintained without unfairly closing the doors to nonradiologists performing imaging procedures. A sample of the credentialing form from the Radiology Department of the Johns Hopkins Medical Institution is demonstrated in Appendix 25-1.

Let's take the example of the neurologist who wants to read magnetic resonance imaging scans of the brain. If you have a DOP form that states that anyone interpreting this study must (1) be fellowship trained in an ACGME-approved neuroradiology program, (2) have interpreted 2000 studies in the past 2 years with an error rate upon peer review of less than 3%, (3) have passed the online hospital magnetic resonance safety module, and (4) have averaged 50 continuing medical education credits in neuroradiology over one's career, you will probably not have turf issues with this individual. Keep in mind, however, that your own people must also meet the high standards you set on your DOP form; otherwise the hypocrisy will reflect poorly on the radiology department and its staff, or worse yet, lead to a legal suit. Remember also that if you have an emergency radiology division that must interpret all cases at night, they too may be restricted in their capacity to officially interpret the same studies.

Allowing nonradiologist physicians in performing activities historically done by radiology professionals can be appropriate when the physician is patient focused, well trained, collaborative, and committed to the success of the entire practice. Unfortunately, this is not the only circumstance where this occurs. At hospitals where the radiology department is politically weak or there are no interventional radiologists to perform said procedures, the likelihood that nonradiologists will be in the catheter laboratories performing peripheral and carotid arteriograms and angioplasties is very high. Furthermore, if no radiologists are present on the credentialing committee it is almost inevitable that watered-down criteria for credentialing may be passed or criteria may even not exist. The radiology advocates must be very careful to scrutinize all the accumulated procedure statements to ensure that radiology procedures are not lost and, at the same time, advocate for reasonable criteria for assessing whether an individual is qualified to perform those procedures.

Besides serving as a battleground for multiple specialties seeking the same patient population, credentialing is a potential source for delays in getting physicians up and running within a radiology practice. At our institution, the typical credentialing procedure lasts between 4 and 6 months. This means that individuals hoping to start on the usual academic year of 1 July 2007 will require beginning the credentialing period in the first quarter of 2007 and certainly before 31 March. If an individual cannot be credentialed in time, then often the practice has to pay that person's salary at a time when they cannot generate revenue at the inpatient facility. You could simply send this person to an outpatient environment and wait for the documentation and approval to be certified, or you could allow the person temporary privileges during the interval between submission of the paperwork and the formal approval by the credentialing committee. For a hospital-based practice, having someone on the payroll who cannot read or perform procedures is obviously a huge deficit to the practice, and some contracts' starting date may be contingent upon obtaining credentials for procedures at the inpatient facility. Many of the teleradiology groups that are providing night call preliminary reports spend an enormous amount of effort in obtaining out-of-state privileges for their remote

facilities. A good credentialing office and office management team can positively affect the financial picture by doing an expeditious job at credentialing.

Core versus Non-Core Privileges

Many departments are beginning to establish privileges that include core practices versus non-core practices. With respect to community hospital general radiologists, core practices may include the performance of fluoroscopic procedures and the interpretation of cross-sectional imaging studies. Simple interventional procedures such as X-ray–guided lumbar puncture or aspiration cytology may also be included in these core privileges.

Non-core privileges may be separated into such specialized procedures as the performance of angiographic or biliary procedures, mammography, nuclear medicine studies, and other invasive therapeutic interventions such as angioplasty, stenting, and ablation procedures.

The advantage of having a set of core privileges is that it streamlines the credentialing procedure and also defines the basis for what makes a radiologist. Any well-trained physician completing a radiology residency should be competent to perform the core procedures. Core privileges may be derived from the graduate medical education directory of the core curriculum for residency programs in radiology.

Most non-core privileges are ones that require additional training or education beyond residency. Nonetheless, particularly for a community hospital–based practice, many neuroradiology and pediatric radiology procedures fall within core privileges. Such is generally not the case, however, for angiographic, biliary, renal, and other visceral invasive procedures. High-risk procedures also are included in non-core privileges. Procedures requiring specialized equipment may also reside in the non-core grouping.

CERTIFICATION

Definition
....

Certification is a process by which physicians are tested and assessed for competence by members of their own specialty. Physicians are policing themselves with increasing frequency and, at the same time, mandating recertification. Some hospitals do not mandate that physicians have been certified and/or have passed their board examinations. This may be for the sake of expediency; alternatively, in some specialties the physicians must have several years of experience in practice before they can even take their board examinations. This is not yet the case for general radiology but does pertain to some subspecialties, including neuroradiology, where a year of practice in the field after fellowship is required before being able to take the neuroradiology examination for subspecialty qualification. Many health plans also do not require subspecialty board certification at initial credentialing, and fewer than half require it at any time.[1,2] Only half of hospitals require recertification as part of their privileging procedures, with almost 70% allowing physicians to retain their privileges even after their time-limited certificate expires.

Since 2002 the 24 member boards of the ABMS have agreed to time-limited maintenance of certification (MOC) requirements and continuing performance assessments. The MOC process requires a knowledge examination, but the ABMS has acknowledged that knowledge is not enough and that the outcomes of patients under the care of physicians should also be interrogated. The physician clinical performance assessment has become popular of late and requires a quantitative assessment based on the outcomes of patient care, patient satisfaction surveys, and the rates at which physicians follow guidelines on the delivery of care determined by evidence-based medicine.

Part of the MOC process in radiology includes the completion of 20 self-assessment modules (SAMs) in the areas of one's core practice (especially if one holds a subspecialty certificate) and 250 category 1 continuing medical education (CME) credit hours over a 10-year period. SAMs are designed to assess an individual's knowledge base and to guide him or her in further continuing self-education in the areas in which there may be weaknesses. Some of the SAMs must be on generic issues in radiology, including radiation safety and other basic patient care issues even for subspecialist radiologists.

The American Board of Radiology (ABR) has embraced the MOC process wholeheartedly with statements such as "Over the next ten years, ABR-MOC will continue to develop into a comprehensive vehicle through which all diplomates can ensure the public and the radiologic community that they are incorporating new information into their practices, thereby delivering excellence in care."

MOC Process

The MOC process really consists of four parts:

Part One: Professional Standing Maintain active unrestricted licenses for all states in which you practice. The ABR will perform spot checks of MOC candidates to make sure licensure is current and will verify all licenses at the time of MOC or initial certification examinations.

Part Two: Lifelong Learning and Self-assessment At least 250 CME credit hours, approved by the Accreditation Council for Continuing Medical Education, are required over the 10-year cycle in Category 1. Some of these hours can include additional specialty-specific material or more general topics such as radiation safety, radiation exposure, informed consent, risk management, ethics, statistics, or quality improvement.

The self-assessment requirement may be satisfied by completing 20 SAMs over 10 years, each of which has been approved by the ABR. These will also be in specialty-specific areas predominantly. A maximum of four SAMs can be performed in a single year.

Part Three: Cognitive Expertise This is the MOC test that is offered during the final 3 years of the 10-year MOC cycle and tests core knowledge in general or subspecialty radiology depending on your initial certificate. The examination includes both general content (20%) and clinical content related to the SAMs taken and practice profile of the registrant (80%). Individualized testing depending on the breakdown of practice composition is planned.

Part Four: Assessment of Performance in Practice The ABR's Practice Quality Improvement program has defined five categories of PQI projects: (1) patient safety, (2) accuracy of interpretation, (3) report turnaround time, (4) practice guidelines and technical standards, and (5) referring physician surveys. Each diagnostic radiologist must complete a project in one of these categories. Most people are working on report turnaround time as the lowest-hanging fruit for now. (Box 25-2 shows the timeline provided by the ABR website.)

Not all credentialing boards have embraced the idea of MOC as a requisite to maintaining practice privileges at their hospitals. However, the expectation is such that recertification may become a standard by which physicians are

---

BOX 25-2

PQI Timeline and Milestone Tracking—Diagnostic Radiology Diplomates

Year of Cycle	What I Must Do Each Year of the 10-Year MOC Cycle	Submit Report/Attestation via the Personal Web Page
1	☐ Learn about PQI process ☐ Select project and metric(s)	Yes
2	☐ Collect baseline data	Yes
3	☐ Analyze the data ☐ Work on improvement plan	Yes
4	☐ Collect data, compare to initial data, summarize results	Yes
5	☐ Modify improvement plan ☐ Implement plan	Yes
6	☐ Collect improvement plan data ☐ If goals achieved, select additional PQI project	Yes
7	☐ Refine improvement plan ☐ Implement plan	Yes
8	☐ Collect improvement plan data	Yes
9	☐ Complete collection of improvement plan data ☐ Analyze data ☐ Summarize data	Yes
10	☐ Prepare a final report of results and conclusions ☐ Sustain the gain of first cycle ☐ Select topic for next cycle	Yes

Notes:
- Projects may be done as part of a practice group, department, institution, or society. Projects may also be done by individuals.
- Outliers in terms of participation may be contacted to produce documentation of participation.
- Diplomates may change project topic if data analysis shows that time may be better spent in improving another area.

From http://www.theabr.org/NEURO_MOC_Req.htm.

---

judged for competency. In the past, just being "board eligible" was one criterion. Now passing the examination tests may become the new bar. In a study by Freed et al[2] of pediatricians being credentialed, 90% of 193 health plans did NOT require general pediatricians to be board certified to be initially credentialed; however, 41% required certification at some point after the initial credentialing. Interestingly, 93% did require successful completion of a pediatrics residency. Among these health plans, 61% had no time frame by which recertification had to be achieved; only 40% required pediatric subspecialty certification at some point after or at the time of credentialing, but 86% require fellowship training. Again just 42% require recertification within a time-specified domain—that is, after initial certification has expired.[1,2]

THE POLITICS OF CREDENTIALING AND RECERTIFICATION

To reiterate, the ABMS is instituting a relatively aggressive and far-reaching policy with respect to certification and recertification of medical specialists. Whereas previously certification was for a lifetime, now that process has limited time frames. For those individuals who are in subspecialties of radiology and who completed their general residency before 2000, the term limit of their subspecialization certification is 10 years; however, their general radiology certification will continue to be timeless. However, for those individuals who have received their ABR general diagnostic radiology certification after 2000, there is a requirement for recertification even for the general radiology knowledge every 10 years. In addition, those individuals who have subspecialty training in radiology for which there are certificates of subspecialty certification (neuroradiology, interventional radiology, pediatric radiology, nuclear medicine), recertification of the subspecialty is also required every 10 years. Therefore, since the certificates of adequate qualifications (CAQs) began in 1994–1995, even those individuals who took their recertification before 2000 in their subspecialty will have to undergo recertification at 10-year intervals.

When the CAQs were initially instituted in 1994 and 1995, part of the justification for pursuing this process was to maintain influence within these subspecialties. Therefore, relatively strict criteria for requisite training before taking the CAQ examinations were created. These required 1 year of educational fellowship training within the subspecialty followed by 1 year (at least) of practice in that one subspecialty in which greater than 50% of the active practice was within that area. Of course, there were grandfather causes for those individuals whose practice consisted of more than 50% in one subspecialty, yet who had never completed fellowship training before 1995. However, the grace period for grandfathering in individuals who had not received full fellowship training has expired, and a fellowship training year in the subspecialty is now required.

The idea was that establishment of a subspecialty certificate of added qualification would lead insurers and payers to demand or require that those subspecialty studies be performed or interpreted by individuals with CAQ certification. In point of fact, the CAQ system has done little to secure turf for radiologists, and it has not strengthened the radiologist's position with respect to things such as medicolegal cases and their expertise. Although it is used in part by lawyers to establish the "medical expert" designation of their individual expert witness, it has not had an impact with respect to the performance and interpretation of imaging studies by general radiologists or nonradiologists. In fact, the general radiologists took umbrage with the notion that they would be restricted from interpreting subspecialty-imaging studies if they did not have these CAQ certifications in that subspecialty. Because the vast majority of radiologists read all types of studies even outside the field in which they may be subspecialty trained, the constituency support for providing the recertification system with more stringent criteria has been lukewarm. This lukewarm support within the ranks has also led to the weakening of its impact with respect to nonradiologists.

Therefore, even though the interventional radiology certificate for added qualification refers to and establishes expertise in the interpretation and performance of vascular imaging in regard to catheter techniques in arteriography, it has not had an impact in preventing vascular surgeons or cardiologists from also performing peripheral vascular or carotid vascular studies. These subspecialties have simply added those studies to their list of procedures required for certification as cardiologists or peripheral vascular surgeons.

It would seem natural that the certification system would prevent overlap of multiple specialties of performing the same studies; however, this has not been the case. Perhaps the precedents had been set by the policies regarding ultrasound with respect to obstetricians and gynecologists and radiologists performing these studies. This battle was lost decades ago.

In a similar vein, it's well known that chest radiographs, orthopedic radiographs, and intravenous urograms are being performed in nonradiologist offices throughout the country, with reimbursement for the interpretation and performance of that study. Strict laws against self-referral have not been evenly applied to all patients and all insurers, often being applied only to government programs under the auspices of the Center for Medicare and Medicaid Services (CMS). It has been interesting to see the publications coming from advocates such as Dr. David Levin showing the much higher number of imaging studies done by nonradiologists as compared with radiologists. This explosion of imaging studies driven by nonradiologist self-referral is one of the reasons that imaging is certainly in the cross hairs of the CMS policy goal to restrict the continued growth of medical care costs. Preauthorization and utilization review with practice guidelines is becoming more widely implemented and controlled by the payers.

The failure of the certification process by the ABR to preserve turf in radiology has led to a shift of the focus to local hospital credentialing committees for preservation of procedure volume. At our institution, the interventional radiology group met with the chief of surgery and vascular surgery to create credentialing guidelines that would apply to vascular surgeons, cardiologists, and radiologists alike. These discussions resulted in a DOP document that specifies the number of different catheter procedures that are required for credentialing at the institution and for maintenance of those credentials in the future. The hope was that these guidelines would ensure patient safety and optimize patient care while maintaining the integrity of the vascular interventional radiology service.

RISK MANAGEMENT AND OVERSIGHT

Some hospitals and practices are performing unannounced audits of their credentialing documents, similar to those performed by JCAHO. Many programs have standardized 100% audits; that is, every file is audited on a quarterly, semiannual, or annual cycle. Through these audits, reviewers have identified annual tuberculosis testing, CME documentation, basic cardiac life support and advanced cardiac life support certification, conscious sedation training, and risk management seminar attendance as the weakest areas of credentialing and reappointment compliance. Making sure all documents are signed and peer references are provided for all appointments is also part of the checklist for compliance. Outside audits may also be used in some institutions.

States hold hospitals accountable for their credentialing procedures, and there have been legal suits naming hospitals, the medical staff officers, committee members, and directors in cases where an unfit or unqualified individual was practicing medicine at a hospital. Accusations of negligent credentialing and/or corporate negligence by hospitals can be separated into various causes as noted in Table 25-2.

Remember that the number of patient complaints that a physician receives is a significant determinant of the relative risk of being sued. These complaints must be investigated closely by the credentialing and recredentialing process. Physician peers that review and discuss the complaints are more effective than administrators at helping practitioners learn from complaints and improve, as appropriate, when complaints are validated.

SITE ACCREDITATION AND PRIVILEGING

The main reasons for site accreditation and privileging rules are to guarantee patient safety, ensure high-quality care, and avoid inappropriate self-referrals. Levin[5] and others have shown in numerous publications that the quality of the imaging suffers while the quantity

Table 25-2 Accusations of Negligent Credentialing and/or Corporate Negligence by Hospitals Separated into Various Causes

Title	Explanation	Remediation
Poor documentation	Approval date and practice dates don't correspond Prolonged temporary credentials Failure to review and reappoint Failure to document training for privileges requested	Good accounting Follow rules to the letter Oversight Expedite only clean records through recredentialing
Failure to follow up on complaints	No action taken after a patient/colleague complaint Failure to follow own procedures	Careful oversight Keep cases on the books for review until completed
Failure to verify basic requirements	Inaccurate data given to credentialing committee and committee doesn't figure it out Malpractice lapses	Must verify all data submitted on forms by third parties National oversight groups JCAHO requires review of 2 years of prior claims
Inadequate review of red flags	Failure to address issues raised	Must review all complaints Detect any patterns Verify information with insurance carriers Request depositions Include lawyers on credentialing committees
Poor oversight and supervision	Failure to mentor physicians in need	Develop confidential mentoring program

From Medical Staff Briefing, June 2006.

of imaging soars in an environment of self-referral, which consequently may lead to an excessive burden on health care costs for our nation.

The privileging programs developed by commercial health plans allow limited ability for nonradiologists to review imaging studies. Hence obstetricians reviewing obstetric ultrasounds and orthopodists reviewing plain radiograms have limited privileges to perform and bill for such work.

ACR site accreditation committees establish protocols and guidelines for facilities that must be met to ensure good-quality imaging that is in a safe environment for the patients. ACR accreditation of sites is a process that many imaging sites both inside and outside hospitals engage in for many of their modalities. Levin

et al[5] report that 18% of facilities that performed imaging studies dropped out of the site accreditation program and therefore could not bill Pennsylvania Blue Shield when asked to fill out a site survey. Among the facilities that filled out the survey, 5% failed the survey and/or image quality review and were dropped. An additional 2% never filled it out and were dropped. The pass rates for a similar review in Massachusetts are recorded in Table 25-3.

Another quality assurance program found that of 92 *nonradiologists'* offices that performed imaging studies, 78% had a major deficiency in one area of image quality, film storage and handling, patient identification, right-left marker usage, and availability of written reports. Nearly 20% either had not been inspected in the previous 12 months by service engineers or had failed

Table 25-3 Blue Shield of Massachusetts Accreditation Survey	
Pass Rate	Specialty
95%	Radiologists, cardiologists
75% to 83%	Obstetricians, orthopedic surgeons
<62%	Internists, chiropractors, podiatrists
17.9%	Refused to participate

Table 25-4 Typical Privileging Afforded by Many Payers to Non-radiologists	
Specialty	Privileges Granted
Cardiology	Nuclear cardiology, echocardiography, chest radiographs
Pulmonary medicine	Chest radiographs
OB-GYN	Fetal and gynecologic ultrasound
Orthopedic surgery	Musculoskeletal radiographs
Otolaryngology	Sinus radiographs
Podiatry	Foot radiographs
Rheumatology	Extremity radiographs
Primary care	Chest, rib, extremity radiographs

to remedy issues with the machinery recommended by those inspectors.

Typical privileging afforded by many payers to nonradiologists is listed in Table 25-4.

CONCLUSIONS

Credentialing and certification may seem a mundane bureaucratic exercise, but the processes are there to ensure quality patient care and compliance with regulatory entities. Radiology practices that excel at monitoring and administering these functions see that their new employees are practicing expeditiously and maintain a track record of physician expertise. Taking action in the politics of credentialing and certification keeps a radiology practice apprised of any turf violations and, if they cannot be avoided, sets the bar for experience and proficiency that leads to the achievement of a high level of patient care by all practitioners. Certification is one way of establishing your "credentials" as knowledgeable in the field, and the recertification process, demanded now by the ABMS, probably arose from public concerns about the quality of care they receive and the high rate of medical errors reported. Credentialing is the public face of a health care entity's attempt to reassure the consumer that the physicians that practice there are being monitored. Certification and recertification are more personal, self-motivated endeavors that, nonetheless, are being required of all physicians as part of a self-improvement process. Embrace these functions!

Dos and Don'ts of the Credentialing and Certification System	
Dos	**Don'ts**
1. Ensure patient safety and quality care	1. Become too rigid and inflexible with individual circumstances
2. Reduce malpractice risk	2. Cause delays in the start-up of new physicians
3. Permit physicians to perform procedures for which they are competent	3. Avoid the difficulties with verifying truthfulness regarding alcohol and drug problems
4. Quickly allow physicians to bill for the work they do	4. Forget that letters of recommendation are solicited by appointees and may be biased
5. Identify oversights in licensing and drug dispensing privileges	5. Allow paperwork to become overwhelming
6. Identify charlatans and scam artists	6. Require too many signatures

Continued

Dos and Don'ts of the Credentialing and Certification System—cont'd	
Dos	**Don'ts**
7. Establish guidelines that help to define "turf" (i.e., specialty responsibilities) 8. Ensure ongoing continuing education and self-assessment 9. Reassure patients and payers that they are in good hands 10. Help in meeting JCAHO standards	7. Forget that one letter that does not verify employment or training can hold up the process for months 8. Forget that often the person completing the verification of training form is far removed temporally from the person's training period and has no data on that person's professional qualities 9. Forget that CME programs may be poorly attended, but the credits are given even to non-attendees 10. Forget that recertification testing incurs cost, inconvenience, and days away from work

REFERENCES

1. Freed GL, Singer D, Lakhani I, et al: Use of board certification and recertification of pediatricians in health plan credentialing policies. JAMA 295:913–918, 2006.
2. Freed GL, Uren RL, Hudson EJ, Lakhani I, Wheeler JR, Stockman JA, 3rd: Policies and practices related to the role of board certification and recertification of pediatricians in hospital privileging. JAMA 295:905–912, 2006.
3. Cassel CK, Holmboe ES: Credentialing and public accountability: a central role for board certification. JAMA 295:939–940, 2006.
4. West RW, Sipe CY: National practitioner data bank: information on physicians. J Am Coll Radiol 1:777–779, 2004.
5. Levin DC, Rao VM: Turf wars in radiology: privileging and site accreditation programs—what they have accomplished for commercial health plans. J Am Coll Radiol 3:534–536, 2006.

APPENDIX 25-1. BYLAWS OF JOHNS HOPKINS HOSPITAL CREDENTIALS COMMITTEE

A. Duties and responsibilities.
   1. Receive from the chiefs of service recommendations for criteria for appointments and delineated clinical privileges, and confirm their compliance with Hospital and regulatory requirements, including licensure, training, and current competence.
   2. Review recommendations from the chiefs of service for appointment, reappointment, and granting of clinical privileges and confirm that the supporting data meet bylaws and regulatory requirements. The Committee is permitted to review appropriate departmental files and to conduct interviews, if necessary, to carry out this function.
   3. Develop procedures and guidelines to facilitate the credentialing system, to coordinate the Hospital and departmental components of the system and to maintain a consistently high level of medical competence across the institution.
   4. Provide written reports concerning actions, evaluations, and recommendations to the Medical Board.
B. Membership
   1. Vice-president for medical affairs
   2. Five or more members of the active medical staff
   3. Dean for graduate medical education
   4. Vice-president for nursing and patient care services
   5. Legal Department representative
   6. Medical staff registrar
C. The Credentials Committee shall meet monthly.

Sample Credentialing Letter:

Date

Name of Requesting Institution
Street Address
City, State, Zip Code

RE: *Fellow Name:* _____
    SS#: _____ - _____ - _____
    DOB: _____
    Training type: _____
    Training dates: _____ *to* _____

To Whom It May Concern:

I am in receipt of your request for a recommendation and/or verification of postgraduate medical education on the above-named individual in reference to application for medical staff appointment and clinical privileges at your Institution. In compliance with the applicant's signed authorization, I am releasing the following information:

Personal Knowledge
I have known the applicant for: Years_____ Months_____

I am related to the applicant: ☐ Yes / ☐ No

The applicant is well known to me: ☐ Yes / ☐ No

My acquaintance with the applicant has continued to date: ☐ Yes / ☐ No

Training / Performance
Has the applicant successfully completed the training program for which he/she was accepted?
☐ Yes / ☐ No   ☐ Still in program   ☐ Expected to complete on: _____

While in this training program, has the applicant received extensive training in the performance (or treatment) of the privileges requested?
☐ Yes / ☐ No

Did this individual ever take a leave of absence or break from his/her training?
☐ Yes / ☐ No

Does the applicant have any physical or mental conditions, including alcohol abuse, that would impair, or could impair, his/her ability to perform the requested privileges?
☐ Yes / ☐ No   Comments:

_____

Does the applicant engage in the use of illegal drugs?
☐ Yes / ☐ No

Has the applicant ever been arrested, fined, charged with or convicted of a crime, indicted, imprisoned, or placed on probation?

☐ Yes / ☐ No   If yes, please explain:

_____

Has the applicant ever had training, staff membership or clinical privileges revoked, suspended, reduced or not renewed?

☐ Yes / ☐ No   If yes, please explain:

_____

Has the applicant ever been placed under investigation, dismissed, placed on probation, or disciplined, or is any disciplinary action pending at the present time?

☐ Yes / ☐ No   If yes, please explain:

_____

Were any limitations or special requirements placed upon this individual because of questions of academic incompetence, disciplinary problems or any other reason?

☐ Yes / ☐ No   If yes, please explain:

_____

Has disciplinary action been taken against the applicant by a licensing agency?

☐ Yes / ☐ No   If yes, please explain:

_____

Has the applicant ever been denied or surrendered a federal or state controlled substance permit?

☐ Yes / ☐ No

Has the applicant ever been warned, censured, disciplined, or had admissions monitored or privileges limited?

☐ Yes / ☐ No

Were any negative reports ever filed by instructors?

☐ Yes / ☐ No If yes, please explain:

_____

Does the applicant have any pending or closed malpractice or lawsuits that you are aware of?

☐ Yes / ☐ No

Has the applicant ever been a defendant in a legal action involving professional liability (malpractice) or had a professional liability claim paid in his/her behalf?

☐ Yes / ☐ No If yes, please explain:

_____

If English is not the native language, I feel this applicant has the ability to adequately communicate in the English language.

☐ Yes / ☐ No If no, please explain: _____

Character

Based on my observation, I believe that the applicant is currently competent in the privileges requested.

□ Yes / □ No

I am very comfortable recommending the applicant for the clinical privileges requested.

□ Yes / □ No

I consider the applicant to be:
Reliable: □ Yes / □ No
Ethical: □ Yes / □ No
Of good character: □ Yes / □ No

Please rate the following:

	Excellent	Good	Average	Adequate	Poor
Professional ability					
Attention to duties					
Breadth of education					
Interpersonal skills					

Comments:
_____
_____
_____

Completion of the following is certification that the information above is an accurate account of this individual's records and is true and correct. The signature line must contain the original signature, or electronic typed signature, of the program director.

_____

Printed Name of Person Completing This Form   Title

_____

Signature   Date

_____/_____/_____

Telephone #   Fax #   Email Address

The Legislative and Working Environment: Clearing the Muddied Waters

Gregory L. Katzman

It is a riddle wrapped in a mystery inside an enigma.
WINSTON CHURCHILL RADIO ADDRESS, OCTOBER 1939

Although Sir Winston Churchill was describing Russia, this feeling also pervades many of our thoughts when contemplating the current legislative environment in which we radiologists practice our profession. Stark laws, Medicare rules, anti-monopoly concerns, kickbacks, intent to fraud, turf wars, appropriate utilization, pay for performance, quality assurance, quality measures, quality improvement, total quality management: what does it all mean? Should we care? The stern answer is "Absolutely!" All of these factors will have a profound effect on the future of our specialty, and unless we understand them, become involved, and anticipate their implementation, we will be at risk.

Think about this cauldron of potential discontent as a complex puzzle similar to Erno Rubik's famous cube. It is intricate and multifaceted; influencing one aspect will probably have untoward effects on others. Yet sufficient effort will lead to a solution, albeit perhaps one that is complex and temporally drawn out. We will first define and discuss subjects separately, assessing interactions and/or synergy, concluding with an eye to the future.

MEDICARE FRAUD

Historically, fraud and abuse in the Medicare reimbursement system have been widespread.[1] Consequently, beginning in the 1990s, the recovery of monies paid by the federal government in the form of Medicare fraud has become an area of intensive investigation and pursuance. In fiscal 1997, federal agencies recovered over $1.2 billion in Medicare overpayments, and the number of individuals and businesses barred from participating in federal health-care programs nearly doubled from the year before to 2700.[2] Astonishingly, the government estimate of improper Medicare billing for that year was more than $20 billion,[1] meaning that they recovered less than 6%.

Over the past few years many high-profile settlements have been reported. This has included nonprofit universities (University of Washington $35 million, University of Pennsylvania $30 million), for-profit providers (Tenet $900 million, Hospital Corporation of America $1.7 billion), and even pharmaceutical companies (Glaxo-SmithKline $150 million, AstraZeneca $343 million).

Most of the Medicare fraud and abuse actions have relied on the federal civil False Claims Act, a statute that traces its origins to the American Civil War.[3] A number of specific actions may establish liability under this act, including:

1. Presenting (or causing to be presented) a false or fraudulent claim to the government for payment or approval
2. Using a false record or statement to get the false or fraudulent claim paid or approved
3. Conspiring to defraud the government to have a false or fraudulent claim allowed or paid

Note that for all of these, a claim does not actually have to be paid to constitute a potential offense, only presented in the form of a bill to the government.[3]

In the process of prosecuting a fraud case, the government must prove that at least one of these actions has been committed "knowingly," which is defined to mean that a person or organization (such as a radiology practice) has actual knowledge of the information, acts in deliberate ignorance of the truth or falsity of the information, or acts in reckless disregard of the truth or falsity of the information.[3] It is very important to understand that legal precedence has been set that no proof of specific intent to defraud is required.[4] In other words, ignorance of the laws/rules cannot be used as an excuse.

Violations under the False Claims Act can result in significant penalties. This includes payment equal to three times the actual amount that was fraudulently billed, up to $11,000 in civil monetary penalties per claim (and the number of claims reported may be in the thousands!), and the defendant may be subject to exclusion from the Medicare program as well as face criminal prosecution.[3] Powerful weapons against fraud were included in the Health Insurance Portability and Accountability Act of 1996, which mandated interagency cooperation among the Federal Bureau of Investigation, the Justice Department, the Civilian Health and Medical Program of the Uniformed Services, the U.S. Postal Service, and the Health Care Financing Administration (HCFA). Additionally, it gave HCFA the authority to contract with private entities to conduct medical necessity reviews, fraud and abuse audits, and investigations for embezzlement.[2]

But what has really given teeth to this initiative is the "*qui tam*" or whistleblower provision (from a Latin phrase, "*Qui tam pro domino rege quam pro se ipso in hac parte sequiter*," which literally means "he who brings the action for the King as well as for himself").[3] The *qui tam* statute allows individuals or organizations outside the government to invoke False Claims Act provisions and receive a significant percentage of monies recovered. The potential of receiving 10% to 30% of judgments, such as the $110 million that National Health Laboratories paid in a 1991 whistleblower case, has emboldened workers to initiate investigations. The U.S. Justice Department has stated that over half of the $1.2 billion recovered from federal health-care fraud activities in fiscal 1997 involved judgments or settlements of cases initiated by whistleblowers.[2] When an individual seeks to bring a *qui tam* action, the federal government has the option of deciding whether it wishes to enjoin the action, in effect converting a private action into a government one.[3] However, even if the government decides against prosecution, *qui tam* allows the whistleblower(s) to retain the right to take their cases to trial with their own attorneys.[2]

Although radiology cases have not drawn the attention of the multimillion, even billion-dollar, settlements, imaging has not gone unpunished. Medaphis, an Atlanta-based billing company, settled with the federal government in 1998 for alleged improprieties in radiology billing. The radiology investigation cost the company $4 million to settle and $12 million to defend during a 3-year investigation. The whistleblower was awarded $1 million.[2] In 1997, St. Luke's Hospital in New Bedford, Massachusetts, agreed to pay $1.3 million to settle claims that it billed for radiograms and ultrasound examinations that had actually been performed, and also billed for, by a separate Brockton, Massachusetts, medical laboratory.[2]

As a rule, it is fraudulent for a radiologist to bill Medicare for services that he or she did not provide. The most common areas of fraud include billing for services not rendered, billing for services not medically necessary, double billing, upcoding, unbundling (using multiple codes rather than a single code so as to obtain greater reimbursement), and fraudulent cost reporting by institutional providers.[1]

In the case of radiologists outside the teaching setting, fraud is present when Medicare is billed for services that were either not performed at all or were performed by another health-care provider who is not eligible to bill Medicare, such as a nurse or technologist, without the supervision or active participation of the billing radiologist.[3]

In the teaching setting, Medicare billing becomes complicated by the presence of trainees, such as residents and fellows. Bear in mind that trainees in graduate medical education (GME)-accredited programs are partially supported by the Medicare program through Medicare payments to their institutions; thus, the federal government views this financial support as payment for the trainees' services to Medicare beneficiaries, making these trainees ineligible to bill for services individually provided in the course of activities related to those accredited programs. Thus, a radiology resident in a GME-accredited program cannot bill Medicare for any procedure or other service that he or she may provide as part of said residency. Attending radiologists supervising residents in a teaching setting may bill Medicare, but only for services they personally render to beneficiaries. This means that the attending radiologist must be present during "key" or "critical" portions of a service or procedure provided by a trainee. In the diagnostic imaging setting, this has been interpreted as requiring that the teaching radiologist either personally interpret a study or review the trainee's interpretation, with the latter requiring more time than merely countersigning an official report. In the setting of an interventional radiology procedure, the teaching physician must be present during all critical portions of the procedure and must be available to immediately furnish services at any time during the entire procedure.[3]

The federal government has aggressively enforced Medicare billing regulations through Physicians at Teaching Hospitals (PATH) audits,[5] where a major focus has been the determination of whether teaching physicians were actually present during procedures performed by trainees and subsequently billed to Medicare.[3] The most notorious example ensuing from a PATH audit occurred at the University of Washington, which ultimately settled at $35 million. Additionally, the chairman of neurosurgery was fined $500,000, was ordered to perform 1000 hours of community service, and became the first physician at a medical school to be convicted of a federal crime stemming from Medicare fraud.[3] He allegedly was billing for multiple operations simultaneously, with the accusation that his trainees were exclusively performing the surgeries themselves.

Previously, the federal government had to identify a serious pattern of upcoding or unnecessary care to prove culpability. However, because of the enactment of newer laws, they now only need show that the procedures were unnecessary, and enforcement may also encompass actions that arise from innocent neglect as well as those that arise from intentional fraudulent actions.[3] As an example of the former, facilities that even inadvertently contract with individuals or entities that have been barred from participating in Medicare (or other federal health insurance programs) may be fined. This includes physicians who order tests and radiologists who perform them.[2]

There are specific policies that can be implemented as protection against unknowingly committing Medicare fraud. Complete documentation is critical to compliance with current Medicare regulations, as well as for obtaining reimbursement from payers, and requires a thorough understanding by all practicing radiologists of the importance of proper documentation. In fact, incomplete documentation or lack of documentation has been shown to be the single most common reason for payment errors; if you didn't document it, you didn't do it.[1] The rationale for each examination must stand alone, meaning that rule-out diagnoses are insufficient and information about symptoms must be obtained.

BOX 26-1

Seven Elements That Have Been Defined for All Effective Compliance Programs

1. Written standards of conduct covering claims submission, coding, and financial relations with other providers, and the procedures that give employees an incentive to comply
2. Designation of a chief compliance officer and/or the creation of a compliance committee
3. Implementation of compliance education and training
4. Presence of feedback mechanisms to receive complaints and procedures to protect anonymity of whistleblowers
5. Established procedures for responding to allegations and disciplining employees
6. A method for continuing audits and risk evaluations to monitor compliance
7. Mechanisms to guard against business dealings with individuals or companies that have been barred from participating in federal health-care programs

Radiologists and radiology groups must have a Medicare compliance program in place to provide an affirmative defense should an allegation ever be made that the practice knowingly engaged in fraud.[3] The federal government considers the presence of a compliance program the single most important factor in the decision to forgo criminal prosecution, or to reduce the civil penalties, because its presence implies that the provider is acting in good faith.[2] There have been seven elements defined for an effective compliance program (Box 26-1); the authority to enforce the program must be delegated to a designated compliance officer (or committee), and the accountability, direction, and focus of the compliance officer's work must be defined in advance.[2] Internal audits have proved to be effective exercises in identifying potential areas for improvement.

Compliance programs at teaching hospitals should include provisions designed to ensure that physicians in GME-accredited training programs routinely receive the supervision required for attending radiologists to legally bill Medicare, and any unsupervised procedure performed by a physician in training (or by any

other individual not eligible to bill Medicare) should not be submitted for professional payment.[3] The technical aspect of the procedure may be billed, however.

Finally, any radiologist (or radiology practice) that receives a Medicare inquiry, or even a hint that a government agency is contemplating launching an investigation into potential billing irregularities, should respond promptly and fully. It is also highly recommended that they consider consulting an attorney who specializes in this area of law. Often, early responses may satisfy an investigator and preempt a full-fledged and costly investigation.[3]

(IN)APPROPRIATE UTILIZATION OF IMAGING, SELF-REFERRAL, AND STARK LAW

These topics go hand in hand, and to understand the intricacies of their interactions one must first have a rudimentary understanding of "Stark law," so named for the congressional sponsor Pete Stark. Although a detailed analysis is beyond the scope of this chapter (in fact entire books and legal practices are based on Stark law), the reader is referred to reviews by Alice G. Gosfield.[6,7] Of course, anyone considering any type of imaging equipment venture will need to consult appropriate legal consul specializing in health-care law.

Stark laws are two separate provisions within the Social Security Act that govern physician self-referral for Medicare and Medicaid patients for specific "designated health services" (DHSs) to any entity for which they, or an immediate family member, have a financial relationship.[6] Although this seems straightforward, in true government fashion there are critical definitions, strict criteria, numerous exceptions, indirect violations, and other obstacles. Here we will summarize those pertinent areas for imaging services.

DHSs of interest covered by Stark law include radiology and imaging services, radiation therapy services and supplies, inpatient and outpatient hospital services, and nuclear medicine.[8] Referrals are defined broadly and include (1) a physician's request for any DHS reimbursable under Medicare Part B, including a request for a consultation and any test or procedure ordered by or performed by that other physician or under the physician's supervision, or (2) a physician's request that includes any DHS, the establishment of a plan of care that includes a DHS, or the certifying or recertifying of the need for a DHS.[8] A "referral" does not include DHSs personally performed or provided by a referring physician; however, it does include referrals within a physician group.[6] A "financial relationship" can be either a direct or indirect "ownership or investment interest" in the entity that furnishes DHSs or a "compensation arrangement" between the physician and the entity.[8] Additionally, there cannot be a financial relationship of any kind between an immediate family member and the entity to which the referral is being made.[6]

It should be noted that Stark is not the same as the anti-kickback statute.[6] Stark pertains only to physician referrals under Medicare and Medicaid; anti-kickback is far broader and affects anyone engaging in business with a federal health-care program. Stark does not require proof of bad intent; anti-kickback requires intent, and it must be specific. Stark is a civil prohibition (not a civil crime) that can only be overcome by complying explicitly with an exception; anti-kickback "safe harbor" regulations describe transactions that may tend to induce referrals but don't necessarily violate the law, and each instance requires evaluation by a prosecutor to make that determination. A Stark violation is

punishable by civil money penalties; an anti-kickback violation is punishable by exclusion from federal health-care programs, criminal penalties of up to $25,000 in fines or up to 5 years in jail (or both), as well as treble damages (three times the illegal remuneration) plus $50,000 civil money penalty for each violation. In every situation where the Stark statute applies, the anti-kickback statute applies too, but not vice versa.

To a certain extent, the intent of Stark should be to the benefit of patients and to the field of radiology, in that it was proposed to inhibit financial incentives for obtaining inappropriate imaging studies. However, the Achilles heels for this intent are the Stark exceptions. Currently, there are approximately 35 exceptions that describe acceptable financial relationships allowing a physician to refer to an entity for the provision of DHSs that would otherwise have been defined as self-referral.[8] Of utmost importance to radiology is the exception allowing referrals for "in-office ancillary services," which includes imaging. To qualify for the exception and refer patients for in-office imaging, four standards must be met (Table 26-1).[6] Scenarios that either adhere to or violate Stark law (based on examples from ref. 6) are illustrated in Table 26-2.

Because of the in-office ancillary services loophole, physicians can install magnetic resonance imaging (MRI), computed tomography

Table 26-1	Four Standards Within Stark Law That Must Be Met to Qualify for the In-Office Exception
Standard	**Description**
1	The medical group must qualify as a "group practice" under the Stark definition.
2	Services must be furnished personally by the referring physician, by a physician in the same group practice, or by individuals who are "directly supervised" by one of those physicians.
3	Services must be provided in a building in which the referring physician or another member of the group practice furnishes physician services unrelated to DHS or in another building that is used by the group practice for "the centralized provision of the group's designated health services."
4	Services must be billed by the physician performing or supervising them, by a group practice of which that physician is a member under a billing number assigned to the group, or by an entity that is wholly owned by the performing physician or group practice.

DHS, designated health services.
From Gosfield AG: The stark truth about the Stark law: Part I. Fam Pract Manag 10(10):27–33, 2003.

Table 26-2   Scenarios That Violate and Do Not Violate Stark Law with Regard to the Self-Referral Exception

Scenario	Rationale
Violations	
A nonradiologist physician invests in an imaging center to which he does not refer Medicare or Medicaid patients; he does refer to a specialist who orders from the center.	This is a violation, because the specialist's order is a downstream referral for a DHS.
Small physician groups form one partnership to share equipment ownership and hire technicians to perform radiologic services, all within the same building. One of the groups bills all of its services under its own individual billing numbers.	All of the radiologic services must be billed through the single partnership billing number.
An internist's wife is a neurosurgeon and investor in an outpatient imaging center for which she receives profit sharing. The internist refers Medicare and Medicaid patients to this group for imaging.	The neurosurgeon and internist are immediate family members.
Nonviolations	
A physician group installs imaging equipment, billing and receiving direct compensation for the technical component of the service, whether or not they were present to supervise. They send all studies to a radiologist, who performs and bills for the professional component.	The technical components are provided incidentally to the physician's treatment of the patient, and there is no requirement that a physician be on premises.
A multispecialty group with several offices establishes a central facility for imaging services that houses no physician offices. All physicians refer patients to it, and services are provided by nonphysicians. Profits are shared among the physician shareholders according to the office in which they work and the number of services each orders as compared to their peers at that location.	The ancillary services office is a centralized location under the Stark statute, and no physician supervision of the services is required. This profit-sharing agreement does not reflect volume or value of referrals for DHS.

DHS, designated health services.
From Gosfield AG: The stark truth about the Stark law: Part I. Fam Pract Manag 10(10):27–33, 2003.

(CT), ultrasound, positron emission tomography, or any other imaging device, in their offices, refer their own patients at will for imaging, and be reimbursed, regardless of their background or training.[9] It is easy to recognize that as physician reimbursement declines, an investment strategy to bolster declining incomes has been to invest in imaging devices.[10,11]

In the early 1990s Hillman et al[12,13] demonstrated that self-referring physicians utilized imaging 1.7 to 7.7 times as frequently as those who referred to radiologists. A study by the U.S. General Accounting Office performed at about the same time confirmed this with nearly identical results.[14] More recent analyses from the Jefferson Center for Research on Utilization of Imaging Services has shown that between 1993 and 2004 the imaging utilization rate per 1000 subscribers among radiologists increased by 12% as compared with 170% among cardiologists; from 2000 to 2003 the rates were 14% and 42%.[9] Contrary to radiologists, who do not have the opportunity to self-refer, cardiologists can either self-refer or refer within group, both Stark exceptions. Some cardiologists have argued that increased imaging utilization reflects a natural progression by substituting for more invasive procedures such as cardiac catheterization.[15] Yet analysis of Medicare Physician Supplier Procedure Summary Master Files data for cardiac catheterization reveals that the utilization rate for cardiac catheterization increased by 19.5% between 1998 and 2002, seemingly invalidating any claim of a substitution effect.[9]

Numerous other studies have shown similar effects of self-referral on the utilization of imaging.[16–20] The evidence is clear; allowing nonradiologist physicians to purchase imaging equipment and then self-refer patients is a conflict of interest and leads to higher utilization. Incredibly, some private health insurance plans have experienced utilization increases as high as 40% to 50% per year.[21]

Regarding Medicare, what most physicians fail to realize is that the financial size of the Medicare pie is fixed, and changes within its payment system each year undergo a "conversion factor" process for allocation. Thus, increased, but inappropriate, utilization takes money out of everyone's pocket[21] by requiring Medicare to cut the slices smaller.

The rapid growth in imaging has been noticed by policy makers, payers, and providers, with recognition that the main culprit is self-referral by nonradiologists.[22] MedPAC has reported[23]:

1. From 1999 to 2002, annualized growth for imaging was 10.1% compared to 5.2% for all fee schedule services. Growth was especially high (15% to 20%), for MRI, CT, and nuclear medicine.
2. From 2002 to 2003, annualized growth for imaging was 8.6% compared to 4.9% for all fee schedule services.
3. A migration occurred from settings that have institutional controls on imaging (e.g., hospitals) to settings in which there is less control (e.g., physician offices).
4. Nonradiologists provided 52% of Medicare imaging services in 2002.

A study of spending patterns for diagnostic imaging as compared to availability has shown that costs are higher in cities with more imaging capacity, and rather than acting as partial substitutes for each other, CT scanners and MRI machines are complementary, meaning that having more MRI capacity is associated with

higher CT use. In fact, areas with more MRI machines also have more CT scanners.[24]

A report from the Lewin Group has asserted that the self-referral exception is justified for the sake of patient convenience.[25] However, analysis of Medicare claims data reveals that only 3% of nonradiologist imaging is billed on the same claims as office visits.[22] Therefore, the imaging procedures are not matching with the office visit 97% of the time; thus they are not occurring at the same time, hence on the same day, invalidating this line of reasoning. Moreover, self-referral is not altruistic[26]; although mammography is in great demand and short supply, few free-standing mammography centers exist, whereas plenty of MRI centers do. The financial returns for mammography are simply too small to be of interest to the self-referring nonradiologist.

Private health plans have taken note, and representatives have stated that "The challenge for health plans, for radiologists, and for referring physicians is how to reduce the use of unnecessary or inappropriate imaging while ensuring access to clinically valuable imaging."[24] According to the Tiber Group (now Navigant Consulting), in 2001 imaging costs rose by 23%, are approaching 10% of every health-care dollar, and are expected to increase 140% by 2014.[27]

Even the American press has recognized a growing problem of inappropriate utilization. A 2004 *New York Times* article entitled "An MRI machine for every doctor? Someone has to pay" reported that MRI scan utilization increases dramatically concurrently with rapid MRI installations.[28] A 2004 *Wall Street Journal* article entitled "Big health insurer to target scan tests as way to cut costs" reported that in the greater Pittsburgh area there were more than 160 MRI scanners installed in 2004, which was more than all of the scanners in Canada. Additionally, for a single large health plan in that area, outpatient imaging expenses rose by 20% for the previous 3 years to more than $500 million annually, with 134 of every 1000 members receiving CT scans.[29]

To battle escalating imaging costs, both government and private health plans have already instituted a variety of responses (Table 26-3). Self-referral is anticompetitive, resulting in imaging procedures that are performed irrespective of quality, cost of service, or medical

Table 26-3   Examples of Governmental and Private Health Care Plan Responses to Escalating Imaging Costs

Entity	Example
Government	Thirty-six states, and the District of Columbia, have enacted certificate-of-need laws. Forty-three states, and the District of Columbia, have some form of medical self-referral laws.
Private health plans	Prior authorization is required for selected nonemergent high-cost examinations while simultaneously monitoring for inappropriate volume and/or utilization. Radiologists contact referring physicians about the appropriateness of a selected modality. Radiologists are paid a fee similar to the reading fee whether or not radiologic procedures are performed, thus incentivizing appropriate utilization. Rigorous quality privileging standards for imaging facilities are being instituted.

necessity, and channels away billions of healthcare dollars from true medical needs.[11,26] It also endangers patients by inappropriately adding unnecessary radiation exposure.[26] The in-office Stark loophole is the greatest contributor to this self-referral abuse, yet the prospects of legislation closing it are unlikely. The American College of Radiology (ACR) has proposed establishing minimum certification and accreditation standards, which could save Medicare-allowed charges $5.9 billion over the period from 2006 to 2015 with a net savings in federal outlays of $4.6 billion.[22]

Perhaps the more promising course of protection from inappropriate self-referral will come from the private sector. The best illustrations of this are the policies implemented by Highmark Blue Cross Blue Shield of Western Pennsylvania in 2004, as reported in the *Wall Street Journal*; any facility receiving reimbursement for CT or MRI must provide at least five different imaging modalities, and the facility must also have a radiologist on site during normal business hours.[30] Intriguingly, as of May 2006, 20 different private payers had adopted a requirement of ACR accreditation.[31]

On individual levels, radiologists must first support the ACR in these efforts, because their legislative voice is the loudest that we have. Second, we must avoid entering into self-referral ventures, as any participation acts as endorsement and hypocrisy.[26] Third, we must rigorously

promote accreditation, certification, and appropriateness, all in the name of optimal patient care by means of improved quality, which will also serve as our best weapon against turf wars. It's also good medicine.

TURF WARS

Turf wars go hand-in-hand with the issue of self-referral. Given space limitations, a thorough discussion of this topic is far beyond the scope of this chapter. Should the reader desire more detail, at the time of this writing Drs. Levin and Rao had produced 12 exceptional papers of a series devoted to "Turf Wars in Radiology" as published in the *Journal of the American College of Radiology*. To date, subjects covered include overutilization from self-referral,[32] overutilization resulting from other causes,[33] quality of nonradiologist interpretations,[34] quality of images from facilities operated by nonradiologists,[35] self-referral remedies available to governments and payers,[36] the battle for peripheral vascular interventions,[37] emergency department ultrasound and radiography,[38] the importance of training standards in imaging,[39,40] radiologists versus cardiologists for cardiac imaging,[41] as well as privileging and site accreditation programs.[42] These are extremely competently researched and well written, and should be read by most, if not all, radiologists.

One example will be discussed as an exemplar of our current and near future environment: cardiovascular imaging (CVI). The American College of Cardiology (ACC) has mounted an intensive effort to promote in-office imaging by cardiologists and has staked several claims:

1. In-office imaging provides "prompt, convenient, reliable results"; hence patients do not have to wait for an appointment at an imaging center.[43] We have already discussed that Medicare data shows that this simply is not true.

2. "The physician most qualified to interpret cardiovascular imaging studies is a cardiologist. It is absolutely necessary to understand how the heart functions to properly interpret the tests."[43] Cardiologists may understand the heart, but they have not been trained in any aspect of CT or MRI, radiation safety, or all the other noncardiac structures appearing on cardiac imaging studies. As an example of the latter, a study presented at the 2004 American Heart Association meeting found that 16% of coronary CT angiograms contain significant noncardiac abnormalities.[44]

3. "There is no credible evidence that in-office imaging is being conducted inappropriately ... or is resulting in inaccurate diagnoses."[43] Several studies, many of them referenced and discussed here, have shown quite the opposite. Clearly, in-office imaging has led to inappropriate utilization and elevated costs, which is recognized by both Medicare and the private sector.

4. "Statistics on in-office imaging growth do not take into account shifts in the site of service. As more specialists offer in-office diagnostic imaging tests, patients are less likely to receive these services in a more expensive hospital setting."[43] Data from the Medicare Physician Supplier Procedure Summary Master Files demonstrate that between 1993 and 2003, in all places of service, the utilization rate of noninvasive diagnostic imaging increased 12% among radiologists as compared with 170% among cardiologists. As this enormous growth by in-use cardiologists is completely independent of the site of service, self-referral becomes the most plausible explanation.[43]

5. "The American College of Radiology acknowledges there is already a shortage of radiologists in the United States, and thus must outsource work to foreign countries. If the current body of radiologists cannot handle the work load, what will happen if in-office restrictions are imposed?"[43] This seems a bit like throwing a rock in a glass house, in that the ACC itself has recognized that there is also a serious shortage of cardiologists. Moreover, the "outsourced work" referred to is for night and weekend coverage so as to provide 24/7 radiology coverage. It is highly doubtful that cardiology in-house imaging will be willing to provide a similar level of service.

Although these statements seem a bit vitriolic, not all cardiologists are of the same opinion. In 2004 the editor-in-chief of the *Journal of the American College of Cardiology* stated: "We ought to guard against providing services for which we have little experience. We invite criticism if we undertake to perform procedures for which we have had little training, scant experience or very low volumes. We should avoid obtaining equipment for our offices for which there is little demonstrated need or advantage. Given the emerging shortage of cardiologists, there would seem to be little reason to work hard at generating business."[45]

The ACR has issued a clinical statement regarding suggested policy for noninvasive CVI that includes qualifications of personnel, safety issues, and equipment recommendations, for both CT and MRI imaging studies.[46] Thus far, it remains to be seen as to its nonradiologic adoption. The ACC has likewise issued a quality initiative that encompasses appropriateness criteria, accreditation, and possibly physician credentialing for CT, MRI, nuclear cardiology, and echocardiography.[47]

CVI has become the 800-pound gorilla in the corner of imaging practice, because it represents nearly one-third (29%) of total noninvasive diagnostic imaging and is growing twice as rapidly as any other type of imaging.[48] This has led to the question as to who should be performing CVI: radiologists or cardiologists. Levin and Rao have argued that this may be an instance where both should work together[41]

Table 26-4 Advantages and Disadvantages of Joint Radiology/Cardiology Ventures for Performing and Interpreting Advanced Cardiovascular Imaging

Examples	Descriptions
Advantages	
Beneficial fund of knowledge overlap	Radiologists train extensively learning multiple imaging techniques for the entire body using all modalities. We learn about PACS, physics, and the effects of radiation on the body. As fellows we hone our expertise for specific modalities or organ systems. Cardiologists learn diagnosis and management of diseases for the entire body. As fellows they focus on one organ—the heart.
Synergistic readouts	Radiologists excel at technical factors for image acquisition and for findings within noncardiac structures. Cardiologists know cardiac anatomy and pathology better and can provide the clinical setting.
Built-in peer review	Assuming that both the radiologist and cardiologist are appropriately trained for interpreting CVI studies, joint readouts provide automatic peer reviewing for 100% of cases.
Patient care	Cardiologists can provide beta blockade to patients for coronary CTA, whereas radiologists oversee image acquisition and radiation safety.
Capital costs	May prevent duplication of equipment costs within the same institution.
Disadvantages	
Fee violations	If both are not actively involved in the interpretations, yet both are participating in a fee-splitting arrangement, this may represent a Medicare anti-kickback or Stark violation.
History	Cardiologists have a proven history of usurping imaging technologies without radiology partners (e.g., coronary angiography and echocardiography).
Interpretation requirements	Radiologists can do these studies without cardiologists, but not vice versa. Cardiologists cannot interpret noncardiac portions of the scans, whereas radiologists can interpret all.
Referral patterns	A significant amount of CVI is ordered by primary care physicians who would probably be more likely to refer to a sole radiology practice, who will not steal their patients, rather than to a cardiology practice.

CTA, computed tomographic angiography; CVI, cardiovascular imaging; PACS, picture archiving and communication systems.
From Levin DC, Rao VM: Turf wars in radiology: should it be radiologists or cardiologists who do cardiac imaging? J Amer Coll Radiol 2(9):749–752, 2005.

(see Table 26-4 for advantages and disadvantages of such a relationship). Bill Bradley would agree, having experienced a successful, fair, and synergistic working relationship after establishing a joint venture at the University of California San Diego (UCSD).[49] In a counterpoint argument, David Levin notes that radiologists must be wary of history repeating itself; as cardiology stole coronary angiography, so could CVI follow.[50] Although a relationship as experienced at UCSD results in good patient care, and is fair to both sides, radiology practices should deem any lesser agreement as unacceptable. At the University of Utah, we have embarked on a joint venture type of model; however, because of its infancy, the jury is still out.

QUALITY

Quality will probably prove to be the new driving legislative force behind health-care planning and decision making for the foreseeable future, and imaging will not be exempt. In this regard, on August 23, 2006, President Bush signed an executive order requiring four federal agencies that oversee large health-care programs (the Defense Department, Department of Health and Human Services, Office of Personnel Management, and the Department of Veterans Affairs) to gather information about the quality and price of care, and to share that information among themselves as well as with program beneficiaries.[51,52] The four agencies, whenever possible, are also to use compatible computer systems and electronic health records to better track a recipient's medical care and condition. Importantly, changes were mandated to be underway in less than 5 months, by 1 January 2007. Because the federal government ultimately pays for as much as 40% of all health-care costs in America, this initiative will probably affect the entire health-care market by setting an example for private insurers to follow.[51,52] A profound governmental emphasis on quality is here to stay, and we are not immune.

Because quality has now been legislated for health care, it behooves us to understand just what quality means with regard to imaging. Quality in radiology has been defined as "a timely access to and delivery of integrated and appropriate radiological studies and interventions in a safe and responsive facility and a prompt delivery of accurately interpreted reports by capable personnel in an efficient, effective, and sustainable manner."[53] Quality improvement (QI) falls under the moniker of total quality management (TQM), a business managerial process that stresses a commitment of an entire organization to excel in all aspects of services or products that are important to customers. When applied appropriately, TQM requires a never-ending process of continual improvement, and whether it's a plan-do-study-act (Demming's PDSA) cycle, Six-Sigma, Kaizen, or some other TQM variant, all have the common feature of continually improving quality over time.[54] Unquestionably, radiologists can only benefit from adopting a quality

"cycle of improvement" concept.[55] As succinctly stated by the Sun Valley Group investigating improved quality in radiology, "Quality is a continuum, and quality improvement is perpetual."[56]

But what are quality improvement measures in radiology? On a professional individual level, proof of competency and hence quality can be found in the form of American Board of Radiology (ABR) certification, subspecialty certificate of added qualification (CAQ), and maintenance of certification (MOC), as well as in ongoing annual continuing medical education. These measures are all relatively easy to obtain, document, and display.

Quality systems for practices, however, are a bit more difficult to define and attain. Accreditation programs on a modality basis exist from several sources, the best known from the ACR. There are even fledgling systemwide QI initiatives, such as the ACR's Medical Excellence in Diagnostic Imaging Campaign, which is working to potentially save taxpayers billions in Medicare costs and improve patient quality by establishing quality standards for advanced medical imaging and limit self-referral.

A departmental QI program should also include peer review, because it provides oversight among colleagues as a means of ensuring quality care for patients, and it is also a requirement of the Joint Commission on Accreditation of Healthcare Organizations (JCAHO).[57] As a process improvement tool, it may aid identification of system deficiencies as well as isolated individual shortcomings, thus also becoming a valuable component of risk management.

PAY FOR PERFORMANCE

Quality, as we discussed in the preceding section, is inextricably intertwined with a profound initiative for reimbursement called "pay for performance" (P4P). Based on quality of care, P4P is already being implemented by both public and private provider sectors.

On 31 January 2005, the Centers for Medicare and Medicaid Services (CMS) released a public statement listing 10 P4P initiatives to encourage improved quality of care in all health-care settings, including physicians' offices, ambulatory care facilities, hospitals, nursing homes, home health care agencies, and dialysis facilities.[58] These can be found at the CMS website (http://www.cms.hhs.gov/apps/media/press/release.asp?Counter=1343).

Without doubt, the CMS views this as the major pathway for our reimbursement future, and the private sector has followed suit, already actively engaging P4P programs. The not-for-profit organization Bridges to Excellence, originated by General Electric, has initiated P4P bonuses to physicians who can earn $100 per patient per year in P4P incentives by meeting objectives in patients with diabetes, $160 per patient for cardiac care, and they can earn $55 per patient per year for implementing specific office-based practice improvements to reduce errors and improve quality.[59] Bridges to Excellence has been licensed nationally to insurers including Blue Cross Blue Shield, Cigna, and United Healthcare,[61] as well as to employers including U.S. corporations such as Proctor & Gamble, Verizon, United Parcel Service, and Ford.[59] The Partners Healthcare System (the parent organization of the Massachusetts General Hospital and the Brigham and Women's Hospital, Boston) has actively pursued contracts with P4P at-risk provisions to push insurance companies to reward higher quality and better utilization management with higher reimbursement.[59] The Integrated Healthcare Association in California, founded by six health plans having over 7 million commercial enrollees, has instituted P4P initiatives whereby the distribution of payments will be 50% for clinical quality, 40% for patient experience, and 10% for investment in information technology (IT).[59]

The Leapfrog Group has quickly drawn significant attention because of its size (more than 160 public and private organizations), membership (including AT&T, Boeing, Exxon, Ford, General Electric, General Motors, Microsoft, PepsiCo, and Xerox), and number of covered lives (more than 34 million).[60,61] In fact, JCAHO estimates that more than 100 P4P programs are in existence, with financial inducements ranging from 1% to 10%, taking the form of either an added bonus or an "at-risk" withholding.[60]

In December 2005, the American Medical Association (AMA) sealed an agreement under which Congress would delay implementation of legislated Medicare cuts, which would have dramatically cut imaging reimbursement, if the AMA produced 140 performance measures for all major specialties by 1 January 2007. The ACR began work with the AMA to develop the performance measures specific to radiology, and the first of these will include radiology measures for stroke and stroke rehabilitation. Future measures could include data regarding call-back rates, repeat rates, referring physician satisfaction,[62] patient satisfaction, investment in IT, upgrading to new or improved imaging equipment, having a high percentage of images interpreted by fellowship-trained radiologists, providing 24/7 emergency department coverage, or even peer review.

On the surface, the P4P future seems optimistically bright. After all, improvement in outcomes benefits patients, their employers, and the public at large. In this optimistic scenario, overall costs are reduced, P4P bonuses are paid, and QI is thus "free."[59] But there is no free lunch, and there are significant concerns regarding P4P structure, especially as it pertains to radiology practice (Box 26-2).

Imaging is usually a minor event in a patient's care, interspersed within a large cascade of diagnostic and therapeutic events that in toto ultimately leads to an outcome. Isolating the specific role of an imaging event, or a specific radiologist, in determining said outcome may be very difficult.[63] A plausible alternative would be to evaluate for "process" or "facility" measures, which could include modality ACR accreditation and/or adherence to ACR Appropriateness Criteria.[63]

As stated by former ACR Chair E. Stephen Amis, Jr., M.D., "It's time to get our collective heads out of the sand. P4P is just around the corner for us."[64] In support of this, P4P took main stage at the 2006 Intersociety Summer Conference, which was entitled "Quality, a Radiology Imperative."[65] In September 2006, the ACR issued a white paper outlining its extensive plans in support of P4P,[66] describing a broad range of initiatives that, if successful, will greatly advance radiology's standing in the P4P playing field.

BOX 26-2

Questions about the Structure of P4P

There is great concern regarding the applicability of P4P measures to radiology, and significant questions regarding P4P structure as it pertains to our practice are listed.

1. Will sufficient monies be available to cover high costs associated with installing information systems and PACS, providing 24-hour in-house radiology coverage, or hiring a sufficient number of fellowship-trained radiologists to interpret examinations by subspecialty?
2. Will a focus on specific quality standards render a number of procedures or even whole modalities (such as mammography) financially nonviable?
3. Will limited, capped funds available make P4P a zero-sum game, with winners and losers? If so, the P4P concept may be self-defeating if providers simply cannot compete, which will result in lower quality and less (or no) service.
4. Will P4P promote "cherry picking"? Physicians may be discouraged from tackling tough cases or caring for the sickest of patients if cost and utilization targets are set incorrectly.
5. How do we reconcile that radiologists practicing in hospital settings often have little input in the hospital-provided support services on which they depend, which nevertheless are an integral component of many already established quality metrics?
6. Because consumer selection on the basis of published quality parameters is cited as a central ingredient of P4P, is this even applicable to radiologists who serve at the request of other physicians?
7. Because most physicians practice at more than one hospital and participate in multiple insurance plans, will P4P programs create an incompatible information system, particularly affecting small practices?
8. Because the poor are much more likely to have lower baseline scores on measures such as breast, cervical, and colorectal cancer screening, hypertension control, and immunization rates, could P4P lead to financial punishment for the physicians and hospitals that care for these patients? This would most certainly asymmetrically affect our nation's academic and primarily urban medical centers.

OFFSHORE TELERADIOLOGY

In 1993, a memorandum was issued by the Office of the Inspector General stating that all radiologic interpretations had to be performed contemporaneously. Faced with the possibility that emergency department (ED) physicians would begin reading and billing cases at night, possibly creating within them a belief that they should also be able to do the same during the daytime, many radiology groups implemented central teleradiology programs to provide hospital coverage.[67] In 2001 the ACR Council passed a resolution that "all radiologic studies performed on ED patients should be promptly interpreted by radiologists."[68] Given a deleterious mix of a growing shortage of radiologists, increasing numbers of nighttime studies, growing complexity of the imaging acquired, and a greater demand for faster "final" interpretation,

the total costs of nighttime coverage have grown significantly. Furthermore, radiologists filling such positions become susceptible to "burnout," and retention has become difficult.[67]

As institutions increasingly began to adopt the use of the picture archiving and communication systems (PACS) and Internet bandwidth expanded rapidly everywhere, it became plausible to be able to view and interpret medical images from anywhere in the world. Thus, images acquired at night in the United States could be interpreted by a radiologist anywhere in the world, where it would still be normal working hours. From all this the concept of offshore teleradiology was born.[67]

It has been argued that, in addition to alleviating diagnostic calls at night, offshore teleradiology may actually improve patient care.[67] In support of this, some studies have documented that sleep deprivation has deleterious effects on clinical performance,[69] mood,[70] and next-day effort.[71]

There are several barriers to establishing, and/or making use of, an offshore teleradiology service. Radiologists must be licensed in the states of service as well as credentialed at each hospital to perform interpretations. Six states (Alabama, Louisiana, North Carolina, Oregon, South Carolina, and Texas) require taking a Special Purpose Examination (which tests basic medical knowledge) to obtain a medical license. All radiologists must have ABR certification. Finally, licensing may also be required in the foreign country within which the interpretation is taking.[67]

Because CMS will not reimburse for interpretation of studies performed outside the United States,[72] only a preliminary report can be issued by offshore teleradiology services. However, because action will be taken on the basis of this report, malpractice insurance is still required for the teleradiologist. Given that, at least on paper, radiologists at the home institution review each study before issuing a final report the next day, an inherent quality assurance (QA) process becomes part of the review. This serves as both an educational tool and a QA instrument for the JCAHO.[67]

Still in evolution, off-shore teleradiology has become a highly emotional topic, hotly debated at nearly every radiology conference, simultaneously felt by many to be boon and by many others bane. In fact, some believe that it may become a threat to the long-term viability of the specialty.[73] They question the message that radiologists send to their referring (and possibly competing) physicians when they sign off at any time to nighthawks, perhaps insinuating that their personal convenience is more important than service to local patients.[73] Once radiologists show a willingness to give up casework, there may not be any great difference between sending studies across the world, or across town perhaps to a nonradiologist.[73]

Because only preliminary interpretations may be issued offshore, the amount of work performed by the local radiologist is unchanged to minimally reduced; thus, the total radiologist work (including that of the nighthawk) is actually increased. Because the nighthawk would presumably otherwise be employed in a more traditional setting, this exacerbates the current radiologist shortage and does not improve global efficiency[73] unless the interpretations

the next day can be performed more rapidly without sacrificing accuracy. Finalized official nighthawk or dayhawk readings by remote radiologists within the United States would provide added value and efficiency.

Moreover, the inspector general has recommended to the Medicare Payment Advisory Commission that only contemporaneous final interpretations be eligible for reimbursement, which would mean a final interpretation would have to be rendered before treatment. If this recommendation becomes law, it would obviate the need for offshore teleradiology, unless their preliminary reports were to become reimbursable, or if they are allowed to issue final reports. In this scenario, the need for local radiologists may be obviated by opening up competition from any foreign radiologist or radiology group at a fraction of even Medicare rates because of a lower cost of living and practicing medicine within their countries. Medicare and other insurers might then seek to base their payments on the rates of offshore radiologists.[73] This has been labeled the "commoditization" of radiology, signifying that our product has become indistinguishable from others like it, and consumers will buy on the basis of price alone. This is a frightening thought.

Legislators have taken notice and have debated federal policies that would regulate the transmission of personally identifiable information outside the United States without consent. Although no proposals have made it out of congressional committee, their introduction indicates an awareness of, and concern about, international transmission of data, including radiologic images. There is also proposed legislation in more than 30 states to prevent outsourcing of state business. Without a doubt, the passage of such legislation, especially at the federal level, would limit or eliminate a significant component of offshore/remote teleradiology services.[73]

Another danger may exist from teleradiology provided in foreign countries: a single qualified radiologist could "oversee" a group of less qualified radiologists. Although most cases would be interpreted by foreign trained radiologists who would not qualify to independently interpret cases in the United States, this single qualified radiologist might claim the work as his or her own.[73] Thus, it behooves anyone contemplating using offshore teleradiology services to carefully investigate the imagers that will be provided, as well as how and where they trained.

It is entirely feasible that ED groups could contract for nighttime offshore teleradiology interpretation themselves, and then hire outpatient radiologists to over-read films during the day.[74] Acceptance of such work is made more likely as offshore teleradiology companies issue initial public offerings and become answerable only to their shareholders for increasing revenue and returns. As well, hospital administrators may take the initiative to contract with offshore/remote nighthawks and/or dayhawks for their entire services, especially in small, rural settings where interventional radiology is not practiced. Hospital administrators might see a significant financial advantage for themselves to take over billing the professional component of radiologic services by contracting with such outside sources.[73] Former ACR Chairman James P. Borgstede has stated that "Nothing is more detrimental to the development of a personal relationship... than the use of after hours teleradiology services. Allowing others to take over our practices at night is a clear statement of our opinion of our importance to patient care. If local radiologists are not necessary at night, why are they necessary during regular business hours?"[75]

Certainly, offshore teleradiology raises challenges to ensuring high-quality patient care, and the ACR issued a report from the ACR Task Force on International Teleradiology in 2005.[76] It detailed several general principles that should be adhered to, as listed in Box 26-3.

There are several considerations a group must assess before contracting with an offshore teleradiology group. Cost may be an issue, as the usual fee ranges from $50 to $70 per study,[67] which may become quite expensive for larger, busier groups. One should find out if there are any objections from the hospital staff or administration, perhaps even approaching ED physicians as a courtesy explaining the potential benefits of such a service including initial interpretation by well-rested radiologists and an automatic double-read of every case.[77] Additionally, discussion should be held with the appropriate executive hospital committee and or executive(s). With attention to detail, some groups have had reported success with satisfaction from referring physicians, hospital administrators, and from within their own group after contracting for offshore teleradiology services.[77]

BOX 26-3

Principles for Using an Offshore Radiology Service

The ACR Task Force on International Teleradiology has issued several general principles that should be adhered to whenever making use of offshore teleradiology.

1. It is critical that its use not reduce quality patient care.
2. International teleradiology should adhere to the ACR Technical Standard for Teleradiology.
3. A physician making an interpretation outside of the country should be licensed in the transmitting state, have liability insurance, be credentialed, and have membership on the medical staff.
4. Physicians should independently interpret teleradiology studies that are read outside the United States and provide the official authenticated written reports.
5. Any group that obtains final interpretations from overseas should ensure that such physicians providing image interpretation have proper liability coverage, state licensure, and credentials.
6. All physicians providing imaging interpretations based both in the United States and abroad should participate in a QA program that must be equivalent to or exceed that of the service hospital.
7. Physicians interpreting emergent cases should be immediately available for consultations. For nonemergent cases, physicians should either be available for consultation or make arrangements to communicate findings.
8. International teleradiology is subject to both U.S. and state privacy laws and regulations. Practices based in the United States that contract teleradiology services should expect to be held jointly responsible for any violations.

From Van Moore A, Allen B, Campbell SC, et al: Report of the ACR task force on international teleradiology. JACR 2(2):121–125, 2005.

With the current radiologist shortage, off-shore radiology is viewed by some as a relief valve that takes both pressure and stress away from what might be otherwise undesirable positions.[78] To this end, it has been reported as a positive factor that has allowed easier group recruitment.[77] Furthermore, offshore teleradiology may be of great assistance to rural radiologists, many of which are in solo practice, who may have no other support locally[79] and who may not have otherwise agreed to practice in rural America.

An alternative is for a radiology group, or a collection of local groups, to consider forming their own offshore teleradiology rotation. A foreign location could be chosen and equipment installed, to be staffed on a rotational basis by group members. In this manner, a group may retain their claim of caring for local service with a dedication to their institution(s) for complete and fully qualified radiologic coverage.[73,77]

CONCLUDING REMARKS

We have discussed several legislative topics including Medicare fraud, inappropriate utilization leading to self-referral, Stark law, turf wars, P4P, and offshore teleradiology. It is notable that a veiled thread within some of these discussions has been that of quality; much like managed care in the 1980s, the era of quality-based decision justification is upon us in the early 21st century, and has already been embraced by the private sector and recently applied by the President to federal payers. We must assess self-referral, inappropriate utilization, and offshore teleradiology by their effects on health-care quality, safety, and cost. In the words of former ACR Chair Dr. Borgstede, "The health care equation is best expressed as quality patient outcome being the product of high quality, increased safety, appropriate utilization, and cost control. If the above equation is applied, control of self-referral will follow."[80] Indeed, verifiable best of quality practice will probably prove to be the winning weapon in the war of turf; whoever is yielding it. We must also be ever vigilant regarding Medicare oversight, documentation, billing, and teaching supervision, and be cautious regarding implementation of offshore teleradiology at the risk of "letting the cat out of the bag." Finally, all readers are again urged to support the ACR, because it is our most effective and loudest voice for legislative matters.

Dos and Don'ts of the Legislative and Working Environment	
Dos	**Don'ts**
1. Ensure your facility has a complete and thorough compliance program. In fact, having a Medicare compliance program in place will provide an affirmative defense should an allegation ever be made.	1. Dismiss compliance as merely a hassle that "other people" need to worry about.
2. Consult appropriate legal consul specializing in health care and Stark law before considering any type of imaging equipment venture.	2. Forget that DHSs of interest covered by Stark law include radiology and imaging services, radiation therapy services and supplies, inpatient and outpatient hospital services, and nuclear medicine.
3. Consider ACR accreditation for all radiologic modalities. As of May 2006, 20 different private payers had adopted a requirement of ACR accreditation.	3. Dismiss P4P as a passing phase. Although its longevity is questionable, it will appear on the immediate horizon, and early adopters may experience a first-mover reimbursement advantage.
4. Combat turf wars with verifiable best of quality practice, with a defined quality patient outcome being the product of high quality, increased safety, appropriate utilization, and cost control. This approach will probably prove to be a winning weapon.	4. Combat turf wars with hubris. Simply stating "because it's radiology" and "we've always done this" will not win the day. A more highly trained and experienced practitioner will win; even if it's a cardiologist.

Dos	Don'ts
5. Consider alternative nighthawk teleradiology coverage. This may be via a self-built program, local group network, commercial provider, or other solution. Regardless of its form, this can be used as a distinct recruiting advantage.	5. Assume that nighthawk teleradiology coverage will be greeted with open arms. A priori, discuss any potential program with as many people as possible, including at a minimum hospital administration and your ED physicians.

REFERENCES

1. Phillips CD, Hillman BJ: Coding and reimbursement issues for the radiologist. Radiology 220(1):7–11, 2001.
2. Brice J: Feds accept no excuses in push to eliminate Medicare fraud. Diagn Imaging (San Franc) 21(2): 35–37, 1999.
3. Smith JJ, Berlin L: Medicare fraud and abuse. Am J Roentgenol 180:591–595, 2003.
4. United States of America v NHC Health Care Corp, 163 F Supp 2d 1051, US Dist LEXIS 15278 2001.
5. Berlin L: Liability of attending physicians when supervising residents. Am J Roentgenol 171:295–299, 1998.
6. Gosfield AG: The stark truth about the Stark law: Part I. Fam Pract Manag 10(10):27–33, 2003.
7. Gosfield AG: The stark truth about the Stark law: Part II. Fam Pract Manag 11(2):41–45, 2004.
8. American Medical Directors Association. Stark law questions and answers. AMDA. Available at http://www.amda.com/advocacy/legal/stark.cfm. 2006.
9. Levin DC: The 2005 Robert D. Moreton Lecture: the inappropriate utilization of imaging through self-referral. J Am Coll Radiol 3(2):90–95, 2006.
10. Phamm HH, Devers KJ, Berenson R: Financial pressures spur physician entrepreneurialism. Health Aff 23(2):70–81, 2004.
11. Fletcher T: The impact of physician entrepreneurship on escalating health care costs. J Am Coll Radiol 2(5): 411–414, 2005.
12. Hillman BJ, Joseph CA, Mabry MR, et al: Frequency and costs of diagnostic imaging in office practice—a comparison of self-referring and radiologist-referring physicians. N Engl J Med 323:1604–1608, 1990.
13. Hillman BJ, Olson GT, Griffith PE, et al: Physicians' utilization and charges for outpatient diagnostic imaging in a Medicare population. JAMA 268:2050–2054, 1992.
14. U.S. GAO.: Referrals to physician-owned imaging facilities warrant HCFA's scrutiny: report to the chairman, Subcommittee on Health, Committee on Ways and Means, House of Representatives (GAO/HEHS-95-2), Washington, DC, US General Accounting Office, 1994.
15. Williams KA: President's message: advocacy for nuclear cardiology—the self-referral issue. J Nucl Cardiol 11:751–753, 2004.
16. Childs AW, Hunter ED: Non-medical factors influencing use of diagnostic x-ray by physicians. Med Care 10:323–335, 1972.
17. Hemenway D, Killen A, Cashman SB, et al: Physicians' response to financial incentives. Evidence from a for-profit ambulatory care center. N Engl J Med 322:1059–1063, 1990.
18. Radecki SE, Steele JP: Effect of on-site facilities on use of diagnostic radiology by non-radiologists. Invest Radiol 25:190–193, 1990.
19. Strasser RP, Bass MJ, Brennan M: The effect of an on-site radiology facility on radiologic utilization in family practice. J Fam Practice 24:619–623, 1987.
20. Oguz KK, Yousem DM, Deluca T, Herskovits EH, Beauchamp NJ. Effect of emergency department CT on neuroimaging case volume and positive scan rates. Acad Radiol 9:1018–1024, 2002.
21. Borgstede JP: Cliffs, marathons, and searches for the silver bullet. J Am Coll Radiol 3(1):2–3, 2006.
22. Moser JW: Getting at the facts on imaging utilization growth. J Am Coll Radiol 2(9):720–724, 2005.
23. Medicare Payment Advisory Commission.: Report to the Congress: Medicare payment policy. Washington, DC, Medicare Payment Advisory Commission, 2005.
24. Rothenberg BM, Korn A: The opportunities and challenges posed by the rapid growth of diagnostic imaging. J Am Coll Radiol 2(5):407–410, 2005.
25. The Lewin Group: Issues in the growth of diagnostic imaging services: a case study of cardiac imaging. Executive summary, Falls Church, VA, The Lewin Group, 2005.
26. Cronan JJ: DEFCON One! Imaging under attack. J Am Coll Radiol 2(3):207–210, 2005.
27. Tiber Group.: Imaging—the race is on, Chicago, Tiber Group, 2004.
28. Abelson R: An M.R.I. machine for every doctor? Someone has to pay. The New York Times (13 March 2004), p. A1.
29. Fuhrmans V: Big health insurer to target scan tests as way to cut costs. The Wall Street Journal (9 August 2004), p. B1.
30. Fuhrmans V: Overuse of medical scans is under fire. The Wall Street Journal (12 January 2005), p D1.
31. Ullrich CG: How you can focus private payers on radiology issues? ACR Leadership Conference—Economics Forum, May 2006.
32. Levin DC, Rao VM: Turf wars in radiology: The overutilization of imaging resulting from self-referral. J Am Coll Radiol 1(3):169–172, 2004.

33. Levin DC, Rao VM: Turf wars in radiology: other causes of overutilization and what can be done about it. J Am Coll Radiol 1(5):317–321, 2004.

34. Levin DC, Rao VM: Turf wars in radiology: the quality of interpretations of imaging studies by nonradiologist physicians—a patient safety issue? J Am Coll Radiol 1(7): 506–509, 2004.

35. Levin DC, Rao VM: Turf wars in radiology: the quality of imaging facilities operated by nonradiologist physicians and the images they produce. J Am Coll Radiol 1(9):649–651, 2004.

36. Levin DC, Rao VM: Turf wars in radiology: possible remedies for self-referral that could be taken by federal or state governments and payers. J Am Coll Radiol 1(11): 806–810, 2004.

37. Levin DC, Rao VM: Turf wars in radiology: the battle for peripheral vascular interventions. J Am Coll Radiol 2(1):68–71, 2005.

38. Levin DC, Rao VM: Turf wars in radiology: emergency department ultrasound and radiography. J Am Coll Radiol 2(3):271–273, 2005.

39. Levin DC, Rao VM: Turf wars in radiology: the past, present, and future importance of training standards in imaging. J Am Coll Radiol 2(7): 602–606, 2005.

40. Levin DC, Rao VM: Turf wars in radiology: training in diagnostic imaging: how much is enough? J Am Coll Radiol 2(12):1016–1018, 2005.

41. Levin DC, Rao VM: Turf wars in radiology: should it be radiologists or cardiologists who do cardiac imaging? J Am Coll Radiol 2(9):749–752, 2005.

42. Levin DC, Rao VM: Turf wars in radiology: privileging and site accreditation programs—what they have accomplished for commercial health plans. J Am Coll Radiol 3(7):534–536, 2006.

43. Levin DC: The statements by the American College of Cardiology on in-office cardiac imaging performed by cardiologists. J Am Coll Radiol 3(1): 6–8, 2006.

44. Shafique I, Shapiro EP, Stafford S, Bush DE: Noncoronary findings on multidetector CT coronary angiography [Abstract]. Circulation 110 (Suppl 3):523, 2004.

45. DeMaria AN: Self-referral in cardiology. J Am Coll Cardiol 43:1500–1501, 2004.

46. Weinreb JC, Larson PA, Woodard PK, et al: ACR clinical statement on noninvasive cardiac imaging. J Am Coll Radiol 2(6):471–477, 2005.

47. Brice J: Cardiac CT sets high bar for physician education. Diagn Imaging (18 July 2006).

48. Levin DC, Rao VM, Parker L, et al: Recent trends in utilization of cardiovascular imaging: how important are they for radiology? J Am Coll Radiol 2(9):736–739, 2005.

49. Bradley WG: Radiologists and cardiologists should work together on advanced cardiac imaging. J Am Coll Radiol 3(5):309–311, 2006.

50. Levin DC: Re: "Radiologists and cardiologists should work together on advanced cardiac imaging." J Am Coll Radiol 3(5):312–313, 2006.

51. Fletcher MA: Bush signs order on health care. Washington Post (Wednesday, 23 August 2006), p A13.

52. Zhang J: Bush's order on health care aims to gauge quality of service. Wall Street Journal (Wednesday, 23 August 2006), p D5.

53. Lau LS: A continuum of quality in radiology. J Am Coll Radiol 3(4):233–239, 2006.

54. Heizer J, Render B: Principles of operations management. Englewood Cliffs, Pearson Prentice-Hall, 2004, pp 187–212.

55. Alpert HR, Hillman BJ: Quality and variability in diagnostic radiology. J Am Coll Radiol 1(2):127–132, 2004.

56. Johnson CD, Swenson SJ, Applegate KE, et al: Quality improvement in radiology: white paper report of the Sun Valley Group Meeting. J Am Coll Radiol 3(7): 544–549, 2006.

57. Halsted MJ: Radiology peer review as an opportunity to reduce errors and improve patient care. J Am Coll Radiol 1(12):984–987, 2004.

58. Centers for Medicare & Medicaid Services.: Medicare "pay for performance (P4P)" initiatives. Press statement release, January 31, 2005.

59. Thrall JH: The emerging role of pay-for-performance contracting for health care services. Radiology 233 (3):637–640, 2004.

60. Swayne LC: Pay for performance: pay more or pay less? J Am Coll Radiol 2(9):777–781, 2005.

61. Pentecost MJ: Pay for performance: at last or alas? J Am Coll Radiol 2(8):655–658, 2005.

62. Van Moore A: P4P—what it means to your practice. American College of Radiology Board of Chancellors letter from the Chairman, 14 July 2006.

63. Hillman BJ: Who gets paid with "pay-for-performance"? J Am Coll Radiol 1(12):891–892, 2004.

64. Amis ES: Leaping frogs, P4PS, and P4P: not so strange bedfellows. J Am Coll Radiol 1(2):79, 2004.

65. Van Moore Jr. A: Quality metrics: value to radiology. J Am Coll Radiol 3(9):641–642, 2006.

66. Moser JW, Wilcox PA, Bjork SS, et al: Pay for performance in radiology: ACR white paper. J Am Coll Radiol 3(9):650–664, 2006.

67. Bradley WG: Offshore teleradiology. J Am Coll Radiol 1(4):244–248, 2004.

68. American College of Radiology: Timely interpretation of emergency radiology studies. Reston, VA, ACR, 2002.

69. Wienger MD, Ancoli-Isreal S: Sleep deprivation and clinical performance. JAMA 287(8):955–957, 2002.

70. Weaver TE: Outcome measurement in sleep medicine practice and research. Part 2: assessment of neurobehavioral performance and mood. Sleep Med Rev 5(3):223–236, 2001.

71. Engle-Friedman M, Riela S, Golan R, et al: The effect of sleep loss on the next day effort. J Sleep Res 12 (2):113–124, 2003.

72. Social Security Act: § 1862(a)(4). 42 USC § 1395y(a) (4).

73. Larson PA, Janower ML: The nighthawk: bird of paradise or albatross? J Am Coll Radiol 2(12):967–970, 2005.

74. Dreisbach JN: Radiology: going, going, gone. J Am Coll Radiol 3(8):572–574, 2006.

75. Borgstede JP: Strategies for the future. J Am Coll Radiol 3(5):305–306, 2006.
76. Van Moore A, Allen B, Campbell SC, et al: Report of the ACR task force on international teleradiology. J Am Coll Radiol 2(2):121–125, 2005.
77. Wagner AL: After-hours coverage: problems and solutions. J Am Coll Radiol 1(5):351–355, 2004.
78. Swayne LC: The private-practice perspective of the manpower crisis in radiology: greener pastures? J Am Coll Radiol 1(11):834–841, 2004.
79. Lamb A: Today's labor market: recruiting radiologists in a time of shortages. J Am Coll Radiol 2(6):520–525, 2006.
80. Borgstede JP: Self-referral: bad health care at any cost. J Am Coll Radiol 1(7):445–446, 2004.

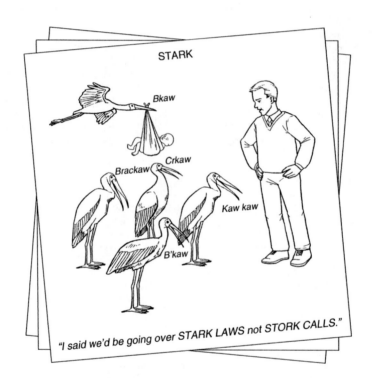

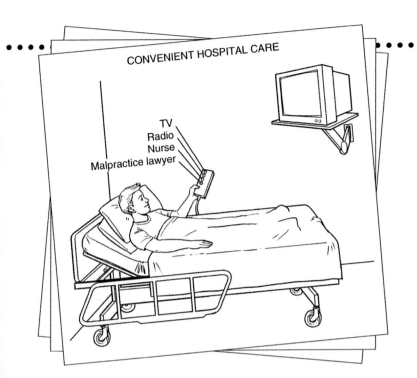

CHAPTER 27

CONVENIENT HOSPITAL CARE

TV
Radio
Nurse
Malpractice lawyer

Medicolegal Issues

David M. Yousem

In this chapter we review some guidelines that will help radiologists practice their craft in a manner that reduces their risk of malpractice litigation as well as discuss the role of the radiologist as a medical expert. There are several important lessons to be learned from the malpractice literature that can affect how a radiologist can avoid litigation. Rather than learning these lessons by going through a court proceeding, a reader can review the past experiences and mistakes made by radiology colleagues so as to change practice patterns in a way that can preempt malpractice suits. Expert witness testimony is one of the best means for understanding the litigation process, as well as reviewing the mistakes made by others and applying the lessons to your own experience.

The Institute of Medicine (IOM) summary, "To Err is Human: Building a Safer Health System," on physician errors published in 1999[1] has led to a significant amount of soul searching about the mistakes made in the medical profession. Limiting the number of mistakes and managing the mistakes that *are* made has become a large focus of individual physicians, group practices, departments, and health-care institutions. It is estimated that medical errors account for 44,000 to 98,000 deaths each year in our country. The cost for treating the effects of these errors is estimated to be between $17 billion and $29 billion per year in hospitals nationwide.

The IOM defined medical errors as "the failure to complete a planned action as intended or the use of a wrong plan to achieve an aim." An adverse event was determined to be "an injury caused by medical management rather than by the underlying disease or condition of the patient."

The types of medical errors cited most frequently by the IOM report are listed in Box 27-1, and one can see that diagnostic errors, for which radiology may be responsible, rank high on the list.

BOX 27-1

Most Frequent Errors Cited in IOM Report

1. Medication errors
2. Wrong surgeries
3. Diagnostic errors
   a. Incorrect choice of therapy
   b. Failure to use an indicated diagnostic test
   c. Misinterpretation of test results
   d. Failure to act on abnormal results
4. Equipment failure
5. Infections, such as nosocomial and postsurgical wound infections
6. Blood transfusion–related injuries, such as giving a patient blood of the incorrect type
7. Misinterpretation of other medical orders

Adapted from Institute of Medicine summary "To Err Is Human: Building a Safer Health System" on physician errors, 1999.

WHY ARE RADIOLOGISTS DISPROPORTIONATELY NAMED IN SUITS?

Radiologists are the seventh most commonly sued medical professional after neurosurgeons, anesthesiologists, obstetricians, orthopedic surgeons, general surgeons, and emergency medicine physicians. Yet radiologists are the third most common specialist to receive unfavorable verdicts. Radiologists are at a distinct disadvantage with respect to malpractice litigation for several reasons (Box 27-2). The evidence for a potential mistake remains retrievable for at least 7 years (with films) and possibly longer (with electronic archiving). With respect to pediatric cases, however, because film must be preserved until the individual reaches a majority age, this

BOX 27-2

Increased "Exposure" to Malpractice by Radiologists

1. Data are retrievable
2. No rapport established with patients
3. Poor communication rampant
4. Absence of clinical data
5. Technology advances exposing new pathology
6. High salaries

exposure of the radiologist may be even longer. Our "data" are open to scrutiny and are time independent.

In the ideal world, all types of practices would be subject to the persistence of the factual evidence of what data were available and how they were evaluated that sets such a high standard for the radiologist. It would be great if this could somehow be matched by other specialties. Specifically, if harm has been done as a result of a physician's inadequate performance, it is appropriate for the patient to have the opportunity to seek funds to address the harm that has occurred. Contrast the radiologist's long-term data availability for second guessing to that of the cardiologist who is sued for missing a heart murmur indicative of aortic insufficiency. He may be able to say that, at the time of his examination, that murmur was not present. He can refer to the medical chart in which he had scribbled in his notes that no murmur was heard. There is no way to go back to determine whether that murmur was missed (or was even listened for) on the basis of a standardized note in the hospital chart. So even if a murmur is heard by another physician several months later, the first physician can deny its prior existence and, provided he recorded his evaluation, is not "exposed" from a medical legal standpoint. In the same fashion the neurologist can say that the "new" hyperreflexia that led to discovery of a patient's spinal cord neoplasm was simply not present on an earlier evaluation 3 months before as demonstrated by a "normal neurologic exam" scribbled in the patient's SOAP note. Even in operative reports the surgeon can use his or her "appendectomy macro" dictation, which states that the cecum and terminal ilium were normal in appearance at the time of the laparoscopic appendectomy. If the patient develops an abscess with evidence of a perforation of the terminal ileum-cecum junction, the surgeon can state that he had looked in this region and recorded that the region was normal in his operative note. Therefore, this could not possibly be from a perioperative complication but must be due to a new process that occurred after the operation, thereby relieving the surgeon of responsibility and possibly potential litigation.

Although these examples may seem somewhat far-fetched, the truth is that radiology, like pathology, is a specialty in which the evidence for the potential malpractice suit cannot be "buried" in an office note. There is no worse feeling than having someone else show you a finding that has been overlooked or misinterpreted with the benefit of 20/20 retrospect. That is the other aspect of radiology that makes it a specialty vulnerable to litigation. The ability to obtain follow-up examinations and see abnormalities in retrospect that otherwise would not have been detected is a wonderful and yet high-risk aspect of our specialty. That very subtle linear density that was interpreted as a vascular structure on the initial chest radiograph can clearly be seen to grow to a 3-cm mass over the course of a 2-year interval when the follow-up chest radiograph is available. We cannot run away from the evidence and, when higher resolution imaging is obtained with each passing year, the conspicuity of our "misses" simply increases and again makes us more vulnerable. That same subtle fracture that was not present on our 2-megapixel home monitor may become much more obvious as we evolve to 5-megapixel monitors and high-resolution digital radiography. Add in the benefits of windowing the study electronically on the picture archiving and communication system (PACS) to show the abnormality as opposed to the overexposed appearance on the film once provided and, once again, our risk of litigation is significantly increased. Our ability to detect the lung nodule may be greatly enhanced through the ultra-thin (0.5 mm) section 64-slice multidetector computed tomography (CT) study compared with the scan-and-shoot 5-mm-thick lung sections that were obtained 5 years ago. Because our technology evolves in a way that improves resolution as well as image quality, lesions may have been missed in the past because of inferior technology and reduced conspicuity rather than because of lack of skill by the radiologist. It takes much less skill for someone to identify a hyperintense stroke on a diffusion-weighted image this year than for someone to have detected the subtle loss of gray-white differentiation on a CT scan that indicated an acute stroke in the 1990s.

To summarize, here are the major vulnerabilities of radiologists:

1. Our misses are observable forever. The bottom line is that there is an image and there is a finding. The challenge is that when an expert witness is asked to evaluate if there was a finding there, his a priori position is that he or she is looking at a study with something on it and the expert has to find it. Often the expert is requested because of that area of expertise, so a person who is established as a stroke expert would investigate to determine if there is evidence for stroke with a more extended search than would be the standard of care in the world of miscellaneous cases. The best lawyers send cases to experts in a blinded fashion, where the only clinical history provided is that which the original radiologist had at the time of examination. In the best of cases, no other records or opinions or discussions that may bias the evaluation occur before the expert review.

2. There is also the effect that lesions grow over time. These lesions are demonstrated with clarity to the jury and with the "retrospectoscope" the original lesion stands out. It is an observer bias. This situation is exacerbated according to the direction in which the technology evolves, so that a lesion that might not have been seen with clarity with the pulse sequences used in the past or displayed without the windowing capabilities of PACS, would have been very difficult to see using original technology.

Another important reason why radiologists are more exposed to malpractice litigation is that we generally do not establish a rapport or relationship with the patient that builds trust or confidence or empathy. In general, we are merely the name at the bottom of the report that a patient reads. We are anonymous. It is very easy, therefore, to characterize us as the villain/enemy when we make a mistake. We have not built the 10 years of trust in the relationship that the practitioner has, taking the children through their various injuries, illnesses, and surgeries as a partner in their health care. We are not the family doctor who provided reassurance and consolation through the chronic illnesses. We don't even see the patient. The establishment of a caring relationship with the patient is one of the best means for avoiding malpractice litigations when a mistake has been made or an unfortunate unexpected consequence has occurred in the provision of medical care.

It is no wonder that mammography has the greatest liability. This is attributed in part to the following:

1. Breast cancer, by its nature, is a highly charged emotional experience in women and therefore has a greater exposure to litigation than other cancers.
2. At the time of the evaluation, these patients are generally healthy people. A properly interpreted screening study would "save" this healthy person. This is different from missing disease in someone who is already manifesting symptoms.
3. In those mammographic practices where close patient contact is not possible, close clinician communication with mammographers functions as a surrogate, but the patient may not appreciate that.
4. The technology with xerography, plain-film mammography, computer radiography, and digital mammography is a moving target.
5. Computer-assisted diagnosis adds another layer of complexity to the doctor-patient-computer relationship.
6. Breast cancer has been on the rise.

How can you explain, however, the numerous suits brought against mammographers for missed breast cancers? In many breast centers the mammographer sees the patient within 6-to 12-month intervals, performs the physical examinations, and reviews the screening mammogram. Considering the huge number of mammograms performed in this country, if we were to calculate the ratio of the number of examinations to the number of malpractice suits, this would probably not be a very noteworthy percentage. Additionally, just as with other high-volume examinations, the ability to detect the cancer increases remarkably in the setting of multiple follow-up examinations. This is also a scenario where things are much more clearly identified in hindsight. Nonetheless, the likelihood of litigation when the study is performed without any interaction between the examiner and the patient is clearly higher than when the mammographer interacts in a positive way with the patient.

As an aside, on the issue of breast cancer detection and mammography, it has recently been ruled in *Gray v. Fairview General Hospital* that computer-aided detection can be used to

bolster a medical expert's testimony but cannot in and of itself validate or refute a radiologist's decision to recall a patient for more extensive evaluation. In other words, computer-aided detection is not a standard of expertise.

EXTENT OF LITIGATION PROBLEM IN RADIOLOGY

Average radiologist liability awards have increased from $120,000 in 1996 to $178,000 in 2004. Plaintiffs, the individuals who bring forward the charge that inadequate care was provided, however, win only about 30% of suits brought to trial. Median medical liability awards increased from $500,000 to over $1,000,000 from 1994 to 2002 nationwide. The average cost to defend a malpractice case that comes to trial is approximately $91,000.[2] The average indemnity payment for radiologists' suits increased from $186,000 to $349,000 between 1995 and 2002, according to the Physician Insurers Association of America.[3]

Overall the percentage of malpractice claims that are attributable to radiology is approximately 10%. Among radiologists, breast imagers are the most exposed of the subspecialties, and mammograms are the studies for which most radiologists are sued. Failure to diagnose or delays in the diagnosis of breast cancer are the most common claims of malpractice. This has led to a reduction in the number of radiologists performing breast imaging in many locales and the closing of mammographic facilities in many settings. The impact on women has been longer wait times for mammograms and sometimes delays in diagnosis due to lack of appointment availability. Compounding this problem is the low reimbursement for screening mammography by the Centers for Medicare and Medicaid Services.

As a result, radiologists can expect, based on past experience, an increase in malpractice insurance premiums of 25% or greater every 3 years. Changing carriers will be required in over one third of practices within a 3-year period, in part because the carriers no longer service radiologists. Current median premiums range from a high of $21,000 in the Northeast to a low of $16,000 out West. State-specific premiums are the highest in Florida at $45,500.

Regarding the escalation of malpractice premiums, the impact of establishing caps on damage levels for malpractice cases remains in controversy. In some states that have implemented punitive/damage caps the insurance premiums have not changed at all. Malpractice lawyers opine that the insurance rates vary most closely with how well the insurance companies' investments in the markets are doing more so than with the number of cases or amounts of awards. If the stock market goes down, malpractice premiums on publicly held insurance carriers probably will rise, they say. Insurance reform that eliminates this source of the variance in premiums imposed on physicians is a useful suggestion for stabilizing the industry.

COMPONENTS OF A MALPRACTICE LAWSUIT

In any malpractice suit certain elements must be fulfilled for the claim to be valid (Box 27-3). Although a person can be sued for frivolous reasons, it is these elements that must be present to justify medicolegal litigation.

Duty

The first element is duty. This means that a physician-patient relationship has been established and there is a duty for the physician to perform a service on the patient. When a radiologist provides an interpretation of an imaging study on a patient, he has established a doctor-patient relationship and has a duty to that patient. In the routine setting of reading cases and dictating reports in the outpatient or hospital setting the establishment of duty is straightforward.

Although the existence of duty may seem intuitive, there are many cases in which a defense has been based on the physician's claim

---

BOX 27-3
Components of a Malpractice Case
1. Duty
2. Breach of standard of care
3. Causation
4. Damage

---

that he or she had no duty to the patient. As an example, suppose a colleague stops you in the hallway and asks your opinion on a case. Has a physician-patient relationship been established in that case? It has been argued that if a curbside consult occurs and a description of the findings of a case are given in very general terms, not specific to an individual patient, a physician-patient relationship has not been established and therefore there is no duty.

"Dave I wonder if I can ask you a question about a case I saw yesterday?"

"Sure."

"There was this case where there was a hyperdense mass in the brain near the sella and had the shape of a peanut."

"Well, I would certainly consider either a hemorrhagic pituitary adenoma or a craniopharyngioma in that instance."

"Wow, I didn't think about a hemorrhagic pituitary adenoma. Thanks for that idea."

In this case, where the final diagnosis turns out to be an internal carotid aneurysm that subsequently bleeds out during the transphenoidal hypophysectomy approach, you could argue that a physician-patient relationship between Dave, the consultant, and the patient has not been established. This is not to say that the defendant might not bring this conversation up at trial to say that even the division chief of neuroradiology at Johns Hopkins Hospital did not consider an aneurysm when the patient had these findings on CT scan. But the consult was nebulous enough, and not specific to the patient, that a specific duty was not established.

On the other hand, if a physician stops Dave in the corridor, and the physician has the films in hand and shows Dave the case on a nearby view box, even if Dave does not dictate a report on the case, he is liable because a physician-patient relationship has been established for that specific case. Although this may be arguable on both sides in court, Dave may be sued because he rendered an opinion on that specific patient that may have been influential in the care of the patient. Duty has been established. It is not at all uncommon for a referring physician to ask you for your "informal opinion," then to dictate in his formal note that "Dr. Yousem was consulted and stated . . . ." This is particularly problematic in that the informal consult may or may not come with available clinical history or prior studies, and these may not be documented when a curbside opinion is obtained. For this reason, our division has established formal "outside/curbside reads" policies (Box 27-4).

Physician-patient relationships may also be established through intermediaries. When a physician's assistant or a nurse practitioner is taking care of the patient in the name of a physician, even if the physician has not personally established a relationship with the patient, the intermediary serves as the conduit to a physician-patient relationship in a duty to perform a service. If a technologist makes an error that injures a patient, it is probable that that technologist's employer or physician director will also be sued, because (1) suits against individually named technologists are not worthwhile unless the technologist is insured, (2) the technologist represents the corporation or entity that is the employer, and (3) the physicians have the big bucks and the larger malpractice insurance. When physicians have malpractice coverage that will not afford the plaintiff the money they need for a lifetime of long-term care ("bad baby outcomes"), the likelihood that the hospital will be included as a plaintiff rises, because this entity has deeper pockets. That means that the nurse and technologist may be named as defendants as a means of bringing the hospital's insurance coverage into the mix.

Vicarious liability is effectively the transfer of liability from one entity to the other. This is most commonly implied in that an employer must be responsible for the activities of its employees and the harm that may come from

---

BOX 27-4

Johns Hopkins Outside Film Review Policy (Draft)

Our department is implementing a policy requiring official interpretations for all outside image consultations. This policy will require a few simple steps:

1. Referring physicians must complete a requisition for the outside image consultation and provide a clinical history. Patients who wish to have their studies reviewed must also fill out a requisition with a referring physician's name and clinical history.
2. Whenever possible the image interpretation report of the outside study should be submitted as well.
3. The outside study, regardless of the submitted format (electronic CD, zip disk, films, paper), and outside study report will be delivered to the Radiology Customer Service Center for input into electronic patient record (EPR) and the electronic archive. Electronic submissions should be in standard DICOM format to assure timely and accurate transfer to the archive.
4. The customer service center will digitize or input the image data, and will add the study to an "outside film" worklist for the appropriate Division or Section. If a specific radiologist is designated to interpret a study, this will be included in the study request but in general is to be discouraged.
5. The outside study will be reviewed and formally interpreted by an accredited physician member of the Department of Radiology.
6. Expected turnaround times are being developed ensuring that this process will provide clinically useful information for the referring physicians before the patient's anticipated or scheduled visits.

Unofficial Curbside Consultations as a Departmental Practice Are Discouraged
This policy is being implemented for the following reasons:

1. Patient safety: A successful precedent was set by the Department of Pathology for outside slide interpretations. Official interpretations by our physicians will either confirm the accuracy of the outside report or suggest recommendations for additional or repeat studies, if needed.
2. Medicolegal considerations: Official reports will become part of the patient record in the electronic patient record instead of "hearsay" notes by referring physicians. Records will be retrievable and reflect the interpreting physicians' official opinion.
3. Quality care: Images will be placed in the electronic archive for permanent storage and retrieval, thus making them part of the patient's official record. Outside studies will no longer be "outside" of the domain of clinicians. They will be available on any PACS workstation.
4. Convenience: Our referring physicians will now have access to the formal interpretations of all studies regardless of where they were performed and in addition to the images in digital format.

the employee's performance. Vicarious liability refers to an indirect legal responsibility of an employer for an employee.

A hospital may be vicariously liable for the behavior and performance of its employees. A radiologist may be vicariously liable for the negligence of his employees, such as technologists and nurses, trainees such as residents or fellows, and contracted nighthawk-teleradiology employees. However, these individuals would not be vicariously liable for the activities of the radiologist. Therefore, radiologists must show concern and maintenance of standards of their employees including having systems for quality improvement, oversight, and risk management. However, the radiologist who is an independently contracted employee at a hospital may not be held responsible for the other hospital employees' actions unless they are under his or her immediate supervision and that supervision was negligent. Nonetheless, the patient is likely to attempt to ascribe blame to all parties when a malpractice suit is levied.

Breach in the Standard of Care

The next element of a successful lawsuit is what is known as the "breach." This means that there has been a deviation of care from that which would be expected of a reasonably competent physician. It is the level of care that a reasonably prudent health-care professional would provide under the circumstances described in the course of patient care in question. The jargon among lawyers would emphasize "reasonable" and "prudent." Most people believe that reasonable is a nebulous word that refers to the expected practice pattern in which the majority of individuals would follow. Reasonable does not mean absolute and does not mean 100%. Reasonable also implies a migration to the mean and not the expert. Expert witnesses realize that a reasonable and prudent interpretation of a film does not mean the interpretation that the world's most noted authority on a topic might render but instead what the average member of the American College of Radiology (ACR) might render.

Expert witnesses are often viewed as physicians who choose to supplement their income either at the expense of colleagues who are performing radiology at the standard of care or at the expense

of patients by defending substandard care. Both are truly inappropriate. Standard of care (SOC) in fact has demonstrated that subtle findings can be missed up to 23% of the time. Very good physicians practicing very good radiology will sometimes miss findings. Has the SOC been breached then? This is to be differentiated from the fact that what is reasonable to one expert witness may be different from what is reasonable to another expert witness, and this is again a source of contention that is often debated at the time of the trial, and decided by a jury.

The breach can occur in any number of settings but, in radiology, breaches of the standard of care are usually in the delayed or missed detection of masses, with breast cancer and lung cancer the most frequently cited breaches. However, the breach may also be in the diagnosis of other conditions, the performance of the study, the communication of the results of the study (another hot topic discussed below), or the treatment of lesions by the radiologist, by his or her team, or by both. Breaches in the standard of care are often referenced to guidelines provided by such austere organizations as the ACR. But standard operating procedures at peer institutions or within the community may also be referenced for potential descriptions of SOC. Once again, the phrase "reasonable expectation" is what is applied often to issues of breaches in the standard of care. The lawyers will refer to what one could reasonably expect to have happen with respect to the interpretation of a film or a performance of a study.

For example, this writer was consulted to be an expert witness in a case in which iodinated contrast dye was injected into a patient's spinal cord during a cervical myelogram. This occurred because the patient moved during the examination, the needle punctured the spinal cord, and the contrast material was injected. Was it a breach of standard of care that the spinal cord was punctured? No. This occurs in a limited percentage of cases during cervical puncture for C1–C2 myelography. Was it a breach in the standard of care that the contrast was injected into the spinal cord? Well, herein lies the debate. In this case the litigation issue revolved around the amount of contrast dye injected into the spinal cord. It would not be malpractice if a small amount of contrast entered the spinal cord when the

469

patient's cord was punctured as a result of the patient's movement during the injection. On the other hand, if the injection of the contrast dye into the spinal cord persisted because no one looked to see if the cord had been punctured or because under fluoroscopy the radiologist did not recognize that he was injecting into the spinal cord, this would represent a breach in the SOC. It is these nuances that determine which way judgments go in trials.

Causation

The next component of a legitimate malpractice suit is the element of causation. This is the linking of the alleged breach in the standard of care to the actual damage that the patient has suffered. In the scenario just described, for example, if a patient suffered cervical myelopathic symptoms such as arm weakness or debilitating paresthesias associated with the injection of contrast dye into the spinal cord and an expert neuroradiologist and neurologist can confirm that the site and location of the contrast dye correspond to the neuronal tissue that innervates the upper extremities, the malpractice claim has fulfilled the criterion of causation. The neurologist should attest to the link between location and symptoms; a neuroradiologist would be well advised to state that he or she is not providing testimony as an expert in structure-function correlation (a smart lawyer will attack him for this). Thus the neuroradiologist localizes the contrast but a neurologist attests to linkage. On the other hand, if the patient's symptom is blurred vision following the cervical myelogram puncture, it is possible that although duty has been fulfilled, a breach in the standard of care has occurred, and the patient has suffered damage (i.e., persistent blurred vision), causation cannot be established. If the cause of that blurred vision cannot be linked to the cervical contrast dye injection, the defendant can win the case based on the causation defense.

This case exemplified a reasonably straightforward example of causation, but there are times when it is not so straightforward. For example, suppose a physician misinterprets a magnetic resonance angiogram performed for headache evaluation and calls it normal but the patient has a left middle cerebral artery (MCA) distribution aneurysm. In retrospect, the film clearly demonstrates an aneurysm, and several witnesses are brought in to confirm that the MCA aneurysm has been missed. Two years later, the patient suffers an MCA distribution infarction after atrial fibrillation with expressive and receptive aphasia and right hemiparesis. Her ability to communicate is gone, and the family is distraught. During the workup the aneurysm is discovered. The patient's family sues on a delayed diagnosis of MCA distribution aneurysm.

In this case arguments can be made that the aneurysm did not predispose the patient to an MCA thrombus, and therefore although duty, breach, and damage have occurred, the condition was not caused by the misinterpretation of the magnetic resonance angiogram. Expert witnesses can be called in to state that the source of the middle artery stroke would more likely have arisen secondary to cardiac source emboli from atrial fibrillation or atherosclerotic disease that the patient had in the carotid circulation. The cardiology expert witness may support the notion that the patient had a source in the left atrium due to the fibrillation unrelated to the MCA aneurysm that was missed. There is no causation.

Of course, for every expert witness on one side, there is the potential for an expert witness on the opposite side, in this case the plaintiff. This expert might posit that the turbulent flow within the MCA distribution aneurysm may have led to a local clot forming that extended intracranially to cause the MCA distribution infarction. Alternatively, the turbulence may have led to a clot from atrial fibrillation lodging at that site, or the MCA aneurysm may have dissected and led to occlusion of the MCA. Vasospasm after subarachnoid hemorrhage may have also led to occlusion of the blood vessel. Potential causation will have thus been established in the jury's mind. In these circumstances the jury must make judgments without the same level of medical knowledge as the physicians and malpractice attorneys, and they produce judgments that sometimes may not seem reasonable. Educating the jury is one of the tasks of the lawyers and their expert witnesses. This responsibility demands considerable effort by the attorneys.

Damage

The final component of a malpractice suit is damage. If the patient had been stuck by the spinal needle and had the contrast dye injected but sustained no long-standing or short-term injury or damage, there would be no cause for a suit. Damages are usually separated into two types: the damage associated with care for the individual after the injury has occurred (economic) and damages associated with the emotional trauma (noneconomic), which may also affect the patient over a long period of time. In addition, one has potential for punitive damages in which the plaintiff is compensated because of the flagrant nature of the error by the physician. In many states a cap on punitive damages is being considered in order to reduce the malpractice premiums that physicians must pay and to provide a more just compensation scheme for plaintiffs injured by malpractice. Even in the case of manufacturing errors, where billions of dollars have been awarded on a punitive basis (this is especially true with cigarette manufacturers), limits are being imposed by the legislature to create a more "reasonable" punitive damage structure.

Thus the patient must have suffered an insult to his or her body or emotional state if that patient is to have a realistic chance of succeeding in a malpractice suit. In many cases neuropsychologists, rehabilitation specialists, actuaries, and other damages experts are brought in to determine the degree of damage that has occurred, the monetary loss that will ensue as a result of the damage, or the monetary outlay that may be required to maintain the health of damaged patients for life.

ANATOMY OF A SUIT

Investigation

A malpractice suit usually begins with an untoward or unfortunate incident that leads to an unhappy patient or patient family member (Box 27-5). The patient or the representative of the patient, the plaintiff, usually has 2 to 4 years for adults and 7 to 10 years for minors (depending on the state and age of the patient) to bring forth a complaint of malpractice from the time the incident was discovered. Wrongful death cases are also usually brought to complaint within 2 years of the death.

The first stop is usually to a plaintiff lawyer, who will review the medical records and often

---

BOX 27-5

Components of a Typical Malpractice Lawsuit

1. Investigation
2. Complaint
3. Discovery
4. Motions
5. Negotiation
   a. Arbitration/mediation
6. Preparation for trial
7. Trial
8. Post-trial motions
9. Appeal

---

consult with medical experts to assess whether the complaint has merit. The lawyers will formally and informally interview potential witnesses about the events surrounding the incident. Some states require that a medical expert and malpractice lawyer jointly file a statement alleging that a breach in the standard of care has occurred and that there is merit in bringing forth a lawsuit.

Summons or Complaint

The lawyer for the plaintiff will then file the lawsuit with the appropriate court, usually in the county where the alleged malpractice occurred. This written complaint may also be called the "original pleading" and is the means by which a legal action is commenced. This may be accompanied by a summons, which is a document prepared by the clerk at the court where the claim has been filed. This is the formal notice that a civil action has been filed against the health professional and is the official statement of being sued. The complaint usually requires a response by the defendant's legal team within a set number of days. The response is called an "answer" to the complaint, and it is filed by the defendant's attorneys with the court. In the answer the defendant will usually deny in part or in whole the plaintiff's allegations, defend his or her behavior, and ask that the suit be dropped.

Discovery

This is the portion of the malpractice case that usually is the most lengthy. At this period the lawyers will continue their meticulous (one would hope) review of the medical record, obtain additional medical charts from physicians who treated the plaintiff or were in some way associated with the alleged incident or incidents before the event, request any additional documents that may have bearing on the case, and submit written interrogatories of key witnesses for written answers. Often the court where the suit is filed will order a preliminary conference with the attorneys for all parties to discuss the materials they have received from each other and request further authorizations, if necessary. This is an opportune time for negotiation for settlement to occur, but often more data are required. The court then authorizes that the formal deposition process begin with testimony to be taken under oath by the various players in the suit. It is important to note that this is a two-way process by which the defendant's lawyer is also investigating previous behavior and health issues of the plaintiff or the patient if the patient is not the plaintiff. Recruitment and depositions of expert witnesses or factual witnesses for both the defendant and the plaintiff are performed. The damage experts will suggest appropriate awards. Review of previous cases to determine if any precedents have been made in similar cases is also the responsibility of the attorneys. When the phase of discovery has been completed, another meeting with the judge is scheduled with all attorneys present (again another potential time when resolution can occur), and the case is certified as ready for trial.

Expert Witness Testimony

The *Daubert v. Merrell Dow Pharmaceuticals Inc.* case required that the conclusions and opinions of expert witnesses be based on sound reasoning and reliable scientific methodology. If these criteria are met, then the scientific evidence provided is admissible. The concept of general acceptance may also be applied to the admissibility of scientific testimony. Thus, even though there may not be good double-blind randomized placebo-controlled studies on the use of steroids in patients with cerebral edema, that the practice is in general acceptance is sufficient to suggest that it constitutes the standard of care. As discussed above, the lack of personal

accountability of physicians to understand what is the expected performance of a peer and not to over- or under-represent this is important.

A defendant is not generally expected to have the knowledge and skills of an expert witness or the most knowledgeable person in the field. The standard of care is based on what a prudent and reasonable physician would be expected to do. This means that the defendant is judged to the average acceptable standard of his peers.

Motions

Motions are requests of the court. The most common motion that is filed is one for a summary judgment by the judge to decide the case without a trial, because the facts are clearly weighted heavily in favor of one side or the other, or because there are other reasons why a suit should not be brought forward (statute of limitations, frivolous nature of the suit, etc). If there is no genuine issue of material fact (i.e., no facts are in dispute by the two sides), then summary judgment can be requested by the moving party to prevail as a matter of interpretation of the law by the judge without the need for a jury to decide on the merits or reliability of the facts. Summary judgments are rarely procured in most legitimate lawsuits. Other motions may include those to move a trial to another location or time. A motion in limine is a request forbidding opposing counsel from referring to or presenting certain evidence at trial that may be prejudicial, irrelevant, or inadmissible. If the court does not grant the motions requested, these may be used as grounds for an appeal in the event of an unfavorable verdict. Appeals courts will review the laws that decide a case (e.g., whether the judge followed the appropriate rules and restrictions trying the case) but not the facts of the case or the jury's decision.

Negotiation

In the best of circumstances there is active communication between the attorneys representing the two parties, as they assess the merits of the case. Justice must be done, and it behooves the plaintiffs and defendants to make a good-faith effort to resolve the case through

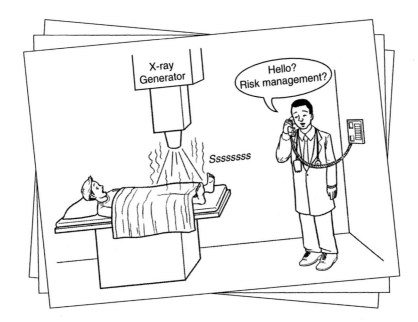

negotiations. Sometimes the judge will order or request the parties to negotiate or to use unbiased third-party mediation. Negotiations can take place at any time in the process, including after a trial has already started. Once a case is settled, if a monetary solution is negotiated, the defendant's insurance company is required by law to make payment within 30 days.

Trial

The trial is the stage that many physicians hope to avoid. You put your career and reputation in the hands of 6 to 12 laypeople in a jury, although occasionally you may have a judge decide the case. This tends to be true when there has been an event in a government-run facility such as a Veterans' Administration or Armed Forces hospital. Typical trials last a week or longer.

Jury selection occurs in a phase of the trial called the voir dire. Voir dire refers to the question-answer interview process of the selection of prospective jurors in which the judge and attorneys try to assess for bias and partiality. The attorneys and judge have an opportunity to exclude a limited number of potential jurors from being appointed to the trial. The goal of the attorneys is to obtain the most unbiased yet favorable person to sit on the jury.

Opening statements provide the basic strategy of the opposing teams and set the stage for the body of the trial. Basic themes may be presented, and the attorneys try to prime the jury to look for the critical (influential) aspects of the trial testimony in their favor. At this point the lawyers are trying to introduce a bias to the jury so that they are favorably disposed to their case.

The lawyers for the plaintiffs first present their case usually starting with factual witnesses about the events that took place and the subsequent impact this had on the patient and/or his or her family. The plaintiff's expert witnesses follow, providing opinions on the issues of duty, breach, causation, and damages of the case. The defendant's lawyers have an opportunity to cross-examine each of these witnesses. Then the defendant's lawyers have the opportunity to present their side of the case with their factual and expert witnesses. Again the plaintiff's attorneys may cross-examine the defendant's witnesses. Rebuttal evidence may be presented by the plaintiff's counsel if new issues are raised by defense testimony.

Closing arguments are presented by counsel for the plaintiff, then the defendant, and finally again by the plaintiff for any additional arguments. The last word is left to the plaintiff. During these summations the attorneys discuss the evidence that has been presented and present their arguments about why they should win the case.

Judgment and Award

The case goes to the jury to determine culpability and/or liability and, if the defendant is found liable, the amount of money to be awarded to the plaintiff. The amount awarded to the plaintiff is composed of different components, usually described as (1) pain and suffering from the date of the malpractice to the date of the verdict, and pain and suffering for the future; (2) lost income in the past and future; (3) expenses related to care for the patient and/or family members in the past and future; and (4) punitive damages for the egregious nature of the malpractice. Taken another way, the awards are separated into economic damages (i.e., medical bills resulting from the harm done by the health-care provider's error and lost wages resulting from the patient's inability to be employed in the manner expected before the malpractice error) and noneconomic damages for pain and suffering, and punitive damages. If the patient is married, the jury may award damages to the spouse of the patient for past and future lost services and consortium (a legal word for what I refer to as sexual satisfaction but they call the "conjugal fellowship of husband and wife in the company, society, cooperation, affection, and aid of the other in every conjugal relationship"). If the suit is for a wrongful death, the jury is asked to evaluate the pain and suffering of the person who died as well as the economic loss to the family caused by the death.

Post-Trial Motions and Appeals

After a verdict has been rendered on a malpractice case, most states allow the potential for appeals. Post-trial motions precede the appeal process and can be categorized as those requesting a completely new trial and those that request that the verdict be set aside and that reverse the verdict. It is rare for a judge to overturn a jury trial consequent to these post-trial motions, but it can happen if the judge feels the jury's decision making was tainted or simply unreasonable. The amount of money awarded to the plaintiff may also be revised by the judge if it is felt that the sum is disproportionate to the injury.

In the post-trial motions, no new information or arguments may be presented. The motions are usually oriented to flaws in the performance or administration of the case rather than an attempt to change people's minds about the

same set of facts and witnesses. Even in the appeal process, no new data can be presented.

The appeal process is not a "right" provided in malpractice cases. In many instances the appellate court will simply refuse to accept the submitted appeal, and the lower court ruling will stand. The grounds of the appeal must be based on errors in the proceeding of the trial court such as admission of nonadmissible evidence, allowing expert witnesses to provide influential testimony beyond the scope of their expertise, allowing hearsay evidence, etc. The appellate court has several options available to it including: (1) summary judgment with no further discussion, (2) letting the verdict and award stand as previously decided, (3) reversal of the decision, (4) reversal and recommendation for retrial, and (5) alteration of the award set forth by the trial court. Some state supreme courts have the discretion to not even accept the case for review.

SOURCES OF SUITS

The sources of malpractice suits are manifold in radiology (Box 27-6).[4]

BOX 27-6

Types of Errors

1. Missed findings
2. Misinterpretation of findings
   a. Fund of knowledge
   b. Incomplete data
3. Miscommunication
4. Clinical issues
5. Technical issues
6. Practice/system-based flaws
7. Improper performance of a study
8. Performing a study when contraindicated
9. Failure to recognize a complication of a study
10. Failure to supervise/monitor a case
11. Failure to appropriately act on findings.

Adapted from Brenner RJ, Lucey LL, Smith JJ, Saunders R: Radiology and medical malpractice claims: a report on the practice standards claims survey of the Physician Insurers Association of America and the American College of Radiology. Am J Roentgenol 1998;171(1):19–22.

Missed Diagnoses

The sources of missed diagnoses may be very different from those revolving around misinterpretation. Missed diagnoses may be on the basis of fatigue, extraneous light or noise, distractions, naivete, or ignorance, but are more commonly attributable to lack of perception. Because most radiology malpractice litigation revolves around the failure to diagnose lung and breast cancer, the ability to detect the lesion among the noise of background quantum mottle and normal tissue is paramount. Radiologists may be fooled by a false sense of satisfaction of search in which the presence of one abnormality leads to a lowering of the guard for the detection of another abnormality. By the same token, many imagers have "blind spots" where they do not focus their attention and may leave a corner of an image unobserved. The availability of prior studies is another critical factor that may aid in the detection of an abnormality, as is the reliability of symmetry between sides (e.g., growth plate fractures in children).

Experience,[5] optimal lighting and concentration settings, lack of distraction, and knowing the telltale signs of cancer are critical, with only the last factor really based on fund of knowledge. Kan et al noted that reading a minimum of 2500 mammographic interpretations per year is associated with better cancer detection rates.[5] Particularly with mammographic screening, there really are two main judgments that must be made on a case-to-case basis:

1. Is it clearly cancer or not?
2. Should there be a recall or a biopsy?

Identifying and perceiving the imaging findings in a screening setting is the key. R. James Brenner notes that absence of detection may be the result of technical errors (image quality) preventing detection (13% to 16% of cases), no imaging features to suggest a lesion, subthreshold features suggestive of malignancy, or observer error.[6] The decision not to perform additional images that might have uncovered a malignancy is cited frequently as a cause of absence of detection.

Double reading of studies, something that is commonly performed in academic institutions where trainees and faculty members will look at studies serially or together, has been shown to improve detection rates of abnormalities by as much as 15%. This may also be a benefit when nighthawk services are used but a final report is not issued. Historical data are also of value when interpreting studies or assessing lesions for pathology.

Misinterpretations

Misinterpretations occur more frequently as a result of a lack of knowledge or poor judgment than from an absence of perception. In these cases, findings are dismissed or credited to other diagnoses that may simply be incorrect. The difference between nondetection and misdiagnosis is like the difference between chest radiography and chest CT scanning. One can easily miss a small cancer hidden amidst the overlapping shadows of the pulmonary vessels on a chest radiogram and experience a "miss" based on nondetection. This same lesion may be readily identifiable on a chest CT study but misattributed to granulomatous disease based on erroneous interpretation of the imaging appearance. In neuroradiology a FLAIR CSF pulsation artifact may be misinterpreted to be a cerebellopontine angle epidermoid.

Educational programs beyond residency and fellowship intuitively and demonstrably improve misinterpretation rate. In one setting the sensitivity for the detection of breast cancer increased from 80% to 87%, and median tumor size and node positivity decreased after an educational program intervention in which 11 radiologists attended 17 breast imaging seminars.[7] Quality improvement initiatives may also improve misinterpretation rates.[7] In a program introduced by ACR, a radiologist examines the interpretation of "old films" as a part of the daily routine. This systematic feedback loop requires minimal additional time and creates an environment of continuous quality improvement.

Communication Breakdowns

The ACR guidelines require direct communication between reporting radiologists and referring physicians in cases of urgent or unexpected findings. This becomes quite a quandary, because many radiologists now provide 24/7 services even for outpatient nonemergency department studies. In an effort to offset Medicare reimbursement declines, many practices are providing evening, night-time, and weekend hours, when clinicians are no longer in their offices to receive communication. Leaving messages with answering services or on voicemail may not be legally compliant with physician notification guidelines.

In a recent article, Leonard Berlin[8] recounted a suit against a radiologist who was evaluating a patient by ultrasound for an epigastric pulsatile mass to rule out aortic aneurysm. In the report in which no aneurysm was seen, the radiologist stated, "Questionable echogenic area in right kidney which may be normal variation, such as prominent column of Bertin, but if clinically indicated a CT can be considered." No follow-up occurred, and a year later the patient was diagnosed with renal cell carcinoma. The patient sued for failure to diagnose the cancer, and the plaintiff's lawyer argued that the radiologist had a duty to call the referring physician (which he did not do) with the "unexpected finding" according to ACR guidelines. Eventually, although the suit never came to trial, the radiologist settled the case on the advice of the claims manager of the insurance company who thought the physician would lose the case. Berlin questioned whether busy radiologists have set the bar too low now with regard to calling in findings even if one thinks that they are inconsequential. What is the standard of care nationwide or regionally?

In a separate case a chest radiograph performed on a patient for chest pain was interpreted by an emergency room physician preliminarily as demonstrating mediastinal adenopathy. In the morning the radiologist reported the same film as suprahilar mass with mediastinal widening, suggestive of bronchogenic carcinoma. The referring physician failed to obtain follow-up scans for 3 months, at which time the woman was diagnosed with lung cancer. The radiologist was called to task for not calling the referring physician because of the "discrepancy" between his final report and the preliminary one. Despite his vociferous objection that the reports were nearly equivalent, the radiologist was advised to settle the case. In this example it was the difference between preliminary and final report readings that were thought to be "inconsequential."

These two cases speak to the current standard in the legal world regarding the need to notify. Communication is key. Both of these cases used the 2001 ACR standard regarding reporting: "In those situations in which the interpreting physician feels that the findings do not warrant immediate treatment but constitute significant unexpected findings, the interpreting physician or his/her designee should communicate the findings to the referring physician ..." and also the statement that "[a]ny significant change between an emergency or preliminary report and the final written report should be promptly reconciled by direct communication to the referring physician."[9]

What about inpatient procedures performed on the day of discharge? Because lengths of stay are becoming shorter and the push to send the patient out expeditiously is becoming more vociferous, these "last day" studies may not make it to the discharge summary and may also not receive the caregiver's attention. If they do, the patient may already be in the taxi home.

A review in 2005 by the ACR of legal cases revolving around communication issues identified four precedents that influence the need for immediate physician-physician communication in radiology[9]:

1. Findings that require immediate intervention
2. Conclusions by a radiologist that differ from a previous interpretation
3. Findings of a condition that may worsen over time if not promptly addressed
4. Findings that are unclear and require close follow-up

The review also concluded that it is the radiologist's responsibility to determine that the clinician has received the report and that the clinician has followed up on its findings. Direct communication has been defined as that which occurs in person or on the telephone. However, in some instances an agent may be used for the delivery (physician aid, assistant trainee) or receipt (nurse, on-call partner, physician's representative) of the imaging findings. Having a speech recognition dictation system that can send a report electronically and immediately to the clinician with an archived return acknowledgment of receipt would be the ideal solution here. Software is available to make this possible. In other circumstances (employment physicals or executive health self-referrals) where there is no designated physician representative, direct communication with the patient is required. At a minimum, we require that the referring physician's contact information be provided; otherwise we reject the study request.

Documentation of direct communication is straightforward when issuing a formal official report on a case. If there are curbside consultations on outside studies or for second opinions on existing studies, the radiologist should attempt to document these interpretations formally in the patient's medical record, by correspondence with the referring physician, or by an outside–curbside read policy described above. The radiologist should stipulate in the report any clinical information provided and the limitations of the outside images. Keeping a personal log of these curbside consultations is another alternative to the radiologist but is less optimal.

All individuals who receive preliminary reports on a patient should be contacted if a final report has a substantive revision or conclusion in comparison with the preliminary report. The responsibility lies with the radiologist to determine who may have acted on the preliminary report even if it is not the initial ordering physician.

Referring physicians, hospitals, and radiologists should work together to determine the preferred means for ensuring adequate delivery of radiology reports. Previous reports and images must be made available for review. Written departmental policies are required to optimize patient care and thus to reduce the liability of the radiologists.

Average awards for malpractice claims based on communication failures are often higher than other errors, in part because they are easy for a jury to understand.[10] When there is a communication lapse in diagnosing a breast cancer, the average indemnity payment is $548,000, whereas for all suits it is $269,000 (Boxes 27-7 and 27-8). If a report goes to the wrong physician (an event that is not uncommon because of inaccuracies or similarities or duplications of referring physicians' names), the courts have ruled by precedent that the receiving physician has no obligation to follow up with the patient (who is not his patient). Thus a report of a lung mass communicated to the wrong physician leaves that physician blameless legally (if not ethically) but the radiology team remains at medicolegal risk. One-way communications without receipt notification also expose the radiologists. The best systems, as stated earlier, are those requiring a reply, with acknowledgment of receipt by the correct individual. Text messages on pagers and cell phone logs are being used more frequently, but documentation of receipt remains problematic.

BOX 27-7

Most Common Communication Errors Leading to Breast Imaging Lawsuits and Average Payouts for Radiologists

1. Failure to directly communicate with treating physician and patient not receiving necessary information for appropriate management ($234K)
2. Communication with referring physician but information not reaching the patient ($228K)
3. Failure to communicate with referring physician but patient receiving information ($105K)
4. Both referring physician and patient receiving information ($15K)

Adapted from Brenner RJ, Bartholomew L: Communication errors in radiology: a liability cost analysis. J Am Coll Radiol 2:428–431, 2005.

BOX 27-8

Factors Involved in Payouts

1. Prognosis
2. Requirement for prolonged care and support
3. Egregious nature of the deviation from standard of care
4. Defendant and expert witness credibility
5. Contribution of patient to delayed diagnosis
6. Assessment of economic and noneconomic damages
7. Caps on pain and suffering by state

Adapted from Brenner RJ, Bartholomew L: Communication errors in radiology: a liability cost analysis. J Am Coll Radiol 2:428–431, 2005.

Improper Performance of a Study

There is some ambiguity surrounding the topic "improper performance of a study." Clearly, if the study was performed in a negligent way and resulted in patient injury, the physician is culpable. Perforated bowel from reductions of intussusception, retroperitoneal hematomas from angiograms, damaged breasts from compression views, fistulas from biliary drainage procedures, and strokes from stent placements account for many suits in this regard. However, these may be known complications of the procedures described in informed consent and do not, by their occurrence, imply negligence on the part of the operator.

What about the scenario when a wrong or an incomplete study is ordered by a referring physician? It happens every day: referring physician orders a head CT scan with the indication, "Facial trauma after MVA [motor vehicle accident]. Rule out orbital fracture." This should be an orbital or maxillofacial CT study, not a head CT. What to do? Naturally it would make sense to change the order to the appropriate study, or the radiologist may fail to make the correct diagnosis because the wrong study will be performed. However, the regulations state that in an outpatient setting and at independent diagnostic testing facilities, radiologists cannot change requesting physicians' orders without contacting the referring physician and getting another order. And we all know how tedious that can be. Medicare rules specifically state that "[t]ests not ordered by the physician who is treating the beneficiary are not reasonable and necessary." "Not reasonable" (buzz word) equals malpractice, although in most instances it would be difficult to show damage. However, studies performed on inpatients and outpatients in a hospital setting are not covered by this regulation, and the requested study can be modified. Why are these rules in place? They were made to prevent overutilization and to prevent aggressive radiologists from tacking on additional studies and thereby committing Medicare fraud. However, in certain instances, reason applies (Box 27-9).[11]

There is some wiggle room for the radiologist to modify a test (1) by changing the number of views to take, (2) if the wrong body part was requested (i.e., a clear error was committed in the order), (3) if the patient's condition is such that he or she could not tolerate the performance of the test, (4) if a diagnostic mammogram is required by virtue of findings on a screening study, (5) if an interventional procedure requires modification based on the ongoing findings, because the interventionalist becomes the "treating physician."[12]

COMPLICATIONS OF RADIOLOGIC PROCEDURES

Communication errors were not the most common sources of litigation in a review of the Canadian Medical Protective Association between

BOX 27-9

Decisions about Additional Imaging

When can a radiologist perform an additional diagnostic test without a new order? Only if all of the following occur[11]:
1. Radiologist was unable to contact treating physician to obtain new order.
2. Radiologist performs the originally ordered test.
3. Radiologist determines that because of an abnormal result an additional diagnostic test is medically necessary.
4. Delaying the additional diagnostic test will adversely affect the patient's health.
5. Radiologist communicated result of test to treating physician.
6. Radiologist documents why the additional test was performed in report.

Adapted from Travis NL, Reisman GD, Zwerling AL: Performing a test in an office setting without an order. J Am Coll Radiol 3:580–583, 2006.

1983 and December 1987. The lawsuits were classified into four major categories: diagnostic errors (40%), complications of radiologic procedures (33%), patient injuries in a department of radiology (7%), and miscellaneous (20%).[13]

Many complications of radiologic procedures may be based in contrast dye incidents. Examples are included in Box 27-10.[14]

BOX 27-10

Potential Sources of Suits Related to Contrast Agents

1. Use of ionic contrast dye in intrathecal studies
2. Failure to take steps to prevent extravasation of power-injected contrast dye
3. Failure to recommend a less invasive or safer test (i.e., MRI)
4. Use of more toxic contrast agent in setting of inflammation
5. Substandard treatment of dye reaction
6. Failure to adequately obtain informed consent
7. Use of high-osmolality contrast media in a patient who would more safely require low-osmolality contrast media

Adapted from Bush WH Jr, Albright DE, Sather JS: Malpractice issues and contrast use. J Am Coll Radiol 2:344–347, 2005.

Informed Consent

Adequate informed consent includes that amount of information that a reasonable physician would provide to the patient (what would a reasonably prudent physician with the same background, training, experience, and practicing in the same community, have disclosed to a patient in the same or similar situation?). This is classified as the "prudent physician" standard. Other states have mandated the "prudent patient" standard, which is defined as the disclosure of information that a reasonable, prudent patient would need to make an informed consent (American rule or materiality standard).

Some states have stipulated that the significant risks that should be discussed with the patient can be defined as those that occur with a prevalence of greater than or equal to 1%. Thus, informing the patient about a potential complication that occurs in 0.01% is not required in some states, because it is not "reasonable." However, the severity of the complication must also be weighed against its frequency. A risk of death, even if extremely uncommon, must be discussed with the patient beforehand for informed consent, although that discussion is unlikely to protect a physician in a juried trial if negligent behavior has occurred.

Recently, in part as a result of the advent of multidetector CT scanning, it has been suggested that the radiation exposure of a procedure and subsequent lifetime risk for future cancer be added to the consent process.[15,16] At the present time, with the exception of pregnant patients, only 15% of academic medical centers discuss radiation risk as part of the consent procedure. This issue has been brought to light in part because of the passing flurry of executive-screening CT scans of the whole body performed and also because of the added radiation dosage occurring with frequent CT scanning. Many emergency departments are instituting protocols that "screen" for pathology in multitrauma settings, even when children are the victims. The increased cancer risk cannot be denied, but does it warrant seeking consent? In the opinion of Lee et al, "the U.S. governing radiologic bodies (should) follow the lead of the European Union and move to develop national policy guidelines regarding screening and diagnostic CT scan informed consent practices, and proper disclosure of radiation dose and possible cancer risks to all patients involved . . . information concerning possible radiation risks among physicians and patients will help the medical community avoid a substantial public health risk and possible malpractice lawsuits."[15]

MITIGATION OF RISK TO MALPRACTICE SUITS

The Personal Touch

What are some steps that can be taken to reduce the likelihood that given an untoward outcome, the patient will sue? After all, it has been noted that only 13% of patients harmed by negligent acts actually file lawsuits, but 84% of claims that are filed have no negligence associated with them.[17]

1. If you are in a position to communicate with patients during their examinations, try as much as possible to establish a rapport. Communication continues to be the best method for establishing a caring relationship and, although patients do sue physicians that they like, this may help in some borderline cases where the patient knows that the intent of the physician was not to harm the patient.

2. If an untoward event occurs, address it immediately, openly, and honestly with the assistance of your legal team. One thing that a juror will detest is the semblance of a coverup or a lack of acknowledgment of a mistake by the physician. Contrition humanizes the medical doctor and is a more effective strategy than denial in the face of numerous medical experts stating that a breach of the standard of care has occurred. At our institution, when an untoward event occurs during the performance of a study, such as dropping a piece of machinery on a patient's limb, our legal team is very proactive about meeting with the patient early—even before a suit has been considered—to offer reparations in a kind, just, and equitable fashion. A $50,000 settlement before an aggressive plaintiff lawyer has whispered in the ear of a disgruntled patient can sometimes prevent a $2 million lawsuit as well as $30,000 in legal fees.

3. Never alter the medical record. Any type of changes to the patient's record after a suit has been started or in an attempt to change the reality of the occurrence is likely to make the physician seem more culpable. "Doctoring" the patient record is worse than bad doctoring with respect to potential liability. An addendum to a report 15 months after a study has been interpreted and 2 months after a suit has been filed may be a greater admission of guilt than any evidence the plaintiff's lawyer may be able to bring to the court.

4. Maintain the relationship with the patient after the untoward event. Even after a suit has been filed, the physician still has a duty to the patient for medical care. Although it is true that most patients who have sued their physician will then seek care from another physician, the maintenance of a good relationship with the patient can be useful at the time of trial or, better yet, before the trial during negotiation for settlement.

5. Do not bring your colleagues into the suit. Too often at the time of depositions or even within the patient record, in order to bolster one's perspective a second physician is mentioned in the interpretation of the study.

   "Well I showed it to my colleague Dr. A when I was reviewing the study for the first time, and he agreed that the study did not show evidence of a stroke. Because he is a subspecialty certified neuroradiologist, I listened to what he said and reported the study as such."
   "Did you show these specific films to Dr. A?"
   "Yes, the entire study."
   Unfortunately, this defense only exposes Dr. A by establishing the duty component of a patient-physician relationship to Dr. A and the patient, thereby potentially allowing Dr. A to be named in the suit as well. In the end, it is the physician whose name is at the bottom of the report, whether he or she has listened to a colleague's opinion or not, who is responsible for the consequences of that report.

6. Reduce the damages. This really applies mostly to interventional procedures where the potential for correcting the harm that occurred during the procedure is possible. For example, if you are performing an arteriogram and an embolism occurs, it may or may not be due to a breach in the standard of care. There is nothing to stop a patient from suing after a stroke during an arteriogram, even though it is a known complication and the patient's having a stroke does not mean that a breach in the standard of care has occurred. Nonetheless, it makes absolute sense if an embolus occurs during an arteriogram that the physician team attempts to safely reduce the damage that may occur secondary to the embolus. This may mean calling in a consultant interventionalist at the time of the study to help resolve the problem.

"I'm Sorry" Laws

Recent "I'm sorry" laws passed by several states have exempted statements of apology or sympathy by providers from being included as evidence of admissions of guilt. In the past it was argued that expressing regret to patients was a positive step in avoiding lawsuits by humanizing the error. Prior experience had shown this to be the case—that is, that patients are more likely to sue if there is no acknowledgment of the untoward outcome or if the mistake is perceived to be covered up.

The issue as to whether to apologize for a mistake that has been made was recently addressed in an *American Journal of Roentgenology* review.[18] In this article, Dr. Berlin strongly recommended following the guidelines requiring the full disclosure of an error that have been espoused by the Joint Commission for the Accreditation of Health Care Organizations and various professional societies including the ACR. Do not cover up the mistake. He suggests that radiologists have several options above and beyond just full disclosure when a mistake has been made (Table 27-1).

Of these options, number 1 is simply unethical even though tempting, option 2 is mandated, and option 3 is probably the most dangerous. It has been shown that a partial apology with no admission of guilt could potentially anger the patient even more than no apology. These partial apologies, which in the past were recommended, consists of the physician saying something akin to "I am so sorry this happened to you" or "I am very sorry that you had this outcome" or "I

Table 27-1 Options for Responding to a Medical Error

Option No.	Action Error	Recommendation
1	Do not disclose to patient	No
2	Disclose error to patient	Yes, mandated
3	Disclose error to patient and make a nonpersonal apology	Yes, but recommend only with caution
4	Disclose error to patient, apologize, and admit guilt	Value not known
5	Disclose error, apologize, admit guilt, and offer compensation	Progressive

apologize that the angiogram resulted in your husband's death." In many cases, the lack of personal admission of guilt makes patients feel like they are being blamed in part for the outcome and that the physicians are not taking responsibility for their role in the patient's care.

By the same token, admitting one's guilt, a statement of fault, is very dangerous and has been shown to be admissible as evidence in court. Any expression of wrongdoing made to a patient outside the courtroom can be used at a later date in the lawsuit, even if done at a highly emotionally charged time. Only one state has passed laws giving immunity to admissions of fault, but many states have passed the impersonal "I'm sorry" laws that allow exemption for admissibility.

Places like Johns Hopkins Hospital have been very proactive in adopting the fifth option ("divulge-admit-compensate"). When a clear case of medical error has occurred, the Johns Hopkins Risk Management Team is aggressive in approaching the patient even before a lawsuit has been considered, and has provided full disclosure, an apology, an admission of guilt, and an offer for monetary or other compensation. In one case of a medical error resulting in an inappropriate intravenous medication administration, the hospital created a special fund and named program for the affected patient, and this has led to research into the field of medical errors. The family has gone country-wide on a crusade to teach physicians about medical errors and to prevent them from occurring elsewhere. In those institutions using option 5, the claim is that they have fewer lawsuits, lower legal expenses, and smaller claims paid.

But will saying "I'm sorry" avert a malpractice case? It depends. It depends on the level of egregiousness of the error, the extent of damages, the pre-existent relationship with the patient (often nonexistent with the radiologist), and the anger of the family. In the end, Berlin recommends consulting with the risk management team for guidance as to whether to apologize and how to frame the apology (Table 27-2).

Other states are adopting legislation designed to deter frivolous lawsuits, often requiring affidavits or certificates of merit from medical experts when malpractice cases are filed. Alternatively, pretrial review panels may be required before a suit can move forward. Still other

Table 27-2 Advantages and Disadvantages of Personal Apologies for Medical Errors

Advantage	Disadvantage
Relieves guilt	Places blame
Honest and open	Exposes physician medicolegally
May prevent a lawsuit	May lead to a lawsuit
Ethically moral	Potentially self-destructive
Builds trust for the future	May lead to censure
May reduce compensation to patient	May increase compensation to patient

states are requiring that mediation be attempted after a period of discovery so that reasonable settlements can be obtained. In Nevada, a screening panel reviews malpractice cases. If there is no finding of malpractice, the plaintiff can still file a suit but must pay the defendant's costs and attorney's fees if the verdict is for the defense.[19] If the panel says that there is merit to the case, the parties are required to attend a settlement conference where the judge decides the reasonable value of the claim.[20] If the defendant rejects the judge's settlement suggestion, and a higher amount is awarded to the plaintiff, the defendant must pay the plaintiff's costs and attorney's fees. If the plaintiff rejects the settlement suggestion and is awarded a smaller amount, the plaintiff must pay the defendant's costs and attorney's fees.

Value of Peer Review Systems and Risk Management

The Joint Commission on Accreditation of Healthcare Organizations mandates radiology departmental peer review but offers flexibility in implementation. Having a strong peer review system may identify potential problems before they arise or may mitigate the exposure of a radiology group. One that shows a mature quality improvement program may influence a jury's impression of the physician participant or of the care taken to reduce errors by a department or practice. As referenced above, some peer review programs use prior reports, which most physicians review as part of ongoing concurrent care, to generate the peer review system. In this scenario, a radiologist reviewing a current study reviews the prior study with its report and merely checks a box to acknowledge that he agrees with that prior interpretation or not. If not, a revision is suggested for the peer review system (if not for the official medical record when it influences patient care). This process has the advantage of being integrated into the work flow and is relevant to patient care rather than adding to the already extensive demands of the physician's workload.

Risk management is the process by which risks to a group's well-being are identified, evaluated, protected against, and prevented. Gunderman[21] defines risk management strategy as the process by which potential losses/negative outcomes can be abated by (1) anticipating and identifying

risks, (2) determining which risks are important to deal with, and (3) implementing strategies to mitigate that risk. To implement an effective risk reduction program requires much thought about process improvement and also a strategy for addressing potential errors that are common, important, and rectifiable. For physicians, risk management may connote malpractice abatement, but a good program actually is designed to prevent any mishaps that can occur in the process of providing care to a patient from clerical errors, to falls, to wrong studies performed, to, yes, incorrect interpretation of the study. Most institutions require attendance at risk management seminars as a requisite of appointment and reappointment, emphasizing the importance of this process. Incident reporting should be encouraged in a blameless framework.

Many programs are including patients and their families in their risk management courses. At Hopkins, one seminar was devoted to a child who died as a result of inappropriate intravenous fluid replacement, and the seminar was conducted by the child's mother. As part of the settlement of the family's case, a risk reduction program named for the child who died was implemented; attendance at the seminar is a powerful influence on all incoming trainees. A patient's perspective on the medical care experience is always enlightening.

Malpractice Insurance Issues

What happens when physicians are no longer insurable or when your insurance company withdraws from the market and the premiums are astronomically high? One option is self-insurance. To self-insure requires having the full commitment of the group members who all participate in the process. It means that peer pressure may be required to change practice patterns of the "higher risk" participants, and everyone is "watching each others' backs." Risk management becomes not just an annual annoyance but an exercise that may lead to the success or failure of the whole program. To determine how much start-up and maintenance money is required to be self-insured, an exhaustive comprehensive review of past claims and expenses to litigate those claims must be made. Self-insured programs require an infrastructure that may be built in part on consultants, but

482

the large cache of money that must be available is usually managed by a dedicated manager and a reputable investment broker. You want the money in the fund to grow and thereby reduce your annual premiums. Coming up short when a claim must be paid is simply not an option. Finally, you should consider adding a claims administrator with both a medical and a legal background to the team.

There are entities known as "captive insurance companies," defined as a company that insures the risks of its owners and is managed and administered by the owners themselves. In fact, the self-insuring academic consortium in which Johns Hopkins Medical Institution participates could be considered a "captive," but it is generally governed by nonemployees. The assets of the captives are owned by the insured. The participants must run the insurance business of claims handling, risk assessment and mediation, litigation, collection of fees, disbursement of claims, and cash management.

CONCLUSION

Everyone makes mistakes. To err is human, and a patient who "forgives and forgets" is divine. Unfortunately, our society believes in punishing imperfections. Many of our errors in radiology are open to public scrutiny and become clear in retrospect. The process of malpractice litigation is lengthy and depressing, so the emphasis must be on prevention of errors. Double reading studies and computer-aided detection are two ways to mitigate the risk, but eventually the number of studies read catches up to the radiologist and mistakes are made. If named in a suit, maintain pristine ethics and work with the lawyers and the risk management team to strategize what an equitable solution to the suit would be. In many cases this means a negotiated settlement, because the outcomes of jury trials are so unpredictable. Use errors as opportunities for learning and growth.

Dos and Don'ts When You Are Sued[22]

Dos	Don'ts
1. Review the records.	1. Discuss the case with friends, associates, or strangers not directly involved with the defense of the case.
2. Collect the records.	2. Contact the plaintiff or the plaintiff's attorney directly.
3. Analyze the case dispassionately.	3. Alter the medical record in any way.
4. Identify experts.	4. Delete, destroy evidence.
5. Identify pitfalls for your defense.	5. Become emotional.
6. Identify fact witnesses.	6. Accept calls from opposing attorneys.
7. Refer to the record when answering questions.	7. Offer additional information to that which is requested.
8. Answer honestly.	8. Answer questions that are incoherent or unclear.
9. Ask for breaks.	9. Accept assumptions by opposing attorneys.
10. Correct errors in your testimony.	10. Answer questions when you do not know the answers.
11. Be sincere, compassionate, and serious.	11. Extend yourself beyond your range of expertise.

Acknowledgment The authors gratefully acknowledge the erudite suggestions of Dr. Leonard Berlin in the writing of this chapter as well as his numerous thoughtful contributions to the academic literature on medicolegal topics. Thanks also go to Kelly Beary for a malpractice lawyer's perspective.

REFERENCES

1. Institute of Medicine summary "To Err Is Human: Building a Safer Health System" on physician errors published in 1999. http://www.nap.edu/books/0309068371/html/.

2. Ellenbogen PH, Hoffman T, Cypel Y: Report of the ACR task force on medical liability reform in radiology. J Am Coll Radiol 1(12):908–915, 2004.

3. Physician Insurers Association of America. Breast cancer study, 3rd ed. Rockville, MD, Physician Insurers Association of America, 2002.

4. Brenner RJ, Lucey LL, Smith JJ, Saunders R: Radiology and medical malpractice claims: a report on the practice standards claims survey of the Physician Insurers Association of America and the American College of Radiology. Am J Roentgenol 171(1):19–22, 1998.

5. Kan L, Olivotto IA, Warren Burhenne LJ, et al: Standardized abnormal interpretation and cancer detection ratios to assess reading volume and reader performance in a breast screening program. Radiology 215(2):563–567, 2000.

6. Brenner RJ.: False-negative mammograms. Medical, legal, and risk management implications. Radiol Clin North Am 38(4):741–757, 2000.

7. Linver MN, Paster SB, Rosenberg RD, et al: Improvement in mammography interpretation skills in a community radiology practice after dedicated teaching courses: 2-year medical audit of 38,633 cases. Radiology 184(1):39–43, 1992.

8. Berlin L: Duty to directly communicate radiologic abnormalities: has the pendulum swung too far. Am J Roentgenol 181:375–381, 2003.

9. Kushner DC, Lucey LL: Diagnostic radiology reporting and communication: The ACR guideline. J Am Coll Radiol 2:15–21, 2005.

10. Brenner RJ, Bartholomew L: Communication errors in radiology: a liability cost analysis. J Am Coll Radiol 2:428–431, 2005.

11. Travis NL, Reisman GD, Zwerling AL: Performing a test in an office setting without an order. J Am Coll Radiol 3:580–583, 2006.

12. Duszak, Jr R: The ordering physician rules. J Am Coll Radiol 3:369–371, 2006.

13. Morrish HF, Messenger OJ: Medicolegal encounters in Canadian radiology. Can Assoc Radiol J 41(5): 259–263, 1990.

14. Bush Jr WH, Albright DE, Sather JS: Malpractice issues and contrast use. J Am Coll Radiol 2:344–347, 2005.

15. Lee CI, Flaster HV, Haims AH, et al: Diagnostic CT scans: institutional informed consent guidelines and practices at academic medical centers. Am J Roentgenol 187(2):282–287, 2006.

16. Lee CI, Haims AH, Monico EP, et al: Diagnostic CT scans: assessment of patient, physician, and radiologist awareness of radiation dose and possible risks. Radiology 231(2):393–398, 2004. Epub 2004 Mar 18.

17. Localio AR, Lawthers AG, Brennan TA, et al: Relation between malpractice claims and adverse events due to negligence. Results of the Harvard Medical Practice Study III. N Engl J Med 325(4):245–251, 1991.

18. Berlin L: Will saying "I'm sorry" prevent a malpractice lawsuit? Am J Roentgenol 187:10–15, 2006.

19. Nev. Rev. Stat. Ann. § 41A.056 1996.

20. Nev. Rev. Stat. Ann. § 41A.059 1997.

21. Gunderman RB, Applegate KE: Managing risk: threat or opportunity? Am J Roentgenol 185(1):43–45, 2005.

22. West RW, Sipe CY: Anatomy of malpractice defense, Part 1: suit through discovery. J Am Coll Radiol 1:383–384, 2004.

APPENDIX 27-1: ACR GUIDELINES ON EXPERT WITNESSES

I. Radiologists are frequently called upon to serve as medical expert witnesses in a variety of legal proceedings and have an obligation to do so in the appropriate circumstances. This obligation includes not only the review of documents, radiographs, or procedures but also the willingness to give sworn testimony by deposition or in court. The public interest requires readily available, objective, and unbiased medical expert testimony. The expert witness should be qualified for the role and follow clear and consistent guidelines. The College recognizes the decisive role of the judge in determining admissibility of expert testimony as well as the difficulty in setting the balance between variations of viewpoints and their reasonableness which fairness requires. This document attempts to assist both the expert witness and the court in achieving that balance.

II. PURPOSE. Medical expert witness testimony is indicated in any legal proceeding in which the court needs an objective physician who is not a party to the case, has no personal interest in the outcome of the case, and has expertise in the matter at hand to help explain the issues.

III. QUALIFICATIONS AND RESPONSIBILITIES OF THE EXPERT WITNESS. The expert witness should be a physician with the following qualifications: At the time of the incident under review was licensed and actively engaged for a reasonable period of time in the practice of the specialty or subspecialty relating to the testimony. Certification in Radiology or Diagnostic Radiology, Therapeutic Radiology, Nuclear Radiology, or Radiation Oncology by the American Board of Radiology, American Osteopathic Board of Radiology, the Royal College of

Physicians and Surgeons of Canada, or Le College des Medecins du Quebec. Education, training, and practical experience, as well as current knowledge and skill concerning the subject matter of the case including in a medical liability case the relevant standard of care.[3] Should the physician defendant be required by federal or state statute to fulfill certain educational or practice experience requirements to interpret an imaging procedure, the expert witness should also meet these same requirements.

IV. REQUISITES OF AN EXPERT WITNESS

A. The role of the expert witness is to help the fact finder analyze the issues in dispute necessary to decide the case. The expert witness is expected and should be able to render an opinion regarding the reasonableness of the conduct of the parties in the circumstances at hand. Depending on the legal issues being tried, this may include an opinion about a defendant doctor's training and experience; the relevant standard of care; the relevance of particular imaging findings, interventional procedures, or radiation therapy treatment to causation of damages, or the adequacy of the technical equipment used. In a medical liability case, the expert opinion should be based on the information available at the time of the incident now under review. Information, facts, and results of imaging studies performed after the incident generally should not be used to formulate an opinion. It should be recognized that physicians have different levels of expertise that are still within the standard of care.

B. Recommended Guidelines for Behavior of the Radiologist Expert Witness

1. Although the nature of legal proceedings is adversarial, the expert witness must be as impartial and objective as possible.

2. In a medical liability case, the expert witness should be familiar with the relevant standard of care.

3. The expert witness should review the relevant materials sufficiently to assure an informed and fair opinion. Original images rather than copies should be used for review.

4. The expert witness should be prepared to explain the basis of his or her opinion and should take care that his or her proffered testimony will be scientifically valid and applicable to the facts at issue, can be or has been tested, and has withstood or reasonably could withstand a peer review. The expert witness should be familiar with and be prepared to address the known or potential limitations regarding his or her opinion, as well as the degree to which that opinion is accepted in the medical community.

5. Compensation of the expert witness should reflect the time and effort involved. Linking compensation for expert testimony to the outcome of the case (contingency fee) is unethical. An individual holding an official capacity with the College who testifies in a legal proceeding must exercise great care to distinguish between his or her personal opinions and the policy positions of the College. The expert witness can be held accountable for statements made during a legal proceeding.

This guideline was developed according to the process described in the ACR Practice Guidelines and Technical Standards book by the Guidelines and Standards Committee of the General and Pediatric Radiology Commission with the assistance of the Medical Legal Committee. Principal Drafter: Harry Zibners, MD, JD.

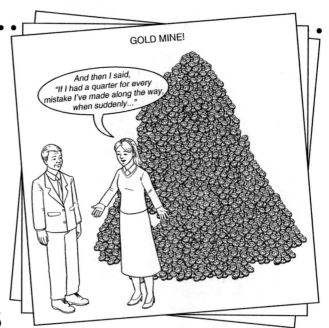

CHAPTER 28

Learning from Others' Mistakes

David M. Yousem

We have come to the final chapter, and perhaps it would be appropriate to impart some final words to the wise. It is a truism that you learn most from your mistakes, or, as Bernard Shaw opined, "The man who has never made a mistake will never make anything else." You are likely to make mistakes as you build your own practice, but remember that mistakes are a natural part of the learning process. Those of us who have contributed to this book have certainly made our own share of mistakes. In the hope of helping you avoid some of the more common mistakes, we would like to outline some of the major areas of potential peril that trip you up. After all, it is well known that the benefit of learning from the mistakes of others is that you could never live long enough to make all of these mistakes by yourself!

Major mistakes, errors, and misjudgments usually involve six key areas:

1. Personnel issues
2. Conflict resolution
3. Communication
4. Customer satisfaction
5. Information technology (IT) issues
6. Leadership issues

PERSONNEL ISSUES

Without question, the worst mistakes you can make in your professional or even your personal life relate to people. The day-to-day relationships in a work environment are critical to maintaining a happy, healthy, productive workplace, and even one "bad apple" amidst a bumper crop of "Gala" workers can create havoc and disharmony. A negative work environment can be diagnosed within a group by (1) frequent turnover, (2) delayed or absent personnel promotion, (3) lack of celebrations of group successes, and (4) inadequate commitment to a shared vision.

How can this type of situation be avoided? It comes down to hiring and keeping the right people, and the three critical areas are (1) getting references on potential employees, (2) conducting meaningful job interviews, and (3) retaining your best workers.

References

It is critical to get reliable unbiased references before hiring individuals at all levels of the work group. Yet because of laws that protect workers from discrimination and incrimination, obtaining reliable and worthwhile recommendations from former employers is becoming more and more difficult. Past employers are frequently unwilling or simply not able to provide negative feedback, often only confirming dates of employment, titles, and salary. Despite these so-called "neutral reference" policies, it is important to confirm what you can, including academic credentials. These "close-mouthed" practices exist to protect employers from claims of former employees asserting that the former employer gave negative information about the candidate that is false. Of course, the side-effect of the practices is to make it difficult for the potential new employer to get information that would be useful to the hiring process. There are a few methods that can be used to try to avoid a former employer's neutral reference policy, although a sharp person receiving these inquiries will recognize them for what they are and continue to provide only the information allowed under the neutral policy.

One standard question that is legally permissible is, "Would you hire this person again?" Another stratagem is to set the rules ahead of time in a way that protects the former boss but gives you some information. You might say, "Please, if you cannot answer favorably to my specific questions, please say 'No comment.'" Or you can say, "Is there anything favorable that you can say about this individual?" If there is a long pregnant pause,

you might want to think about aborting the recruitment, so to speak. Or another favorite of mine, "How would you compare this person to X (a mutually known good, fair, or bad employee) as a candidate?"

One lesson we have learned in dealing with candidates for employment is to obtain multiple references for every candidate and to get them from individuals who are not hand-picked by the candidate. When prospective employees provide a list of references, clearly the applicant has chosen those individuals who he/she thinks will give a favorable review. You should call those individuals to make sure there are no obvious red flags, but a standard question to ask a reference should be, "Who in your group got along least well with this individual?" Do not ask for the contact information for that person, so there is no implication of collusion by the positive reference and no assumption that you will subsequently contact the "negative reference." But do call this potential negative reference. If the former employer has done a good job at protecting himself or herself from potential liability, the call to the new reference may be short. He or she may simply refer you to the designated office official to respond to reference inquiries. But many employers fail to require that kind of a designation or have employees who routinely violate the requirement.

If you do get through, you might have to reassure the new reference that you will not share any of the comments with the candidate, and again ask the standard questions, "Would you rehire this individual?" "Do you have anything positive to say about this person?" Sometimes they will volunteer negative comments "off the record" and one should surely not record or write down any negative comments that might "expose" a reference. At the end of the new reference call ask again, "Is there anyone that you know who did not have a favorable opinion of this individual?" This then hopefully will lead to a trail of potential opinions that can provide a "total" picture of the candidate. Continue down this "negative" trail until the only people who are subsequently referenced as negative toward the candidate are people to whom you have already spoken. With a strong candidate, this will be a very short list. To be clear, I am in no way suggesting that you trick the reference provider into doing something illegal. Rather, these comments are to facilitate your getting the very best input you can before hiring a new employee.

Time spent in considering an applicant thoroughly before he or she is hired is time well spent, since getting rid of an employee who does not work out is not always a simple task.

As far as providing references, when the shoe is on the other foot, the safest legal practice is to follow strictly a neutral-reference policy and to demand that your employees do the same. There should be one and only one person assigned to respond to reference requests, a policy prohibiting anyone else from responding, and appropriate action taken when an employee strays from that policy. The neutral information should be limited to name, dates of employment, and maybe salary. To maintain the strongest protection from legal action, *nothing* else should be said because nothing said means nothing for the former employee to sue over. If you do find yourself in a conversation, obviously do not say anything negative. Even your silence, hesitations, or backhanded compliments may send a message that, while helpful to the potential new employer, still subjects you to a risk of litigation. I remember a legal friend of mine said that she liked hearing the reference about a lazy colleague, "It'd be fantastic if you got this person to work for you!" I have stated about one former employee, "He is really very very strong on the research side of things!" I didn't even have to be asked whether I was implying that he was weak clinically. If asked, I'd simply reply, "Research really is his strongest suit."

Employment Interviews

Most managers are terrible at employment interviews. They tend to meander about, asking about long-term career goals and vague lists of strengths and weaknesses. A good employment interview focuses on specific behaviors, skills, and values that will help you determine whether the candidate is a good fit or not. Ask the candidate to give you specific examples of times he or she demonstrated a particular behavior, skill, or value, and don't be satisfied if you get a vague and generalized answer in reply. Ask again if you don't get the specific example you want. Of course, this assumes that you know what behaviors, skills, and values are good predictors of a successful employee.

There are also some potential negatives that you should probe for in an interview. We've learned from experience to ask our potential employees whether there are any lawsuits, both malpractice or related to a candidate's job performance, that are pending or ongoing. This question should be asked toward the end of the interview, but it should not be omitted. Please note that you, as a potential employer could be sued for retaliation for failing to hire an applicant if the applicant has a protected lawsuit (discrimination, sexual harassment, etc.) against a current or prior employer. These are not the lawsuits you want to probe because if a candidate is involved in such a lawsuit and is not hired, you have to have very good, objective reasons for not hiring the candidate. Only ask about lawsuits that relate to the candidate's job performance, like malpractice and "work-environment" lawsuits about the candidate's behavior.

Asking for attendance records from prior employees is often useful as well. Ask a potential employee, "If I were to review your attendance records from the past 5 years, how often do you think I would find you absent from work per month?" You may get mixed reactions in answers to this question. Some may suspect that you already have access to their attendance records and will answer honestly with explanations such as, "It was a very bad year for illness with my little children, and I had to take sick days to be off with them" or "I had a death in the family and had to take time off to deal with their effects" or "I was going through a very rough time with my spouse and needed some days off to deal with court issues." Be careful about getting too specific with these questions because of the potential to get into areas protected by the Americans with Disabilities Act. The Equal Employment Opportunity Commission specifically permits some questions but the agency prohibits the question, "How many days were you sick" and any others that might reveal the existence of a disability. Likewise, if the candidate responds that he or she was absent many days because of an illness, the interviewer should avoid the temptation to pursue that issue because the questions likely would be potentially disability-related and therefore prohibited. Do not ask questions about whether the person was ill or injured and do not pursue the details if the candidate offers that information in response to a permissible question or else you may run afoul of the ADA. Before making an offer, an employer may ask questions about the ability to perform job-related functions or ask the candidate to describe or demonstrate how, with reasonable accommodation, he/she will perform those functions.

There is an old joke that has the business owner complaining, "I hired some *employees,* but then some *people* showed up to work in their place." Your employees are people first and employees second, and they bring with them all the joys and sufferings and the good days and bad that all people have in their lives. Nevertheless, it is one thing to stand by a long-time employee who is going through a difficult time, and it is another to hire someone who is going to be a problem from day one.

The interview is a time to get as much information as possible that will help you in the hiring of the right person. The interview must focus on those issues that are relevant to future job performance and ability to work with colleagues. You must not actively pursue personal information that is protected. However, it is appropriate to listen closely to how the candidate manages relationships inside and outside of work; much can be learned from careful listening. For example, emotional intelligence that is central to forming strong personal relationships also fosters effective leadership and collaboration at work.

We try to obtain a sense of how a person will fit in with our staff by asking, "Describe the worst boss you have ever had, or if you've never had a bad boss, describe what you would imagine one to be like." "Who has been your worst co-worker to date, and why?" We also ask, "Describe the ideal boss, the ideal work environment for you." "Describe the perfect day at the office." "Describe what would be your worst possible day at the office." If some of these negative scenarios fit you, the boss, to a T, you may want to consider whether this candidate is a good match for your organization.

Asking a candidate to list his or her most negative attributes never is useful. Invariably the answers tend toward, "I'm too modest" or "I'm too trusting" or "I'm a workaholic." This line of questioning is simply not fruitful.

Retention

Although it is no doubt critical to avoid recruiting problem employees, it is equally imperative to retain the best people—the top performers—already on your team. Why is this important? Think of how much time and effort it will take to interview, hire, and train the replacement. Think of all the lost productivity as one of your best employees is replaced by a new person who can only slowly begin to pick up the workload of the former employee.

If you are the boss, this means several things. It means recognizing good employees and acknowledging them. Too often we assume that such people know how valuable they are and do not bother to let them know how much their work is appreciated. One senior manager we know had a pop-up alert on the computer flash this message, "Acknowledge someone's good work today." It was a cue to send a short note (e-mail is good, but a handwritten note is better because it has more significance) to an employee who had done something extraordinary that week. This was very effective and gained a lot of favor in the division.

Be careful not to overdo it. For our senior manager friend, the notes worked well until one of the team members recognized that the calls, e-mails, and notes were received every Friday at 2 PM. She also, unfortunately, observed the pop-up reminder on the computer one day when the office was unoccupied. Because it was a "scheduled event," its meaning was diminished for the team. Nonetheless, it is still a good idea to make note of exceptional performance when it happens. What people want most from their boss is recognition, respect and the opportunity to do interesting and challenging work.

Fight for promotions, upgrades, awards, and titles for your employees. In many cases you should lead the charge for recommending a submission for a new pay grade or promotion for your direct reports. Don't wait for them to bring it up. You lead the effort—sincerely. Seek aggressively to advance their careers. Suggest additional education in the fields of management, counseling, web design, and so on for your employees, so that they can move up the corporate ladder. You do not want your employees to be complacent, stagnant, or bored.

Another department head has a research coordinator he has worked with for more than 15 years, and she is one of the keys to his academic success. When he meets with her at the regularly scheduled review periods (and sometimes in between), he will often say to her, "You are so valuable to our division. Is there a way for us to get you up another pay grade? What additional responsibilities or job duties are necessary to move you up in pay or job title? Even if we have to be a bit creative to fit you into that upgrade, let's submit the paperwork and give it a shot." At times he succeeds in getting that pay raise and at times he fails, but at least she knows that he is out there willing to fight to get her the compensation and recognition that she deserves.

Sometimes the bureaucracy and the paperwork to get this done will seem daunting, but replacing your top employees will take much, much more effort and may result in worse performance. So fight for your best employees.

Push for your best direct reports to accept the next major challenge, even if it means that they may leave you prematurely. If you get a reputation as a boss who is an advocate for your people, the better people will gravitate to you and you will obtain greater loyalty from all your workers.

One of the biggest mistakes you can make is allowing an excellent employee to leave or to feel underappreciated. Always counteroffer. The counteroffer works best if it is personal, "I don't want you to leave. I really want you to stay. You are very important to us here." It is amazing what a positive impact one can have on an employee when one looks him or her in the eye and says that one would be very sad if he or she left. Before even going through the issues or the circumstances or the terms of the other job, you want the employee to know that you are miserable at the idea of losing him or her. Nonetheless, sometimes it's the right time for a great employee to try something else, even if he or she has to leave you. As a boss you need to understand that.

Sometimes employees come in to the boss to say that they are leaving, hoping against hope that the boss will provide a reason why they should stay. They really want to stay, but they are attracted to another job for some reason.

And, mistakenly, the boss just assumes that it is a *fait accompli* and never counteroffers or expresses remorse over the employee's decision. The employee then leaves the job convinced more than ever that he or she was never valued and that the boss didn't care whether the employee left or not.

One foreign employee we know of had visa issues that led him to pursue a potential job with the Veteran's Administration, which would virtually guarantee him a green card. His current institution couldn't match the green card guarantee of the V.A., but was ultimately able to retain him through a combination of (1) acknowledging how critical he was to the success of the team, (2) stating how hard the institution would work with him to sponsor a waiver for his J-1 visa and support a green card application, (3) paying for his annual O-1 visa and lawyers' fees, and (4) stressing the importance of academia in his career.

Counteroffer. To the end, counteroffer. Go down swinging. Let the person know that you are trying in every way possible to find the right combination of strategies to retain the excellent employee. When other employees recognize your faithfulness and dedication to that employee, they see that your words of encouragement and praise through the years were and are sincere. Repair that which is broken. Ask the employee straightforwardly, "What will it take for you to stay here? What can I do to make you reconsider?" If it is revealed that this is a spousal decision or a social one or a non-work-related move issue, at least you have made it clear that you are flexible about negotiating. Perhaps the work can be done via telecommuting. Perhaps the work can be done at home. Perhaps the work can be done on a part-time basis. Counteroffer. Be persistent. Let that employee tell potential new hires how tirelessly you tried to keep him or her and how dedicated you are to keeping excellent team members. Know also that it's not always about the salary. Among the non-salary items you might consider offering: parking expenses, commuting expenses, train tickets, secretarial support, grant writers, physician's assistants, front office help, legal expenses, new office computers, home computers, direct access to the chairman, the office with the window (for a radiologist?!!), real estate broker names, cell phone expenses, cable network charges, wireless cards, or recurring airfare expenses to Arkansas and Texas.

All that said, it is still better to tell your best employees how valuable they are *before* they come to you with a competing job offer, and let them know you are fighting for them throughout their time with you, not just at the end.

CONFLICT RESOLUTION

Forms and Sources of Conflict

Box 28-1 lists the forms and sources of conflict in the workplace and outlines strategies for dealing with them. One source of conflict that needs to be addressed in particular is sexual

---

BOX 28-1

Sources of Conflict and Strategies for Addressing It

Sources

1. Communication: What you mean is often not what is understood, especially with multiethnic and multicultural staff members.
2. Emotions: The second layer of communication
3. Values: Personal beliefs about ethics, integrity
4. Structure: Framework of decision making
5. History: "Baggage" brought to a conflict, precedents made
6. Identity Issues: What the conflict reflects about you and your view of yourself

Strategies to Deal with Conflicts

1. Avoidance—for minor low-impact annoyances
2. Organizational/structural change
3. Repression/punishment
4. Sharpening—open discussion of smoldering conflicts
5. Productive action, principles-based management
6. Creative design—construction of resolutions satisfactory to all by mutual assent

Adapted from Harolds J, Wood BP: Conflict management and resolution. J Am Coll Radiol 3: 200–206, 2006; Mayer B: The dynamics of conflict resolution: a practitioner's guide. San Francisco, Jossey-Bass, 2000.

---

harassment, which can be very damaging to your employees and your organization.

Sexual Harassment

Sexual harassment is defined as unwelcome sexual advances, requests for sexual favors, and other verbal or physical conduct that unreasonably interferes with an individual's work or study performance or creates an intimidating, hostile, or offensive working environment based on sex. Note the important terms: (1) unwelcome, (2) sexual, (3) verbal (there need not be physical contact), (4) physical (of any type), (5) unreasonably (what might a reasonable, rational, ordinary person expect), (6) interferes (this implies damage), (7) work or study performance (implying a colleague at work or a student who may not be employed), (8) creates (hence achieving causation as per medical malpractice), (9) intimidating (which may not be hostile), (10) hostile (violence or harm is implied), (11) offensive (very subjective—what is offensive to one may not be to another; hence the use of "reasonably"), (12) working environment (implies a limitation to behavior in the workplace but it may be a carryover from behavior outside of work or from behavior at work to outside of work—there need not be a specific incident between specific individuals if the working environment is deemed intimidating, hostile, or offensive), (13) based on sex (which is not necessarily the same as item 2 above because conduct can be based on sex even if it is not sexual in nature, as in the case where a manager routinely assigns the female employees to menial tasks and the male employees to the more prestigious work).

In running your own practice, you need to worry about sexual harassment on two different levels: (1) as a professional, in your own relationships with your co-workers, and (2) as a manager, dealing with complaints brought to you about other people's behaviors. Both can cause everyone tremendous trouble.

As a Professional First let's deal with your own behavior as a professional.

Sexual harassment is a serious and widespread problem. Intimidation on the basis of gender has been reported to occur in up to 75% of residency programs. It has been

BOX 28-2

Steps for Dealing with Sexual Harassment

- State emphatically that the behavior is unwanted and inappropriate.
- Document repeated events and obtain witnesses.
- Consult an authority in the institution early and often (review the institution's sexual harassment policy to know which authority should receive your report).
- Refer to an institution's sexual harassment policy for its definition.
- Document the "damage" that has occurred by the behavior.
- File a complaint.
- Obtain legal advice if the pattern continues.

Adapted from Berlin L: To deal with sexual harassment. Am J Roentgenol 187:288–293, 2006.

estimated that unwanted sexual advances occur in as many as 10% of training programs. Unfortunately, like child abuse, this is a violation in which the victim must often suffer alone, too afraid to divulge the provocation because of the hierarchical nature of the medical profession. Even professors have reported harassment, suffering in silence for years before coming forward to express their difficulties.

How does a victim of sexual harassment deal with the offensive behavior? The typical steps are listed in Box 28-2.

One of the most sensitive areas of employee relations is that of consensual romantic relationships within an office environment. Since people spend most of their waking hours at work, it is natural for people to form friendships and relationships with their co-workers. When those relationships are of a romantic nature, the employer can have problems when the relationships end. However, even more difficult problems arise when individuals not at the same level of training or stature in a department become romantically involved. In those relationships, a power play becomes intrinsic to the relationship. This may occur at the level of (1) a chief resident (who determines the monthly schedule) and a more junior resident, (2) a trainee and a faculty member, and/or (3) a boss and a subordinate outside of the training

relationship role. Any relationship at work is fraught with the potential for intimidation, but one between non-equals is especially dangerous to all involved and to the individuals in that environment, even if they are not in the relationship. For someone heading up a practice, this is a position of power in the work environment, and a relationship with anyone in a subordinate role is inappropriate—consensual or not, reciprocated or not.

A person's position in the department has a tremendous impact on what behaviors are perceived as appropriate. One newly promoted section chief discovered that his jokes and remarks, which worked so well in his old hospital where he was just one of many faculty members, were offending people. The irreverence and satire were no longer coming from the ranks but from the boss. People were insulted and hurt and misunderstood the humor. The lesson to be learned is that with leadership comes responsibility and "gravity." As the "boss," you simply cannot engage in the same activities that you can as a rank-and-file employee.

Remember that the key phrases in our definition of sexual harassment include "intimidating, hostile, or offensive working environments based on sex." Sex or sexual favors need not be involved at all. Trouble can also arise if someone feels intimidated or just consistently treated less favorably because they happen to be of a particular sex.

An attending was once reprimanded by a resident for his behavior toward her because, after warning her four times that she was mishandling a catheter and was putting the patient at risk, he grabbed her arm and removed the catheter from her hand. The attending admonished the resident that her behavior was exposing the patient to danger. At the end of the day the resident approached the attending and complained that she felt that she had been physically manhandled. Even though the act was clearly not of a sexual nature, she felt intimidated and uncomfortable.

As a Manager So what do you do when *you* are the section chief and someone comes to you and complains about sexual harassment by a coworker? There are a number of things you *should* have done before the complaint arose, and we'll get to those in a second. There are also things you need to do right now, when the employee comes to you with the complaint. Your reaction to the complaint is extremely important to your department. First, deal with the perceived harassment so your employee no longer feels threatened and assure her that her concern is taken seriously. Next, call your human resources representative and have them involved in the discussion. They deal with similar issues frequently, so they likely will have valuable advice on how to handle the complaint. Document all discussions and include witnesses to those discussions if the complainant will allow it. "I know that this is a very personal issue, but would you feel comfortable if I pulled Michelle from human resources into the discussion? She has a lot of knowledge on these situations." In some work environments, human resources may actually take over the discussion and coordinate the investigation and response process.

The best time to deal with a sexual harassment complaint, though, is before it ever happens. It is up to you as a manager to create a working environment that is open, comfortable, and professional. People should know that there are clear standards of expected behavior. People should be able to come to work knowing they will not be bothered by an environment that is in any way hostile, intimidating, or offensive.

The "corporate culture"—those unwritten rules that everyone has in their heads about "how things are done around here"—is everything in the fight to build a healthy working environment. You have the power to set the tone for the whole department.

1. Don't assume that everyone knows the official policy on sexual harassment. Make a point of handing out the written policy to the entire staff every 6 to 12 months. Do it in a staff meeting, where you can reinforce the policy verbally while you give them the written policy. Most people will ignore something stuffed in their mailboxes. It also is a good idea to have each member of the staff sign an acknowledgement of receipt of the policy.

   Although sexual harassment may be the most well-known type of discriminatory harassment, it also is illegal to harass on the basis of race, religion, and other protected characteristics. The harassment policy should therefore not be limited to sexual harassment.

2. Set a good example. Avoid telling off-color jokes, and watch those off-hand comments. If you hear someone else do it, ask them quietly and privately to be more careful in their comments.

3. Talk to people throughout the department. Ask them if they feel the working environment is the best it can be. Ask for their help in educating their coworkers on proper behavior.

4. Remember that sexual harassment is not just man-to-woman, but also woman-to-man, man-to-man, and woman-to-woman.

Be careful how you treat an employee after a complaint has been registered. Keep things confidential and continue to apply institutional policies evenly and fairly to all employees. Remember our admonition about references for employees. Retaliation claims are one of the most dangerous claims for employers and these days virtually anything can be pointed to as alleged retaliation.

COMMUNICATION

There are more mistakes due to communication than to any other cause. These can be generalized into several categories, as listed Table 28-1. Of the topics and consequences listed here, some of the more common mistakes made in a professional environment involve direct communications, through e-mail and in-person meetings, and indirect communications, where you talk with someone about an absent third person.

E-mail Usage

A new section chief arrived one day, and he pledged that he would keep his faculty very well informed. He felt that the best way to do this was to send group e-mails to division members, keeping them current with the various events or issues that were occurring on a day-to-day basis in the division. One day it might be the weekly report turnaround time numbers, the next day

Table 28-1   Communication Errors

Error	Outcome
Not communicating at all	Colleagues feel out of touch and distant.
Not communicating enough	Colleagues feel confused and misdirected.
Not communicating in the right format	Colleagues take material out of context, are late in receiving information, or feel exploited.
Using a condescending tone	Colleagues feel belittled and disrespected.
Making assumptions	People won't know the basis for your statements and think you or they are out of touch.
Not prefacing one criticism with even 7 compliments	Colleagues will not be receptive to hearing constructive feedback.
Not using reflective speech	Colleagues will feel that you are not listening or hearing them.
Not being inquisitive about others	People like to believe that you find them fascinating; it guarantees they will like you.
Inappropriate topics	Be culturally sensitive. What may be appropriate in western society may be inappropriate in eastern culture.

the revenue picture for the month, the next day a message from the chairman of surgery asking for more help in reviewing outside cases, another day the grants office promoting a particular grant, and so on. This practice led to team members receiving group e-mails two or three times a day. Mistake! The team began to think of these messages as a form of spam. More and more, the new chief found that even though he had sent a message out repeatedly, the faculty seemed to retain less and less. They were ignoring the messages and becoming *less* informed about the events in the division. At the same time, his summaries of division and department faculty meetings that his subordinates were supposed to attend met with great approval, but led to a significant drop in attendance at those same meetings. "Why should we show up for 90 minutes?" they asked, "when we can get your summary that boils it down to a few paragraphs and 5 minutes of reading?" Aaaaaarrrgghhh! No administrator can tolerate that!

Bottom line: overutilization of e-mail can harm communications. People don't like the clutter, and important messages can get missed in an avalanche of relatively unimportant trivia. Use the e-mail stream judiciously, and if some

bit of data is not urgent, post the message in a weekly newsletter rather than as a daily blog entry.

E-mail gaffes can occur at the highest level. It takes only a simple accidental click on the "Reply to All" button for your ill-thought comments, meant only for a close friend, to be broadcast to everyone in the organization. One new chairman recounts the story that he was a bit overwhelmed at the start of his new job. He had a faculty member who was somewhat persistent in his divisional demands right from the beginning. In response to an e-mail seeking the immediate attention of the chairman, the chair e-mailed a new administrator and requested that he help get this "irritating person" to relax long enough for the chair to get his feet wet in the new position. In an attempt to help, the administrator sent an e-mail to the faculty member offering to help out in place of the chairman. Unfortunately, he left the e-mail trail with the chairman's comments attached as well!

This happens extremely often and is a frequent source of frustration with e-mail communication. There it is in writing! Not only did this not do much to encourage the person to put his issue on hold out of trust for the new leader, but it was also embarrassing to be seen so early as being critical of a faculty member. This story also highlights another dangerous aspect of e-mail: once you send it, you have no control over what the person receiving it is going to do with it. As for those concerned about legal suits, e-mail is a discoverable communication and, because of long-term servers and modern-day computer forensics work, may last a lot longer in the webosphere than one might think. Indeed, some computer forensic experts say that electronic communications are *never* really deleted. Hence the evidence that can be found in some of the recent business fraud suits.

Occasionally life becomes busy and the pressure causes you to not be adequately respectful. First, when under stress or irritated, do not send e-mail. Second, if it cannot be put in the newspaper for all to read, do not e-mail it.

In-Person Communication

E-mail is less efficient than "in person" or "telephone" communication. E-mail is great for broadcasting information to multiple recipients, because it avoids the need to call each person or to waste paper sending out multiple memos. But there is no substitute for sitting across from someone and discussing a topic. There is no delay in waiting for a response, no wondering whether a computer transmission or reception failed, no frustration because of downtimes. Besides, one-on-one communication is richer and more complete.

As an example, supervising doctor A sent an e-mail regarding an unsafe biopsy technique that went awry. To the sender, the content seemed to make it clear that the message was laced with sarcasm, with the phrase, "Well, that certainly was effective!" Unfortunately, the sarcasm was not perceived by doctor A's colleagues, and they *all* began to use the same ill-fated technique. When doctor A questioned a colleague he saw repeating the same mistake, the colleague replied, "I thought that was what you wanted us to do." "But didn't you read my e-mail?" doctor A asked. The colleague said, "Of course I did." And he had, but the use of sarcasm was lost on him. The lesson is this simple rule: E-mail should be clear and should say exactly what you mean.

It's been said that more than 50% of communication is nonverbal. It is body language, inflection, and eye contact. All of that is lost in e-mail. More miscommunications have been made via e-mail than any other medium. Besides, people are much more aggressive behind the curtain of e-mail than they are in person. It is much easier to dismiss a proposal with a quick e-mail blurb than to look someone in the eye and say no. A Brazilian research fellow was making no progress with a neuropathologist, who had been ignoring her e-mails for a month. He would not provide her with a digital image of a histology slide for a case report she was writing. She was given this advice: "Go up to his office, introduce yourself, shake his hand, smile, and ask him for the image. Do not use e-mail. It is too impersonal. In person he will not turn you down." She came back from meeting him with the image on a CD.

We are all much more charming in person. For the Brazilian research fellow, the nonverbal communication made the difference: (1) her willingness to walk to his office, (2) her undemanding request for the image, (3) her winsome smile, and (4) her personal thank you and obvious appreciation. None of that was available in the e-mail.

Well, in-person communication is obviously better than e-mail, but what about those times when even in-person communication gets murky? This is especially true when emotions are involved. One good technique is to use "I feel" terms. The idea here is that you really have little visibility into the emotions or motivations of the person you are talking to; you only know about your own emotions and motivations. Acknowledge your feelings, let the other person express his or her feelings, and you are halfway toward solving the problem. When you are angry with someone, avoid accusations and use the "I feel" technique promoted by the Harvard negotiating team and other emotional intelligence experts. Say, "When you took my idea and published it before me, it made me feel angry and sad. I felt betrayed." Be honest, but instead of overreacting with insults or character assassination and saying something like, "You are a lying cheating scumbag. You stole my idea and ripped me off," try keeping it in the realm of the consequences of the action and how it made you feel. Research has shown that by avoiding personal attacks and instead informing

495

the other person of the impact of the infraction, you will elicit a more open response.

Psychologists often advise not to assume intent but instead to inform people of the impact of their actions. They may not have realized the consequences of their actions, and we shouldn't hasten to assume malevolent intent. For example, suppose one day a colleague comes to you and says, "You know, Dr. Jones doesn't even read the reports that you guys provide on your CTAs and MRAs. He says that when you say there's an aneurysm, angiography often shows that there is no aneurysm. And if you say there's no aneurysm, he often finds that on angiography there is an aneurysm. So he says your reports are worthless."

It might seem natural to take that as a personal attack. Here someone was telling a colleague of yours that you are incompetent—that your reports could not be trusted. Well, in the end, your anger and indignation may not be justified. Suppose that Dr. Jones was really saying that he finds that the techniques of CTA and MRA are not as reliable as conventional angiography. His complaint may not have been about your interpretation of the study but with the modality itself. It could have been the technique he didn't trust, rather than the reader. You would have ascribed malevolent intent to Dr. Jones erroneously. The other lesson is that hearsay testimony is not as reliable as direct, first-person testimony. In-person communication is key. Immediate clarification will prevent any potential misunderstanding between you and "Dr. Jones."

Do not ascribe blame. Ascribe contribution. Nothing makes a person more defensive than a culture of blame. "The reason we were late to the meeting was that you came to the parking lot 15 minutes past our agreed upon departure time. It was your fault. You are always so selfish." Convert this to "Although I could have reminded you earlier about the deadline, your extra time in arriving at the parking lot contributed to our being late for the executive committee and missing the vote." Your colleague may reply, "Actually it was because I had to take our friend Joan's call. Her mother was admitted to the hospital. I couldn't just hang up. It was an acute M.I. and she needed advice, so that contributed to my delay." That exchange transformed the paradigm and avoided the argument. Accept some of your own contribution to

the issue. It is true that most miscommunications are due to contributions by both or all or unapparent parties. Ascribing blame only leads to resistance and defensiveness. Adding a generalized attack on the person's self-image ("You are always so selfish") will only compound the defensiveness and add to the hurt.

Be Faithful to the Absent

Nothing can damage your employees' confidence in you more than to hear you disparage someone who is not present. There is a story about a junior faculty member who was mentored by one of the senior faculty. The senior liked to denigrate his competition, and because he felt comfortable with the junior member, he invited the junior member into his inner circle. The junior member came to know exactly how the senior felt about every person in the department, yet he was shocked to see how suave and supportive the senior faculty member could seem when working with the very person he had been dismissing only the hour before. If you are a trifle insecure, and most of us are, you would probably wonder, as the junior faculty member did, what the senior was saying about you when you weren't in the room. The junior faculty member never felt absolutely comfortable that this person was his advocate, and he wondered if he too were being "played." Not being faithful to those who are absent can lead to these a lack of trust in you by those who are present.

If you have to be critical of a person who is not present, criticize the behavior or the action or the event, not the person. Frame the discussion in terms of, "I would not have approached the technologist about the mislabeled film in that fashion" rather than "She is so rude to the employees." If other employees perceive you as the type that makes such personal attacks, they will fear you and distrust you. Those are not the feelings you want in the workplace.

CUSTOMER SATISFACTION

Jump on Problems Immediately

One of the most important lessons you can learn is to address customer issues as soon as they arise. "Customer" in this case obviously means "patient," but it can also apply to colleagues and co-workers who are dealing with patient-related issues and any number of other people in the patient care and revenue process. Letting a complaint languish without your attention for more than a short period of time is an invitation to escalate the issue out of the simple "damage control" category to the "natural disaster" level. Do not procrastinate on patient care or other issues. Treat each issue as if it is going to be a difficult problem if not solved immediately, even if it may seem trivial to you, because there is a good chance it may be some influential person's pet peeve.

On the other hand, some nonessential, non–patient care issues do have to play themselves out before the right decision or action can be made. It can take time for all the right facts to come to light or for consensus to be reached on an issue. In that case, it is still good to reassure the complainant that you take the issue seriously and want to make sure you have the facts right. Remember your "I feel" strategy for conflict resolution? A similar strategy here is to use "I hear" phrases and then validate the importance of the issue to them: "I hear that you are frustrated with this problem. This is obviously an important issue for you, and I will investigate it. Can I call you back when I have learned more?"

Waiting for a cool-down period when you are angry with another person is an excellent idea. Don't just hurry, wait! This has been called the 3-11 rule. Wait 3 days before replying to someone who has angered you. Wait 11 days before replying in writing, if a written record is necessary. It's amazing how a little quiet time can put a whole new perspective on a problem.

Treat even the smallest problem as important, solving it with a friendly attitude, and you may find that it helps smooth over some of the bigger problems that come your way. One story has a referring physician who used to contact the section chief every time his secretary was unable to retrieve a requested film from the film library (this was before picture archiving and communications systems became common). Although some might have found this an annoyance, it led to the development of fairly good rapport between the section chief, the referring physician, and the film library staff.

Although the long-term solution was to have a reliable film library and/or a reliable PACS system that could address his needs, the referring physician came to view the section chief as a problem solver, and this perception prevented him from escalating many other more substantive issues over the head of the section chief to the dean or chief executive officer, which might have led to a less flattering position.

Important Customers Are Important

All customers are important, but your highest volume customers must get the "white-glove" treatment. One practice had one of its most frequently referring ear-nose-throat surgeons call to request a biopsy on one of his patients. He said the patient, who was a nurse, was very anxious. Because he was such a good referrer, the practice rescheduled some appointments to accommodate the patient the next day. As promised, the patient was very nervous, demanding sedation with ever-increasing doses of fentanyl and Versed. She was consoled and reassured that the procedure would go smoothly, but she was clearly anxious to the point of hysteria. She was coaxed through four passes with a 22-gauge needle and one pass with a biopsy gun system. Still, the on-site cytology team was not able to provide a diagnosis with the specimens obtained. A second core biopsy could not be cajoled out of her—she was too uncomfortable. This was a disappointment to everyone, but the team continued attending to the patient, despite a growing line of other patients waiting for the CT, as the procedure passed into the second hour. Important customers are important.

Not unexpectedly, the surgeon called the head of the practice two days later. The surgeon said that the final reading was "nondiagnostic" and that when he called the patient to tell her that an open biopsy was required, she complained to him that the team was inattentive to the pain she experienced. The head of the practice was able to document for him the steps taken before, during, and after the procedure to alleviate her anxiety and pain. The data were all there. The team had listened to her and tried to address her every need. In the end, the surgeon admitted that she was a difficult patient to manage in his own experience and that he was not relishing the issues he would have to face in treating her lesion. This brings up another point in dealing with customer complaints: document what you do. A factual, written log of events and actions taken, written as they occur or shortly after, can prevent a lot of trouble.

Not Apologizing Compounds the Mistake

Most radiologists know that the emergency department and pediatric trauma services tend to be the most vocal customers. One radiology department learned the importance of reading the ED cases first when coming on service when a faculty member failed to call a referring physician over a missed case. This led to a crisis in which a patient was called back to the hospital for additional images. When the referring physician was not addressed in a timely, respectful manner, and did not receive a personal apology for the gaffe, what followed was a 14-month campaign to have the emergency department cases read by the radiology faculty 24 hours a day, 7 days a week, instead of by the trainees who normally provided such round-the-clock preliminary response support. Fortunately, the radiology department had data that suggested that the trainees had an error rate of approximately 0.2% on emergency department studies. Having that kind of data carried the day, but for a long period the referring physicians pushed the issue again and again, all because one faculty member was disrespectful that one time.

Such situations can be avoided by immediately and openly calling referring physicians when mistakes are made, acknowledging the mistakes, and addressing the consequences. Calling an emergency patient back in for repeat or additional images is far less costly than allowing a mistake that may lead to avoidable morbidity or mortality on the part of the patient.

INFORMATION TECHNOLOGY ISSUES

Blind Reliance on Information Technology Personnel

People tend to trust the information coming out of a computer. The numerical precision

498

and the superhuman speed make the results seem almost magical. Always remember that computers are built by people, programmed by people, and installed by people. Computers can therefore be as fallible as people—perhaps even more so, because they can take a single, simple human mistake and replicate it hundreds of thousands of times in the blink of an eye.

One radiology department discovered this when it converted to a new radiology information system (RIS), installed by a large team of vendor support people and the hospital's own in-house IT group. Before the new system went "live," the department had several brief trial runs, all of which were accomplished with only a few, easily corrected hitches. In fact, when the department went live with the system after these trial runs, everyone was pleasantly surprised by the smoothness of the transition and the relative ease of transfer of the data. That made what came next even more of a shock.

Two months later, after the typical 40 to 60 days in accounts receivable, the initial billing numbers showed a disparity between the charges and the revenues, suggesting a collection rate far lower than with the previous RIS. While this was a concern, the department assumed that the deficit was in large part a result of starting the RIS in June and having new faculty in July, who because of delays in getting insurance provider numbers could not have the bills officially submitted. Another month passed. The department saw a huge increase in its workload, so it expected to see a 12% increase in revenue over the previous year. When the third month's numbers also did not reflect the appropriate billings and collections, the department began an intensive investigation.

It took six weeks to discover what had happened. *All* of the bills for outside films interpretations, neurointerventional spine procedures, and vascular interventional procedures were being electronically excluded from submission for payment because of a programming error. Yes, the department had tested the system before going live, but the testing had relied largely on plain films and cross-sectional imaging, because that constituted the vast majority of the bills being sent out by the department. The higher relative value unit (RVU) procedural/surgical work was not tested, and this was the source of the billing error.

Rebilling for studies 4 to 6 months after their performance was extremely troublesome; collecting from payers was even more difficult. The department spent several months trying to regain the revenue that had been lost. Each month, the department continued to see stellar growth in the number of procedures performed and amount of charges submitted, but it failed to meet budget, with a variance greater than 10%. The department was working harder and receiving less remuneration. With each month, another batch of studies that were unexpectedly left off the charge-capture system was discovered: portables, intraoperative cases, lumbar punctures under fluoroscopy, research scans. It was a nightmare.

Implement Accountability Programs and Check and Recheck

One lesson to be learned from this imbroglio is the necessity of having safeguards that can determine whether there is a disconnect between the hospital-technical component of your work and the professional fees. Until this fiasco with the new IT system, the department was not motivated to make sure that, for every charge that the hospital sent, there was a comparable professional fee bill sent for the interpretation (so called technical-professional reconciliation for those radiology groups that do not bill a global fee). Although this is unique to a hospital practice where one entity owns the equipment and another entity interprets the studies and sends a pro-fee bill, it may also apply to those practices where third parties own the equipment. With these safeguards in place, the department can now tell if there is a disparity between increases in technical fee charges and increases in professional fee charges, which may be a good alarm system for a disjunction of charges.

The other lesson is to make sure that all modalities are represented in your sample of studies that are tested for your new RIS or PACS or any other computer system used in your practice. Testing beforehand should be supplemented with continuing to test these same modalities during the first 2 to 3 months of the implementation. That it works in the nth trial run does not mean it will work in "real world" conditions. And the longer the delay in diagnosing a mistake, (1) the lower you can expect your collection rate to be, (2) the greater your days in accounts receivable, and (3) the higher your bad-debt write-offs.

Make Sure You Have Adequate Physician Representation for PACS-RIS Selection

Another radiology department is now implementing a new PACS system after sinking more than $4 million into their "failed" first system. This is not unusual. Many radiology groups are either unhappy with their current PACS system or are on their second or third versions. In some cases the "early adopters" are suffering from implementing an immature product that has not been upgraded and has fallen behind the crowd. In part this is because the cost of implementing a PACS is barely justifiable even under the best of circumstances; the cost of upgrading that PACS is often not something that can be shown to generate additional revenue. In some cases, the original vendor that first sold the RIS-PACS product is either no longer in business (creating a "legacy product") or has been bought out by another company as the industry has consolidated. In either case the outlay of money to "fix" the system is often quite formidable.

In this case, the problems with the first system were largely due to under-representation of physicians in the PACS-RIS selection process. The physicians were not involved for a number of reasons, the most important of which are time and money. The time commitment for sampling the various PACS systems and for traveling to the various institutions to observe the systems at work is huge. In a department where RVUs and physician productivity are highly scrutinized, there are few physicians who are both willing and qualified to assess multiple PACS systems. Unless a percentage of effort is applied to someone whose salary is reimbursed by a department for this type of work, it is hard to get a committed group of physicians who will be able to compare products for what is best for that individual practice. Also, it may be that the best PACS for a largely plain films division is not the same as that for ultrasound or nuclear medicine or CT-MRI or interventional procedures, so to make the right choice you need a physician

499

who understands the full range of work done by the department.

Shrugging it off and leaving it to your IT personnel is a huge mistake. They do not know the operational needs of the interpreting physician. They may be left-handed and not understand the needs of a right-handed person who has a Dictaphone in one hand and mouse in the other. They certainly cannot assess the quality of images projected onto the monitor the way a trained radiologist can. The IT professionals should play an advisory role but should not be the major players in, for example, selecting physician viewing stations for clinicians or radiologists.

The first PACS selected was chosen because it met the needs of the IT group, which liked it because it was modifiable (thereby voiding the service contract and making it difficult to work with the vendor architects of the system). The physicians reading the cases were exasperated with the cumbersome functionality of the first PACS, and they were stuck with it for more than 5 years. With the new PACS, the physicians were closely involved in the selection. The new PACS stood a better chance at acceptance/satisfaction when the people using the system were involved in the purchase decision. Still, do you know the joke? What's the best PACS system? Anyone's but mine.

Simplify, Simplify, Simplify

Another invitation to an IT nightmare is the perception that the more features, functions, add-ons, and customization, the better the product. That a system can, with several clicks of the mouse, accomplish something that is required three times a year should not be a cause for admiration. It is the actions you take on every case (like windowing) that make the real difference, and if they are clumsy and problematic to perform then the system is going to cause headaches. It is best to start with a "dumbed-down" version of a product, based on a simple model that all physicians can use, than to have a system that can be designed for each individual. The upkeep on all of these individualized formats is hellacious. Instead, having a standard platform with a universal set of software that can be easily pulled in and out and replaced with little work for the IT group is best. One excellent strategy is to use bare-bones

workstations that cost less than $500, so that the IT group can swap them in and out at home and in the office at the drop of a coin. With this simple approach, physicians can always be working and functioning with minimal downtime, and they all know how to use the system because it is standardized. For these bare-bones workstations, they should be locked down—no software can be added. They do not replace someone's personal laptops or desktops, but they are available for the basic functions that all faculty require.

Simplify the design. Try to reduce clicks. Try to have the default mode be one where you can reduce the interaction you require with the computer. This means reducing the variability in the "hanging protocols" of viewing stations such that anyone can take a seat in front of the monitor and figure out how to use the workstations. Apple had it right when they designed a computer to be intuitive. Having systems in place that need extensive training to use and require lengthy IT support and education negates the improved efficiency that IT systems are supposed to create. This is particularly true for people such as fellows, who are only in the department for 1 year but might require 3 months to "get the hang of" a complicated system. Lost productivity due to IT! Therefore, standardize protocols and systems design such that one can complete 95% of the tasks that one does each day on the basic setup. This is particularly true of things like basic cross-referencing or magnification.

Simplify workflow. Try to apply the same workflow design to numerous modalities so that a technologist moving from CT to MR to ultrasound knows how to do the same registration and networking functions. In this way, absences due to illness, vacation, or the like can be readily ameliorated by moving technologists, clerks, patient service personnel from one site to another without requiring arduous retraining. If operations can remain functional with only a day's turnover, it means a more robust business.

Do Not Replace the Functions of Low-Paid Employees with High-Paid Employees

The driving force behind most new information technology is a quest for greater productivity:

doing more work with fewer people. The standard approach is to put in a new computer system and reduce the number of people who are needed to do a job. Sometimes this works, but sometimes it is a mistake. Take voice recognition dictation (VRD). Some people argue that using VRD converts the highest paid employees in the radiology department (i.e., the physicians) into glorified transcriptionists. If the VRD system is not Six Sigma accurate, the physicians will spend excessive time having to correct the mistakes of the computer-generated reports instead of spending full time reviewing and interpreting the images. Transcriptionists are relatively low cost compared to physicians. Does it really make economic sense to eliminate the role of transcriptionist and force physicians to take on the work?

The argument can be made that converting low-wage file clerks into high-wage IT digital specialists also is problematic. In this scenario it is to be hoped that you can get more productivity from an individual as an IT specialist than what he could do as a film clerk. Are you just creating an expense or truly promoting development of the individual and enhancing job satisfaction as advertised? How can you expect to reap savings from going filmless if you treble the wages of the "clerks" when you train them to be IT support personnel?

This sort of thing is not limited to technology either, and the costs are not always purely economic. One section chief adopted the policy of eliminating fellows in the division to replace them with junior faculty. Even though an assistant professor-instructor made three times the salary of a fellow, it was felt that the productivity gains would be worth the trade-off. Now, once again you had the highest paid individuals taking on the work responsibilities of what were formerly the duties of lower paid members of the department. Faculty members now had to cover all injections, on-call responsibilities, consent taking, and so on, disrupting workflow. Worse yet, because teaching the fellows was eliminated as a function, this change violated the educational mission of the division. For the section chief this was an advantage, but for those faculty whose raison d'etre in academics was the teaching mission, the policy was a disservice. This policy was quickly and happily reversed once a new division chief was selected.

Prepare for the Future, Understanding Financial Concepts

A chief once requested that every year she would receive a minimum of 10% of capital equipment install base commitment to her department to reinvest in radiology capital. In the discussions she did not feel it necessary to state that this money would be used to acquire new equipment nor that the hospital would cover the cost associated with construction. She also did not feel it necessary to clarify that the install base would be calculated from nondepreciated value. So for example, on a $50 million install base, she would receive $6 million calculated off the nondepreciated value. Unfortunately, the hospital's initial support offer included depreciation. Thus, on a 5-year depreciation cycle, each piece of equipment lost 20% of its value per year. Thus, the $6 million dropped to approximately $3.5 million. Subtract construction costs, and she could only possibly install a PLAYSTATION 3 videogame machine.

Now, fortunately, her department had become very profitable and she subsequently had made the case that investing in radiology, with its 14- to 18-month return on investment, was where the administration should be investing. The correct answer is that the reinvestment should be closer to 15% and not include depreciation. The lesson learned is to think about the financial nuances, take as much time as you need to put clarity into any agreement, and make sure that everyone is working under the same set of assumptions.

LEADERSHIP

Don't Forget the Mission

Never forget the basic mission of the team. If academia argues in favor of the tripartite values of clinical service, education, and research, then stressing a teleradiology program whose sole purpose is to generate revenue at the expense of the other values is destructive to morale.

501

Many chairs use the argument that having some ventures whose main purpose is money making is the only way to have the funds to support the research and education mission ("no margin, no mission"). Although this may be true, obtaining consensus to devote the time and effort to this chore—when many academicians are already feeling the stress to publish or perish or to obtain extramural funding or to spend additional time teaching the trainees—may be difficult to achieve. It may be necessary to rely on some clinical associates whose main task is revenue generation instead of the traditional academic types.

The Triple-Threat Conundrum

Trying to convert all members of the faculty into "triple threats"—good at clinical duties, good at education, and good at research—is another mistake. People tend to be very good at one or two things and somewhat mediocre at the third. With a global view of the team as the "whole," you can construct a model whereby the people who are heavily weighted to clinical duties are offset by others whose main aptitude is teaching or research. It is less important to have each *individual* "in balance" on the tripartite mission than having the whole department or *team* in balance. Forcing a researcher to attend all the teaching conferences of the department will lead to hostility and probably decreased productivity. By the same token, there are some people who are just not interested in hypothesis-driven research. To have them try and fail to obtain research grants will just lead to frustration. Feed the strengths of individuals. If you take a mediocre researcher who is a brilliant clinician, and force her to become a better researcher, she still will be only in the "middle of the pack" among your researchers. Instead, let her improve her clinical skills and become the best clinician that ever was.

There is certainly still a role for observational research in radiology. Innovation need not just be based on grants. The classic example of a division that usually is not research oriented is the interventional group. These people by their very nature are more interested in patient care and often are less interested in spending months preparing the necessary paperwork and statistical references for a submission to the National Institutes of Health. Nonetheless, some academic institutions can count on several funded interventionalists who enjoy the challenge of the laboratory, animal studies, and grantsmanship. This mold is changing with time.

Leadership Fallacies

Richard Gunderman provided a perspective in an *American Journal of Roentgenology* article about seven leadership mistakes that people in authority can make and how to fix them. His perspective is summarized in Table 28-2.

CONCLUSIONS

Medical errors are made every day. These revolve around patient care and require clinical training and quality assurance programs as described in Chapter 15. If you fail to resolve recurring patient care errors, you may need to review Chapter 27 on medicolegal issues. The topic of the present chapter, leadership and judgment errors, can damage a workplace environment and require equal vigilance. The mistakes that are made in managing a practice and handling colleagues are nefarious in that they may have impact far removed from the immediate scene. In the end, operating your business with integrity, compassion, and consideration for others while remaining loyal to the agreed-upon mission and vision of the team will serve the group to best advantage. When mistakes in judgment occur, acknowledge them, repair the damage, and set policies in place that prevent their recurrence.

Table 28-2 Seven Leadership Fallacies and How to Correct Them

Leadership Fallacy	Explanation	Correction
Irrelevance	Viewing leadership as an unknown, unachievable, irrelevant force	Educate physicians on leadership skills, place them in positions of responsibility
Disqualification	Thinking one lacks leadership qualifications, avoiding leadership opportunities	Encourage participation, develop leadership skills training program, mentor
Tyranny	Trying to overwhelm any opposition, convincing others of your way alone, imposing your will	Care about workers, invite diversity of opinion, listen to others, seek to understand
Technique	Constantly strategizing about the best way to get your way, focusing on techniques to manipulate	Focus on the mission and the direction, be adaptable to different methodologies, focus on ends—not the means
Vanity	Assuming you are better because you lead, taking undue credit, being self-absorbed	Serve others, grant credit and responsibility to others, share, strive to make a difference for others
Ease	Assuming leadership is easy when it takes years of practice, training	Study the organization, the people, the environment; do not take role lightly
Sacrifice	Feeling that taking on a leadership role means giving up something else in your life, losing out on other roles to be a leader, giving up ethics/values to lead	Remain focused and well balanced, keep foot in every pot, develop oneself fully as a leader, grow as a person, and use values to be effective, successful; use leadership to affect ethics, maintain morality

Adapted from Gunderman RB: Seven leadership fallacies and how to correct them. Am J Radiol 184:1065–1068, 2005.

Dos and Don'ts to Avoiding Major Mistakes

Dos	Don'ts
1. Practice good communication skills.	1. Be lackadaisical on hiring and firing issues.
2. Avoid delegating critical decisions.	2. Overuse or misuse e-mail.
3. Become involved in operations that affect you—especially PACS/RIS issues.	3. Speak when you should be listening.
4. Show employees appreciation.	4. Be critical in a personal way instead of directed to actions.
5. Promote and reward strong performers.	5. Assume intent without getting verification.
6. Be aggressive about personal references for employment candidates.	6. Complicate instead of simplifying.
7. Keep sexual, racial, and edgy humor or comments out of the workplace.	7. Allow co-workers or direct reports too far into your personal life.
8. Be faithful to the absent: practice no gossip.	8. Set policy before consensus has been reached.
9. Stick to the mission.	9. Ignore the lessons of prior mistakes.
10. Lead by example.	10. Fail to implement two new ideas you learned from this book!

Note: Page numbers followed by *f* indicate figures; those followed by *t* indicate tables; those followed by *b* indicate boxes.

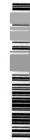

Edwards Brothers Malloy
Ann Arbor MI. USA
April 24, 2012